Handbook of Self-Regulation

Handbook of Self-Regulation

Research, Theory, and Applications

Edited by

ROY F. BAUMEISTER
KATHLEEN D. VOHS

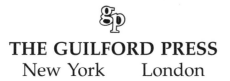

THE GUILFORD PRESS
New York   London

© 2004 The Guilford Press
A Division of Guilford Publications, Inc.
72 Spring Street, New York, NY 10012

Printed in the United States of America

This book is printed on acid-free paper.

Last digit is print number: 9 8 7 6 5 4 3 2 1

Library of Congress Cataloging-in-Publication Data
Handbook of self-regulation : research, theory, and applications / edited by Roy F. Baumeister, Kathleen D. Vohs.
     p. cm.
Includes bibliographical references and index.
  ISBN 1-57230-991-1 (alk.paper)
  1. Self-control. I. Baumeister, Roy F. II. Vohs, Kathleen D.
  BF632.H262 2004
  153.8—dc22
                                                    2003020013

For Dale and Warren—gone, but not forgotten

About the Editors

Roy F. Baumeister, PhD, holds the Eppes Professorship in the Department of Psychology at Florida State University. He also has taught and conducted research at the University of California at Berkeley, Case Western Reserve University, University of Texas, University of Virginia, the Max-Planck Institute in Munich (Germany), and Stanford's Center for Advanced Study in the Behavioral Sciences. Dr. Baumeister has contributed nearly 300 professional publications (including 15 books), spanning such topics as self and identity, performance under pressure, self-control, self-esteem, finding meaning in life, sexuality, aggression and violence, suicide, interpersonal processes, social rejection, the need to belong, and human nature. His research on self-regulation has been funded for many years by the National Institute of Mental Health.

Kathleen D. Vohs, PhD, holds the Canada Research Chair in Marketing Science and Consumer Psychology at the University of British Columbia. She has conducted research on self-regulation at the University of Utah and Case Western Reserve University under a grant from the National Institute of Mental Health. Dr. Vohs has over 50 professional publications that focus on understanding processes related to self-regulation, self-esteem, interpersonal functioning, and bulimic symptomatology. Her research has been extended to the domains of chronic dieting, sexuality, and personal spending and savings.

Contributors

Ozlem Ayduk, PhD, Department of Psychology, University of California at Berkeley, Berkeley, California

Austin S. Baldwin, BS, Department of Psychology, University of Minnesota, Minneapolis, Minnesota

Jane F. Banfield, PhD, Institut für Psychologie, Otto-von-Guericke-Universität Magdeburg, Magdeburg, Germany

John A. Bargh, PhD, Department of Psychology, Yale University, New Haven, Connecticut

Russell A. Barkley, PhD, College of Health Professions, Medical University of South Carolina, Charleston, South Carolina

Roy F. Baumeister, PhD, Department of Psychology, Florida State University, Tallahassee, Florida

Jeanne Brooks-Gunn, PhD, Department of Human Development, Teachers College, Columbia University, New York, New York

Susan D. Calkins, PhD, Department of Psychology, University of North Carolina at Greensboro, Greensboro, North Carolina

Charles S. Carver, PhD, Department of Psychology, University of Miami, Coral Gables, Florida

Daniel Cervone, PhD, Department of Psychology, University of Illinois at Chicago, Chicago, Illinois

Natalie J. Ciarocco, PhD, Department of Psychology, Florida Atlantic University, Treasure Coast, Florida

Colleen Corte, PhD, Department of Psychiatry, Division of Substance Abuse, University of Michigan, Ann Arbor, Michigan

Marisol Cunnington, BA, National Center for Children and Families, Teachers College, Columbia University, New York, New York

Nancy Eisenberg, PhD, Department of Psychology, Arizona State University, Tempe, Arizona

Lesa K. Ellis, PhD, Department of Psychology, Westminster College, Salt Lake City, Utah

Ronald J. Faber, PhD, School of Journalism and Mass Communication, University of Minnesota, Minneapolis, Minnesota

Gráinne M. Fitzsimons, MA, Department of Psychology, New York University, New York, New York

Kentaro Fujita, BA, Department of Psychology, New York University, New York, New York

Peter M. Gollwitzer, PhD, Department of Psychology, New York University, New York, New York

James J. Gross, PhD, Department of Psychology, Stanford University, Stanford, California

Todd F. Heatherton, PhD, Department of Psychological and Brain Sciences, Dartmouth College, Hanover, New Hampshire

C. Peter Herman, PhD, Department of Psychology, University of Toronto, Toronto, Ontario, Canada

Andrew W. Hertel, BA, Department of Psychology, University of Minnesota, Minneapolis, Minnesota

E. Tory Higgins, PhD, Department of Psychology, Columbia University, New York, New York

Travis Hirschi, PhD, Department of Sociology, University of Arizona, Tucson, Arizona

Jay G. Hull, PhD, Department of Psychological and Brain Sciences, Dartmouth College, Hanover, New Hampshire

Randy J. Larsen, PhD, Department of Psychology, Washington University, St. Louis, Missouri

Mark R. Leary, PhD, Department of Psychology, Wake Forest University, Winston-Salem, North Carolina

Donal G. MacCoon, MS, Department of Psychology, University of Wisconsin–Madison, Madison, Wisconsin

C. Neil Macrae, PhD, Department of Psychological and Brain Sciences, Dartmouth College, Hanover, New Hampshire

Lisa A. McCabe, PhD, Cornell Early Childhood Program, Department of Human Development, Cornell University, Ithaca, New York

Walter Mischel, PhD, Department of Psychology, Columbia University, New York, New York

Nilly Mor, PhD, Department of Psychology, University of Maryland, College Park, Maryland

Thomas F. Münte, PhD, Institut für Psychologie, Otto-von-Guericke-Universität Magdeburg, Magdeburg, Germany

Joseph P. Newman, PhD, Department of Psychology, University of Wisconsin–Madison, Madison, Wisconsin

Susan Nolen-Hoeksema, PhD, Department of Psychology, University of Michigan, Ann Arbor, Michigan

Kevin N. Ochsner, PhD, Department of Psychology, Columbia University, New York, New York

Gabriele Oettingen, PhD, Psychologisches Institut II, Universität Hamburg, Hamburg, Germany

Heather Orom, MA, Department of Psychology, University of Illinois at Chicago, Chicago, Illinois

Janet Polivy, PhD, Department of Psychology, University of Toronto, Mississauga, Ontario, Canada

Michael I. Posner, PhD, Department of Psychology, University of Oregon, Eugene, Oregon

Zvjezdana Prizmic, PhD, Department of Psychology, Washington University, St. Louis, Missouri

Mary K. Rothbart, PhD, Department of Psychology, University of Oregon, Eugene, Oregon

Alexander J. Rothman, PhD, Department of Psychology, University of Minnesota, Minneapolis, Minnesota

M. Rosario Rueda, PhD, Department of Psychology, University of Oregon, Eugene, Oregon

Adrienne Sadovsky, PhD, Department of Psychology, Arizona State University, Tempe, Arizona

Michael A. Sayette, PhD, Department of Psychology, University of Pittsburgh, Pittsburgh, Pennsylvania

Brandon J. Schmeichel, MA, Department of Psychology, Florida State University, Tallahassee, Florida

Walter D. Scott, PhD, Department of Psychology, University of Wyoming, Laramie, Wyoming

William G. Shadel, PhD, Department of Psychology, University of Pittsburgh, Pittsburgh, Pennsylvania

Laurie B. Slone, BS, Department of Psychological and Brain Sciences, Dartmouth College, Hanover, New Hampshire

Cynthia L. Smith, PhD, Department of Psychology, Arizona State University, Tempe, Arizona

Scott Spiegel, PhD, Department of Psychology, Columbia University, New York, New York

Tracy L. Spinrad, PhD, Department of Family and Human Development, Arizona State University, Tempe, Arizona

Kathleen D. Vohs, PhD, Sauder School of Business, University of British Columbia, Vancouver, British Columbia, Canada

John F. Wallace, PhD, Carroll Regional Counseling Center, Carroll, Iowa

Michael W. Wiederman, PhD, Department of Human Relations, Columbia College, Columbia, South Carolina

Carrie L. Wyland, BA, Department of Psychological and Brain Sciences, Dartmouth College, Hanover, New Hampshire

Preface

Why do people eat too much? Why is it so hard to quit smoking or get one's alcohol consumption under control? Why can people not save their money for a rainy day? Why is there an epidemic of unwanted pregnancy despite the ready availability of more and better contraceptives than the world has ever seen before?

These and similar questions reflect the wide-ranging importance of self-regulation, the ability to change oneself and exert control over one's inner processes. As such, it is an important key to success in life, whether this is understood at the cultural level (of discharging one's social roles and achieving wealth, fame, and other signs of social approval) or the biological level (of adapting to one's circumstances and achieving harmony with one's environment).

For decades now, social scientists have flocked to the study of self and identity. That study is a large tent with many subtopics, and over these recent decades, the favored focus has shifted repeatedly. Self-concept, self-esteem, self-presentation, social roles, identity crisis, group and ethnic identity, and other such topics have garnered widespread attention at different times. Is self-regulation merely the currently reigning darling of "self" topics?

On the contrary, we think there are important reasons why self-regulation is special. Almost everything the self is or does is tied in some way to self-regulation. This began to dawn on leading researchers in the 1980s and swept the field by the 1990s. The phrase "is or does" is revealing too, because as researchers began to shift their focus from what the self is to what it does, self-regulation caught their attention more and more. To do anything, the self has to keep its own inner house in order, such as by organizing its actions toward goals, avoiding swamps of emotional distress, obeying laws, and internalizing society's standards of good (both moral and competent) behavior.

This handbook reflects the widespread recognition of the central importance of self-regulation, both to the practicalities of everyday life and to the advancement of psychological theories about self and identity. We started out with a sense that self-regulation is studied in many different ways and contexts, with the use of different approaches and methods, but that this diversity of approaches was based on a common, underlying acceptance that the topic is indispensable to much other work. Our goal, therefore, was to draw together the many strands of self-regulation research. Self-regulation was simply too large, diverse, and important a topic not to have a handbook.

Much of the encouragement to get going on this project came from Seymour Weingarten, Editor-in-Chief of The Guilford Press. Seymour is well known and widely respected among authors in psychology, so we relied heavily on his wisdom. His enthusiasm stimulated us to move forward with putting the book together, even though the timing of the book coincided with heavy demands on both of us. We are grateful for his encouragement and advice. Carolyn Graham, at Guilford, was also crucial to the success of this volume, and her guidance made this project continue smoothly and on schedule.

We invited psychological researchers from across the spectrum of self-regulation research to participate. Essentially, they were all given the same task: Tell us about your approach to the study of self-regulation, and tell us what you, and people like you, have learned. We wanted a comprehensive collection of up-to-date, state-of-the-art summaries of as many different approaches to self-regulation research as we could fit into one big book.

At first, we thought the editing task would be a long series of heavy chores. But as the chapters began to come in, our excitement about the project increased. The chapter authors are leading experts in various areas, and they seemed to share our sense that this book was a specially important chance to assemble in one volume the many different ideas, methods, and findings about this fascinating and profoundly important topic. They labored to make their own contributions shine, which in turn made our editorial task more satisfying and less tedious than is the norm.

We hope this book will be read by social scientists of every stripe. Self-regulation is relevant to nearly all forms of social behavior. To be sure, some fields are better represented in these pages than others, but probably this only means that researchers in some fields have not yet fully realized what an understanding of self-regulation can do for them. We hope that scholars from those fields will consult these pages with a sense of opportunity and challenge: They may both gain and contribute by filling in the gaps they find in our knowledge about self-regulation. For other fields, in which self-regulation is already recognized and respected as a crucial aspect of human life, scholars may consult these pages with the confidence that they can come away with a solid and fundamental understanding of what is known in the field and where it stands.

The study of self-regulation is also diverse in the width of its approaches, and here too, we are especially pleased with what this book has to offer. Some researchers study it at the most general of levels: How do people set goals for themselves; how do they keep track of their progress and evaluate where they stand; and so forth? Others study self-regulation in specific problem domains: How do people keep to a diet, recover from addiction, control their anger, or practice safe sex?—or, conversely, why do they sometimes fail at these concrete and highly desirable efforts? Our book begins with the most general of self-regulation processes and moves steadily toward the applications and implications for specific problems.

The chapters are self-contained, so readers may read them in any order or pick and choose which ones are most relevant to their interests. Still, we encourage readers who are new to the study of self-regulation to spend at least some time on every chapter. Readers will not be disappointed, and, indeed, we anticipate that they will come away with much of the same, satisfying intellectual excitement that has characterized the entire project.

Contents

1. Understanding Self-Regulation: An Introduction   1
Kathleen D. Vohs and Roy F. Baumeister

I. Basic Regulatory Processes

2. Self-Regulation of Action and Affect   13
Charles S. Carver

3. Affect Regulation   40
Randy J. Larsen and Zvjezdana Prizmic

4. The Cognitive Neuroscience of Self-Regulation   62
Jane F. Banfield, Carrie L. Wyland, C. Neil Macrae, Thomas F. Münte, and Todd F. Heatherton

5. Self-Regulatory Strength   84
Brandon J. Schmeichel and Roy F. Baumeister

6. Willpower in a Cognitive–Affective Processing System: 99
The Dynamics of Delay of Gratification
Walter Mischel and Ozlem Ayduk

7. Self-Regulation and Behavior Change: Disentangling Behavioral   130
Initiation and Behavioral Maintenance
Alexander J. Rothman, Austin S. Baldwin, and Andrew W. Hertel

II. Cognitive, Physiological, and Neurological Dimensions of Self-Regulation

8. Automatic Self-Regulation   151
Gráinne M. Fitzsimons and John A. Bargh

9. Promotion and Prevention Strategies for Self-Regulation: 171
A Motivated Cognition Perspective
E. Tory Higgins and Scott Spiegel

10. Self-Efficacy Beliefs on the Architecture of Personality: 188
    On Knowledge, Appraisal, and Self-Regulation
    Daniel Cervone, Nilly Mor, Heather Orom, William G. Shadel,
    and Walter D. Scott

11. Planning and the Implementation of Goals   211
    Peter M. Gollwitzer, Kentaro Fujita, and Gabriele Oettingen

12. Thinking Makes It So: A Social Cognitive Neuroscience Approach   229
    to Emotion Regulation
    Kevin N. Ochsner and James J. Gross

III. Development of Self-Regulation

13. Effortful Control: Relations with Emotion Regulation, Adjustment,   259
    and Socialization in Childhood
    Nancy Eisenberg, Cynthia L. Smith, Adrienne Sadovsky,
    and Tracy L. Spinrad

14. Attentional Control and Self-Regulation   283
    M. Rosario Rueda, Michael I. Posner, and Mary K. Rothbart

15. Attention-Deficit/Hyperactivity Disorder and Self-Regulation: 301
    Taking an Evolutionary Perspective on Executive Functioning
    Russell A. Barkley

16. Early Attachment Processes and the Development   324
    of Emotional Self-Regulation
    Susan D. Calkins

17. The Development of Self-Regulation in Young Children: 340
    Individual Characteristics and Environmental Contexts
    Lisa A. McCabe, Marisol Cunnington, and Jeanne Brooks-Gunn

18. Temperament and Self-Regulation   357
    Mary K. Rothbart, Lesa K. Ellis, and Michael I. Posner

IV. The Interpersonal Dimension of Self-Regulation

19. The Sociometer, Self-Esteem, and the Regulation   373
    of Interpersonal Behavior
    Mark R. Leary

20. Interpersonal Functioning Requires Self-Regulation   392
    Kathleen D. Vohs and Natalie J. Ciarocco

V. Individual Differences and Self-Regulation

21. Gender and Self-Regulation   411
    Susan Nolen-Hoeksema and Colleen Corte

22. Self-Regulation: Context-Appropriate Balanced Attention   422
    Donal G. MacCoon, John F. Wallace, and Joseph P. Newman

VI. Everyday Problems with Self-Regulation

23. Self-Regulatory Failure and Addiction   447
   Michael A. Sayette

24. Alcohol and Self-Regulation   466
   Jay G. Hull and Laurie B. Slone

25. The Self-Regulation of Eating: Theoretical and Practical Problems   492
   C. Peter Herman and Janet Polivy

26. To Buy or Not to Buy?: Self-Control and Self-Regulatory Failure   509
   in Purchase Behavior
   Ronald J. Faber and Kathleen D. Vohs

27. Self-Control and Sexual Behavior   525
   Michael W. Wiederman

28. Self-Control and Crime   537
   Travis Hirschi

Author Index
                                                                             553

Subject Index
                                                                             571

Handbook of Self-Regulation

1

Understanding Self-Regulation

An Introduction

KATHLEEN D. VOHS
ROY F. BAUMEISTER

This handbook offers a vast overview of the state of the art of research into one of the most exciting and challenging topics in all of human behavior. Self-regulation refers to the many processes by which the human psyche exercises control over its functions, states, and inner processes. It is an important key to how the self is put together. Most broadly, it is essential for transforming the inner animal nature into a civilized human being.

We deliberately cast a very wide net in putting this book together. We wanted cognitive processes and motivational ones. We wanted basic research and practical applications. We wanted research on children and adults. We wanted deliberate, conscious processes and automatic, nonconscious ones. Rather than try to promote a particular theory or approach to the topic, we sought to include every available perspective. In fact, our only regrets about this experience center on the two chapters we failed to obtain, because they would have added two more views. As it was, however, we were thrilled with the positive response we received: Almost every author we invited accepted.

WHAT IS SELF-REGULATION?

Our diversity of perspectives necessarily entails that the chapters do not share the same definition of self-regulation, but some common themes have emerged, so that we can define our topic. Some definition is certainly necessary insofar as "self-regulation" and "self-control" are used in different ways by different authors. We use the terms "self-control" and "self-regulation" interchangeably, though some researchers make subtle distinctions between the two (such as by using "self-regulation" more broadly to refer to goal-directed behavior or to feedback loops, whereas "self-control" may be associated specifically with conscious impulse control).

Connotations aside, "regulation" carries the meaning of "control" with a hint of regularity. In that sense, self-regulation refers to the exercise of control over oneself, especially with regard to bringing the self into line with preferred (thus, regular) standards. Such processes can be found deep in nature. For example, the body's homeostatic processes can be considered a form of self-regulation insofar as the human body performs various functions to maintain a constant temperature. If the body gets overheated or chilled, its inner processes seek to return it to its regular temperature.

The term "self-regulation" has in psychology also taken on the connotation of regulation *by* the self (thus, not just *of* the self). The psychological self is not usually much involved in regulating body temperature, but it may be called into strenuous action to resist temptation or to overcome anxiety. The importance of regulation by the self has helped elevate self-regulation to become one of the central interests of researchers who study the self (see Carver & Scheier, 1981, 1998).

Thus, one definition of "self-regulation" encompasses any efforts by the human self to alter any of its own inner states or responses. We have previously described self-regulation in terms of people regulating their thoughts, emotions, impulses or appetites, and task performances. Based on this volume, we amend that list to include attentional processes as another domain of regulated responses.

Another definitional issue is whether "self-regulation" should be restricted to conscious processes. On this matter, the field has evolved from a tentative answer of "yes" to a firmer "no." There is still an emphasis on conscious, deliberate efforts at self-regulation, and some chapters focus almost exclusively on such processes (e.g., the inner struggle to resist temptation). But evidence has increasingly accumulated to show the importance of automatic or nonconscious processes in self-regulation, and some of the chapters in this volume specifically review such contributions. For purposes of definition, therefore, it is important to recognize both conscious and nonconscious processes, and to appreciate their differences even while recognizing that some experts will continue to use the term "self-regulation" to refer primarily or even exclusively to the conscious processes.

Differences of emphasis are also prominent. Research on self-regulation was greatly influenced by cybernetic theory, which showed how even inanimate mechanisms can regulate themselves by making adjustments according to programmed goals or standards. Much of this thinking was motivated by the attempt to design weapon systems, such as missiles, that could be made more accurate if they adjusted their course while in flight. A more common, everyday example is the thermostat that controls a heating and cooling system to maintain a desired temperature in a room. Carver and Scheier's (1981) landmark treatment of self-awareness as self-regulation emphasized these applications of cybernetic theory (especially the feedback loop) to how people monitor their states in relation to goals or other standards, and the influence of this work has kept feedback loops and other self-monitoring processes at the center of much work on self-regulation. Meanwhile, though, other workers have emphasized processes of change (the "operation" phase of the feedback loop), for example, by examining how people bring about an improvement in their current state (e.g., Baumeister, Bratslavsky, Muraven, & Tice, 1998; Vohs & Schmeichel, 2003). Although, superficially, these two approaches may seem to be talking about vastly different phenomena, we regard them as quite compatible. Ultimately self-regulation cannot succeed unless it is successful both at monitoring the state in relation to the goal and at making the changes and adjustments as desired.

WHY STUDY SELF-REGULATION?

Self-regulation has two sides: an applied side and a theoretical side. Although the "two sides" description is true of many topics in psychology, the study of self-regulation (perhaps unlike some other topics) is influential only when it contributes to both theory and practice. It is not surprising, then, that the chapters in this volume provide not only general models that can be used to predict behavior scientifically but also give insightful instructions as to how to better one's life.

A recognition of the practical significance of self-regulation brings about the realization of its profound impact on people's everyday struggles. From our perspective, nearly every major personal and social problem affecting large numbers of modern citizens involves some kind of failure of self-regulation, albeit in the context of broader social influences. Alcoholism, cigarette smoking, and drug addiction reflect the failure to subdue one's escalating appetites for these pleasure-giving substances. Some obesity and some eating disorders reflect the inability to keep one's eating (especially of fatty foods) down to a sensible level. The failure to control one's use of money is sometimes implicated in problems people have with debt, excessive spending, and failure to save money (whether for emergencies or for anticipated future expenditures such as the children's education, or even for retirement). Crime and violence often reflect the failure to control one's aggressive impulses. Emotional problems generally involve the failure to avoid or to recover from unwanted feelings. Many health problems stem from failure to exercise or to eat healthy foods when they are available. Underachievement in work and school may stem from a lack of regulation to make oneself study. Procrastination, which leads to increased stress and inferior performance quality, stems from a failure to keep one's work moving on a proper schedule. Even such complex problems as the spread of sexually transmitted diseases and the prevalence of unwanted pregnancy could be reduced by taking simple, often-neglected precautionary steps. Self-regulation also may play a mediating role in some clinical phenomena such as attention-deficit/hyperactivity disorder (see Barkley, 1997). Thus, a broad range of bad outcomes can be linked to self-regulatory factors.

The second route into self-regulation research emphasizes theory rather than practical applications. Self-regulation holds a pivotal place in self theory and, thus, is a key to understanding many different aspects of psychological functioning. Psychologists have been studying self and identity for decades, but in the last two decades, they have come to appreciate that no account of the self can be anywhere near complete without an understanding of how the self maintains control over itself and makes the adjustments that it deems best to maintain harmony with its social and physical environment.

The theoretical importance of self-regulation is likely to grow further. In recent decades, there has been an increasing effort by psychologists to situate the phenomena they study in the broad contexts of evolutionary biology and cultural influence (movements that will increase psychology's ties to related fields such as biology and anthropology). We think that the evolution of self-regulation will prove to be one of the defining features of human evolution, contributing some of the central abilities that have made human beings distinctively human. It is also crucial for culture insofar as self-regulation allows the basic animal nature to be brought into line with the demands and ideals of vastly different cultures. Indeed, the argument that natural selection shaped human nature specifically for participation in culture (Baumeister, in press) holds that self-regulation is one of the most important factors in making it possible for human beings to live as they do. All cultures require self-regulation and punish its failures, even though they may differ as to what impulses must be regulated and when (or which) lapses may be permitted.

OVERVIEW OF THIS VOLUME

This volume brings together preeminent social, personality, consumer, clinical, and developmental psychologists who have devoted their careers to the study of goal pursuit, all manner of controlled processes, and the (primarily unanticipated) consequences of self-control failure. We have divided the chapters into six sections, featuring basic processes; cognitive, physiological, and neural dimensions; development of self-regulation; interpersonal components of self-regulation; individual differences and psychopathologies; and consequences of self-regulatory failure. We feel that these sections nicely demonstrate the range of self-regulatory effects, while also providing a fundamental framework with which many researchers resonate in terms of their understanding of how self-regulation works.

In Part I we have amassed authors whose work is the bedrock of self-regulation science. Carver's seminal work on the cybernetic aspects of self-regulation is revisited in Chapter 2. Carver uses his new ideas on action to understand better the role of affect in self-regulation. He pursues the idea that affect, in the context of regulatory goals, serves as a signal as to how well or poorly one is doing at achieving one's goals.

Larsen and Prizmic (Chapter 3) also focus on affect in their contribution, but they approach the topic from a broader perspective, providing a rich and detailed overview of the research on affect regulation. They effectively point out the history of affect regulation research, the differences between downregulating negative affect and upregulating positive affect, various models used to predict affect regulation styles, and they conclude by noting some essential paths that future research in affect regulation should take.

The basic processes of self-regulation are represented in the brain, according to the chapter on neuroscientific properties of self-control by Banfield, Wyland, Macrae, Münte, and Heatherton. Their chapter is devoted to outlining the function and structure of the prefrontal cortex in the frontal lobes, which is the control center of the brain, then linking the operations of the prefrontal cortex to regulatory constructs such as attention, decision making, planning, and inhibition.

Turning to a different approach to studying self-regulation, Schmeichel and Baumeister (Chapter 5) give a thorough overview of their research program on self-regulation as a limited resource. Whereas others pursue self-regulation in terms of feedback loops (Carver, Chapter 2), patterns of brain activation (Banfield et al., Chapter 4), or as a cognitive–affective control system (Mischel & Ayduk, Chapter 6), this chapter concentrates on the internal processes governing the action of getting from here to there. This model has led to steady advances in predicting how and when people are apt to be unsuccessful in regulating themselves.

In Chapter 6, Mischel and Ayduk's account of self-regulation emphasizes effortful control and willpower. Drawing from a wealth of data, such as data gleaned from the myriad studies on delay of gratification effects, as well as sophisticated models of cognition, affect, and neuroscience, this chapter encapsulates the concept of willpower as both an individual difference and as a set of internal processes. Mischel and Ayduk also call on researchers to understand better whether effortful control can be taught, which in their view is a question of utmost importance as we head into the new century.

Rounding out the first section on basic processes, Chapter 7 on behavioral change is by Rothman, Baldwin, and Hertel. This chapter provides a unique viewpoint on behavioral change by specifying that the initiation and maintenance of behavioral change efforts are guided by different underlying systems. Rothman et al. demonstrate that although people may start their regulatory endeavors because of the outcomes they wish to obtain, their continuation of these acts depends mainly on their satisfaction with perceived progress. Data from smoking, eating, and other health-relevant studies confirm their ideas.

Part II features chapters on the cognitive, neural, and physiological aspects of self-regulation. Fitzsimons and Bargh lead the way in Chapter 8 by asserting that self-regulation need not be consciously intended or guided. This model of nonconscious, automatic self-regulation has opened up avenues of research previously not imagined by showing that people's behaviors and responses are sometimes aimed at goals they themselves did not realize, because the goals were activated outside of awareness. Their studies are perfect exemplars of the idea that the theory–practice dichotomy can be bridged in one research stream.

People can be said to have two different types of goals: nurturance-related and safety-related. According to Higgins and Spiegel (Chapter 9), these two types of goals have vastly different consequences in terms of the responses they set into motion, the cues for which one is vigilant, and the outcomes to be achieved. Drawing on the regulatory focus model, Higgins and Spiegel show how chronically activated promotion (nurturance-related goals) or prevention (safety-related goals) mindsets, or situational features that prime either mindset, influence judgment processes. Their chapter also highlights a new area of research, the idea of transfer of value from fit. This model, which emphasizes a match between people's current means of goal pursuit and their chronic orientation toward goal achievement, is sure to have a great impact on regulation research for decades to come.

The role of expectations in goal pursuit is addressed by Cervone, Mor, Orom, Shadel, and Scott in Chapter 10 on self-efficacy. Using a social-cognitive–affect model, Cervone and colleagues place self-efficacy in the context of both enduring goal structures and dynamically occurring goal pursuits, which ties together disparate types of research into one cohesive model.

The idea of expectations is also echoed in the work of Gollwitzer, Fujita, and Oettingen (Chapter 11), albeit in a slightly different fashion. Their research on implementation intentions underscores the need for privately endorsed rules that establish a line of action to facilitate goal implementation, particularly in the face of obstacles or difficult regulatory tasks. Gollwitzer's research has shown that effective self-regulation is greatly enhanced by the use of implementation intentions, which set up a series of "if . . . then" contingencies to help grapple with situations that may inadvertently alter one's behaviors away from the intended goal.

The theme of cognitive, physiological, and neuroscientific dimensions of self-regulation is fully incorporated by the last chapter in this section. Ochsner and Gross (Chapter 12) discuss a social-cognitive neuroscience approach to emotion regulation. This chapter is in a sense a counterpart to the entry by Banfield and colleagues (Chapter 4), in that both draw links between brain activations and self-regulatory ability. Ochsner and Gross, however, go over in detail the reciprocal relations among neural activity, emotion regulation strategies, situational features triggering or impeding affect regulation, and the combined psychological and physiological consequences of these various influences.

Part III is one of the strongest and most integrated among the approaches and domains in which these authors place their work. Chapter 13 by Eisenberg, Smith, Sadovsky, and Spinrad features their research on effortful control in the context of age and environment. This model has been particularly useful in portraying children's effortful control abilities as having meaningful consequences for their social development.

Rueda, Posner, and Rothbart's developmental approach (Chapter 14) is to focus on another domain of self-control among young people: attentional control. Their chapter, along with a few others in this volume, brought to our attention (no pun intended) the vital importance of allocating attention in the pursuit of intentions. Rueda and colleagues' contribution gives hope to the question of whether self-regulation can be assisted in development (see Mischel & Ayduk, Chapter 6).

The developmental implications of self-regulation failure are exemplified in Chapter 15 by Barkley on attention-deficit/hyperactivity disorder (ADHD). Barkley's thesis about executive functioning and metacognition in the role of ADHD revolves around the notion that these processes aid in the formation of bonds with other members of one's social group. This social-evolutionary approach takes the concept of ADHD and links it with broader, higher order constructs such as attention and social control.

Social bonds are also highlighted in the work by Calkins (Chapter 16), who underscores the operation of attachment-related processes in development. Calkins posits that attachment processes, which are outgrowths of early interactions with parents, serve emotion regulation functions. Attachment security in Calkins's model is shown to have autonomic and physiological implications, as well as repercussions for emotion regulation, and is particularly important in dyadic relationships.

In Chapter 17, McCabe, Cunnington, and Brooks-Gunn also focus on young children's development, this time from the perspective of a bioecological model. In this approach, self-regulation is seen as resulting from the person x environment interaction, which is examined from macro- and microlevel contexts. On the latter, McCabe and colleagues note some cultural differences in self-regulation development (e.g., between Chinese and U.S. children) and include this aspect of investigation as being on the forefront of future child regulation research.

Rothbart, Ellis, and Posner (Chapter 18) conclude our section on development. Their thesis involves the idea of temperament as a personality construct that is based in reactivity (onset, intensity, and duration of emotional, motor, and attentional reactions) and is intimately connected with self-regulation. Self-regulation is defined by Rothbart et al. as modifications of reactivity, of which fear-based inhibitions that control behavior play a large part. This sophisticated model integrates many of the diverse aspects of childhood self-regulation and provides a nice encapsulation of the research in this burgeoning area.

Part IV represents an up-and-coming research area. The definition of "self-regulation" is expanded in these chapters to include social variables as inputs and outputs of regulatory behaviors. Leary, in Chapter 19 on the sociometer model, posits that the self monitors for signs of interpersonal exclusion and alters behaviors if one appears to be headed toward rejection. Although the sociometer has been largely connected to the concept of self-esteem, it fits within the rubric of self-regulation just as well, because it displays the dynamism of the self in response to conscious and nonconscious cues of goal failure. Chapter 20 by Vohs and Ciarocco is also about the interplay between self-regulation and social functioning, but instead of focusing on one topic, they provide a general overview of the myriad interpersonal phenomena that have self-regulatory functions at their core. Their model shows how interpersonal functioning can be affected by previous self-regulatory endeavors and can also affect subsequent acts of self-control.

Part V begins with a discussion of the role of gender in self-regulation. In Chapter 21, Nolen-Hoeksema and Corte review gender differences in emotion regulation, especially by way of rumination. Rumination tendencies are much stronger and more prevalent among women than among men, which these authors believe may help explain women's higher rates of depression and anxiety. Turning to a completely different individual difference, MacCoon, Wallace, and Newman (Chapter 22) discuss psychopathic individuals' self-regulatory capacities, using cognitive and neurological evidence to inform their response modulation hypothesis, in which self-regulation failures follow from failures to shift attention to nondominant cues that indicate the need for the self to alter its momentary responses.

We conclude the volume with Part VI, six chapters that illustrate the vast and serious ramifications of self-regulation failure. In Chapter 23, Sayette begins this section with a review of the literature on addiction. He parses problems with self-regulation that lead or contribute to drug problems as being due to either *underregulation* or *misregulation*. The former refers to a failure to exert control over oneself, whereas the latter refers to exerting control, but control that leads to an undesirable response. He focuses on smoking as a particularly good exemplar of addictive processes, and reviews the laboratory and naturalistic studies on smoking addiction and control processes.

Hull and Slone (Chapter 24) discuss a specific drug, alcohol, and its relation to self-regulation. They contend that alcohol impairs the cognitive operations needed for effective self-regulation. According to them, people who are low in self-control capacity are more likely to have alcohol use and abuse problems, which is one way that alcohol is problematic for self-control. A second way is that people often indulge in alcohol as a method of controlling their social, emotional, or other psychological difficulties. Their ideas about specific mechanisms suggest avenues for future research.

Eating may perhaps be one of the most commonplace—yet least well-understood—self-regulated domains; at last count, over 50% of Americans are overweight (which prompted comedian Jay Leno to note that it is now "normal" to be overweight). Therefore, understanding the self-regulation of eating is increasingly imperative, and it is a topic that Herman and Polivy (Chapter 25) have tackled for their entire careers. Reviewing evidence on dieting, social norms, the effects of others on food intake, and eating as emotion control, these two eminent researchers show that although the self-regulation of eating may be complex, it need not be convoluted. Herman and Polivy's elegant experimental designs reveal the how far we have come in understanding this pernicious regulation problem.

Personal spending is another domain in which people have great difficulty trying to curb their impulses. In Chapter 26, Faber and Vohs undertake the issue of financial control and examine three basic patterns of (mis)regulated spending: self-gifting, impulsive spending, and compulsive spending. The three concepts are related to one another via problems with self-control, but each also reflects the influence of other factors that are revealed by other theories of psychology and economics. For instance, Faber and Vohs posit that compulsive spending results from processes related to self-regulation failure, as well as escape from the self. Their review sheds light on the idea of financial self-regulation as a consequential arena in which to examine regulatory processes.

Wiederman's chapter on sexuality is an eye-opener, perhaps mostly because it illuminates a massive gap in the study of self-regulation. Wiederman (Chapter 27) astutely notes that although societies throughout the world and across eras have attempted to control their peoples' sexuality, research on the influence of personal self-regulation standards has been largely overlooked. Given that sexuality is one of the most basic aspects of human interaction and also (not coincidentally) a primary domain in which relationships can fall apart, Wiederman's pleas for more research should not go unheard.

Our last chapter in this volume is on the link between self-regulation and criminality. Hirschi's contribution (Chapter 28) lays out his and Gottfredson's theory (see Gottfredson & Hirschi, 1990) of crime and self-control. Their influential model places self-control abilities at the heart of acts of crime, and posits that virtually all criminal acts are linked together by the fact that they provide short-term benefits but incur long-term costs. Hirschi demonstrates the utility of this model in predicting and describing criminal behavior and smartly shows how much variability in criminal acts can be accounted for by one basic internal process (self-control).

In summary, we have collected a stellar group of self-regulation researchers, who have laid out the underlying processes, cognitive and physical operations, and emotional repercussions of self-regulation; demonstrated the developmental trajectories of self-regulation and effortful control processes, and their associated outcomes; highlighted the far-ranging effects of self-regulation in terms of personal relationships, addictions, and consumption; and have shown how people differ in their basic abilities and styles of self-control. We are enormously pleased with the amount and sophistication of information on how self-regulation works, and we are particularly excited to have much of it here in this volume.

PROGRESS AND PROSPECTS

Research on self-regulation has made more progress in some areas than in others (which is probably true of any field or topic). We can briefly highlight some areas in which progress has been rapid and others in which it has lagged.

Applied research has in some cases led the way. Research on control of eating, drinking, smoking, and similar topics has long had to recognize the importance of self-regulation and the sources of self-regulation failure. Basic researchers have built onto this substantial amount of information and have begun to develop more elaborate and general theoretical models. Hence, one priority in the coming years is that the basic research models go back to the applied settings for testing.

At the core of any scientific enterprise is the effort to understand the causal sequence of processes that produce any effect, and in self-regulation, the development of such microlevel theories seems crucial and promising. Until recently, self-regulation was itself considered an explanation for other processes and behavioral outcomes, but now, the field is starting to take the next step and unpack how self-regulation succeeds and fails in terms of the intrapsychic events.

Emotion plays multiple roles in self-regulation. This handbook does not have a separate section devoted to emotion, partly because emotion comes up in different ways in each of the other sections. Emotion contributes mightily to both successes and failures of self-regulation. How this seemingly contradictory, paradoxical pattern can be true is a fascinating challenge for further work, though, already, there have been important steps in that direction.

Not surprisingly, most models of self-regulation have focused on what happens inside the individual psyche. The past few years have, however, seen a rising recognition that interpersonal relations affect, and are affected by, self-regulation. The interpersonal dimension of self-regulation is still underappreciated and seems likely to attract further study in the coming years.

The 1990s was the "decade of the brain" and in fact was a great stimulus for the study of physiological and neurological processes. Researchers have scarcely begun to map out the brain processes and other physiological determinants of self-regulatory processes. It seems a safe bet that the growing field of social-cognitive neuroscience will devote increasing effort to understanding these aspects of self-regulation.

Another fascinating development is the beginning recognition that people must often juggle multiple goals and other self-regulatory projects simultaneously. A given Saturday afternoon can be devoted to work, repairing relationship damage, or exercising, all of which involve self-regulation, yet cannot all be done simultaneously. Moreover, if the capacity for self-regulation is limited, then people must operate with a shifting system of priorities as to what behaviors are most urgent to regulate.

Integration across subdisciplines is an important, promising area, although the structures of academic life make such integration difficult and uncertain. Developmental psychologists believe that they were the first to recognize the importance of self-regulation, in their studies of how children become socialized and learn to control themselves for the sake of social participation. Neuroscientists similarly believe that they led the way in their studies of executive function. Clinical psychologists, especially those who deal with addiction and eating disorders, recognized the central importance of self-regulation long before laboratory researchers had any inkling of how to study it. Social psychologists, especially those interested in the self, claim priority insofar as they alone have the general understanding of how self-regulation fits into the operation of the self. Personality psychologists also point out that they have long recognized individual differences in ego strength and conscientiousness. Finally, cognitive psychologists have for decades examined how limited resources in attention are allocated and, indeed, how processes of metacognition regulate cognitive performance.

All these claims are valid, and all areas have something to offer. It is our hope that this volume contributes to such integrative understanding and cross-fertilization of ideas. In any case, the next decade promises to be an exciting and productive one in the understanding of self-regulation!

REFERENCES

Barkley, R. A. (1997). *ADHD and the nature of self-control.* New York: Guilford Press.

Baumeister, R. F. (in press). *The cultural animal: Human nature, meaning, and social life.* New York: Oxford University Press.

Baumeister, R. F., Bratslavsky, E., Muraven, M., & Tice, D. M. (1998). Ego depletion: Is the active self a limited resource? *Journal of Personality and Social Psychology, 74,* 1252–1265.

Carver, C. S., & Scheier, M. F. (1981). *Attention and self-regulation: A control theory approach to human behavior.* New York: Springer-Verlag.

Carver, C. S., & Scheier, M. F. (1998). *On the self-regulation of behavior.* New York: Cambridge University Press.

Gottfredson, M., & Hirschi, T. (1990). *A general theory of crime.* Stanford, CA: Stanford University Press.

Vohs, K. D., & Schmeichel, B. J. (2003). Self-regulation and the extended now: Controlling the self alters the subjective experience of time. *Journal of Personality and Social Psychology, 85,* 217–230.

I

Basic Regulatory Processes

2

Self-Regulation of Action and Affect

CHARLES S. CARVER

This chapter outlines the fundamentals of a viewpoint on self-regulation in which behavior is seen as reflecting the processes of cybernetic control. I develop the argument that two layers of control manage two different aspects of behavior. I argue further that, taken together, these layers of control permit the human being to handle multiple tasks in its life space. More specifically, they help transform the simultaneous concern with many different goals into a stream of actions that shifts repeatedly from one goal to another over time.

The view described here has been identified with the term "self-regulation" for a long time (e.g., Carver & Scheier, 1981, 1990, 1998, 1999a, 1999b). This term, however, means different things to different people. When using it, I intend to convey the sense that the processes are purposive, that self-corrective adjustments are taking place as needed to stay on track for whatever purpose is being served, and that the corrective adjustments originate within the person. These points converge in the view that behavior is a continual process of moving toward (and sometimes away from) goal representations, and that this movement embodies characteristics of feedback control. Although this chapter makes additional points, these ideas lie at its heart.

Certainly the processes described here are not the *only* processes behind behavior. Other chapters in this volume examine aspects of self-regulation that differ substantially from this. Failure to include full discussion of those ideas should not be taken to mean that I think they are unimportant. Quite the contrary. Furthermore, I believe many of them are quite compatible with the broad principles described here. These principles might be thought of as a rough exoskeleton on which a number of more subtle processes can be hung. It is a view of the structure of behavior that accommodates diverse ways of thinking about what qualities of behavior matter and why. For this reason, it complements a wide variety of other ideas about what goes on in human self-regulation.

BEHAVIOR AS GOAL DIRECTED AND FEEDBACK CONTROLLED

I begin this discussion with the goal concept. My use of goals as a starting point resonates with a renewed interest in goal constructs in today's personality and social psychology (Austin & Vancouver, 1996; Elliott & Dweck, 1988; Pervin, 1982, 1989; Read & Miller, 1989). Writers have used a variety of labels, reflecting differences in emphasis—for example, *current concern* (Klinger, 1975), *personal striving* (Emmons, 1986), *life task* (Cantor & Kihlstrom, 1987), *personal project* (Little, 1989), *possible self* (Markus & Nurius, 1986), and *self-guide* (Higgins, 1987, 1996). All these constructs contain overall goals and subgoals, with ample room for individualization; that is, most goals can be reached in many ways. People choose pathways that are compatible with other aspects of their situations and their personalities.

Theorists who use these various terms—and others—have their own emphases (for broader discussions, see Austin & Vancouver, 1996; Carver & Scheier, 1998, 1999b; Pervin, 1989), but they have many points in common. All assume that goals energize and direct activities (Pervin, 1982). All convey the sense that goals give meaning to people's lives, that understanding the person means understanding the person's goals. Indeed, it is often implicit in such views that the self consists partly of the person's goals and the organization among them (cf. Mischel & Shoda, 1995).

Feedback Loops

How are goals used in acting? Answers to this question can be framed at several levels of abstraction. The answer I pursue here is that goals serve as reference values in feedback loops. The feedback loop is an organized system of four elements (MacKay, 1966; Miller, Galanter, & Pribram, 1960; Powers, 1973; Wiener, 1948). The elements include an input function, a reference value, a comparator, and an output function (Figure 2.1).

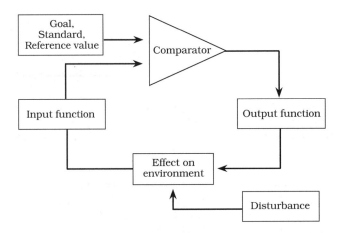

FIGURE 2.1. Schematic depiction of a feedback loop, the basic unit of cybernetic control. In a discrepancy-reducing loop, a sensed value is compared to a reference value or standard, and adjustments occur in an output function (if necessary) that shift the sensed value in the direction of the standard. In a discrepancy-enlarging loop, the output function moves the sensed value away from the standard.

An input function (which I'll treat as equivalent to perception) brings information from a sensor into the system. A reference value is a second source of information, derived from within the system. In the loops discussed here, I'll treat reference values as equivalent to goals.

A comparator is a mechanism that compares the input to the reference value, yielding one of two outcomes. Either the values being compared are discriminably different, or they are not. The degree of discrepancy detected by the comparator is sometimes referred to as an "error signal." Greater discrepancy implies greater error. (The idea that error detection is fundamental to living systems is echoed in recent evidence that negative events [implying discrepancies] draw more attention than positive ones; Baumeister, Bratslavsky, Finkenauer, & Vohs, 2001.)

Next comes an output function. I'll treat this as equivalent to behavior, though sometimes the behavior is internal. If the comparison yields "no difference," the output function remains as it was. This may mean that there is no output (if there was none before), or it may mean that an ongoing output continues. If the comparison yields a judgment of "discrepancy," the output function changes.

There are two different kinds of feedback loops, which diverge in their overall functions. In a discrepancy-reducing loop (also called a negative [for negating] feedback loop), the output function acts to reduce or eliminate any discrepancy noted between input and reference value. Such an effect is seen in human behavior in the attempt to attain a valued goal, or to conform to a standard.

The second kind of loop is a discrepancy-enlarging loop (also called a positive feedback loop). The reference value here is one to avoid. It may be convenient to think of it as an "anti-goal." A psychological example of an anti-goal is a feared or disliked possible self (Carver, Lawrence, & Scheier, 1999; Markus & Nurius, 1986; Ogilvie, 1987). Other examples are traffic accidents, having your date make a scene in public, and being seen by others as a prototypical mental patient (Niedenthal & Mordkoff, 1991). A discrepancy-enlarging loop senses existing conditions, compares them to the anti-goal, and acts to enlarge the discrepancy. Consider the rebellious adolescent who abhors the possibility of resembling his parents. He senses his behavior, compares it to his parents' behavior, and tries to make his own behavior different from theirs in some way.

The action of discrepancy-enlarging processes in living systems is typically constrained by discrepancy-reducing processes. To put it differently, acts of avoidance often lead into other acts of approach. An avoidance loop tries to increase distance from an anti-goal. But there may be one or more approach goals in near psychological space. If a goal is noticed and adopted, the tendency to move away from the anti-goal is joined by a tendency to move toward the goal. The approach loop pulls subsequent behavior into its orbit. The rebellious adolescent, trying to differ from his parents, soon finds other adolescents to conform to, all of whom are being different from their parents.

The use of the word "orbit" in the previous paragraph suggests a metaphor that some find useful. One might think of these loops as metaphorically equivalent to gravity and antigravity. The discrepancy-reducing loop exerts a kind of gravitational pull on the input it is controlling, bringing that input closer to it. The positive loop has a kind of antigravitational push, moving sensed values away. Remember, this is a metaphor. There is more here than a force field, though precisely how much more is somewhat up in the air (see Carver & Scheier, 2002).

I should say explicitly that feedback processes do more than create and maintain steady states, because this point is often misunderstood. Some reference values (and goals) *are* indeed static end states. But others are dynamic and evolving (e.g., the goal of taking a month's vacation in Europe, the goal of writing a book chapter). In such cases, the goal changes character as the person traverses the path of activity. Thus, feedback processes apply perfectly well to moving targets (Beer, 1995).

Goals also vary in abstractness. You can have not only the goal of being a caring person, but also the goal of parking your car straight (which entails the even more concrete goal of turning the steering wheel with just the right pressure). Thus, it is often said that goals form a hierarchy (Carver & Scheier, 1998; Powers, 1973; Vallacher & Wegner, 1987). Abstract goals are attained by attaining the concrete goals that help to define them. This issue is very important in some contexts (see, e.g., Carver & Scheier, 1998, 1999a, 1999b, 2003), but not to the themes of this chapter.

Other Phenomena of Personality–Social Psychology and Feedback Control

The goal concept, in its various forms, represents one place in which the constructs of personality and social psychology intersect with the logic of the feedback loop. I want to note briefly, however, that the intersection is much broader. The notion of reducing sensed discrepancies has a long history in social psychology, in behavioral conformity to norms (Asch, 1955) and in models of cognitive consistency (Festinger, 1957; Heider, 1946; Lecky, 1945). The self-regulatory feedback loop, in effect, is a metatheory for such effects.

Another literature that appears to fit the feedback loop picture is that of social comparison (e.g., Buunk & Gibbons, 1997; Suls & Wills, 1991; Wood, 1996). I have argued elsewhere (Carver & Scheier, 1998) that upward comparisons often are part of the process by which people formulate desired reference points and pull themselves toward them (discrepancy reduction). Downward comparisons sometimes help people to push themselves farther away from anti-goals represented by groups who are worse off than they are (discrepancy enlargement).

FEEDBACK PROCESSES AND AFFECT

Thus far I have considered behavior—the process of getting from here to there. There is much more to the human experience than action. Another important part of experience is feelings (indeed, feelings turn out to be an important element in action). Two fundamental questions about affect are what it consists of and where it comes from. It is widely held that affect pertains to one's desires and whether they are being met (e.g., Clore, 1994; Frijda, 1986, 1988; Ortony, Clore, & Collins, 1988). But what exactly is the internal mechanism by which feelings arise?

Answers to these questions can take any of several forms, ranging from neurobiological (e.g., Davidson, 1984, 1992, 1995) to cognitive (Ortony et al., 1988) and beyond. The answer we posed (Carver & Scheier, 1990, 1998, 1999a, 1999b) focuses on some of the functional properties that affect seems to display in the behaving person. Again we use feedback control as an organizing principle. But now the feedback control bears on a different quality than it did earlier.

We have suggested that feelings arise as a consequence of a feedback process that operates automatically, simultaneously with the behavior-guiding process, and in parallel to it. Perhaps the easiest way to convey what this second process is doing is to say that it is checking on how well the first process (the behavior loop) is doing at reducing *its* discrepancies. Thus, the input for this second loop is some representation of the *rate of discrepancy reduction in the action system over time*. (I limit myself at first to discrepancy-reducing loops, then turn to enlarging loops.)

An analogy may be useful. Action implies change between states. Thus, consider behavior as being analogous to distance. If the action loop controls distance, and if the affect loop assesses the progress of the action loop, then the affect loop is dealing with the psychological analogue of velocity, the first derivative of distance over time. To the extent that this analogy is meaningful, the perceptual input to the affect loop should be the first derivative over time of the input used by the action loop.

Input by itself does not create affect (a given rate of progress has different affective effects in different circumstances). I believe that, as in any feedback system, this input is compared to a reference value (cf. Frijda, 1986, 1988). In this case, the reference is an acceptable or desired rate of behavioral discrepancy reduction. As in other feedback loops, the comparison checks for deviation from the standard. If there is one, the output function changes.

Our position is that the error signal from the comparison in this loop is manifest phenomenologically as affect, a sense of positive or negative valence. If the rate of progress is below the criterion, negative affect arises. If the rate is high enough to exceed the criterion, positive affect arises. If the rate is not distinguishable from the criterion, no affect arises.

In essence, the argument is that feelings with a positive valence mean you are doing better at something than you need to, and feelings with a negative valence mean you are doing worse than you need to (for more detail, including a review of evidence on the link between this "velocity" function and affect, see Carver & Scheier, 1998, Chs. 8 and 9). One fairly direct implication of this line of thought is that the affective valences that might potentially arise regarding any given action domain should fall along a bipolar dimension. That is, for a given action, affect can be positive, neutral, or negative, depending on how well or poorly the action is going.

Two Kinds of Behavioral Loops, Two Dimensions of Affect

Now consider discrepancy-enlarging loops. The view that I just outlined rests on the idea that positive feeling results when a behavioral system is making rapid progress in *doing what it is organized to do*. The systems considered thus far are organized to reduce discrepancies. There is no obvious reason, though, why the principle should not apply as well to systems organized to enlarge discrepancies. If that kind of a system is making rapid progress doing what it is organized to do, there should be positive affect. If it is doing poorly, there should be negative affect.

The idea that affects of both valences can occur would seem comparable across both approach and avoidance systems. That is, both approach and avoidance have the potential to induce positive feelings (by doing well), and both have the potential to induce negative feelings (by doing poorly). But doing well at moving *toward an incentive* is not quite the same as doing well at moving *away from a threat*. Thus, the two positives may not be quite the same, nor may the two negatives.

Based on this line of thought, and drawing as well on insights from Higgins (e.g., 1987, 1996) and his collaborators (see Higgins & Spiegel, Chapter 9, this volume), I have argued (Carver, 2001; Carver & Scheier, 1998) for two bipolar affect dimensions (Figure 2.2). One dimension relates to the system that manages the approach of incentives, the other to the system that manages the avoidance of, or withdrawal from, threat. The di-

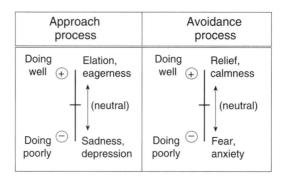

FIGURE 2.2. Two behavioral systems and poles of the affective dimensions held by Carver and Scheier (1998) to relate to the functioning of each. In this view, approach processes yield affective qualities of sadness or depression when progress is very poor; they yield qualities such as eagerness, happiness, or elation when progress is very high. Avoidance processes yield anxiety or fear when progress is very poor; they yield relief, calmness, or contentment when progress is very high. From Carver and Scheier (1998), *On the self-regulation of behavior.* Copyright 1998 by Cambridge University Press. Adapted by permission.

mension related to approach ranges (in its "purest" form) from affects such as elation, eagerness, and excitement to sadness and dejection. The dimension related to avoidance ranges (in its "purest" form) from fear and anxiety to relief, serenity, and contentment.

Merging Affect and Action

This viewpoint implies a natural link between affect and action. That is, if the input function of the affect loop is a sensed rate of progress in action, the output function must be a change in rate of that action. Thus, the affect loop has a direct influence on what occurs in the action loop.

Some changes in rate output are straightforward. If you are lagging behind, go faster, try harder. Sometimes the changes are less straightforward. The rates of many "behaviors" are defined not by a pace of physical action but in terms of choices among potential actions, or entire programs of action. For example, increasing your rate of progress on a project at work may mean choosing to spend a weekend working rather than skiing. Increasing your rate of being kind means choosing to do an action that reflects that value when an opportunity arises. Thus, adjustment in rate must often be translated into other terms, such as concentration, or reallocation of time and effort.

The idea that two feedback systems are functioning in concert with one another is something we more or less stumbled into. It turns out, however, that such an arrangement is quite common in a very different application of feedback concepts. This other application is the literature of control engineering (e.g., Clark, 1996). Engineers have long recognized that having two feedback systems functioning together—one controlling position, the other controlling velocity—permits the device in which they are embedded to respond in a way that is both quick and stable (i.e., prevents overshoots and oscillations).

The combination of quickness and stability in responding is valuable in the kinds of electromechanical devices with which engineers deal, but its value is not limited to such devices. A person with very reactive emotions is prone to overreact and to oscillate behaviorally. A person who is emotionally nonreactive is slow to respond even to urgent events. A person whose reactions are between the two extremes responds quickly but without undue overreaction and oscillation.

For biological entities, being able to respond quickly yet accurately confers a clear adaptive advantage. We believe this combination of quick and stable responding is a consequence of having both behavior-managing and affect-managing control systems. Affect causes people's responses to be quicker (because this control system is time-sensitive) and, provided that the affective system is not overresponsive, the responses are also stable.

DIVERGENT VIEW OF THE DIMENSIONAL STRUCTURE OF AFFECT

The theoretical elements outlined up to this point have an internal conceptual coherence. However, there are also ways in which this model differs from other theories. At least two of the differences appear to have interesting and important implications.

One difference concerns the dimensional structure of affect (Carver, 2001). A number of theories, including ours, conceptualize affects as aligned along dimensions (though it should also be noted that not all theorists make this assumption; cf. Izard, 1977; Levenson, 1994, 1999). As just described, our dimensional view holds that affect relating to approach and affect relating to avoidance both have the potential to be either positive or negative. Most dimensional models of affect, however, assume a different arrangement.

The idea that eagerness, excitement, elation, and so on should relate to an approach process is intuitive. It is also intuitive that fear, anxiety, and so on should relate to an avoidance process. Both of these relations are noted commonly (Cacioppo, Gardner, & Bernston, 1999; Watson, Weise, Vaidya, & Tellegen, 1999). Both are also represented in a variety of neurobiological theories bearing on affect (e.g., Cloninger, 1988; Davidson, 1992, 1998; Depue & Collins, 1999; Gray, 1990, 1994a, 1994b).

But attention must also be given to the opposite poles of these two dimensions. Here is where the consensus breaks down. For example, Gray (e.g., 1990, 1994b) has taken the position that the inhibition (or avoidance) system is engaged by cues of both punishment and frustrative nonreward. It is thus tied to negative feelings in response to either sort of cue. Similarly, he holds that the approach system is engaged both by cues of reward and by cues of escape or avoidance of punishment. It thus is tied to positive feelings in response to such cues.

In Gray's view, then, each system is responsible for the creation of affect of one, and only one, hedonic tone (positive in one case, negative in the other). This theory yields a picture of two unipolar affective dimensions (running neutral to negative, and neutral to positive), each of which is linked to the functioning of a separate behavioral system. A similar position has been taken by Lang and colleagues (e.g., Lang, 1995; Lang, Bradley, & Cuthbert, 1990), by Cacioppo and colleagues (e.g., Cacioppo & Berntson, 1994; Cacioppo et al., 1999), and by Watson and colleagues (1999). In this respect, this version of a dimensional view (which now dominates discussions of dimensional models of affect) is quite different from our view.

Evidence of Bipolar Dimensions

Which view is more accurate? There is not a wealth of information on this question, but there is a little. Consider affect when "doing well" in threat avoidance. In one study (Higgins, Shah, & Friedman, 1997, Study 4), people received either an approach orientation to a laboratory task (try to attain success) or an avoidance orientation to it (try to avoid failing); they then experienced either goal attainment or nonattainment. After the task outcome (which was manipulated), several feeling qualities were assessed. Among persons given an avoidance orientation, success caused elevation in calmness, and failure caused elevation in anxiety. Effects on calmness and anxiety did not occur, however, among persons given an approach orientation. This pattern suggests that (consistent with Figure 2.2) calmness is linked to doing well at avoidance, rather than doing well at approach.

Another source of information, though more ambiguous, is data reported some years ago by Watson and Tellegen (1985). In their analysis of multiple samples of mood data, they reported "calm" to be a good (inverse) marker of negative affect in the majority of the data sets they examined. In contrast, "calm" never emerged as one of the best markers of positive affect. This suggests that these feelings may be linked to the functioning of a system of avoidance.

There is more evidence linking certain kinds of negative affect to "doing poorly" in approaching incentives. Some of that evidence comes from the study by Higgins and colleagues (1997) just described. The conditions I focused on in the previous paragraph were those that led to feelings of calmness and anxiety. However, the study also provided data on sadness. Among persons with an approach orientation, failure caused elevated sadness, and success caused elevated cheerfulness. These effects did not occur, however, among participants who had an avoidance orientation. The pattern suggests a link between sadness and doing poorly at approach, rather than doing poorly at avoidance.

Another source of evidence on sadness is a laboratory study (Carver, in press) in which participants were led to believe they could obtain a desired reward if they performed well on a task. The situation involved no penalty for doing poorly—just the opportunity of reward for doing well. Participants had been preassessed on a self-report measure of the sensitivity of their approach and avoidance systems, a measure that has been validated with regard to affective responses to cues of impending incentive and threat (Carver & White, 1994). All participants were given false feedback indicating they had not done well; thus, they failed to obtain the reward. Reports of sadness and discouragement at that point related significantly to premeasured sensitivity of the approach system, but not to sensitivity of the avoidance system.

Another source of information is the literature on self-discrepancy theory. Several studies have shown that feelings of depression relate uniquely (i.e., controlling for anxiety) to discrepancies between people's actual selves and their ideal selves (see Higgins, 1987, 1996, for reviews). Ideals are qualities that a person intrinsically desires to embody: aspirations, hopes, positive wishes for the self. There is evidence supporting the view that pursuing an ideal is an approach process (Higgins, 1996). Thus, this literature also suggests that sad affect stems from a failure of approach.

Yet one more source of evidence, though again ambiguous, is the data reported by Watson and Tellegen (1985). They reported "sad" to be a good (inverse) marker of positive affect in the majority of the data sets they examined, whereas it never emerged as one of the top markers of negative affect in those data sets. This pattern suggests a link between sad feelings and approach. The ambiguity about this particular finding derives from the fact that "sad" usually relates more strongly to the negative-affect factor (despite not being among the best indicators of that factor) than to the positive-affect factor.

There is also evidence linking the approach system to the negative affect of anger. Harmon-Jones and Allen (1998) studied individual differences in trait anger. Higher trait anger related to higher left frontal activity (and to lower right frontal activity). This pattern suggests a link between anger and the approach system, because the approach system has been linked to activation of the left prefrontal cortex (e.g., Davidson, 1992). On the other hand, an important qualification on this finding is that it pertains to trait rather than state anger. More recently, Harmon-Jones and Sigelman (2001) induced a state of anger in some persons but not others, then examined cortical activity. Consistent with the findings described thus far, they found elevations in relative left frontal activity, suggesting that anger relates to greater engagement of the approach system.

One more source of evidence on anger is research in which participants indicated the feelings they experienced in response to hypothetical events (Study 2) and after the destruction of the World Trade Center (Study 3; Carver, in press). Participants had been preassessed on a self-report measure of the sensitivity of their approach and avoidance systems (Carver & White, 1994). Reports of anger related significantly to premeasured sensitivity of the approach system, whereas reports of anxiety related to sensitivity of the avoidance system.

In summary, there are good reasons to believe that certain kinds of negative affect relate to an approach system. There is also some reason to suspect that certain kinds of positive affect relate to an avoidance system.

I have devoted a good deal of space to this issue. Why does it matter so much? It matters because it appears to have major implications for the search for a conceptual mechanism underlying affect. Theories that argue for two unipolar dimensions appear to assume that greater activation of a system translates directly to more affect of that valence (or greater potential for affect of that valence). If the approach system instead relates to both positive and negative feelings, this direct transformation of system activation to affect is not tenable. How, then, can theories assuming such a transformation account for the negative affects?

A conceptual mechanism would be needed that naturally addresses both positive and negative feelings within the approach function (and, separately, the avoidance function). One such principle is the one described here (Carver & Scheier, 1990, 1998). There may be others, but this one has advantages. For example, its mechanism fits nicely with the fact that feelings occur continuously throughout the attempt to reach an incentive, not just at the point of its attainment. Indeed, feelings rise, wane, and change valence as progress varies from time to time along the way forward.

COUNTERINTUITIVE IMPLICATIONS

Another potentially important issue also differentiates this model from most other viewpoints on the meaning and consequences of affect. Recall that this theory sees affect as reflecting the error signal from a comparison process in a feedback loop. This idea has some very counterintuitive implications—in particular, implications concerning positive affect (Carver, 2003b).

If affect reflects the error signal in a feedback loop, affect is therefore a signal to adjust rate of progress. This would be true whether the rate is above the mark or below it, that is, whether affect is positive or negative. For negative feelings, this is not at all controversial. This line of thought is completely intuitive. The first response to negative feelings is to try harder. (For now, I disregard the possibility of giving up effort and quitting the goal, though that possibility clearly is important; I return to it later.) If the person tries harder, and assuming that more effort (or better effort) increases the rate of intended movement, the negative affect diminishes or ceases.

For positive feelings, however, the implications of this line of argument are very counterintuitive. In this model, positive feelings arise when things are going better than necessary. But the feelings still reflect a discrepancy (albeit a positive one), and the function of a negative feedback loop is to minimize discrepancies. Thus, the system "wants" to see neither negative nor positive affect. Either quality (deviation from the standard in either direction) would represent an "error" and lead to changes in output that would eventually reduce the error.

This view argues that people who exceed the criterion rate of progress (i.e., who have positive feelings) will reduce subsequent effort in this domain. They are likely to "coast" a little (cf. Frijda, 1994, p. 113)—not necessarily stop, but ease back, such that subsequent rate of progress returns to the criterion. The impact on subjective affect would be that the positive feeling is not sustained for very long. It begins to fade. The fading may be particularly rapid if the person does turn from this activity to another domain of behavior (Erber & Tesser, 1992).

Let me be clear that expending greater effort to catch up when behind, and coasting when ahead, are both presumed to be specific to the goal domain to which the affect is attached. Usually (though not always), this is the goal that underlies the generation of the affect in the first place (for exceptions, see Schwarz & Clore, 1983). I am not arguing that positive affect creates a tendency to coast *in general*, but rather that it creates a tendency to coast with respect to this activity.

There is an analogy that fits this theory nicely. This is a kind of "cruise control" model of the origins and consequences of affect. That is, the system just described operates much the same as a car's cruise control. If your behavior is progressing too slowly, negative affect arises. You respond by increasing effort, trying to speed up. If you are going faster than needed, positive affect arises, and you coast. A car's cruise control is very similar. Coming to a hill slows you down; the cruise control responds by feeding the engine more gas, and you speed back up. If you cross the crest of a hill and roll downward too fast, the system cuts back the gas, dragging the speed back down.

The analogy is intriguing partly because both parts have an asymmetry in the consequences of deviation from the reference point. That is, both in a car and in behavior, addressing the problem of going too slow requires adding effort and resources. Addressing the problem of going too fast does not. Indeed, quite the opposite. It requires only reducing resources. The cruise control does not apply the brakes, it just cuts back the fuel. The car coasts back to the velocity set point. Thus, the effect of the cruise control on a high rate of speed depends in part on external circumstances. If the hill is steep, the car may exceed the cruise control's set point all the way to the valley below.

In the same fashion, people usually do not react to positive affect by actively trying to make themselves feel less good (though there are exceptions—Martin & Davies, 1998; Parrott, 1993). They simply pull back temporarily on the resources devoted to the domain in which the affect has arisen. The positive feelings may be sustained for a long time (depending on circumstances) as the person coasts down the subjective analogue of the hill. Eventually, though, the reducing of resources would cause the positive affect to diminish. Generally, then, the system would act to prevent great amounts of pleasure as well as a great amount of pain (Carver, 2003b; Carver & Scheier, 1998).

Coasting

The idea that positive affect leads to coasting, which would eventually result in reduction of the positive affect, strikes some people as being unlikely at best. Many believe that pleasure is instead a sign to continue what one is doing or even to immerse oneself in it more deeply (cf. Fredrickson, 2001; Messinger, 2002). On the other hand, the latter view creates something of a logical problem. If pleasure increases engagement in the ongoing activity, leading thereby to more pleasure and thus more engagement, when and why would the person ever cease that activity?

The notion that positive feelings induce coasting may seem unlikely, but we are not the only ones to have suggested such a thing. In discussing joy, Izard (1977) wrote,

> If the kind of problem at hand requires a great deal of persistence and hard work, *joy may put the problem aside before it is solved.* . . . If your intellectual performance, whatever it may be, leads to joy, the joy will have the effect of *slowing down performance* and removing some of the concern for problem solving. This change in pace and concern may postpone or in some cases eliminate the possibility of an intellectual or creative achievement. . . . If excitement causes the "rushing" or "forcing" of intellectual activity, a *joy-elicited slowing down* may be exactly what is need to improve intellectual performance and creative endeavor. (p. 257, emphasis added)

More recently, Izard and Ackerman (2000) wrote, "Periodic joy provides *respite from the activity* driven by intense interest" (p. 258, emphasis added).

Does positive affect lead to coasting? I know of no data that address the question unambiguously (though suggestive evidence was reported by Mizruchi, 1991). To do so, a study must assess coasting with respect to the same goal as that underlying the affect. Many studies have been done in which positive affect is created in one context and its influence is assessed on another task (e.g., Isen, 1987, 2000; Schwarz & Bohner, 1996). Those who conduct such studies typically work hard to make the two contexts appear unrelated. Thus, this question seems to remain relatively open.

Coasting and Multiple Concerns

One reason for doubting the idea that positive affect induces coasting is that it is hard to see why a process could possibly be built-in that limits positive feelings—indeed, that reduces them. After all, a truism of life is that people supposedly are organized to seek pleasure and avoid pain.

I believe that a basis for the adaptive value of the tendency to coast lies in the fact that people have multiple concerns at the same time (Carver, 2003b; Carver & Scheier, 1998; Frijda, 1994). Given multiple concerns, people do not optimize their performance on any one of them, but rather "satisfice" (Simon, 1953)—do a good-enough job on each concern to deal with it satisfactorily.

A tendency to coast would virtually define satisficing regarding that particular goal. That is, reducing effort would prevent the attainment of the best possible outcome. A tendency to coast would also foster satisficing regarding a broader set of several goals. That is, if progress toward goal attainment in one domain exceeds current needs, a tendency to coast in that particular domain (satisficing) would make it easy to shift to another domain at little or no cost. This would help ensure satisfactory goal attainment in the other domain and, ultimately, across multiple domains.

Continued pursuit of the present goal without letup, in contrast, can have adverse effects. Continuing a rapid pace in one arena may sustain positive affect in that arena, but by diverting resources from other goals it also increases the potential for problems elsewhere. This would be even more true of an effort to *intensify* the positive affect, because doing that would entail further diverting of resources from other goals. Indeed, a single-minded pursuit of yet-more-positive feelings in one domain can even be fatal, if it causes the person to disregard threats looming elsewhere.

A pattern in which positive feelings lead to easing back and to an openness to shifting focus, would minimize such adverse effects. It is important to note that this view does not *require* that people with positive feelings shift goals. It simply holds that openness to a shift in goals is a potential consequence—and a potential benefit—of the coasting tendency. This line of thought would, however, begin to account for why people do eventually turn away from what are clearly pleasurable activities.

A provocative finding in this regard is that smiling infants engaging in face-to-face interactions with their mothers periodically avert their gazes from their mothers, then stop smiling. Infants are more likely to do this (and to avert their gaze longer) when they are smiling intensely than when the smiles are less intense (Stifter & Moyer, 1991). This pattern hints that the experience of happiness creates in the infant an openness to shifting focus, or at least a tendency to coast with respect to the interaction with the mother, letting the affect diminish before returning to the interaction.

PRIORITY MANAGEMENT
AS A CORE ISSUE IN SELF-REGULATION

The line of argument just outlined begins to implicate positive feelings in a broad function within the organism that deserves much further consideration. This function is the shifting from one goal to another as focal in behavior (cf. Shallice, 1978). This basic and very important function is often overlooked. Humans usually pursue many goals simultaneously (cf. Atkinson & Birch, 1970; Murray, 1938), and only one can have top priority at a given moment. Yet from one time to the next, there clearly are changes in which goal has the top priority.

The problem of priority management among multiple goals was addressed many years ago in a creative and influential article by Herb Simon (1967). He pointed out that any entity that has many goals needs a way to rank them for pursuit, and a mechanism to change the rankings as necessary. Most of the goals we are pursuing are largely outside awareness at any given moment. Only the one with the highest priority has full access to consciousness. Sometimes events that occur during the pursuit of that top-priority goal create problems for another goal that now has a lower priority. Indeed, the mere passing of time can sometimes create a problem for the second goal, because the passing of time may make its attainment less likely. If the second goal is important, an emerging problem for its attainment needs to be registered and somehow taken into account. If the situation evolves enough to seriously threaten the second goal, some mechanism is needed for changing priorities, so that the second goal replaces the first one as focal.

Negative Feelings and Reprioritization

Simon (1967) reasoned that emotions are calls for reprioritization. He suggested that emotion arising with respect to a goal that is outside awareness eventually induces people to interrupt their behavior and give that goal a higher priority than it had. The stronger the emotion, the stronger is the claim being made that the unattended goal should have higher priority than the current focal goal. The affect is what pulls the out-of-awareness into awareness. Simon did not address negative affect that arises with respect to a current focal goal, but the same principle seems to apply. In that case, negative affect seems to be a call for an even greater investment of resources and effort in that focal goal than is now being made.

Simon's analysis is applied easily to negative feelings such as anxiety. If you are following driving instructions that take you into a dangerous part of town, the focal goal is getting to your destination. Anxiety that arises concerns a second issue—a threat to your safety. If you promised your spouse you would go to the post office this afternoon and you have been too busy to go, the creeping of the clock toward closing time can cause an increase in anxiety. The anxiety is not about the work you've been occupied with, but about the second issue: an angry spouse. Anxiety arises when a threat is coming closer, whether the threat comes from an ongoing action (e.g., entering a bad area of town) or arises through the passage of time. The greater the threat, the stronger the anxiety. The stronger the anxiety, the more likely it is that the anti-goal from which it stems will rise in priority, until it comes fully to awareness and itself becomes the focal reference point for behavior.

Positive Feelings and Reprioritization

Simon's discussion of shifting priorities focused on cases in which a nonfocal goal demands a higher priority than it now has and *intrudes* on awareness. By strong implication, his discussion dealt only with negative affect. However, there is another way in which priority ordering can shift: The currently focal goal can *relinquish its place*. Simon noted this possibility obliquely. He pointed out that goal completion results in termination of pursuit of that goal. However, he did not address the possibility that an as-yet-unattained goal might also yield its place in line.

Consider the possibility that positive feelings represent a cue regarding reprioritization, but a cue to *reduce* the priority of the goal to which the feeling pertains. This possibility appears to do no violence to the sense of Simon's analysis. Rather, it simply suggests that the function he asserted for affect is relevant to affects of both valences. Positive affect regarding an avoidance act (relief or tranquility) indicates that a threat has dissipated, no longer requires as much attention as it did, and can now assume a lower priority. Positive feelings regarding approach (happiness, joy) indicate that an incentive is being attained. If it *has* been attained, effort can cease, as Simon noted. If it is not yet attained, the affect is a signal that you could temporarily put this goal aside, because you are doing so well. That is, it's a sign that this goal can assume a lower priority (Carver, 2003b).

If a focal goal diminishes in priority, what follows? In principle, this is a less directive situation than the one in which a nonfocal goal demands an increase in priority (which is very specific about what goal should receive more attention). What happens next in the case of positive affect depends partly on what else is waiting in line. It also depends partly on whether the context has changed in any important way while you were busy with the focal goal. That is, opportunities to attain incentives sometimes appear unexpectedly, and people often put aside their plans to take advantage of such unanticipated opportunities (Hayes-Roth & Hayes-Roth, 1979; Payton, 1990). It seems reasonable that people experiencing positive affect should be most prone to shift goals at this point if something else needs fixing or doing (regarding a next-in-line goal or a newly emergent goal) or if an unanticipated opportunity for gain has appeared.

Sometimes the next item in line is of fairly high priority in its own right. Sometimes the situation has changed and a new goal has emerged for consideration. On the other hand, sometimes neither of these conditions exists. Often the situation has not changed enough that a new goal has emerged for consideration, and no pressing goal is waiting in line. In such a case, no change in focal goal would occur, because the downgrade in priority of the now-focal goal does not render it lower than the priorities of the alternatives. Thus, positive feeling does not *require* that there be a change in direction. It simply sets the stage for such a change to be more likely.

Given the nature of this line of reasoning, it seems likely that when the priority of the focal activity drops, there ensues a scanning for potential next actions (cf. Vallacher & Kaufman, 1996). Such scanning would use internal information about goals waiting in line and also information from the environment. Unless the latter took place, there would be no chance to recognize and act on unexpected opportunities.

Evidence That Positive Affect Promotes Shifting

Aspects of this line of reasoning have a good deal in common with ideas recently proposed about circumstances under which people do and do not engage in self-esteem-protective behavior. Maintaining self-esteem is an important human goal (e.g., Tesser, 1988). When people are in good moods, however, self-esteem enhancement becomes less likely (Tesser, Crepaz, Collins, Cornell, & Beach, 2000). Tesser et al. argued from this that self-esteem maintenance follows the principle of satisficing. That is, it does not happen all the time in people's behavior. As long as the self-image is above a threshold of positivity, there is no effort to build it higher. Only if it falls below the threshold is effort engaged to prop it back up (cf. Reed & Aspinwall, 1998).

This line of argument was specific to self-evaluation maintenance. But it is consistent in theme with the ideas just presented about coasting and shifting as a way of satisficing with respect to multiple concerns. The effects that Tesser and colleagues (2000) discussed appear very much like the behaviors of people who are doing well enough for the time being with respect to one important goal (self-esteem), and are free to turn to something else that might benefit from their attention.

Indeed, a variety of other evidence appears to fit the idea that positive feelings make people more open to alternate goals, particularly desired goals that seem threatened. Trope and Neter (1994) had participants complete two ostensibly unrelated sessions in succession. In the first, positive affect was induced or not. In the second, participants took a social sensitivity test and were told that they performed well on two parts of it but poorly on a third. They then indicated their interest in reading more about their performances on the various parts of the test. Positive-mood participants showed more interest in the part they had failed than did controls. I interpret this as indicating that the positive feeling (arising from a behavioral context unrelated to the target task) rendered people more open to fixing a problem that needed fixing—the poor performance on the target task.

Trope and Pomerantz (1998) conceptually replicated this effect. In a first session, participants experienced either success or failure. In an ostensibly unrelated second session, they were offered feedback about their ability to attain life goals that varied in self-relevance. The feedback would pertain to either self-assets or self-liabilities. After success, greater self-relevance of the goal related to greater participant interest in feedback about self-liabilities pertaining to that goal.

Reed and Aspinwall (1998) also conceptually replicated this effect. Participants completed a measure on which they had an opportunity to affirm their kindness (or a control measure). They then had an opportunity to read information that either asserted or discounted a potential health threat from caffeine. The key finding occurred among participants who were high caffeine users, and thus had the greatest reason to be threatened by the threat assertion. The prior affirmation of positive self-image (kindness) made these persons more open to the information about how caffeine poses a health threat.

These studies all represent cases in which people confronted a personally relevant situation in need of repair. Other researchers have created situations in which someone else needed help. A substantial body of research shows that people in good moods are more willing to help another than are those in less-good moods (Isen, 1987, 2000). I interpret this as reflecting a tendency to fix a salient problem (for more detail, see Carver 2003b).

Psychological Resource Models

Effects such as these have contributed to the emergence of the view that positive experiences represent psychological resources. Trope and Pomerantz (1998) wrote that experiences such as a success or a positive mood often serve as means to other ends, rather than as ends themselves. Reed and Aspinwall (1998) suggested that positive self-beliefs and self-affirmations act as resources that permit people to confront problematic situations such as health threats (see also Aspinwall, 1998; Isen, 2000; Tesser et al., 2000; for even broader resource models, see Hobfoll, 1989, 2002; Muraven & Baumeister, 2000).

This line of thought is not quite the same as that underlying the position I am taking, but some of its connotations are very similar. Either line of thought suggests that when the situation seems to be in good shape in the focal domain (via a success, or recall of good times, or positive feelings, or self-affirmation), people are more likely to take up a salient problem in another domain. Although the findings described are consistent with this line of reasoning, most of the studies were conducted to investigate self-protective tendencies per se, rather than shifts in goal or task. My line of reasoning holds that such shifts should be observable for a wide range of alternative activities, rather than just for those related to self-improvement, health maintenance, helping, or the like (although repairing problems for oneself would certainly be very high-priority targets for such shifts).

Opportunistic Shifting

On the other hand, the idea that positive feelings act as psychological resources need not be limited to cases in which resources permit people to turn to problems. For example, secure infant attachment is widely seen as a resource that promotes exploration (Bowlby, 1988). Such a view also seems implicit in Fredrickson's (1998) position that positive feelings promote play.

The idea that positive affect serves as a resource for exploration resembles in some ways the idea that positive feelings open people to noticing and taking advantage of emergent opportunities, to being distracted into enticing alternatives—to opportunistic behavior. Some evidence is consistent with this idea. Kahn and Isen (1993) reported studies in which people had opportunities to try out choices within a food category. Those in whom positive affect had been induced switched among choice alternatives more than did controls. Isen (2000, p. 423) interpreted this as indicating that positive affect promotes "enjoyment of variety and a wide range of possibilities," which seems almost a description of opportunistic foraging.

Another source of evidence worth brief mention, although there are also reasons to view it with caution, is the behavior of persons in manic or hypomanic states. Mania is characterized by positive feelings, and also by a high degree of distractibility (American Psychiatric Association, 1994). This pattern is consistent with the idea that the positive feelings render these persons especially susceptible to cues indicating opportunities for gain that lie outside the framework of their current goal pursuit.

Priority Management and Depressed Affect

One more aspect of priority management that should be addressed here concerns the idea that in some circumstances, goals are not attainable and are better abandoned. We have long argued that sufficient doubt about goal attainment results in an impetus to disengage from efforts to reach the goal, and even to disengage from the goal itself (Carver & Scheier, 1981, 1998, 1999a, 1999b). This is certainly a kind of priority adjustment, in that the abandoned goal now has a lower priority than it had before. How does this sort of reprioritization fit into the picture sketched in the preceding sections?

At first glance, the idea that doubt about goal attainment (and the negative feelings associated with that doubt) causes reduction in effort seems to contradict Simon's (1967) position that negative affect is a call for higher priority. I believe, however, that there is an important distinction between two kinds of negative affective experiences associated with approach (Carver, in press). (A parallel line of reasoning can be applied to avoidance, but I limit myself here to approach.) One set of negative affects related to approach coalesce around frustration and anger. The other set coalesces around sadness, depression, and dejection.

In presenting the Carver and Scheier (1998, 1999b) view on affect earlier (Figure 2.2), I described the approach-related affective dimension as ranging from elation to depression. That depiction accounts for feelings of sadness, but it ignores frustration and anger. In reality, however, although Figure 2.2 conveys the sense that approach-related affect can be either positive or negative (or absent), it has only a rough fit to the conceptual model on which it was based.

Theory holds that falling behind—progress below the criterion—creates negative affect, as the incentive seems to be slipping away. Inadequate movement forward (or no movement, or reverse movement) gives rise to feelings such as frustration, irritation, and anger. The lagging of progress (or the affect thereby created) prompts enhanced exertion, in an effort to catch up. Thus, the function of these feelings (or of the mechanism that underlies them) is to engage effort more completely, to overcome obstacles and reverse the inadequacy of current progress. If the situation is one in which more effort (or better effort) can improve progress, such effort allows the person to move toward the incentive at an adequate rate, and attaining the incentive seems likely. This case fits the priority management model of Simon (1967).

Sometimes, however, continued efforts do not produce adequate movement forward. Indeed, if the situation involves loss, movement forward is precluded, because the incentive is gone. In a situation in which failure seems (or is) assured, the negative affect has a different tone. Here the feelings are sadness, depression, despondency, dejection, grief, and hopelessness (cf. Finlay-Jones & Brown, 1981). Accompanying behaviors also differ in this case. The person tends to disengage from—give up on—further effort toward the incentive (Klinger, 1975; Wortman & Brehm, 1975; for supporting evidence, see Lewis, Sullivan, Ramsay, & Allessandri, 1992; Mikulincer, 1988).

I know of two published studies that obtained patterns of emotions consistent with this portrayal (Mikulincer, 1994; Pittman & Pittman, 1980). In each, participants received varying amounts of failure, and their emotional responses were assessed. In both cases, reports of anger were most intense after small amounts of failure, and lower after larger amounts of failure. Reports of depression were low after small amounts of failure, and intense after larger amounts of failure.

As just described, approach-related negative feelings in these two kinds of situations are presumed to link to two very different effects on ongoing action. Both have adaptive properties. In the first situation—when the person falls behind but the goal is not seen as lost—feelings of frustration and anger accompany an increase in effort, a struggle to gain the incentive despite setbacks. Consistent with this view, Frijda (1986, p. 429) has argued that anger implies having the hope that things can be set right (see also Harmon-Jones & Allen, 1998). This struggle is adaptive (thus, the affect is adaptive) because the struggle fosters goal attainment.

In the second situation—when effort appears futile—negative feelings of sadness and depression accompany *reduction* of effort. Sadness and despondency imply that things cannot be set right, that further effort is pointless. Reduction of effort in this circumstance can also have adaptive functions (Carver & Scheier, 2003; Wrosch, Scheier, Carver, & Schulz, 2003; Wrosch, Scheier, Miller, Schulz, & Carver, in press). It serves to conserve energy rather than to waste it in futile pursuit of the unattainable (Nesse, 2000). If reducing effort also helps to diminish commitment to the goal (Klinger, 1975), it eventually readies the person to take up pursuit of another incentive in place of this one. That is, it is hard to turn to a new goal until one disengages from the unattainable goal and is no longer preoccupied by it.

The variations in effort described in the preceding paragraphs are portrayed in Figure 2.3, which elaborates on the left panel of Figure 2.2 (and is an adaptation of a figure from Carver, in press). The left side of Figure 2.3 portrays the hypothesized reduction in effort when velocity exceeds the criterion, discussed earlier. The right side portrays both the strong engagement implied by frustration and anger, and the disengagement of sadness and dejection.

I want to make two additional points about the portion of Figure 2.3 to the right of the criterion rate. First, this part of Figure 2.3 has much in common with several other depictions of variations in effort when difficulty in moving toward a goal gives way to loss of the goal (for details, see Carver & Scheier, 1998, Ch. 11). Perhaps best known is Wortman and Brehm's (1975) integration of reactance and helplessness. They described a region of threat to control, in which there is enhanced effort to regain control, and a region of loss of control, in which efforts diminish. Indeed, the figure they used to illustrate those regions greatly resembles the right side of Figure 2.3.

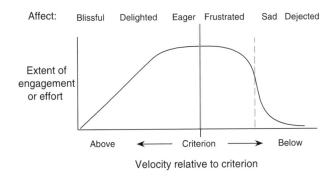

FIGURE 2.3. Approach-related affects as a function of doing well versus doing poorly compared to a criterion velocity, building on the left panel of Figure 2.2, which has been rotated 90° at the left. Additional affects are named here, and a second (vertical) dimension indicates the degree of behavioral engagement posited to be associated with affects at different degrees of departure from neutral. From Carver (in press). Copyright by the American Psychological Association. Adapted by permission.

Second, the right side of Figure 2.3 is drawn with a rather abrupt shift from frustration to sadness. The degree of abruptness of the transition in this figure is arbitrary. I believe there are cases in which the transition is abrupt, and also cases in which it is not. The two sets of cases may be distinguished by their relative importance. Importance is a variable that I have ignored in this discussion, but it is one that obviously must play a very large role in the intensity of affective experience. Although there is not space here to address this issue adequately, discussions of it can be found elsewhere (Carver & Scheier, 1998, 1999a, 1999b).

This aspect of Figure 2.3 illustrates how these ideas can be linked to another set of ideas that are increasingly influencing thought in psychology: the concepts of dynamic systems theory (Vallacher, Read, & Nowak, 2002). The transition from engagement to disengagement can be seen as a gradual movement along a dimension, but it can also be seen as a qualitative shift, even the bifurcation of a cusp catastrophe (Carver & Scheier, 1998, Chs. 14–16). In theory, situations that create aggravation versus despondency move subsequent behavior in divergent directions: further efforts versus giving up. The idea that behavior under adversity bifurcates into the two classes of effort versus giving up has been an aspect of our conceptual model for decades (Carver & Scheier, 1981).

TWO MORE ISSUES

I would like to mention briefly two more issues that remove us from the main points of this chapter, but also bear on the viability of these ideas. Both suggest ways in which these ideas must incorporate additional flexibility.

Conflict and Self-Control

One issue concerns conflict. Conflict occurs whenever two values are engaged at the same time (for pursuit or avoidance), and responses to one create problems for the other. Conflict has been an important concept in psychological theory for generations (Miller, 1944). The theoretical model outlined here seems well suited to the general notion of conflict (for details, see Carver & Scheier, 1998, 1999a, 1999b).

Of particular interest to many people in recent years have been cases in which a person is both motivated to do something and motivated to restrain that impulse (Carver, 2003a). Impulse restraint is a common problem in life outside the laboratory, and one with serious practical implications in contexts that include dieting, substance abuse, restraint of aggression, and many others. Partly for this reason, this class of situations has become the focal case for many discussions of conflict. Indeed, some writers have gone so far as to use the term "self-regulation" as synonymous with "self-control," referring to the overcoming of an impulse (Baumeister & Heatherton, 1996).

Self-control often is difficult, and sometimes the restrained impulse breaks free. Consider binge eating. The binge eater wants to eat but also wants to restrain that desire. If self-control lapses, the person stops trying to restrain, and binges. Baumeister and Heatherton (1996) have noted that mental fatigue plays a role in this, but fatigue is rarely the sole factor. There often is a point where the person says "Enough," and stops trying to self-control. We've suggested that confidence plays a role here, as elsewhere in behavior (Carver & Scheier, 1998). The person who is confident continues the struggle to restrain. The person whose confidence has sagged is more likely to give up. As in Figure 2.3, there is a bifurcation among responses: continued resistance versus giving up.

Muraven, Tice, and Baumeister (1998; Muraven & Baumeister, 2000) extended this line of thought to argue that self-control involves a resource that is limited and can become depleted by extended self-control efforts (see also Schmeichel & Baumeister, Chapter 5, and Vohs & Ciarocco, Chapter 20, this volume). When the resource is depleted, the person becomes vulnerable to a failure of self-control. This view suggests further that the pool of self-control resources is shared, so that exhausting resources with one kind of self-control (e.g., concentrating hard for many hours on a writing assignment) can leave the person vulnerable to a lapse in a different domain (e.g., eating restraint). This model of competition for limited energy, which evokes the competition between id and ego, is a reminder that behavioral self-regulation occurs in a living biological body that has its own constraints (e.g., energy depletion through exertion).

Much of the recent literature on this issue focuses on situations in which the person is restraining a self-destructive or socially destructive impulse. As noted earlier, the practical implications of such cases make them particularly salient. Yet the structure of these conflicts does not seem inherently different from the structures of other conflicts. The desire to eat without restraint conflicts with the desire to control one's weight. The desire to lash out in anger at one's boss conflicts with the desire to keep one's job. In each case, pursuing one desire creates problems for the other one.

There does appear to be one peculiarity in the case of impulse restraint that makes it at least somewhat different from other cases, and this peculiarity may be important in its own right. What I have described as an impulse under restraint is often literally impulsive. That is, it is not planful, thought out, or premeditated. The act of restraint, in contrast, typically is an effort to attain or maintain a somewhat more abstract or long-term goal, which usually is more premeditated and planful. A number of theorists in personality–social psychology and elsewhere have asked how impulsive and planful actions differ. Some theorists have argued that there are two distinct systems of self-regulation, with two sorts of operating characteristics (cf. Chaiken & Trope, 1999; Epstein, 1985, 1994; Lieberman, Gaunt, Gilbert, & Trope, 2002; Metcalfe & Mischel, 1999; Shastri & Ajjanagadde, 1993; Sloman, 1996; Smith & DeCoster, 2000).

This is an interesting idea that has many implications. For example, it helps to make sense of the finding that a loss of self-awareness (via deindividuation or alcohol ingestion) causes behavior to become more impulsive and responsive to cues of the moment (e.g., Diener, 1979; Hull, 1981; Prentice-Dunn & Rogers, 1989; Steele & Josephs, 1990; see also Hull & Slone, Chapter 24, this volume). In this pattern, it seems as though an effortful, planful system is functioning less, leaving in charge an impulsive system with only short-term goals. Indeed, some kinds of impulsive behavior cause further reduction in self-awareness, thereby exacerbating the impulsive and unrestrained character of the behavior (Baumeister & Heatherton, 1996; Heatherton & Baumeister, 1991; see also Carver & Scheier, 1998, Ch. 13). This line of thought undoubtedly will receive much further consideration.

Self-Organization and Dynamic Systems

Another issue I want to raise briefly concerns the emerging influence of a set of ideas often labeled dynamic systems theory (Nowak & Vallacher, 1998; Vallacher & Nowak, 1994, 1997; Vallacher et al., 2002). The details of dynamic systems theory would require a long discussion (for basic introductions to some of the themes, see Carver & Scheier, 1998, 2002; for more elaborate treatments, though still based in the topics of social psychology, see Vallacher & Nowak, 1994, 1997; Vallacher et al., 2002). For present purposes, I wish only to raise some of the central premises of dynamic-systems thinking and to consider their implications for feedback models.

Dynamic systems models allow for stability (regions of behavioral space termed "attractors"), but their hallmark is that they describe how systems change over time (e.g., shifts from one attractor basin to another). One way to link the concepts of dynamic systems to the ideas discussed here is to think of goals as attractors, and the reprioritization of goals that people undergo as representing shifts from one attractor basin to another (Carver & Scheier, 2002).

The dynamic-systems view of behavior and the control-process view of behavior are in many ways complementary. However, there are different emphases in the ways the models have been applied to psychological phenomena. In describing the feedback-based view earlier, I implied that when a goal is adopted, the process of moving toward it is guided by a representation of the goal, and managed and controlled by some sort of "executive" or intentional process.

In contrast, the dynamic-systems model does not rely on assumptions about top–down guidance, or even structure. Rather, attractors are said to arise from the intrinsic dynamics of the system as it operates in its world over an extended period of time. Complex systems are said to have a *self-organizing* character (Kelso, 1995; Prigogene & Stengers, 1984). The various forces interweave in ways that are not determined by any one of them alone, but rather by their mutual influences on each other. Patterns emerge spontaneously.

The principle of self-organization has some fairly obvious applications to human behavior (Carver & Scheier, 2002). People's perceptions appear to coalesce in Gestalt patterns from the bits and pieces that underlie them (Read, Vanman, & Miller, 1997). People's actions are sometimes shunted to an unintended path because of slight variations in the circumstances they encounter. People occasionally discover what they are doing as they find themselves doing it. Far more than we might think, our actions are influenced by incidental stimulus qualities that we happen to encounter along the way (Bargh, 1997).

How can such different emphases be reconciled? One possibility returns us to the idea of there being two different systems with somewhat different operating characteristics (Carver & Scheier, 1998, 2002). There is good reason to believe that self-organizing, emergent rhythms and cycles in behavior exert influences that have not been well appreciated. There is reason to suspect that people drift or stumble into patterns of action (or thought) they have not experienced before. Yet it also seems reasonable to suggest that as emergent patterns stabilize over repeated occurrences, the patterns are coded into memory in a form that permits them to be invoked for re-creation by an intentional process. To put it differently, a bottom–up process of self-organized pattern development may consolidate in a way that leaves an entry point for top–down control.

Does such consolidation occur? Clearly, something like this happens in skill learning. Something changes, as behaviors—even self-organized coordinations—are repeated over and over. Indeed, there is evidence that different parts of the brain are involved to different degrees when a behavior is relatively new versus being well practiced (Gazzaniga, Ivry, & Mangun, 1998). Two modes of creating behavior may be at work, one operating bottom–up, the other top–down. Executive use of compiled capabilities cannot happen without a solid record of what the capabilities are; one way for such a record to exist would be through an earlier emergence and consolidation of lower order, self-organized coordinations.

CONCLUDING COMMENTS

The ideas just outlined are more than just a little speculative, and they raise many questions. Indeed, many questions about human behavior have been ignored altogether here. For instance, what about will? What about self-determination? Even the top–down effortful processes outlined earlier were described in ways that seem rather automatic, devoid of self-determination. These questions, though important, remain untouched in this chapter. They are discussed in depth in other places (e.g., Bargh, 1997; Deci & Ryan, 2000; Ryan & Deci, 2001; Wegner, 2002). As I said at the chapter's outset, however, the ideas outlined here cover only parts of the puzzle. Creating models of self-regulation, as is true of all of psychology, remains a work in progress.

ACKNOWLEDGMENT

Preparation of this chapter was facilitated by Grant Nos. CA64710, CA78995, and CA84944 from the National Cancer Institute.

REFERENCES

American Psychiatric Association. (1994). *Diagnostic and statistical manual of mental disorders* (4th ed.). Washington, DC: Author.

Asch, S. E. (1955). Opinions and social pressure. *Scientific American, 193*, 31–35.

Aspinwall, L. G. (1998). Rethinking the role of positive affect in self-regulation. *Motivation and Emotion, 22*, 1–32.

Atkinson, J. W., & Birch, D. (1970). *The dynamics of action*. New York: Wiley.

Austin, J. T., & Vancouver, J. B. (1996). Goal constructs in psychology: Structure, process, and content. *Psychological Bulletin, 120*, 338–375.

Baumeister, R. F., Bratslavsky, E., Finkenauer, C., & Vohs, K. D. (2001). Bad is stronger than good. *Review of General Psychology, 5*, 323–370.

Bargh, J. A. (1997). The automaticity of everyday life. In R. S. Wyer, Jr. (Ed.), *Advances in social cognition* (Vol. 10, pp. 1–61). Mahwah, NJ: Erlbaum.

Baumeister, R. F., & Heatherton, T. F. (1996). Self-regulation failure: An overview. *Psychological Inquiry, 7*, 1–15.

Beer, R. D. (1995). A dynamical systems perspective on agent–environment interaction. *Artificial Intelligence, 72*, 173–215.

Bowlby, J. (1988). *A secure base: Parent–child attachment and healthy human development*. New York: Basic Books.

Buunk, B. P., & Gibbons, F. X. (Eds.). (1997). *Health, coping, and well-being: Perspectives from social comparison theory*. Mahwah, NJ: Erlbaum.

Cacioppo, J. T., & Berntson, G. G. (1994). Relationship between attitudes and evaluative space: A critical review, with emphasis on the separability of positive and negative substrates. *Psychological Bulletin, 115*, 401–423.

Cacioppo, J. T., Gardner, W. L., & Berntson, G. G. (1999). The affect system has parallel and integrative processing components: Form follows function. *Journal of Personality and Social Psychology, 76*, 839–855.

Cantor, N., & Kihlstrom, J. F. (1987). *Personality and social intelligence*. Englewood Cliffs, NJ: Prentice-Hall.

Carver, C. S. (2001). Affect and the functional bases of behavior: On the dimensional structure of affective experience. *Personality and Social Psychology Review, 5*, 345–356.

Carver, C. S. (2003a). *Impulse and constraint: Converging lines of thought from diverse aspects of psychology.* Unpublished manuscript.

Carver, C. S. (2003b). Pleasure as a sign you can attend to something else: Placing positive feelings within a general model of affect. *Cognition and Emotion, 17,* 241–261.

Carver, C. S. (in press). Negative affects deriving from the behavioral approach system. *Emotion.*

Carver, C. S., Lawrence, J. W., & Scheier, M. F. (1999). Self-discrepancies and affect: Incorporating the role of feared selves. *Personality and Social Psychology Bulletin, 25,* 783–792.

Carver, C. S., & Scheier, M. F. (1981). *Attention and self-regulation: A control-theory approach to human behavior.* New York: Springer-Verlag.

Carver, C. S., & Scheier, M. F. (1990). Origins and functions of positive and negative affect: A control-process view. *Psychological Review, 97,* 19–35.

Carver, C. S., & Scheier, M. F. (1998). *On the self-regulation of behavior.* New York: Cambridge University Press.

Carver, C. S., & Scheier, M. F. (1999a). Several more themes, a lot more issues: Commentary on the commentaries. In R. S. Wyer, Jr. (Ed.), *Advances in social cognition* (Vol. 12, pp. 261–302). Mahwah, NJ: Erlbaum.

Carver, C. S., & Scheier, M. F. (1999b). Themes and issues in the self-regulation of behavior. In R. S. Wyer, Jr. (Ed.), *Advances in social cognition* (Vol. 12, pp. 1–105). Mahwah, NJ: Erlbaum.

Carver, C. S., & Scheier, M. F. (2002). Control processes and self-organization as complementary principles underlying behavior. *Personality and Social Psychology Review, 6,* 304–315.

Carver, C. S., & Scheier, M. F. (2003). Three human strengths. In L. G. Aspinwall & U. M. Staudinger (Eds.), *A psychology of human strengths: Fundamental questions and future directions for a positive psychology* (pp. 87–102). Washington, DC: American Psychological Association.

Carver, C. S., & White, T. L. (1994). Behavioral inhibition, behavioral activation, and affective responses to impending reward and punishment: The BIS/BAS scales. *Journal of Personality and Social Psychology, 67,* 319–333.

Chaiken, S. L., & Trope, Y. (Eds.). (1999). *Dual-process theories in social psychology.* New York: Guilford Press.

Clark, R. N. (1996). *Control system dynamics.* New York: Cambridge University Press.

Clore, G. C. (1994). Why emotions are felt. In P. Ekman & R. J. Davidson (Eds.), *The nature of emotion: Fundamental questions* (pp. 103–111). New York: Oxford University Press.

Davidson, R. J. (1984). Affect, cognition, and hemispheric specialization. In C. E. Izard, J. Kagan, & R. Zajonc (Eds.), *Emotion, cognition, and behavior* (pp. 320–365). New York: Cambridge University Press.

Davidson, R. J. (1992). Anterior cerebral asymmetry and the nature of emotion. *Brain and Cognition, 20,* 125–151.

Davidson, R. J. (1995). Cerebral asymmetry, emotion, and affective style. In R. J. Davidson & K. Hugdahl (Eds.), *Brain asymmetry* (pp. 361–387). Cambridge, MA: MIT Press.

Davidson, R. J. (1998). Affective style and affective disorders: Perspectives from affective neuroscience. *Cognition and Emotion, 12,* 307–330.

Deci, E. L., & Ryan, R. M. (2000). The "what" and "why" of goal pursuits: Human needs and the self-determination of behavior. *Psychological Inquiry, 11,* 227–268.

Depue, R. A., & Collins, P. F. (1999). Neurobiology of the structure of personality: Dopamine, facilitation of incentive motivation, and extraversion. *Behavioral and Brain Sciences, 22,* 491–517.

Diener, E. (1979). Deindividuation, self-awareness, and disinhibition. *Journal of Personality and Social Psychology, 37,* 1160–1171.

Elliott, E. S., & Dweck, C. S. (1988). Goals: An approach to motivation and achievement. *Journal of Personality and Social Psychology, 54,* 5–12.

Emmons, R. A. (1986). Personal strivings: An approach to personality and subjective well being. *Journal of Personality and Social Psychology, 51,* 1058–1068.

Epstein, S. (1985). The implications of cognitive–experiential self theory for research in social psychology and personality. *Journal for the Theory of Social Behavior, 15*, 283–310.

Epstein, S. (1994). Integration of the cognitive and the psychodynamic unconscious. *American Psychologist, 49*, 709–724.

Erber, R., & Tesser, A. (1992). Task effort and the regulation of mood: The absorption hypothesis. *Journal of Experimental Social Psychology, 28*, 339–359.

Festinger, L. (1957). *A theory of cognitive dissonance.* Evanston, IL: Row, Peterson.

Finlay-Jones, R., & Brown, G. W. (1981). Types of stressful life event and the onset of anxiety and depressive disorders. *Psychological Medicine, 11*, 803–815.

Fredrickson, B. L. (1998). What good are positive emotions? *Review of General Psychology, 2*, 300–319.

Frederickson, B. L. (2001). The role of positive emotions in positive psychology: The broaden-and-build theory of positive emotions. *American Psychologist, 56*, 218–226.

Frijda, N. H. (1986). *The emotions.* Cambridge, UK: Cambridge University Press.

Frijda, N. H. (1988). The laws of emotion. *American Psychologist, 43*, 349–358.

Frijda, N. H. (1994). Emotions are functional, most of the time. In P. Ekman & R. J. Davidson (Eds.), *The nature of emotion: Fundamental questions* (pp. 112–126). New York: Oxford University Press.

Gazzaniga, M. S., Ivry, R. B., & Mangun, G. R. (1998). *Cognitive neuroscience: The biology of the mind.* New York: Norton.

Gray, J. A. (1990). Brain systems that mediate both emotion and cognition. *Cognition and Emotion, 4*, 269–288.

Gray, J. A. (1994a). Personality dimensions and emotion systems. In P. Ekman & R. J. Davidson (Eds.), *The nature of emotion: Fundamental questions* (pp. 329–331). New York: Oxford University Press.

Gray, J. A. (1994b). Three fundamental emotion systems. In P. Ekman & R. J. Davidson (Eds.), *The nature of emotion: Fundamental questions* (pp. 243–247). New York: Oxford University Press.

Harmon-Jones, E., & Allen, J. J. B. (1998). Anger and frontal brain activity: Asymmetry consistent with approach motivation despite negative affective valence. *Journal of Personality and Social Psychology, 74*, 1310–1316.

Harmon-Jones, E., & Sigelman, J. D. (2001). State anger and prefrontal brain activity: Evidence that insult-related relative left-prefrontal activation is associated with experienced anger and aggression. *Journal of Personality and Social Psychology, 80, 797–803.*

Hayes-Roth, B., & Hayes-Roth, F. (1979). A cognitive model of planning. *Cognitive Science, 3*, 275–310.

Heatherton, T. F., & Baumeister, R. F. (1991). Binge eating as escape from self-awareness. *Psychological Bulletin, 110*, 86–108.

Heider, F. (1946). Attitudes and cognitive organization. *Journal of Psychology, 21*, 107–112.

Higgins, E. T. (1987). Self-discrepancy: A theory relating self and affect. *Psychological Review, 94*, 319–340.

Higgins, E. T. (1996). Ideals, oughts, and regulatory focus: Affect and motivation from distinct pains and pleasures. In P. M. Gollwitzer & J. A. Bargh (Eds.), *The psychology of action: Linking cognition and motivation to behavior* (pp. 91–114). New York: Guilford Press.

Higgins, E. T., Shah, J., & Friedman, R. (1997). Emotional responses to goal attainment: Strength of regulatory focus as moderator. *Journal of Personality and Social Psychology, 72*, 515–525.

Hobfoll, S. E. (1989). Conservation of resources: A new attempt at conceptualizing stress. *American Psychologist, 44*, 513–524.

Hobfoll, S. E. (2002). Social and psychological resources and adaptation. *Review of General Psychology, 6*, 307–324.

Hull, J. G. (1981). A self-awareness model of the causes and effects of alcohol consumption. *Journal of Abnormal Psychology, 90*, 586–600.

Isen, A. M. (1987). Positive affect, cognitive processes, and social behavior. In L. Berkowitz (Ed.), *Advances in experimental social psychology* (Vol. 20, pp. 203–252). San Diego, CA: Academic Press.

Isen, A. M. (2000). Positive affect and decision making. In M. Lewis & J. M. Haviland-Jones (Eds.), *Handbook of emotions* (2nd ed., pp. 417–435). New York: Guilford Press.

Izard, C. E. (1977). *Human emotions.* New York: Plenum Press.

Izard, C. E., & Ackerman, B. P. (2000). Motivational, organizational, and regulatory functions of discrete emotions. In M. Lewis & J. M. Haviland-Jones (Eds.), *Handbook of emotions* (2nd ed., pp. 253–264). New York: Guilford Press.

Kahn, B. E., & Isen, A. M. (1993). The influence of positive affect on variety-seeking among safe, enjoyable products. *Journal of Consumer Research, 20,* 257–270.

Kelso, J. A. S. (1995). *Dynamic patterns: The self-organization of brain and behavior.* Cambridge, MA: MIT Press.

Klinger, E. (1975). Consequences of commitment to and disengagement from incentives. *Psychological Review, 82,* 1–25.

Lang, P. J. (1995). The emotion probe: Studies of motivation and attention. *American Psychologist, 50,* 372–385.

Lang, P. J., Bradley, M. M., & Cuthbert, B. N. (1990). Emotion, attention, and the startle reflex. *Psychological Review, 97,* 377–395.

Lecky, P. (1945). *Self-consistency: A theory of personality.* New York: Island Press.

Levenson, R. W. (1994). Human emotion: A functional view. In P. Ekman & R. Davidson (Eds.), *The nature of emotions: Fundamental questions* (pp. 123–126). New York: Oxford University Press.

Levenson, R. W. (1999). The intrapersonal functions of emotion. *Cognition and Emotion, 13,* 481–504.

Lewis, M., Sullivan, M. W., Ramsay, D. S., & Allessandri, S. M. (1992). Individual differences in anger and sad expressions during extinction: Antecedents and consequences. *Infant Behavior and Development, 15,* 443–452.

Lieberman, M. D., Gaunt, R., Gilbert, D. T., & Trope, Y. (2002). Reflection and reflexion: A social cognitive neuroscience approach to attributional inference. In M. Zanna (Ed.), *Advances in experimental social psychology* (Vol. 34, pp. 199–249). San Diego, CA: Academic Press.

Little, B. R. (1989). Personal projects analysis: Trivial pursuits, magnificent obsessions, and the search for coherence. In D. M. Buss & N. Cantor (Eds.), *Personality psychology: Recent trends and emerging directions* (pp. 15–31). New York: Springer-Verlag.

MacKay, D. M. (1966). Cerebral organization and the conscious control of action. In J. C. Eccles (Ed.), *Brain and conscious experience* (pp. 422–445). Berlin: Springer-Verlag.

Markus, H., & Nurius, P. (1986). Possible selves. *American Psychologist, 41,* 954–969.

Martin, L. L., & Davies, B. (1998). Beyond hedonism and associationism: A configural view of the role of affect in evaluation, processing, and self-regulation. *Motivation and Emotion, 22,* 33–51.

Messinger, D. S. (2002). Positive and negative: Infant facial expressions and emotions. *Current Directions in Psychological Science, 11,* 1–6.

Metcalfe, J., & Mischel, W. (1999). A hot/cool-system analysis of delay of gratification: Dynamics of willpower. *Psychological Review, 106,* 3–19.

Mikulincer, M. (1988). Reactance and helplessness following exposure to learned helplessness following exposure to unsolvable problems: The effects of attributional style. *Journal of Personality and Social Psychology, 54,* 679–686.

Mikulincer, M. (1994). *Human learned helplessness: A coping perspective.* New York: Plenum Press.

Miller, G. A., Galanter, E., & Pribram, K. H. (1960). *Plans and the structure of behavior.* New York: Holt, Rinehart & Winston.

Miller, N. E. (1944). Experimental studies of conflict. In J. McV. Hunt (Ed.), *Personality and the behavior disorders* (Vol. 1, pp. 431–465). New York: Ronald Press.

Mischel, W., & Shoda, Y. (1995). A cognitive-affective system theory of personality: Reconceptualizing the invariances in personality and the role of situations. *Psychological Review, 102,* 246–268.

Mizruchi, M. S. (1991). Urgency, motivation, and group performance: The effect of prior success on current success among professional basketball teams. *Social Psychology Quarterly, 54,* 181–189.

Muraven, M., & Baumeister, R. F. (2000). Self-regulation and depletion of limited resources: Does self-control resemble a muscle? *Psychological Bulletin, 126,* 247–259.

Muraven, M., Tice, D. M., & Baumeister, R. F. (1998). Self-control as a limited resource: Regulatory depletion patterns. *Journal of Personality and Social Psychology, 74,* 774–789.

Murray, H. A. (1938). *Explorations in personality.* New York: Oxford University Press.

Nesse, R. M. (2000). Is depression an adaptation? *Archives of General Psychiatry, 57,* 14–20.

Niedenthal, P. M., & Mordkoff, J. T. (1991). Prototype distancing: A strategy for choosing among threatening situations. *Personality and Social Psychology Bulletin, 17,* 483–493.

Nowak, A., & Vallacher, R. R. (1998). *Dynamical social psychology.* New York: Guilford Press.

Ogilvie, D. M. (1987). The undesired self: A neglected variable in personality research. *Journal of Personality and Social Psychology, 52,* 379–385.

Ortony, A., Clore, G. L., & Collins, A. (1988). *The cognitive structure of emotions.* New York: Cambridge University Press.

Parrott, W. G. (1993). Beyond hedonism: Motives for inhibiting good moods and for maintaining bad moods. In D. M. Wegner & J. W. Pennebaker (Eds.), *Handbook of mental control* (pp. 278–305). Englewood Cliffs, NJ: Prentice-Hall.

Payton, D. W. (1990). Internalized plans: A representation for action resources. In P. Maes (Ed.), *Designing autonomous agents: Theory and practice from biology to engineering and back* (pp. 89–103). Cambridge, MA: MIT Press.

Pervin, L. A. (1982). The stasis and flow of behavior: Toward a theory of goals. In M. M. Page & R. Dienstbier (Eds.), *Nebraska Symposium on Motivation* (Vol. 30, pp. 1–53). Lincoln: University of Nebraska Press.

Pervin, L. A. (Ed.). (1989). *Goal concepts in personality and social psychology.* Hillsdale, NJ: Erlbaum.

Pittman, T. S., & Pittman, N. L. (1980). Deprivation of control and the attribution process. *Journal of Personality and Social Psychology, 39,* 377–389.

Powers, W. T. (1973). *Behavior: The control of perception.* Chicago: Aldine.

Prentice-Dunn, S., & Rogers, R. W. (1989). Deindividuation and the self-regulation of behavior. In P. B. Paulus (Ed.), *Psychology of group influence* (2nd ed., pp. 87–109). Hillsdale, NJ: Erlbaum.

Prigogene, I., & Stengers, I. (1984). *Order out of chaos.* New York: Bantam.

Read, S. J., & Miller, L. C. (1989). Inter-personalism: Toward a goal-based theory of persons in relationships. In L. Pervin (Ed.), *Goal concepts in personality and social psychology* (pp. 413–472). Hillsdale, NJ: Erlbaum.

Read, S. J., Vanman, E. J., & Miller, L. C. (1997). Connectionism, parallel constraint satisfaction processes, and Gestalt principles: (Re)introducing cognitive dynamics to social psychology. *Review of Personality and Social Psychology, 1,* 26–53.

Reed, M. B., & Aspinwall, L. G. (1998). Self-affirmation reduces biased processing of health-risk information. *Motivation and Emotion, 22,* 99–132.

Ryan, R. M., & Deci, E. L. (2001). On happiness and human potentials: A review of research on hedonic and eudaimonic well-being. *Annual Review of Psychology, 52,* 141–166.

Schwarz, N., & Bohner, G. (1996). Feelings and their motivational implications: Moods and the action sequence. In P. M. Gollwitzer & J. A. Bargh (Eds.), *The psychology of action: Linking cognition and motivation to behavior* (pp. 119–145). New York: Guilford Press.

Schwarz, N., & Clore, G. L. (1983). Mood, misattribution, and judgments of well-being: Informative and directive functions of affective states. *Journal of Personality and Social Psychology, 45,* 513–523.

Shallice, T. (1978). The dominant action system: An information-processing approach to consciousness. In K. S. Pope & J. L. Singer (Eds.), *The stream of consciousness: Scientific investigations into the flow of human experience* (pp. 117–157). New York: Wiley.

Shastri, L., & Ajjanagadde, V. (1993). From simple associations to systematic reasoning: A connectionist representation of rules, variables, and dynamic bindings using temporal synchrony. *Behavioral and Brain Sciences, 16,* 417–494.

Simon, H. A. (1953). *Models of man.* New York: Wiley.

Simon, H. A. (1967). Motivational and emotional controls of cognition. *Psychology Review, 74,* 29–39.

Sloman, S. A. (1996). The empirical case for two forms of reasoning. *Psychological Bulletin, 119,* 3–22.

Smith, E. R., & DeCoster, J. (2000). Dual-process models in social and cognitive psychology: Conceptual integration and links to underlying memory systems. *Personality and Social Psychology Review, 4,* 108–131.

Steele, C. M., & Josephs, R. A. (1990). Alcohol myopia: Its prized and dangerous effects. *American Psychologist, 45,* 921–933.

Stifter, C. A., & Moyer, D. (1991). The regulation of positive affect: Gaze aversion activity during mother–infant interaction. *Infant Behavior and Development, 14,* 111–123.

Suls, J., & Wills, T. A. (Eds.). (1991). *Social comparison: Contemporary theory and research.* Hillsdale, NJ: Erlbaum.

Tesser, A. (1988). Toward a self-evaluation maintenance model of social behavior. In L. Berkowitz (Ed.), *Advances in experimental social psychology* (Vol. 21, pp. 181–227). New York: Academic Press.

Tesser, A., Crepaz, N., Collins, J. C., Cornell, D., & Beach, S. R. H. (2000). Confluence of self-esteem regulation mechanisms: On integrating the self-zoo. *Personality and Social Psychology Bulletin, 26,* 1476–1489.

Trope, Y., & Neter, E. (1994). Reconciling competing motives in self-evaluation: The role of self-control in feedback seeking. *Journal of Personality and Social Psychology, 66,* 646–657.

Trope, Y., & Pomerantz, E. M. (1998). Resolving conflicts among self-evaluative motives: Positive experiences as a resource for overcoming defensiveness. *Motivation and Emotion, 22,* 53–72.

Vallacher, R. R., & Kaufman, J. (1996). Dynamics of action identification: Volatility and structure in the mental representation of behavior. In P. M. Gollwitzer & J. A. Bargh (Eds.), *The psychology of action: Linking cognition and motivation to behavior* (pp. 260–282). New York: Guilford Press.

Vallacher, R. R., & Nowak, A. (Eds.). (1994). *Dynamical systems in social psychology.* San Diego, CA: Academic Press.

Vallacher, R. R., & Nowak, A. (1997). The emergence of dynamical social psychology. *Psychological Inquiry, 8,* 73–99.

Vallacher, R. R., Read, S. J., & Nowak, A. (Eds.). (2002). The dynamical perspective in personality and social psychology [Special issue]. *Personality and Social Psychology Review, 6*(4).

Vallacher, R. R., & Wegner, D. M. (1987). What do people think they're doing? Action identification and human behavior. *Psychological Review, 94,* 3–15.

Watson, D., & Tellegen, A. (1985). Toward a consensual structure of mood. *Psychological Bulletin, 98,* 219–235.

Watson, D., Wiese, D., Vaidya, J., & Tellegen, A. (1999). The two general activation systems of affect: Structural findings, evolutionary considerations, and psychobiological evidence. *Journal of Personality and Social Psychology, 76,* 820–838.

Wegner, D. M. (2002). *The illusion of conscious will.* Cambridge, MA: MIT Press.

Wiener, N. (1948). *Cybernetics: Control and communcation in the animal and the machine.* Cambridge, MA: MIT Press.

Wood, J. V. (1996). What is social comparison and how should we study it? *Personality and Social Psychology Bulletin, 22,* 520–537.

Wortman, C. B., & Brehm, J. W. (1975). Responses to uncontrollable outcomes: An integration of reactance theory and the learned helplessness model. In L. Berkowitz (Ed.), *Advances in experimental social psychology* (Vol. 8, pp. 277–336). New York: Academic Press.

Wrosch, C., Scheier, M. F., Carver, C. S., & Schulz, R. (2003). The importance of goal disengagement in adaptive self-regulation: When giving up is beneficial. *Self and Identity, 2,* 1–20.

Wrosch, C., Scheier, M. F., Miller, G. E., Schulz, R., & Carver, C. S. (in press). Adaptive self-regulation of unattainable goals: Goal disengagement, goal re-engagement, and subjective well-being. *Personality and Social Psychology Bulletin.*

3

Affect Regulation

RANDY J. LARSEN
ZVJEZDANA PRIZMIC

A literature search 15 years ago on the terms "emotion," or "mood," or "affect" and "regulation" or "management" would have produced scant results concentrated mostly in the area of developmental psychology (e.g., Kopp, 1989). An important exception to this was an influential, early article by Morris and Reilly (1987), who presented a review of a few broad mood regulation strategies and summarizxed research relevant to mood management in adulthood. Their article marked the start an era of intense interest in, and active research on, the topic of affect regulation in adulthood. Consequently, if one were to enter the same terms in a PsychINFO search today, over 3,000 references would be retrieved, at least, as of this writing.

Our purpose in this chapter is to describe research on affect regulation that has emerged since the Morris and Reilly (1987) article. Our intention is not to provide an exhaustive review, but rather to summarize some of the key concepts and issues in this area, and to cover topics important to research, including measures and models of affect regulation. We also discuss several specific affect regulation strategies. However, we begin by discussing what is regulated, and toward what purposes, in affect regulation.

DEFINING AFFECT REGULATION

There are many proposed definitions of affect regulation, but most include the notion that, in the process of monitoring and evaluating affective states, individuals take action either to maintain or to change (enhance or suppress) the intensity of affect, or to prolonged or shorten the affective episode (Gross, 1999; Parkinson, Totterdell, Briner, & Reynolds, 1996; Thompson, 1994). "Affect" refers to the feeling tone a person is experiencing at any particular point in time. Feeling tones vary primarily in terms of hedonic valance, but they can also differ in terms of felt energy or arousal. If the feeling tone is strong, has a clear cause, and is the focus of conscious awareness, then we use the term "emotion" to refer to those feelings. However, if the feeling tone is mild, does not have a clear cause or referent, and is in the background of awareness, then we use the term "mood." Although some authors have used the term "emotion regulation" (e.g., Davidson, 2000; Gross & John, 2002) and others, the term "mood regulation" (e.g., Parkinson et al., 1996), we prefer the more general term "affect regulation" to subsume the management of subjective feeling states in general. Also, in this chapter, we are mostly concerned with effortful or controlled affect regulation rather than automatic processes, yet we acknowledge that many forms of affect regulation might involve either or both (Forgas & Ciarrochi, 2002).

Why regulate affect? Affective states influence subsequent behavior, experience, and cognition, especially in terms of social consequences (e.g., Bless & Forgas, 2000). So one function of affect regulation is to limit the residual impact of lingering emotions and moods on subsequent behavior and experience. Certainly, feelings provide important information to a person and serve to direct subsequent thought and behavior in mostly adaptive ways; therefore, the goal of affect regulation is not to prevent or short-circuit *all* affect. Rather, this goal of effective affect regulation is akin to hanging up the phone after receiving a message. For example, if a woman is angry at her spouse because he did not listen to her side in an argument, then that experience of anger should tell her that this issue is important to her. Effective anger regulation would allow her to have the information that her angry feelings convey, yet also use these feelings to energize an effective response, thereby limiting the residual maladaptive interpersonal effects that often follow in the wake of anger.

Affect regulation, according to this view, refers primarily to the modulation of feeling states, mostly in terms of the valance of those states, but people seek to regulate energy level as well (Thayer, 2001). Researchers in the stress and coping tradition have primarily emphasized the downregulation of negative affect (e.g., Bushman, 2002; Tamres, Janicki, & Helgeson, 2002). However, other researchers are considering the upregulation of positive affect as well (Davidson, 2000; Fredrickson, 2000; Lucas, Diener, & Larsen, 2003; Lyubomirsky, 2001). Whereas the emphasis on positive or negative affect differs somewhat across investigators, the importance of affect regulation for adaptive functioning in everyday life has also received much attention (e.g., Fichman, Koestner, Zuroff, & Gordon, 1999). For example, researchers have discussed the role of affective regulation in organizational settings (e.g., Judge & Larsen, 2001), in families (e.g., Gottman, Katz, & Hooven, 1997), in relationships (e.g., Eisenberg, Fabes, Guthrie, & Reiser, 2000), and in old age (e.g., Carstensen, 1993).

Another important outcome of affect regulation is its relation to physical and mental health. Research on neural correlates of emotion, which shows that disruption in the ability to regulate the duration of negative affect and to suppress (or inhibit) it, may be crucial in explaining depression and other mood disorders (Davidson, 2002a; Davidson et al., 2002a; Schaefer et al., 2002). Yet another example concerns the effects of affect suppression on physiological functioning (Gross & Levenson, 1997), though the connection between affect regulation and long-term health is still an open question (Davidson, Jackson, & Kalin, 2000).

The main outcome variables of interest mentioned so far include how regulation influences the residual or downstream consequences of feeling states, how regulation functions in adapting to the challenges of daily life, and how affect regulation relates to health. In addition to these purposes, we believe that people regulate affect to achieve another superordinate goal: to maintain a global sense of subjective well-being (SWB; Larsen, 2000a). SWB, according to most experts (e.g., Diener & Seligman, 2002), has two affective components at its core, both of which are considered as aggregates, or averages, over relatively long time periods. These two components are average levels of positive affect (PA) and negative affect (NA). Thus, people influence their SWB by regulating the "Big Two" affective states: PA and NA.

AFFECT REGULATION FOR SUBJECTIVE WELL-BEING

It is tempting to think in terms of a full factorial model of affect regulation, with a two (PA and NA)-by-two (increase, decrease) model. The most obvious regulation strategies are to increase PA and to decrease NA. There are, however, times when people want to increase NA (e.g., increase sadness after a loss or increase anger after having been wronged), or to decrease PA (e.g., to decrease happiness after some successful experience to get back to some mundane task). Although these more counterintuitive versions of affect regulation do exist (Parrott, 1993) and are worthy of study, they are most likely rare and play a peripheral role in terms of affecting the outcomes mentioned earlier. Consequently, we focus on those mechanisms directly related to minimizing NA or maximizing PA.

Minimizing and maximizing affects also have multiple meanings. These efforts can be directed toward influencing the felt *intensity* of the respective affect states. For example, in terms of NA, efforts might be directed toward transforming absolute distress into common misery. Alternatively, efforts might be directed toward the temporal *duration* of the affective states. For example, one might regulate affect to shorten an episode of distress. Overall, volitional efforts involve hastening the adaptation to negative events and slowing the adaptation to positive ones.

STRATEGIES AND BEHAVIORS FOR AFFECT REGULATION

Rippere (1977) was perhaps the first to generate a list of behaviors and cognitive strategies designed to relieve negative emotions. Since then, there have been several proposals for classifying affect regulation strategies. Borrowing and adapting a scheme from the literature on stress and coping, Morris and Reilly (1987) classified techniques for the self-regulation of mood into four broad categories: management of the mood, modification of the meaning or significance of the problem, problem-directed action, and affiliation. Other researchers have sought to develop more empirically based classification schemes. Based on factor analyses of self-reported frequency and effectiveness of strategy use, Thayer, Newman, and McClain (1994) reported six categories of mood regulation: (1) active mood management; (2) seeking pleasurable activities and distraction; (3) passive mood management; (4) social support, venting, and gratification; (5) direct tension reduction; and (6) withdrawal/avoidance. Using a different approach, Parkinson and Totterdell (1999) developed a classification system based on a hierarchical cluster analysis of the conceptual distinctions among 162 different strategies and behaviors. Their comprehensive work on mapping affect regulation strategies identified two main distinctions: (1) cognitive versus behavioral strategies, and (2) engagement versus diversionary strategies.

Larsen (1993, 2000b) reported results of applying an act-frequency approach to eliciting behaviors used in the regulation of emotion. After eliminating redundancies and combining similar acts, Larsen (2000b) reported on an organizing scheme for presenting 24 behaviors into a two-by-two table: The acts are either behavioral or cognitive and are focused on changing the situation or the emotion. This list of affect-regulating acts, many of which we discuss here, has been formed into a measure—called the Measure of Affect Regulation Styles (MARS)—that has proved useful to researchers (e.g., Fichman et al., 1999; Lerner & Larsen, 2002). We discuss this measure later and present an updated version in Figure 3.1. Although more taxonomic work will undoubtedly be useful, it appears that most of the variation in affect regulation behaviors is captured in the lists mentioned so far, and researchers can proceed with more substantive questions.

An important substantive question is, which of the affects—PA or NA—is more important or more fundamental in terms of regulation efforts? Given the two routes to SWB (increase PA and decrease NA), which is more efficacious? What should psychologists recommend that someone do first, concentrate on promoting, PA or concentrate on remediating NA?

INSTRUCTIONS FOR STATE ASSESSMENT

Did you do any of the following behaviors in an attempt to influence your feelings, either to increase positive moods or to decrease negative moods? Check all that apply.

INSTRUCTIONS FOR TRAIT ASSESSMENT

In the space preceding each item, place a number from the following scale to indicate how frequently you use that behavior to influence your feelings, either to increase positive moods or to decrease negative moods.

Not at all	Hardly ever	Sometimes	Moderate amount	Often	Very often	Almost always
0	1	2	3	4	5	6

____ I took action to solve the problem causing my mood

____ I tried to understand my feelings by thinking and analyzing them

____ I made plans or a resolution to avoid such problems in the future

____ I ate something to get over my bad mood

____ I wrote about my feelings in a diary, letter, or e-mail

____ I withdrew from or avoided the situation

____ I tried to not let my feelings show, to suppress any expression

____ I talked to someone about my feelings

____ I tried to be grateful for the things in my life that are going well

____ I thought about something to distract myself from my feelings

____ I drank coffee or caffeinated beverages

____ I did something fun, something I really enjoy

____ I prayed, put my faith in God, or did something religious

____ I watched TV, read a book, etc., for distraction

____ I used alcohol to get out of a bad mood

____ I talked to an advisor or mentor

____ I socialized to forget my mood

____ I tried to reinterpret the situation, to find a different meaning

____ I tried to accept it as my fate, what will be, will be

____ I let my feelings out by venting or expressing them

____ I kept to myself, I wanted to be alone

____ I treated myself to something special

____ I tried to put things in perspective

____ I tried to think about those things that are going well for me

____ I laughed, joked around, tried to make myself or others laugh

____ I compared myself to people who are worse off

____ I tried to find something good in the situation

____ I worked on something or stayed busy to forget my mood

____ I played sports, exercised

____ I slept or took a nap

____ I went out of my way to help someone

____ I daydreamed of the time when I will not have this problem

FIGURE 3.1. Measure of Affect Regulation Styles (MARS). Copyright by R. Larsen and Z. Prizmic.

Negative Affect Regulation May Be More Important Than Positive Affect Regulation

A good deal of literature suggests that negative life events have a stronger impact on subjective feelings than do positive events (Baumeister, Bratslavsky, Finkenauer, & Vohs, 2001). Larsen (2002) presented data showing that negative events have a stronger gain function than do positive events in terms of producing affective reactions, that negative events produce more subjective consequences than do equally strong positive events, that strong NA reactions last longer than strong PA reactions, and that the cognitive system is designed to prioritize the processing of negative compared to positive information. Larsen argues that NA is two to three times as strong as PA, such that, one bad day must be outweighed by two or three good days to maintain average levels of subjective well-being. Because NA is so much stronger than PA, we begin our discussion of specific affect regulation strategies with those that seem most appropriate for remediating unpleasant emotions. We acknowledge, however, that the distinction between strategies for negative and positive affect regulation is more conceptual than absolute.

Distraction, Getting One's Mind Off Negative Events or Emotions, Avoiding Rumination

Distraction can involve disengagement from the problematic situation, or avoidance of thinking about the problem. The behaviors employed may involve engaging in somewhat low-effort but preoccupying activities (e.g., watching television, listening to music) or in more difficult activities (e.g., working on a hobby, reading an involving book) in an effort to get one's mind off of a negative event or emotion. A somewhat different slant on this strategy is to focus on the future, when this problem is resolved. One can also reallocate resources, by thinking about something that occupies attention, or engage in a demanding task.

In his study of emotion regulation in everyday life, Larsen (1993) reported that, among a sample of college students, distraction was the single most frequently mentioned mood regulation strategy. Out of all occasions when mood regulation strategies were used, students mentioned distraction 14% of the time. However, the effects of distraction were short-lived; mood on the occasion of distraction was slightly better than expected, though in the next report period (between 6 and 12 hours later), it was no different than average.

To the extent that distraction is effective for affect regulation, it mostly likely works by interrupting or preventing rumination. Although most people respond to negative life events with a negative mood, those who are prone to depression or other emotion disorders have difficulty "getting over" or recovering from negative events (Larsen & Cowan, 1988). Rumination, viewed as a breakdown in negative affect regulation caused by focusing on feelings and enhancing negative cognitions, predicts depressive disorders, the onset of depressive episodes, and anxiety symptoms (see Nolen-Hoeksema & Corte, Chapter 21, this volume). Being able to control one's own thoughts through volitional effort to avoid thinking about some unpleasant event is the way to avoid rumination. Whereas this is often easier said than done, perhaps one approach to short-circuiting rumination is to engage, at least temporarily, in distraction.

Venting, Expressing the Negative Affect, Catharsis

Freud taught that negative emotions, when not expressed, build up tension and ultimately produce symptoms. Consequently, the discharge of negative emotions through expression was thought to rid the psychological system of tension. Psychoanalysis is sometimes viewed as a form of venting therapy, because patients are encouraged to reexperience the emotions associated with past traumas, a process known as "catharsis."

Catharsis theory is most often associated with the management of anger. However, reviews of relevant research (e.g., Geen & Quanty, 1977) conclude that venting or expressing anger does not reduce aggressive behavior. In recent studies, Bushman (2002; Bushman, Baumeister, & Phillips, 2001) provided strong experimental evidence that angered participants are more, not less, aggressive if they are encouraged to "let off steam" by hitting a punching bag in the time between becoming angry and having an opportunity to aggress against the person who angered them. Bushman concluded that venting anger (e.g., hitting a punching bag) makes people angrier and more likely to be aggressive.

What about venting as a regulation strategy for other negative emotions? In a daily experience-sampling study, in which subjects reported on their moods and affect regulation behaviors three times a day, Larsen (1993) found that venting was not an effective strategy for regulating sadness. In fact, occasions when a person expressed or vented sadness (e.g., by having a good cry) tended to be followed by occasions of elevated sadness. Expressions of sadness appeared to perpetuate the sad feelings into the next reporting occasion.

Emotion feedback theories (e.g., facial feedback) suggest that the outward expression of an emotion serves to amplify the subjective impact or feeling of the emotion. Larsen, Kasimatis, and Frey (1992) demonstrated how inducing a furrowed brow produces stronger negative affect in response to unpleasant images compared to looking at the same images with relaxed brow muscles. The authors argued that the facial expression serves to amplify ongoing emotion. From this perspective, venting, at least in the short term, would work to amplify subjective feelings. As such, venting would probably be more useful in the upregulation of positive emotions; that is, according to this line of thinking, smiling, laughing, or even postural adjustments, such as sitting up tall or holding one's shoulders back, can be used to increase positive feelings. We discuss this further later.

Suppression, Keeping the Negative Affect from Being Expressed

In contrast to venting, "suppression" refers to inhibiting the expression of the negative emotion. Emotional containment, or suppression, has been programmatically studied by Gross (see Ochsner & Gross, Chapter 12, this volume). In a typical experiment, as participants watch an emotion-inducing film (e.g., an arm amputation), some of them are instructed to suppress outward signs of any emotion they might experience. Subjects in the suppression condition do report less disgust than the control group. However, the suppression group also exhibits increased physiological activation compared to the control group. Using a similar paradigm (viewing emotionally loaded slides), Buck (1977; Buck, Miller, & Caul, 1974) reported conceptually similar findings two decades earlier. Buck and colleagues reported that, when looking at similar emotional images, less expressive subjects exhibited the most autonomic arousal. Buck argued then, as Gross and colleagues do now, that because the act of suppression takes work or effort, it is associated with increased physiological arousal. This outlay of energy may interfere with adaptive functioning.

Other researchers question this conclusion and suggest that the inhibition of negative emotions may not always be associated with poor outcomes. For example, Consedine, Magai, and Bonanno (2002) argued that it is a mistake to believe that emotional inhibition is inherently unhealthy. They suggest that the capacity to inhibit emotional expression evolved because it is beneficial, in some instances, to be able to do so. Consedine and colleagues argued for a more contextualized view of emotional inhibition, suggesting that much depends on the specific emotion being inhibited, the time course of the emotion, which component of emotion is being inhibited, and the degree of volition involved in the inhibition. In addition, emotional suppression or inhibition may have different short- and long-term consequences.

Cognitive Reappraisal, Finding Meaning in Negative Events

This strategy involves the attempt to find meaning in, or develop a positive interpretation of, a problematic situation. Many terms have been used to describe this strategy, including "positive reappraisal," "cognitive restructuring," and "cognitive reframing" (Tamres et al., 2002). Tennen and Affleck (2002) used the term "benefit finding" to refer to the search for benefits in adversity, the so-called "silver lining" in every dark cloud. They reviewed an impressive amount of research showing that perception of benefits in otherwise negative experiences is associated with more adaptive long-term outcomes. For example, Davis, Nolen-Hoeksema, and Larson (1998) asked people who had recently lost a spouse, a parent, a child, or a sibling whether they could find anything positive in the experience. Seventy-three percent of the subjects reported that something positive could be found, such as finding supportive others, strengthening family bonds, or providing a new perspective on life. Six months later, those who had found some benefit to their loss were less distressed than those who did not find such benefits.

The self-disclosure research by Pennebaker and colleagues (e.g., Niederhoffer & Pennebaker, 2002) is relevant to this strategy. Pennebaker and others have shown that persons who are induced to write about a traumatic experience over a period of time tend to fare better—in terms of physical health, immune function, and psychological health—than those who spend the same period of time writing about a mundane experience. Pennebaker's original explanation for this effect concerned the effort it takes to inhibit a traumatic experience, something akin to keeping a secret. His more recent interpretation of the effect, however, is more along the lines of self-disclosure as cognitive reappraisal. By writing about a negative experience, he argues, people construct a story, a reinterpretation of the event that facilitates a sense of resolution.

Gross (2001) makes the important observation that cognitive reappraisal can occur even before a negative emotion is evoked. As such, this strategy is useful even when negative emotions are anticipated. For example, before a job interview, candidates might try to convince themselves that the main purpose of the interview is to gather information about the prospective employer. By keeping the upcoming job interview in this perspective, they potentially avoid the anxiety of seeing the situation in purely social evaluation terms.

Downward Social Comparison

This strategy concerns comparing oneself to others and, if the comparison is favorable to the self, then positive affective consequences accrue. After a negative event, comparing oneself to others who have experienced a more severe negative event can serve to put one's problem into perspective. So a professor receiving a poor teacher rating might be seen as a bad event. But if he can find other professors who have received worse ratings, then his own rating might not seem so bad. No matter what, there are always people who are worse off, and making the comparison explicitly may serve to put one's problem into perspective.

Social comparison research occupies a very large domain within social psychology (see Suls, Martin, & Wheeler, 2002, for a review), so generalizations are risky. Nevertheless, research shows that people play an active role in using comparison information, and that they do so in part for emotional reasons (Suls & Wheeler, 2000). Correlational studies have shown that dispositionally happy persons are less affected by unfavorable social comparison information (Lyubomirsky & Ross, 1997; Lyubomirsky, Tucker, & Kasri, 2001). Lockwood (2002) has demonstrated that the impact of downward comparison on self-evaluation is dependent on factors such as similarity to the comparison other and the likelihood that his or her fate might become one's own (perceived vulnerability). Although there is much to learn about social comparison processes, it is clear that people often look for worse-off others with whom to compare fates, thereby enhancing their own affective states.

Problem-Directed Action or Planning to Avoid Problems in the Future

This strategy involves thinking about and acting on the problem responsible for the unpleasant mood. For example, asking to be transferred to a different unit at work to avoid an unpleasant coworker would be problem-directed action. Or the situation, if it cannot be avoided, might be modified with an effort toward changing the problematic aspect. For example, if one could not transfer to a different unit, then he or she might make an effort toward modifying how he or she interacts with the troublesome coworker. Another way to regulate the situation is for a person to control how he or she directs attention, picking and choosing what parts of the situation receive attention.

Problem-focused and emotion-focused coping have been prominent for several decades in the coping literature (e.g., Lazarus & Folkman, 1984). Whereas emotion-focused coping is any attempt to reduce negative emotion, problem-focused coping involves concrete actions designed to solve the problem causing the person to feel unpleasant. The emphasis in this distinction is on the actions taken to solve the problem in problem-focused but not emotion-focused coping. However, Larsen (1993) reported that planning how to avoid similar problems in the future is a frequently used strategy. Moreover, this strategy is associated with concurrent and subsequent improvements in mood. Because some problems, like water under the bridge, cannot be recalled and fixed, it would seem that efforts expended on planning to *avoid* similar problems in the future might be useful. As such, after an unpleasant event, an improvement in mood might follow on the heels of explicitly planning to avoid such events in the future.

Self-Reward, Thinking about or Doing Pleasant Activities

A common feature of behavioral approaches to self-management is the frequent use of self-reward. These techniques grow out of a tradition that views emotion disorders, especially depression, as being caused by a lack of appropriate reinforcing experiences, especially self-administered reinforcement. Along these lines, researchers have found that depressed persons display a low frequency of self-reinforcing activities (Heiby, 1983). Experimental studies, in which some subjects are encouraged to increase the number of pleasant events they provide themselves, and to focus on the pleasantness of those events, indicate that this method is associated with lessened depression (Dobson & Joffe, 1986).

Studies of daily experience have similarly shown that frequency of pleasurable activities is correlated with increased positive affect (Parkinson et al., 1996), though the causal direction (is mood causing the selection of more pleasant activities, or vice versa?) is still unknown. Nevertheless, in another study of daily experience, Fichman and colleagues (1999) found that engaging in pleasant, rewarding activities is the most successful strategy for reducing negative affect. For the remediation of negative states, it would seem that self-reward is an obvious and anecdotally frequent response. Faber and Vohs (Chapter 26, this volume) propose the notion of self-gifting as a method of affect regulation, prolonging PA or diminishing NA.

Self-rewarding experience can be an actual event (e.g., going shopping) or a more cognitive pleasure (e.g., taking a few minutes off to recall some pleasant experience). One strategy is to imagine the future, when the current problem has faded. Pleasant anticipations and pleasant memories may serve the same purposes. Josephson, Singer, and Salovey (1996) demonstrate how, after being induced to a sad mood, then required to list two memories, many participants listed positive memories. Moreover, when asked why they elected memories of that valence, most participants mentioned mood repair as their motivation. Similar results using positive memories to regulate negative moods are reported by Rusting and DeHart (2000).

Fredrickson's theory of positive affect (Fredrickson, 1998, 2000) holds that the function of positive affect is, in part, to hasten recovery from negative events. In experimental studies, she has shown that, following a stressor, persons induced to a positive mood show faster cardiovascular recovery than those in a control condition (Fredrickson & Levenson, 1998). Such results suggest that the deliberate attempt to self-induce positive affect through self-reward may be especially useful in speeding recovery from negative events.

Exercise, Relaxation, Eating, and Other Physical Manipulations

Thayer (2001) provides an important review and integration of information on the affective consequences of exercise and eating. The empirical literature is large, is dispersed across different disciplines, and is replete with ostensibly contradictory findings. For example, moderate exercise appears positively correlated with pleasant affect in some samples but not in others. Extremely fit persons who are regular exercisers appear to get less of an energy boost from exercise compared to persons who are only modestly fit. Thayer's own research (1987) indicates that moderate exercise, such as taking a brisk, 20-minute walk, is a reliable method for the average person to change a bad mood and boost felt energy.

It may seem ironic that the use of energy (to exercise) actually elevates energy, but the impact of exercise on affect and felt energy has been reliably demonstrated in a number of studies (e.g., Ekkekakis, Hall, Van Landuyt, & Petruzzello, 2000). In other research (Stevens & Lane, 2001) with a group of athletes, exercise was rated as the most effective strategy for regulating anger, depression, fatigue, and tension. One possible explanation why exercise might be judged so positively, especially among athletes, is that it not only serves as a distraction from the negative affect they are trying to regulate, but it also is seen as a good and positive behavior in its own right, independent of its affect-regulating impact.

When it comes to food, emotional effects are complicated by a variety of factors, including gender, culture, obesity, and psychopathology. There is a great deal of research on the effects of prior mood on subsequent eating (reviewed in Thayer, 2001). Of the studies on the other causal direction, there appears to be reliable evidence that the intake of sweets (refined sugar) leads to increased fatigue or tension (Thayer, 1987). Also, people appear to use stimulants, such as coffee, tea, or nicotine, in explicit attempts to self-regulate energy level (Adan, 1994). Research that directly examines the effects on mood of ingesting various substances is relatively sparse. It seems likely, however, that substances that influence blood glucose, hormones, or neurotransmitters (especially dopamine and serotonin) are likely to produce alterations in affective state. Similarly, activities such as exercise or meditation (Davidson, 2002b), or even napping or going to sleep earlier than usual (Parkinson et al., 1996), that affect these important biochemicals are also likely to be associated with consequent changes in affective states.

Socializing, Seeking Comfort, Help, or Advice from Others

One characteristic that almost always correlates with happiness is the number, quality, and frequency of relationships (Diener & Seligman, 2002). Happy people spend time with others; they join groups, have many friends and loving relationships, build social support networks, and generally find the presence of others to be both a satisfaction and a motive for further social activity. Although such correlational evidence does not prove that spending time with others causes one to be happy, such findings are at least consistent with such a conclusion.

In a daily study of affect regulation in salespersons (who have frequent disappointments), Larsen and Gschwandtner (1995) found that social activity was among the most frequently used regulation strategies among female salespersons. As pointed out by Tice and Baumeister (1993), an important aspect of socializing for mood regulation concerns not socializing with persons who are in the same mood. To socialize with a bunch of angry people would probably not be a good choice for one trying to get over his or her anger. Socializing may work to relieve negative affect through a variety of processes. For example, telling one's story to someone else provides the opportunity to reframe the situation cognitively, allowing for a reappraisal and reinterpretation. It also provides distraction, changes the situation, and potentially elicits positive emotions.

Withdrawal, Isolation, Spending Time Alone

It may seem contradictory that both socializing and isolation might be useful affect regulation strategies. Nevertheless, isolation appears on the list of strategies presented by several researchers (Larsen, 1993; Morris & Reilly, 1987; Parkinson et al., 1996). This strategy refers to removing oneself from social activities during a negative emotional experience. We have all heard someone say, "Leave me alone, I'm in a bad mood." Larsen (1993), in his study of daily mood regulation patterns, reported that although this strategy is not uncommon, it is also not very successful in remediating negative affect. This basic finding was replicated by Fichman and colleagues (1999), who reported that spending time alone correlated with dispositional self-criticism (a component of depressive style) and also was unrelated to mood improvement in their study of daily mood. Thus, spending time alone is often employed or endorsed as a mood regulation strategy, yet its overall effectiveness for general NA relief remains doubtful.

Perhaps the one type of NA for which withdrawal or self-isolation is adaptive is anger. It would seem that when one is angry, especially when on the verge of "flooding" or losing self-control, withdrawal from the situation is an appropriate strategy. For example, if a parent becomes so angry at a child that he or she is on the verge of abusive physical action, then leaving the scene can be an adaptive response. However, for most other negative emotions, including sadness, anxiety, or shame, findings in the literature suggest that spending time alone may not be adaptive.

Positive Affect Regulation

At first glance, it would seem that when people are feeling positive, they do not need to regulate their affect. However, in a study of affect regulation strategies used in daily life, 91% of subjects reported that they had tried effortful strategies to induce or maintain a positive mood (Prizmic, 1997). Based on these results, and on recent work from the positive psychology movement (e.g., Snyder & Lopez, 2002), we discuss three specific PA regulation strategies.

Gratitude, Counting One's Blessings, or Focusing on Areas of Life That Are Going Well

This strategy is a bit like ruminating on the positive. It involves keeping a focus on one's strengths, or the events in life for which one can be thankful. Emmons and McCullough (2003) have reported two experiments in which participants were randomly assigned to one of three conditions: listing their hassles, listing things for which they were thankful, or listing mundane daily activities. Participants made these lists either weekly for 10 weeks (Study 1) or daily for 21 days (Study 2). Participants also kept records of their moods, coping behaviors, health behaviors, and physical symptoms. Across the studies, gratitude-outlook groups exhibited heightened well-being on most of the outcome measures relative to the control groups. The effect of counting one's blessings was not only particularly strong for measures of positive affect but it also produced interpersonal and self-reported health benefits.

Emmons and Shelton (2002) provide an interesting review of both philosophical and spiritual perspectives on gratitude, and the small but growing scientific literature on this topic. Typically, gratitude is expressed for positive events. However, finding something in a negative event that is positive and worth being grateful for is a way of taking control over the event, thereby choosing to extract some benefit by perceiving the event as a gift. Most of the current research on gratitude nevertheless focuses on documenting the positive consequences of regularly reminding oneself of the good in one's life. The "examined life" is one in which a person regularly inventories those things for which he or she is thankful.

How does gratitude work as an affect regulation strategy? One potential mechanism is that it may slow down adaptation to positive events. People habituate or adapt even to instances of great good fortune, such as winning a lottery (Brickman, Coates, & Janoff-Bulman, 1978). Gratitude may work to slow adaptation by consistently reminding one or refreshing the experience of the good event. Another potential mechanism whereby gratitude may work is by reminding the person of areas of his or her life that are going well. This may be especially useful in times of stress, or following particularly negative events. The process may be similar to Linville's (1985) self-complexity notion. By reminding oneself that there are things in life to be thankful for, one can buffer the effects of negative events.

Helping Others, Committing Acts of Kindness

Altruism and emotion have been widely studied. However, the predominant causal direction of interest in almost all experiments conducted to date has been the effects of emotion on subsequent helping. A few studies have focused indirectly on the effects of helping on the emotional state of the helper. For example, Wegener and Petty (1994) examined the anticipated consequences of helping and found that persons in a happy mood (compared to sad) based their decision to help on the anticipated affective consequences of helping. In another example, Rosenhan, Salovey, and Hargis (1981) found that happy persons were more likely to help and to anticipate positive consequences for helping. However, actual measures of affect obtained after helping behavior were not obtained. Nevertheless, many psychologists assume it is a forgone conclusion that helping produces positive effects on affective state (e.g., Salovey, Mayer, & Rosenhan, 1991).

A lot of indirect evidence suggests that helping may influence PA. For example, Simmons, Hickey, and Kjellstrand (1971) showed that persons who donated a kidney to a relative were more likely to be happier than other relatives who did not donate. Lucas (2000) found, in a daily experience sampling study, a substantial correlation between the percentage of time participants spent helping other people and their scores on a global well-being measure. And several researchers have demonstrated a link between dispositional happiness and the propensity to be generous, altruistic, and charitable (e.g., Feingold, 1983; Williams & Shiaw, 1999).

Humor, Laughter, Expressing Positive Emotions

Older theories of humor viewed the phenomenon as a form of disguised hostility or as a defensive release of tension. More recent theories (e.g., Lefcourt, 2002) view humor as an evolved mechanism that facilitates social interaction. Whatever the theory, most researchers agree that there are several different forms of humor, including derisive/disparaging, self-depreciating, and self-directed or mature humor, where a person laughs at his or her own disappointments or failings, or those of human nature in general. The latter is thought to be the most positive and beneficial form of humor (Vaillant, 1977).

Researchers have demonstrated that people who smile or laugh frequently also have more positive life outcomes. Much of the research shows that this effect is especially strong during periods of stress. For example, Bonanno and Keltner (1997) reported that bereaved persons who could smile and laugh as they spoke about their deceased spouse were rated as more attractive and appealing by the interviewers. They interpret this finding to mean that laughing and smiling after a traumatic event serve as a social signal that the stressed individual is ready to reengage in normal social interaction. Correlational studies show that persons with a sense of humor cope better with stress and illnesses, recover faster from illnesses, and appear to have enhanced immune system responses compared to low-humor persons (Lefcourt, 2002). Of the few true experiments conducted on the topic, in which laughter was induced in one group but not another (the control), results also suggest that laughter attenuates certain physiological responses to stress (e.g., Newman & Stone, 1996).

In terms of coping with stress, Taylor, Kemeny, Reed, Bower, and Gruenewald (2000) have shown that periods of self-conscious PA induction can be quite useful in overcoming the deleterious effects of chronic stress. For example, among caretakers for HIV patients, they found that many of the better copers reported efforts to self-induce laughter and humor, such as taking time to tell jokes or watch a humorous movie. The key to how laughter works may lie in the fact that it is an overt expression of a pleasant state, and expression may be the key. Kuiper and Martin (1998) demonstrated that laughter, not unexpressed pleasant emotions, moderated the relation between stress and distress. Expressions may amplify or extend the effects of the positive emotion. Duclos and Laird (2001) argued that emotional experiences can be controlled through the deliberate control of emotional expressions.

MODELS AND MEASURES OF AFFECT REGULATION

Models of Affect Regulation

Several researchers have proposed models for the process of affect regulation. Models are useful, because they identify the key elements or parts of a process and explain mechanism for how those parts work together. In one model of affect regulation, proposed by Carver and Scheier (1982, 1990), progress toward one's goals is regulated (see Carver, Chapter 2, this volume). Affect is seen as a useful by-product in terms of providing feedback to the system in a self-correcting or control theory model of goal pursuit. Larsen (2000b) provides a similar control theory model, the main difference being that affect is directly regulated in his model; that is, Larsen proposed that people have a set point for how they typically desire to feel. They then compare their current state to this set point on a regular basis. When they notice discrepancies, they take action to regulate affect. One valuable aspect of Larsen's model is that it posits several points at which individual differences might become apparent in the system. Many researchers view individual differences in affect regulation with great interest, because these may offer insight into both normal personality functioning and disorders of emotion.

Another model, the process model of emotion regulation, proposed by Gross (1999), divides emotion regulation into two phases: strategies that may be engaged before the emotion is evoked, and strategies that may occur after the emotional response. In this model, antecedent-focused emotion regulation includes factors such as situation selection, situation modification, and attention deployment. Cognitive reappraisal might be one form of antecedent-focused emotion regulation, if the effort to interpret the situation benignly occurs before the emotional response. After the emotional response there is response-focused emotion regulation, which includes strategies that diminish the intensity or shorten unpleasant emotional experiences. The strategy that has received most of Gross's attention is suppression or inhibition of expression of negative affect, which we discussed earlier.

Measures of Affect Regulation

State Conceptions

Several studies of affect regulation have employed the experience sampling method, where subjects make repeated reports, perhaps several times a day, for fairly long time periods. In such studies the assessment of affect regulation typically occurs using a checklist format, where subjects check off whether or not they engaged in a particular behavior or cognitive strategy during the time period over which they are reporting. The assessment instrument first developed by Larsen (1993) was based on the list of mood regulation strategies presented by Morris and Reilly (1987) and contained 11 strategies in a checklist format. This checklist was adopted and modified by Fichman and colleagues (1999) in the form of a checklist used in their study of daily mood regulation and depression.

This checklist was recently updated and used in a study of daily affect regulation (Prizmic, 2000). The 24 affect regulation items on that checklist were also presented in a theoretical paper by Larsen (2000b). We present the latest version of the MARS checklist in Figure 3.1. This checklist, which consists of 32 affect regulation items, is a rapid way to assess state affect regulation by asking participants whether they have engaged in any of the behaviors or strategies described by the items. The MARS contains all of the strategies discussed earlier, plus several others that might be of more specialized interest, such as prayer, denial, or use of alcohol or drugs.

The MARS is probably most useful in prospective studies, in which the interest lies in assessing ongoing affect regulation in everyday life. For example, it could be used to assess the frequency with which people engage in each strategy over a fairly long time period. One could also assess the relative effectiveness of each strategy by assessing ongoing affect and examining changes that follow the enactment of specific strategies. By combining both within- and between-person variations, even more complex questions can be asked about affect regulation. For example, one might imagine that most people would frequently use those strategies that are most effective. However, some persons (perhaps those high on neuroticism) might persist in using ineffective strategies.

The MARS can be used in a variety of ways besides simply assessing current behavior. It might be used, for example, to assess participants' recollections of past behaviors, in an effort to assess the recollected frequency of use, or it might be used to have participants judge the relative effectiveness of each strategy in their own experience. Perhaps one of the more interesting applications of the MARS is to use its items to code open-ended content for mood-regulating styles. For example, Lerner and Larsen (2002) asked participants to write down what they did in the wake of the September 11, 2001, tragedy to manage their affective reactions. The open-ended responses were then content-coded according to the items on the MARS. The most widely use strategies in response to the September 11 tragedy were socializing and information gathering, though cognitive reappraisal, withdrawal, helping others, and distraction were the next most frequent strategies used. Subjects in the Lerner and Larsen sample were then categorized according to whether or not they engaged in any strategies found by Larsen (1993) to be relatively ineffective (i.e., distraction, withdrawal, venting, ingesting mood-altering substances, fatalism, intellectualizing, and active forgetting). Subjects who engaged in ineffective affect regulation styles had more physical and psychological symptoms following September 11 than subjects who engaged in the more effective affect regulation styles. Other researchers have also formulated checklists and rating scales for assessing affect regulation. In particular, interested readers should consult the taxonomies of Parkinson and Totterdell (1999) and Thayer and colleagues (1994).

Trait Conceptions

Several researchers have focused on the assessment of affect regulation as an individual-difference characteristic. As such, several personality trait–type measures exist. For example, Gross and John (2002) presented a 10-item measure, the Emotion Regulation Questionnaire, that assesses the affect regulation strategies of suppression and cognitive reappraisal. The items are statements to which the person either agrees or disagrees on a 7-point Likert-type scale. Although this scale shows promising levels of validity (e.g., Richards & Gross, 2000), it is limited to two regulation strategies, and the degree of overlap (or lack of discriminant validity) with existing personality traits (such as emotional expressivity) is of some concern.

Another trait measure of affect regulation, developed by Garnefski, Kraaij, and Spinhoven (2001), the Cognitive Emotion Regulation Questionnaire, is a 36-item inventory that taps into a person's style of responding to stressful events. The inventory yields nine subscales for specific affect regulating styles (e.g., Cognitive Reframing, Positive Focus, Rumination, Planning for the Future, Self-Blame, Acceptance of Fate). The scales have acceptable psychometric properties, and some have been shown to moderate the relationship between stress and symptoms.

Mayer and Stevens (1994) developed the 7-item Meta-Regulation scale, which assesses the three conscious affect regulation strategies of repair, dampening, and maintenance. This scale has been used by several researchers (e.g., Kokkonen & Pulkkinen, 2001). Mayer and Salovey (1997) combined their interests to develop the concept of emotional intelligence, which includes the concept of effective affect regulation. Although their conceptual definition of affect regulation as an ability is lauded, the specific measure they published (Mayer, Salovey, & Caruso, 2000) has been criticized on a number of grounds (e.g., Davies, Stankov, & Roberts, 1998; Lerner & Larsen, 2002). Moreover, the affect regulation components of emotional intelligence inventories typically yield one score; thus, they do not provide much in the way of differential abilities or specific styles of affect regulation. At this point, if one wanted a thorough assessment of the many and various styles of affect regulation, then a version of the MARS (see Figure 3.1), with instructions worded in terms of trait responding, might be the most discriminating approach to assessment of individual differences.

ISSUES FOR FUTURE RESEARCH

Frequency and Efficacy of Regulation Strategies

One important question concerns how frequently the strategies are employed. In the study by Thayer and colleagues (1994), results were based on people's recollected judgments of which strategies they used in the past to change a bad mood. The most frequently reported strategies included call, talk to, or be with someone; think positively; concentrate on something else; avoidance; listen to music; and try to be alone. In a daily study of a sample of trainee teachers, participants prospectively reported on their use of mood-regulation strategies every 2 hours for 2 weeks (Totterdell & Parkinson, 1999). Results showed that the most frequently used strategies were the diversionary strategies (e.g., distraction, rationalization, cognitive avoidance, and self-reward), which exceeded the frequency of more engagement-type strategies (e.g., reappraisal, seeking social support). Another study by same researchers (Parkinson & Totterdell, 1996), examining a sample of undergraduates, found that the most frequently used strategies were the engagement strategies. In our daily study of undergraduates, using items from the MARS (Prizmic, 2000), the most frequently used strategies were the more active, engagement-type strategies of reappraisal and interacting with others. The question about frequency appears to be influenced by which persons are being studied, and under what circumstances.

Efficacy of strategies will likely prove to be a challenging topic to study. Preliminary findings suggest that efficacy depends on numerous factors, such as the situations that elicit the use of strategies (i.e., context-related regulation), individual differences, and the effects of previously used mood-regulation strategies (i.e., individual experience; Kokkonen & Pulkkinen, 2001; Parkinson et al., 1996; Rusting & DeHart, 2000). One particular difficulty will be judging whether persons are poor at enacting affect regulation strategies, or whether they really have no problematic affects to regulate. For example, both depressed and nondepressed persons might show low frequency of affect regulation; the depressed, because they do not have the abilities, and the normals, because they do not have the need to regulate.

Few studies have directly tackled the question of efficacy. Thayer and colleagues (1994) assessed recollected effectiveness of strategies to change a bad mood, enhance energy, and reduce tension. Their results showed that people believed that the most effective strategy for changing a bad mood, judged both by self-ratings and by psychotherapists, was exercise, whereas controlling thoughts, reappraisal, and religious or spiritual activity were rated best to raise energy and reduce tension. When strategy effectiveness is based on actual prospective data, results show that different strategies are useful for regulating different affective states. For example, in Totterdell and Parkinson's (1999) daily study of affect regulation, both engagement (e.g., reappraisal) and diversionary (e.g., distraction) strategies increased cheerfulness and calmness, but only engagement was associated with increases in energy. Pleasant activities and relaxation were best for enhancing calmness, whereas active and energetic activities were best for enhancing energy.

In our own research (Prizmic, 2000), in which undergraduates reported their moods and use of regulation strategies three times a day for 4 consecutive weeks, we were able to assess efficacy as the degree to which negative affect was lower than would be expected by chance on occasions following strategy use. Cognitive reappraisal correlated with lower NA, whereas passive strategies, such as distraction and avoidance, correlated with higher NA after their use. In addition, Prizmic (2000) found that the most frequently used strategies were also the most effective strategies (i.e., cognitive reappraisal, socializing, focusing on feelings).

Origin and Maintenance of Affect Regulation Styles

How do people develop effective affect regulation styles? If affect regulation is an ability, from where does it come? Is there a genetic contribution? How much is learned? Could schools develop and incorporate classes or interventions that teach affect regulation? Might affect regulation produce biological changes that allow affective styles to be maintained? This is just a sampling of questions about the origin and maintenance of affect regulation styles.

Davidson proposed increasing positive affect through meditation, which can potentially influence plastic changes in brain circuits controlling emotion (Davidson, 2000; Davidson et al., 2000). Further questions about maintenance concern whether more automatic forms of emotion regulation are associated with actual structural changes in the brain (Davidson et al., 2000). In other words, when affect regulatory behaviors or strategies have long durations or occur with great frequency, changes in the central circuitry of emotion may actually occur. Individual or state differences in prefrontal activation may play role in affect regulation, and may potentially be detectable with neuroimaging technology (Davidson, 2000).

Short- and Long-Term Consequences

Another potentially important topic for research concerns understanding the short- and long-term consequences of affect and affect regulation. Clearly, emotions are part of a cascade of responses, ranging from very fast central nervous system changes to somewhat slower autonomic nervous system changes, to slower neurochemical and hormonal changes, and to even slower changes in health status. Moreover, negative affect and stress responses may accumulate over time to build up what has come to be called "allostatic load" (e.g., Cacioppo & Gardner, 1999), the total physiological burden that has accrued over a person's lifetime. Total allostatic load may be one of the important concepts that explain the long-term consequences of affect. Effective affect regulation may lessen the buildup of allostatic load.

Another example of how short- and long-term consequences might be different concerns effects of venting. It may turn out that venting, or the physical expression of negative emotions, is, in the short term, associated with a perpetuation of emotion and thereby runs counter to effective regulation. On the other hand, emotional expression may have beneficial long-term consequences in terms of health and relationship benefits. Understanding the different processes that might be associated with short- versus long-term processes involved in affect regulation remains a challenge for future researchers.

Affect Specificity and Person Specificity in Affect Regulation

It seems likely that different affect-regulating behaviors or strategies work differentially for the different affective states. This might be assessed in terms of frequency (e.g., do people more frequently engage in downward social comparison when they are sad compared to when they are angry?), or the affect specificity might be assessed more in terms of efficacy (e.g., inhibition of expression is more effective for controlling affects with clear expressiveness components, such as anger, compared to affects that are not clearly expressive, such as loneliness).

Person specificity is also very likely to be found in affect regulation. Sex differences are an obvious first place to look. We might predict, for example, that women may more frequently and successfully use strategies that rely on social interaction, whereas men may be more likely to use and find effective those strategies that are less social, such as exercising, seeking pleasure, or ingesting mood-altering substances. Age and cultural differences might also be found to be instances of person specificity. For example, persons from Asian cultures may be more likely to employ inhibition of expression strategies to control affect.

Another very likely source of specificity is in terms of personality. Are certain personality traits associated with using specific strategies either more effectively or more frequently? For example, do extraverts engage in more active socializing, helping others, and talking to friends or mentors than introverts? Do subjects who score high on neuroticism, for example, persist in engaging strategies that are generally ineffective? Addressing the person- and affect-specificity questions may bring a new level of complexity to research on affect regulation.

CONCLUSIONS

Research on affect regulation has grown tremendously over the last 20 years. Whereas once it was almost the exclusive domain of developmental psychology, it is now a large and active field of research, linking social, clinical, biological, and personality psychology to affective science. The field of affect regulation has matured to the point that several taxonomies have been published, and several measures exist for researchers interested in studying the topic. Moreover, a preliminary body of knowledge about the nature and role of affect regulation in daily function exists, especially in terms of coping with negative life events, and the roles of upregulating positive emotions and downregulating negative ones. Yet much still remains to be learned about affect regulation. In this chapter, we have tried to highlight developments in this area, to share our enthusiasm for this field and our perspective on key issues, and to suggest several questions for future research.

ACKNOWLEDGMENT

Preparation of this chapter was supported by Grant No. RO1-MH63732 from the National Institute of Mental Health

REFERENCES

Adan, A. (1994). Chronotype and personality factors in the daily consumption of alcohol and psychostimulants. *Addiction, 89,* 455–462.

Baumeister, R. F., Bratslavsky, E., Finkenauer, C., & Vohs, K. D. (2001). Bad is stronger than good. *Review of General Psychology, 5,* 323–370.

Bless, H., & Forgas, J. P. (2000). *The message within: The role of subjective experience in social cognition and behavior.* Philadelphia: Psychology Press.

Bonanno, G. A., & Keltner, D. (1997). Facial expressions of emotion and the course of conjugal bereavement. *Journal of Abnormal Psychology, 106,* 126–137.

Brickman, P., Coates, D., & Janoff-Bulman, R. (1978). Lottery winners and accident victims: Is happiness relative? *Journal of Personality and Social Psychology, 36,* 917–927.

Buck, R. (1977). Nonverbal communication of affect in preschool children: Relationships with personality and skin conductance. *Journal of Personality and Social Psychology, 35,* 225–236.

Buck, R., Miller, R. E., & Caul, W. F. (1974). Sex, personality, and physiological variables in the communication of affect via facial expression. *Journal of Personality and Social Psychology, 30,* 587–596.

Bushman, B. J. (2002). Does venting anger feed or extinguish the flame? Catharsis, rumination, distraction, anger, and aggressive responding. *Personality and Social Psychology Bulletin, 28,* 724–731.

Bushman, B. J., Baumeister, R. F., & Phillips, C. M. (2001). Do people aggress to improve their mood?: Catharsis beliefs, affect regulation opportunity, and aggressive responding. *Journal of Personality and Social Psychology, 81,* 17–32.

Cacioppo, J. T., & Gardner, W. L. (1999). Emotion. *Annual Review of Psychology, 50,* 191–214.

Carstensen, L. L (1993). Motivation for social contact across the life span: A theory of socioemotional selectivity. In J. E. Edwards (Ed.), *Nebraska Symposium on Motivation: Developmental perspectives on motivation* (pp. 209–254). Lincoln: University of Nebraska Press.

Carver, C. S., & Scheier, M. F. (1982). Control theory: A useful conceptual framework for personality-social, clinical, and health psychology. *Psychological Bulletin, 92,* 111–135.

Carver, C. S., & Scheier, M. F. (1990). Origins and functions of positive and negative affect: A control-process view. *Psychological Review, 97,* 19–35.

Consedine, N. S., Magai, C., & Bonanno, G. A. (2002). Moderators of the emotion inhibition–health relationship: A review and research agenda. *Review of General Psychology, 6,* 204–228.

Davidson, R. J. (2000). Affective style, psychopathology, and resilience: Brain mechanisms and plasticity. *American Psychologist, 55,* 1196–1214.

Davidson, R. J. (2002a). Anxiety and affective style: Role of prefrontal cortex and amygdala. *Biological Psychiatry, 51,* 68–80.

Davidson, R. J. (2002b). Toward a biology of positive affect and compassion. In R. J. Davidson & A. Harrington (Eds.), *Visions of compassion: Western scientists and Tibetan Buddhists examine human nature* (pp. 107–130). London: Oxford University Press.

Davidson, R. J., Jackson, D. C., & Kalin, N. H. (2000). Emotion, plasticity, context, and regulation: Perspectives from affective neuroscience. *Psychological Bulletin Special Issue: Psychology in the 21st Century, 126,* 890–909.

Davidson, R. J., Lewis, D. A., Alloy, L. B., Amaral, D.G., Bush, G., Cohen, J.D., et al. (2002). Neural and behavioral substrates of mood and mood regulation. *Biological Psychiatry, 52,* 478–502.

Davies, M., Stankov, L., & Roberts, R. D. (1998). Emotional intelligence: In search of an elusive construct. *Journal of Personality and Social Psychology, 75,* 989–1015.

Davis, C. G., Nolen-Hoeksema, S., & Larson, J. (1998). Making sense of loss and benefiting from the experience: Two construals of meaning. *Journal of Personality and Social Psychology, 75,* 561–574.

Diener, E., & Seligman, M. E. P. (2002). Very happy people. *Psychological Science, 13,* 81–84.

Dobson, K. S., & Joffe, R. (1986). The role of activity level and cognition in depressed mood in a university sample. *Journal of Clinical Psychology, 42,* 264–271.

Duclos, S. E., & Laird, J. D. (2001). The deliberate control of emotional experience through control of expressions. *Cognition and Emotion, 15,* 27–56.

Eisenberg, N., Fabes, R. A., Guthrie, I. K., & Reiser, M. (2000). Dispositional emotionality and regulation: Their role in predicting quality of social functioning. *Journal of Personality and Social Psychology, 78,* 136–157.

Ekkekakis, P., Hall, E. E., Van Landuyt, L. M., & Petruzzello, S. J. (2000). Walking in (affective) circles: Can short walks enhance affect? *Journal of Behavioral Medicine, 23,* 245–275.

Emmons, R. A., & Shelton, C. M. (2002). Gratitude and the science of positive psychology. In C. R. Snyder & S. J. Lopez (Eds.), *Handbook of positive psychology* (pp. 459–471). New York: Oxford University Press.

Emmons, R. A., & McCullough, M. E. (2003). Counting blessings versus burdens: An experimental investigation of gratitude and subjective well-being in daily life. *Journal of Personality and Social Psychology, 84,* 377–389.

Feingold, A. (1983). Happiness, unselfishness, and popularity. *Journal of Psychology, 115,* 3–5.

Fichman, L., Koestner, R., Zuroff, D. C., & Gordon, L. (1999). Depressive styles and the regulation of negative affect: A daily experience study. *Cognitive Therapy and Research, 23,* 483–495.

Forgas, J. P., & Ciarrochi, J. V. (2002). On managing moods: Evidence for the role of homeostatic cognitive strategies in affect regulation. *Personality and Social Psychology Bulletin, 28,* 336–345.

Fredrickson, B. L. (1998). What good are positive emotions? *Review of General Psychology, 2,* 300–319.

Fredrickson, B. L. (2000). Cultivating positive emotions to optimize health and well-being. *Prevention & Treatment, 3* [Online], Article 1. Retrieved November 11, 2002, from *http://journals.apa.org/prevention/volume3/pre0030001a.html*

Fredrickson, B. L., & Levenson, R. W. (1998). Positive emotions speed recovery from the cardiovascular sequelae of negative emotions. *Cognition and Emotion, 12,* 191–220.

Garnefski, N., Kraaij, V., & Spinhoven, P. (2001). Negative life events, cognitive emotion regulation and emotional problems. *Personality and Individual Differences, 30,* 1311–1327.

Geen, R. G., & Quanty, M. B. (1977). The catharsis of aggression: An evaluation of a hypothesis. In L. Berkowitz (Ed.), *Advances in experimental social psychology* (Vol. 10, pp. 1–37). New York: Academic Press.

Gottman, J. M., Katz, L. F., & Hooven, C. (1997). *Meta-emotion: How families communicate emotionally.* Mahwah, NJ: Erlbaum.

Gross, J. J. (1999). Emotion regulation: Past, present, future. *Cognition and Emotion [Special issue: Functional accounts of emotion], 13,* 551–573.

Gross, J. J. (2001). Emotion regulation in adulthood: Timing is everything. *Current Directions in Psychological Science, 10,* 214–219.

Gross, J. J., & John, O. P. (2002). Wise emotion regulation. In L. Feldman Barrett & P. Salovey (Eds.), *The wisdom in feeling: Psychological processes in emotional intelligence* (pp. 297–318). New York: Guilford Press.

Gross, J. J., & Levenson, R. W. (1997). Hiding feelings: The acute effects of inhibiting negative and positive emotion. *Journal of Abnormal Psychology, 106,* 95–103.

Heiby, E. M. (1983). Assessment of frequency of self-reinforcement. *Journal of Personality and Social Psychology, 44,* 1304–1307.

Josephson, B. R., Singer, J. A., & Salovey, P. (1996). Mood regulation and memory: Repairing sad moods with happy memories. *Cognition and Emotion, 10,* 437–444.

Judge, T., & Larsen, R. J. (2001). Dispositional sources of job satisfaction: A review and theoretical extension. *Organizational Behavior and Human Decision Processes, 86,* 67–98.

Kokkonen, M., & Pulkkinen, L. (2001). Examination of the paths between personality, current mood, its evaluation, and emotion regulation. *European Journal of Personality, 15,* 83–104.

Kopp, C. B. (1989). Regulation of distress and negative emotions: A developmental view. *Developmental Psychology, 25,* 343–354.

Kuiper, N. A., & Martin, R. (1998). Laughter and stress in daily life: Relation to positive and negative affect. *Motivation and Emotion [Special issue: Positive affect and self-regulation], 22,* 133–153.

Larsen, R. J. (1993, August). Mood regulation in everyday life. In D. M. Tice (Chair), *Self-regulation of mood and emotion.* Symposium conducted at the 101st annual convention of the American Psychological Association, Toronto.

Larsen, R. J. (2000a). Maintaining hedonic balance: Reply to commentaries. *Psychological Inquiry, 11,* 218–225.

Larsen, R. J. (2000b). Toward a science of mood regulation. *Psychological Inquiry, 11,* 129–141.

Larsen, R. J. (2002). Differential contributions of positive and negative affect to subjective well-being. In J. A. Da Silva, E. H. Matsushima, & N. P. Riberio-Filho (Eds.), *Annual Meeting of the International Society for Psychophysics* (Vol. 18, pp. 186–190). Rio de Janeiro, Brazil: Editora Legis Summa Ltda.

Larsen, R. J., & Cowan, G. S. (1988). Internal focus of attention and depression: A study of daily experience. *Motivation and Emotion, 12,* 237–249.

Larsen, R. J., & Gschwandtner, L. B. (1995, March). A better day. *Personal Selling Power,* pp. 41–49.

Larsen, R. J., Kasimatis, M., & Frey, K. (1992). Facilitating the furrowed brow: An unobtrusive test of the facial feedback hypothesis applied to unpleasant affect. *Cognition and Emotion, 6,* 321–338.

Lazarus, R. S., & Folkman, S. (1984). *Stress, appraisal, and coping.* New York: Springer.

Lefcourt, H. M. (2002). Humor. In C. R. Snyder & S. J. Lopez (Eds.), *Handbook of positive psychology* (pp. 619–631). New York: Oxford University Press.

Lerner, C., & Larsen, R. J. (2002). *Emotional intelligence and mood regulation following September 11.* Unpublished manuscript, Washington University, St. Louis, MO.

Linville, P. W. (1985). Self-complexity and affect extremity: Don't put all of your eggs in one basket. *Social Cognition, 3,* 94–120.

Lockwood, P. (2002). Could it happen to you?: Predicting the impact of downward comparisons on the self. *Journal of Personality and Social Psychology, 82,* 343–358.

Lucas, R. E. (2000). *Pleasant affect and sociability: Towards a comprehensive model of extraverted feelings and behaviors.* Unpublished doctoral dissertation, University of Illinois, Urbana.

Lucas, R., Diener, E., & Larsen, R. (2003). The measurement of positive emotions. In C. R. Snyder & M. Lopez (Eds.), *Handbook of positive psychological assessment* (pp. 201–218). Washington, DC: American Psychological Association.

Lyubomirsky, S. (2001). Why are some people happier than others?: The role of cognitive and motivational processes in well-being. *American Psychologist, 56,* 239–249.

Lyubomirsky, S., & Ross, L. (1997). Hedonic consequences of social comparison: A contrast of happy and unhappy people. *Journal of Personality and Social Psychology, 73,* 1141–1157.

Lyubomirsky, S., Tucker, K. L., & Kasri, F. (2001). Responses to hedonically conflicting social comparisons: Comparing happy and unhappy people. *European Journal of Social Psychology [Special issue: New directions in social comparison research], 31,* 511–535.

Mayer, J. D., & Salovey, P. (1997). What is emotional intelligence? In P. Salovey & D. Sluyter (Eds.), *Emotional development and emotional intelligence: Educational implications* (pp. 3–39). New York: Basic Books.

Mayer, J. D., Salovey, P., & Caruso, D. R. (2000). *Test manual for the MSCEIT V.2.0: The Mayer, Salovey, and Caruso Emotional Intelligence Test.* Toronto: Mental Health Systems.

Mayer, J. D., & Stevens, A. A. (1994). An emerging understanding of the reflective (meta)experience of mood. *Journal of Research in Personality, 28,* 351–373.

Morris, W., & Reilly, N. (1987). Toward the self-regulation of mood: Theory and research. *Motivation and Emotion, 11,* 215–249.

Newman, M. G., & Stone, A. A. (1996). Does humor moderate the effects of experimentally-induced stress? *Annals of Behavioral Medicine, 18,* 101–109.

Niederhoffer, K. G., & Pennebaker, J. W. (2002). Sharing one's story: On the benefits of writing or talking about emotional experiences. In C. R. Snyder & S. J. Lopez (Eds.), *Handbook of positive psychology* (pp. 573–583). New York: Oxford University Press.

Parkinson, B., & Totterdell, P. (1996). Deliberate affect-regulation strategies: Preliminary data concerning reported effectiveness and frequency of use. In N.H. Frijda (Ed.), *Proceedings of the Ninth Meeting of the International Society for Research on Emotion* (pp. 401–405). Storrs, CT: International Society for Research on Emotion.

Parkinson, B., & Totterdell, P. (1999). Classifying affect-regulation strategies. *Cognition and Emotion, 13,* 277–303.

Parkinson, B., Totterdell, P., Briner R. B., & Reynolds, S. (1996). *Changing moods: The psychology of mood and mood regulation.* London: Longman.

Parrott, W. G. (1993). Beyond hedonism: Motives for inhibiting good moods and for maintaining bad moods. In D. M. Wagner & J. W. Pennebaker (Eds.), *Handbook of mental control* (pp. 278–305). NJ: Prentice-Hall.

Prizmic, Z. (1997). [Mood regulation strategies for positive mood]. Unpublished raw data.

Prizmic, Z. (2000). *Mood regulation strategies and subjective health.* Unpublished doctoral dissertation, University of Zagreb, Croatia.

Richards, J. M., & Gross, J. J. (2000). Emotion regulation and memory: The cognitive costs of keeping one's cool. *Journal of Personality and Social Psychology, 79,* 410–424.

Rippere, V. (1977). What's the thing to do when you're feeling depressed: A pilot study. *Behaviour Research and Therapy, 15,* 185–191.

Rosenhan, D. L., Salovey, P., & Hargis, K. (1981). The joys of helping: Focus of attention mediates the impact of positive affect on altruism. *Journal of Personality and Social Psychology, 40,* 899–905.

Rusting, C. L., & DeHart, T. (2000). Retrieving positive memories to regulate negative mood: Consequences for mood-congruent memory. *Journal of Personality and Social Psychology, 78,* 737–752.

Salovey, P., Mayer, J. D., & Rosenhan, D. L. (1991). Mood and helping: Mood as a motivator of helping and helping as a regulator of mood. In M. S. Clark (Ed.), *Prosocial behavior* (pp. 215–237). Thousand Oaks, CA: Sage.

Schaefer, S., Jackson, D., Davidson, R., Aquirre, G. K., Kimperg, D. Y., & Thompson-Schill, S. L. (2002). Modulation of amygdalar activity by the conscious regulation of negative emotion. *Journal of Cognitive Neuroscience, 14,* 913–921.

Simmons, R. G., Hickey, K., & Kjellstrand, C. M. (1971). Donors and non-donors: The role of the family and the physician in kidney transplantation. *Seminars in Psychiatry, 3,* 102–115.

Snyder, C. R., & Lopez, S. J. (Eds.). (2002). *Handbook of positive psychology.* London: Oxford University Press.

Stevens, M. J., & Lane, A. M. (2001). Mood-regulating strategies used by athletes. *Athletic Insight: Online Journal of Sport Psychology, 3*(3). Retrieved October 12, 2000, from *http://www.athleticinsight.com/vol3iss3/Moodregulation.htm*

Suls, J., Martin, R., & Wheeler, L. (2002). Social comparison: Why, with whom, and with what effect? *Current Directions in Psychological Science, 11,* 159–163.

Suls, J., & Wheeler, L. (Eds.). (2000). *Handbook of social comparison.* New York: Kluwer Academic/Plenum Press.

Tamres, L. K., Janicki, D., & Helgeson, V. S. (2002). Sex differences in coping behavior: A meta-analytic review and an examination of relative coping. *Personality and Social Psychology Review*, 6, 2–30.

Taylor, S. E., Kemeny, M. E., Reed, G. M., Bower, J. E., & Gruenewald, T. L. (2000). Psychological resources, positive illusions, and health. *American Psychologist*, 55, 99–109.

Tennen, H., & Affleck, G. (2002). Benefit-finding and benefit-reminding. In C. R. Snyder & S. J. Lopez (Eds.), *Handbook of positive psychology* (pp. 584–597). New York: Oxford University Press.

Thayer, R. E. (1987). Energy, tiredness, and tension effects of a sugar snack versus moderate exercise. *Journal of Personality and Social Psychology*, 52, 119–125.

Thayer, R. E. (2001). *Calm energy: How people regulate mood with food and exercise.* London: Oxford University Press.

Thayer, R. E., Newman, J. R., & McClain, T. M. (1994). Self-regulation of mood: Strategies for changing a bad mood, raising energy, and reducing tension. *Journal of Personality and Social Psychology*, 67, 910–925.

Thompson, R. A. (1994). Emotion regulation: A theme in search of definition. *Monographs of the Society for Research in Child Development*, 59, 25–52.

Tice, D. M., & Baumeister, R. F (1993). Controlling anger: Self-induced emotion change. In D. M. Wegner & J. W. Pennebaker (Eds.), *Handbook of mental control* (pp. 393–409). Upper Saddle River, NJ: Prentice-Hall.

Totterdell, P., & Parkinson, B. (1999). Use and effectiveness of self-regulation strategies for improving mood in a group of trainee teachers. *Journal of Occupational Health Psychology*, 4, 219–232.

Vaillant, G. E. (1977). *Adaptation to life.* Boston: Little, Brown.

Wegener, D. T., & Petty, R. E. (1994). Mood management across affective states: The hedonic contingency hypothesis. *Journal of Personality and Social Psychology*, 66, 1034–1048.

Williams, S., & Shiaw, W. T. (1999). Mood and organizational citizenship behavior: The effects of positive affect on employee organizational citizenship behavior intentions. *Journal of Psychology*, 133, 656–668.

4

The Cognitive Neuroscience
of Self-Regulation

Jane F. Banfield
Carrie L. Wyland
C. Neil Macrae
Thomas F. Münte
Todd F. Heatherton

A fundamental human capacity is the ability to regulate and control our thoughts and behavior. Recent developments in neuroscience have increased our understanding of the neural underpinnings of self-regulation. Our goal in this chapter is to describe areas in the brain that appear to be involved in the self-regulation of thought and action. Self-regulation is viewed here as the higher order (i.e., executive) control of lower order processes responsible for the planning and execution of behavior. For our purposes in this chapter, self-regulation refers not only to executive processes such as working memory, attention, memory, and choice and decision making, but also to the control of emotion (covering issues of affect, drive, and motivation). The primary brain region responsible for these control functions is the prefrontal cortex (PFC), the anterior portion of the frontal lobes.

The PFC can be viewed as the seat of consciousness; it is the only area of the brain that receives input from all sensory modalities; therefore, it is the area in which inputs from internal sources conjoin with information received from the outside world. For these reasons, the PFC has been labeled the "chief executive" (Goldberg, 2001) that is responsible for subjective reactions to the outside world and exernal behaviors that shape our "personalities" (e.g., Bechara, Damasio, Damasio, & Anderson, 1994; Damasio, 1994; Stuss, Gow, & Hetherington, 1992; Stuss & Levine, 2002; Stuss, Picton, & Alexander, 2001).

THE FRONTAL LOBES
AS A SUPERVISORY ATTENTIONAL SYSTEM

A useful framework for understanding self-regulation is provided by Norman and Shallice (1986). Their seminal model concerning the role of attention in automatic and willed action describes two processes for the control of behavior. According to the model, well-learned, simple actions may be executed via the contention scheduling system, without conscious input. On the other hand, more complex behaviors that require attentional input are carried out via the supervisory attentional system (SAS). The contention scheduling system works via lateral activation and inhibition among selected schemas for action. Schema activation within this system does not rely on attentional control but is simply based on the determination of the activation values of the schemas. Norman and Shallice use the example of typing a word on signal; this action sequence is represented by a set of schemas that trigger the appropriate finger, hand, and arm movements, and can be carried out within the contention scheduling system without attentional input.

However, the model also allows for the conscious control of more novel or complex tasks, a function of the SAS. This system mediates attention, which in turn can control the activation or inhibition values of behavioral schemas and bias the selection of the contention scheduling system. This higher order control provided by the SAS is required only for complex, novel, or dangerous tasks (e.g., a task that requires error correction or planning), or tasks that require planning or overriding temptation. In other words, the SAS is required when there is no available schema to achieve control of the desired behavior. As mentioned earlier, the initiation and execution of routine action sequences do not require input from the SAS.

Support for the notion that action sequences can be executed without conscious attentional control is provided in part by the investigation of action slips. An example of an action slip would be putting shaving cream on a toothbrush (see Norman, 1981; Reason, 1979; Reason & Mycielska, 1982). Such errors arise now and then precisely because the contention scheduling system is capable of selecting and initiating actions schemas without attentional control. Occasionally, a schema for an inappropriate action may become more strongly activated than the correct schema within the contention scheduling system, resulting in an action slip. One of the key functions of the SAS is to inhibit such prelearned responses when the context is inappropriate (see Baddeley, 1986, 1996; Damasio, 1994; Luria, 1966; Shallice, 1988), so action slips are particularly likely to occur if the supervisory system is directed elsewhere at the time (i.e., if the mind is otherwise engaged). In summary, although it is possible to apply attention to consciously modulate behaviors, it is not necessary for the execution of routine actions. The concept of "will," in this sense, corresponds to the output of the SAS and the inhibition or activation of behavioral schemas.

What happens, then, when this willful control is disrupted by damage to certain parts of the brain (e.g., control and inhibition are impeded or no longer possible)? Does damage to the PFC in effect equate to a damaged SAS? Norman and Shallice (1986) proposed precisely this possibility: They maintained that the functions assumed for the SAS correspond to the prefrontal areas described by Luria (1966) as responsible for the execution and regulation of behavior. Patients with frontal lobe damage provide support for this contention. For example, in the same way that routine behaviors can be executed without input from the SAS, basic functions (e.g., speaking or using objects) are usually left unimpaired in persons with damage confined to prefrontal structures. Yet patients with frontal lobe damage (particularly those with damage to the dorsolateral PFC, as out-lined later in the chapter) *do* have problems with tasks that are novel or that require plan-ning or error correction (see Walsch, 1978)—precisely the role of the SAS in the Norman and Shallice model. Frontal lobe patients often appear to have lost their supervisory con-trol—their guide to complex or novel behavior. Rather, the cues that activate their behav-ior are often environmentally driven, automatic, and immediate (Shallice, 1988; Stuss et al., 1992). Therefore, such individuals are unable either to direct or to regulate their behavior successfully.

Stimulus-based behavior is clearly evident in "utilization behavior," which is the compulsive need to act out the actions normally associated with everyday objects, even if not appropriate to the current context—for example, drinking from an empty cup, or get-ting into bed whenever one enters a bedroom (see Brazzelli, Colombo, Della Sala, & Spinner, 1994; Lhermitte, Pillon, & Serdaru, 1986). A less common but more arresting example of action error can be seen in alien hand syndrome, which is often the result of damage to the supplementary motor area (SMA) or the corpus callosum. In this disorder, one hand appears to have a will of its own, or is even seen as belonging to someone else. The result of this loss of agency is that the alien hand performs uncontrollable and dis-turbing movements—for example, one hand will undo every button that the other hand does up (see Della Sala, Marchetti, & Spinnler, 1991; Ramachandran & Blakesee, 1998). These types of behavior are often described as "environment-driven exploratory re-sponses," and can occur following lesions to the medial or orbital frontal lobes, as out-lined later in this chapter. Clearly, these disorders represent a severe breakdown in self-regulation, in that the individual is unable to achieve an intended goal.

Because patient data and observations appeared to be consistent with Norman and Shallice's viewpoint, Cooper and Shallice (2000) further explored the notion of routine and complex action schemas by developing a computational model in which action schemas are hierarchically organized within a network, and the selection of routine ac-tions is based on competitive activation within this network. Cooper and Shallice pro-posed that both everyday lapses and the more severe cases resulting from neurological damage can be explained in this way. One explanation for frontal behaviors (such as uti-lization behavior) is a loss of top–down input in the system (i.e., a loss of supervisory control; Shallice, 1982; Shallice, Burgess, Schon, & Baxter, 1989). Another explanation is offered by Schwartz and colleagues (1995), who proposed that these deficits may arise from a lack of distinction between contention scheduling and supervisory attention with-in the action system itself.

In simulating the contention scheduling system in detail, Cooper and Shallice (2000) were able to vary the amount of top–down and environmental influence, and to apply the model to a specific task—for example, the "coffee preparation domain." They found that the model was capable of producing hierarchically structured argument and action selec-tions. For this particular task, 12 actions were performed (e.g., picking up the coffee, tearing open the packet). The model could account for both everyday action sequences and, with noise used to mimic a lesion, action disorganization or utilization behaviors in neurological patients, providing support for the selection of routine actions based on competitive activation within a hierarchical network of action schemas.

Shallice and Burgess (1996) further refined Norman and Shallice's (1986) original model by proposing that the SAS is in fact a modular system that can be divided into dif-ferent subprocesses. In line with Norman and Shallice, and earlier work (Shallice & Bur-gess, 1991), the authors propose that the SAS is functionally analogous to the PFC. How-ever, this differs from previous accounts in that, here, the SAS is viewed as being responsible for a number of varied processes when confronted with a novel situation. Shallice and Burgess suggested that to deal with a novel situation, a new, temporary, schema must be constructed and implemented to take the place of the source schema triggered by environmental cues. The temporary schema is then responsible for the control of lower level schemas needed to achieve the task at hand. In extending the original role of the SAS, this model takes into account the wide range of deficits that patients with frontal damage exhibit.

However, Hart, Schwartz, and Mayer (1999) provided an alternative angle on the routine–complex distinction that is fundamental to Norman and Shallice's model and the influence of the SAS. They provided examples of patients with traumatic brain injury who made action errors not only on complex and novel tasks but also on familiar and basic tasks. This, they maintained, is because action errors originate from a nonspecific consequence of brain damage, which is not necessarily connected entirely to frontal lobe function. Rather, they saw the cause for impairment as an overall reduction in attention and capacity that correlated with the severity of the cerebral damage.

Whether or not supervisory control is restricted entirely to the frontal lobes, these ideas provide a useful framework for understanding issues of self-regulation and self-regulation failure. Norman and Shallice's model is important in highlighting the different means by which actions can be executed, sometimes with the need for higher level processing, yet often at a level outside conscious control, via the contention scheduling system. The model allows for variety in how we experience actions and, therefore, regulate our behavior, depending on the amount of supervisory or attentional input that occurs within the execution of a particular action sequence.

A CLOSER LOOK AT THE FRONTAL LOBES

Three main PFC circuits have been implicated in executive function: the ventromedial–orbitofrontal cortex (OFC), the dorsolateral prefrontal cortex (DLPFC), and the anterior cingulate cortex (ACC) (see Chow & Cummings, 1999; Kaufer & Lewis, 1999). It has been well documented for some time that these areas are responsible for the executive control of behavior (e.g., Goldstein, 1944; Jastrowitz, 1888; Luria, 1973). Unusual case studies dramatically highlight the importance of the frontal lobes in the execution of everyday behavior. In this chapter, we discuss issues of self-regulation in terms of brain regions within the PFC deemed to be responsible for executive control (DLPFC) and emotion regulation (VPFC and ACC), and also particular psychological concepts such as working memory, self-awareness, and choice.

Dorsolateral Prefrontal Cortex

The DLPFC is implicated in spatial and conceptual reasoning processes, and has been associated with planning, novelty processing, choice, working memory, and language function (see D'Esposito et al., 1995; Dronkers, Redfern, & Knight, 2000; Fuster, Brodner, & Kroger, 2000; Goldman-Rakic, 1987). These are traditionally viewed as "cold" executive functions (Grafman & Litvan, 1999). More anterior functions of the DLPFC include attentional switching, selective attention, and sustained attention (e.g., Chao & Knight, 1998; D'Esposito & Postle, 1999; McDonald, Cohen, Stenger, & Carter, 2000; Stuss & Benson, 1984). Moreover, evidence suggests that the DLPFC is active in behavioral self-regulation tasks, for example, the selection and initiation of actions (Spence & Frith,

1999). It has been suggested that the DLPFC is important for mental control, in that it provides top–down input for task-appropriate behaviors, whereas the ACC monitors when this control needs to be implemented (McDonald et al., 2000), an issue we address later in this chapter.

This idea is further supported by evidence that damage to DLPFC often results in apathy, as well as diminished attention, planning, temporal coding, judgment, metamemory, and insight (Dimitrov et al., 1999). Individuals with damage to this area may also exhibit motor programming deficits (e.g., apraxia or aphasia), and often show diminished self-care. If the damage to the DLPFC is bilateral and advanced, the patient may display perseveration (the uncontrollable repetition of a verbal or a motor response) and "primative reflexes" such as snouting, grasping, rooting, or sucking (e.g., Knight & Grabowecky, 2000). These behaviors are also commonly evident in patients with frontotemporal dementia, known as Pick's disease (e.g., Ringholz, 2000), and clearly illustrate a breakdown in self-regulation and an inability to direct behavior. Individuals with DLPFC damage often find it extremely difficult to initiate behavior, but perversely, once behavior has been initiated, they find it equally difficult to stop it.

Other characteristics linked to DLPFC damage include inertia, aggression, and increased use of spoken profanities and loss of drive (Blumer & Benson, 1975; Pandya & Barnes, 1987). Moreover, damage to areas that are richly interconnected with the frontal lobes, for example, the cingulate, the thalamus, or the striatum, may also result in decreased drive and motivation (Damasio & Van Hoesen, 1983; Habib & Poncet, 1988; Laplane, 1990). It seems that a crucial component of self-regulation—the ability to compare the achieved outcome to the intended goal—is either gone or severely disrupted in many patients with DLPFC damage.

Those with DLPFC damage may suffer from "dorsolateral syndrome," characterized by a sense of indifference and a generalized flatness of affect. One consequence of this disorder is a change in the perception of pain. Patients who still report the sensation of severe pain but are no longer *bothered* by it provide an extreme example of this disorder. Those given frontal lobotomies in the 1940s and 1950s were described in this way. Freeman and Watts (1950) attested that although the patients were capable of experiencing pain, they did not react to it in the usual manner. Indeed, they appeared to have lost the fear of pain altogether. Although this may perhaps appear to be a positive outcome of the lobotomy, it should be noted that these individuals also lost depth of any emotion or feeling (Freeman & Watts, 1950; Hurt & Ballantine, 1974). It has been suggested that this alteration in the experience of pain as most people know it is caused by a disruption of higher order regulation of lower order processes (see Goldberg, 2001), or, with reference to Norman and Shallice's model, disruption of the SAS.

In summary, although the DLPFC is most strongly associated with cold executive function processes, it is clear that successful self-regulation would not be possible without them. Processes such as emotional and behavioral self-regulation are, like many other processes, underpinned by working memory, choice, novelty detection, and language functions, and are therefore vital to the processes outlined in the rest of this chapter.

Ventromedial Prefrontal Cortex

The VPFC is strongly interconnected with the limbic structures involved in emotional processing (Pandya & Barnes, 1987). The VPFC appears to be particularly important for what is commonly viewed as the crux of self-regulation—how we control our behavioral and emotional output, and how we interact with others (i.e., our "personality"; Dolan,

1999). The OFC, a part of VPFC, is particularly implicated in emotional processing (Pandya & Barnes, 1987), reward and inhibition processes (Elliott, Dolan, & Frith, 2000; Rolls, 2000; Volkow & Fowler, 2000), real-life decision making (Damasio, 1994; Damasio, Tranel, & Damasio, 1991), self-awareness (Levine, Freedman, Dawson, Black, & Stuss, 1999; Stuss, 1991; Stuss & Levine, 2002), and strategic regulation (Levine et al., 1998). Damage to this area may therefore be associated with striking, and sometimes aggressive, behavioral changes (e.g., Rolls, Hornak, Wade, & McGrath, 1994) and a startling disregard or "myopia" with respect to the future (Bechara et al., 1994).

Perhaps the most famous case of damage to this part of the brain is that of Phineas Gage, who underwent an extreme personality change after an explosion pushed an iron tamping bar through his frontal lobes (Harlow, 1868). However, there are many other disturbing examples of how damage to the VPFC and the polar frontal cortex can bring about dramatic personality changes (see Stuss & Benson, 1986). Damage to the OFC usually results in personality changes such as indifference, impaired social judgment, impaired pragmatics and social responsiveness, poor self-regulation, and inability to associate situations with personal affective markers (Damasio, 1994; Nauta, 1973). Damage in this area has also been associated with deficits in creativity and reasoning (Eslinger & Damasio, 1985; Milner, 1982), and can therefore severely disrupt everyday behavior.

Damage to the OFC may result in "orbitofrontal syndrome." Unlike dorsolateral syndrome, which results in a flattening of emotional affect, orbitofrontal syndrome may be characterized by lack of impulse control and emotional disinhibition, distractibility, poor judgment and insight, lack of social skills, and inappropriate affect (Stuss & Alexander, 2000). Therefore, emotional expression and control is often severely impaired (e.g., Stone, Baron-Cohen, & Knight, 1998; Tranel & Damasio, 1994). Often, an individual with damage to this area cannot inhibit the urge for instant gratification and, as a result, may engage in behaviors such as shoplifting, or display sexually aggressive behavior. These individuals, who apparently feel no obligation to abide by rules, etiquette, or even laws, are often described by others as selfish, boastful, immature, or sexually explicit (e.g., Blumer & Benson, 1975; Grafman et al., 1996).

Strikingly, patients with damage to the OFC are often quite able to judge whether a behavior is moral or immoral; acceptable or unacceptable, but they are unable to act on this knowledge in order to adjust or guide their own behavior appropriately. Many years ago, Luria (1966) noted this discrepancy between rhetorical knowledge and the ability to use this knowledge as a guide to behavior in individuals with frontal lobe damage. Anderson, Bechara, Damasio, Tranel, and Damasio (1999) investigated the acquisition of complex social norms and moral rules. Interestingly, they found that whereas persons who acquired brain damage later in life were aware of what was inappropriate and what was not (even if they could not act on this information), it appeared that the acquisition of such rules was impaired in those who sustained early-onset (prior to age 16 months) damage to the PFC. They reported that such early damage could lead to a lack of morality akin to psychopathy.

For these reasons, damage to the OFC is often associated with criminal behavior, or "frontal lobe crime." A case study reported by Blair and Cipolotti (2000) describes an individual, J.S., with damage to the right frontal lobes, including the OFC, who became extremely aggressive and showed a "callous disregard" for others following his injury. In their study, J.S.'s performance on several scales was compared to that of another patient displaying dysexecutive syndrome and five prison inmates with developmental psychopathy. What made J.S.'s "acquired sociopathy" different, the authors argued (see also Damasio, Tranel, & Damasio, 1990), was in part due to J.S.'s inability to respond to others' negative (particularly angry) emotional reactions. He was unable to use these emotional cues, as most of us do, to regulate his everyday behavior. Blair and Cipolotti (2000) argued that the OFC is particularly important in generating these expectations (i.e., responding to social–emotional signals) to guide behavior or to suppress inappropriate behavior. Emotions and emotional signals are thought to play a large role in a wide variety of executive processes, including decision making.

In his somatic marker hypothesis, in which reasoning and emotion are integral to one another, Damasio (1994) proposed that the brain creates associations between body states and emotions. For example, an association may be formed between the object *tiger* and the emotion *fear* following repeated exposure to tigers. According to Damasio, this feedback from our bodies is then stored as an emotional marker, or a biasing device (although once the decision has been made, we do not necessarily link our choice to the reason that these associations were formed in the first place). Somatic markers, he argued, are crucial in the process of future decision making in terms of reducing options and selecting actions. In this way, somatic markers work like an emotional alarm system, producing our "gut feelings" that steer us toward, or pull us away from, certain courses of action. In this sense, emotions comprise an integral part in decision making and other aspects of self-regulation.

In defining more specific roles for the medial and lateral OFC, Elliott and colleagues (2000) suggested that the OFC in general is implicated in monitoring reward values, and the lateral OFC is particularly involved in suppressing a response that has been previously associated with a reward (e.g., gambling; see also Damasio, 1994; Rogers et al., 1999). Moreover, the lateral OFC is involved in responding to angry facial expressions, perhaps because they serve as a cue to inhibit inappropriate behavior in social contexts. The anterior area of the OFC, they pointed out, has strong connections with the DLPFC, a stucture that is also implicated in processes of inhibition. More posterior regions of the OFC (which have the strongest connections to the amygdala, the insula, and the temporal pole), the authors argued, are concerned with making risky decisions and choices, perhaps because these choices involve overriding the risk of punishment with the possibility of reward. In summary, the VPFC is strongly implicated in many overt aspects of behavioral self-regulation, particularly in terms of emotional processing and the expression or inhibition of inappropriate responses.

Anterior Cingulate Cortex

The ACC, located on the medial surface of the frontal lobes, is interconnected with cortical and subcortical brain regions, including limbic and motor systems. The ACC interacts with the PFC in monitoring and guiding behavior (Gehring & Knight, 2000) and is thought to be part of a circuit that regulates both cognitive and emotional processing (Bush, Luu, & Posner, 2000). As such, it is strongly implicated in issues of self-regulation (Awh & Gehring, 1999; Botvinick, Nystrom, Fissell, Carter, & Cohen, 1999; Carter et al., 2000; Posner & Rothbart, 1998), as well as more traditional executive functions, such as the division of attention or the selection of appropriate responses (e.g., as required in the Stroop task, see Bush et al., 1998). Thus, whereas the more posterior section of the ACC is responsible for processing cognitive information, the anterior section is implicated in affective and regulatory processing (see Bush et al., 2000, for review).

As Paus (2001) points out, the ACC is involved in behavioral control in three main ways. Dense projections from the ACC to the motor cortex and the spinal cord implicate the structure in aspects of motor control. The ACC is also strongly interconnected with the PFC, particulary the DLPFC, implicating the area in cognitive processing. Finally, links with the thalamus and brain-stem nuclei suggest that arousal and drive states are important for ACC function. Paus argues that it is the powerful functional overlap of these three domains, particulary the strong connections between motor and cognitive systems, that provides the ACC with capabilities to translate intentions into actions. As such, he argues that the ACC is essential for the willed control of action, not only to initiate actions but also to overcome competing, well-established tendencies (see Paus, 2001, for supporting patient data and a full review), processes heavily involved in self-regulation. Note that some of these functions that Paus outlined are conceptually similar to those assigned by Norman and Shallice (1986) to the SAS. In summary, Paus concluded that the ACC is implicated in the modulatory or regulatory influence of several brain systems operating at different levels and is important for the interactions between cognition, motor control, emotion, and motivation.

In line with the notion that the ACC is important in regulation, Badgaiyan and Posner (1998) suggested that the ACC is best viewed as an executive attentional system that is needed whenever any kind of supervisory input is required (see Rueda, Posner, & Rothbart, Chapter 14, this volume), for example, when a task requires the resolution of conflict, planning, and decision making, or when the task is novel, dangerous, or requires overcoming a habitual response—precisely the conditions outlined by Norman and Shallice (1986) in describing the role of the supervisory attentional system (see also Posner & DiGirolamo, 1998). Is the ACC our closest anatomical equivalent to the SAS? There has been some controversy surrounding the precise role of the ACC, as it appears to be involved in several different aspects of executive and regulatory function, although it is widely accepted that the ACC is somehow implicated in the processing of conflicting information.

Research has implicated the role of the ACC in decision making and monitoring (Bush et al., 2002; Elliott & Dolan, 1998; Liddle, Kiehl, & Smith, 2001), initiating the selection of an appropriate novel response from several alternatives (Raichle et al., 1994), performance monitoring (MacDonald, Cohen, Stenger, & Carter, 2000), action monitoring (Gehring & Knight, 2000; Paus, 2001), detecting or processing response conflict (Gehring & Fencsik, 2001); detecting and processing errors (Carter et al., 1998; Kiehl, Liddle, & Hopfinger, 2000; Menon, Adleman, White, Glover, & Reiss, 2001), error outcome and predictability (Paulus, Hozack, Frank, & Brown, 2002), internal cognitive control (Wyland, Kelley, Macrae, Gordon, & Heatherton, in press) and reward–punishment assessment (Knutson, Westdorp, Kaiser, & Hommer, 2000). Recent research reflects a shift toward the idea that the ACC not only assumes a role in conflict resolution but is also involved in the *degree* and *nature* of conflict. Moreover, it has been suggested that the conflict itself may be resolved in other parts of the brain, particularly the PFC (see Botvinick et al., 1999; Carter, Botvinick, & Cohen, 1999; Cohen, Botvinick, & Carter, 2000; MacDonald et al., 2000; Ruff, Woodward, Larens, & Liddle, 2001).

The ACC is further involved in attentional processes necessary for the successful self-regulation of behavior, including the division of attention between tasks (Corbetta, Miezin, Dobmeyer, Shulman, & Petersen, 1991), attention for action or target selection (e.g., Posner, Petersen, Fox, & Raichle, 1988), working memory (e.g., Petit, Courtney, Ungeleider, & Haxby, 1998), as well as various processes less directly relevant to self-regulatory processing, such as motor response selection (e.g., Badgaiyan & Posner, 1998) and pain perception (Devinsky, Morrell, & Vogt, 1995). Clearly, dysfunction within the ACC can disrupt self-regulatory processes at several different levels.

Interestingly, different areas of the ACC appear to show increased activity in response to different types of cognitive tasks (Badgaiyan & Posner, 1998) and may therefore be implicated in different aspects of regulation and executive processing. It has been proposed that two pathways for control within the ACC system respond to conflict detection (Cohen et al., 2000). One is responsible for general preparatory function, and the other has a more selective influence on task demands and is modulated by the PFC. Accordingly, ACC dysfunction has been associated with obsessive–compulsive disorder (OCD) and schizophrenia (e.g., Johannes et al., 2001; Tamminga et al., 1992), disorders that exemplify a severe lack of inhibitory control. In relation to OCD, it is argued that the process of comparing current status with the expectation of achieving a goal is disrupted. Recently, Shidara and Richmond (2002) reported that in monkeys, one third of the single neurons recorded in the ACC had responses that progressively changed strength with reward expectancy. This, they proposed, could account for the changes in activity recorded in the ACC for persons with OCD, or those experiencing drug abuse problems—conditions that are heavily characterized by disturbances in reward expectancy. Other problems associated with damage to the ACC include mutism, diminished self-awareness, motor neglect, depression, emotional instability, apathy, loss of regulation of autonomic function, and severe disruption to social behavior (e.g., Devinsky et al., 1995), all of which point to the vital function of ACC in self-regulation.

THE FRONTAL LOBES AS AN INTEGRATED STRUCTURE

Although the PFC circuit appears to be responsible for the executive control of different tasks, it is important to note that damage to the frontal lobes can be described as a bottleneck—the point of convergence of the effects of damage anywhere else in the brain (Goldberg, 2001). Precisely because of the rich interconnections the frontal lobes share with the rest of the brain, damage to the frontal lobes has widespread consequences. Similarly, damage to any other region of the brain can disrupt normal brain activity in the frontal lobes. Damage to the upper brain stem in a "mild" closed head injury can result in frontal lobe dysfunction, or "reticulofrontal disconnection syndrome" (see Goldberg, Bilder, Hughes, Antin, & Mattis, 1989). Moreover, it has been reported that in depression, blood flow to the frontal lobes is markedly disrupted (Nobler et al., 1994). Indeed, frontal lobe damage does not, for the most part, reflect direct damage to these areas but is often the consequence of damage to other parts of the brain. Furthermore, damage to adjacent parts of the cortex can produce similar cognitive deficits, suggesting that adjacent areas of the neocortex are capable of performing similar functions.

An approach based entirely on localizations is incomplete, because the brain is a complex and integrated system (Stuss, 1992). As such, the notion of a gradual, continuous trajectory within the cortices, as opposed to a fully modular system, has become more popular in recent years. This is reflected in the practice of describing frontal lobe processes as psychological constructs, as opposed to purely anatomically localized functions. Although it is clear that certain regions of the brain are more implicated in psychological processes than others, terms such as "executive control function" (Lezak, 1983; Milner & Petrides, 1984; Stuss & Benson, 1986; Stuss & Gow, 1992), "supervisory system" (Norman & Shallice, 1986; Shallice, 1988), and "dysexecutive syndrome" (Baddeley & Wilson, 1988) reflect the move toward investigating psychological processes rather than focusing on pure anatomical specificity. In the remainder of this chapter, we therefore focus on several critical psychological processes related to aspects of self-regulation. Many of these are more closely associated with the function of a particular brain area, such as the DLPFC, the VPFC, or the ACC, but all are underpinned by a complex interplay among not only different brain regions but also other social and cognitive factors.

KEY CONCEPTS IN SELF-REGULATION

Attention and Working Memory

Working memory is a key function of the PFC and is vital to maintain information in the mind for the execution and sequencing of mental operations (Baddeley, 1986; Fuster & Alexander, 1970). Moreover, because attention and working memory systems rely on the shifting of attentional resources, it has been proposed that increased working memory load results in a decrease in the ability to suppress inappropriate responses (Engle, Conway, Tuholski, & Shisler, 1995; Roberts, Hager, & Heron, 1994). Some debate exists about whether working memory and behavioral inhibition rely on the same or different areas within the PFC. It has been suggested that DLPFC is implicated in working memory processes, whereas VPFC is implicated in behavioral inhibition (see Fuster, 1997). However, other researchers have suggested that the distinction is not so clear, because the processes are heavily dependent on one another (e.g., May, Hasher, & Kane, 1999), or are subserved by the same areas in the brain (Miller & Cohen, 2001).

Recent evidence points toward partially segregated networks of brain areas responsible for different attentional functions. Specifically, Corbetta and Shulman (2002) argue for the existence of two attentional systems. One system is involved in top–down (goal-directed) selection and processes, and is dependent on parts of the intraparietal cortex and superior frontal cortex. The second system is largely lateralized to the right hemisphere (temporoparietal cortex and inferior frontal cortex), is dorsally driven, and works in detecting behaviorally relevant stimuli, especially those that are particularly salient or unexpected (as described later in this chapter).

In a study that highlights the role of working memory in the suppression of behavioral responses, Mitchell, Macrae, and Gilchrist (2001) demonstrated that failures of action control can result from frontoexecutive load. By measuring oculomotor movements, they found that antisaccadic errors increased in response to an *n*-back task (in which participants were presented with a series of items and were asked to determine whether each item matched the item that preceded *n*-back in the series). However, these effects were restricted to the inhibitory component of the task, suggesting that working memory and inhibitory processes work in union to regulate prepotent behavioral responses, arguably one of the key ways in which we regulate our behavior. Attention, then, is a key process in the regulation of cognition and behavior, as seen in the following sections regarding inhibition, novelty, and decision making.

Inhibition

Arguably one of the most important functions of the attentional system, and a key component of self-regulation, is to select and inhibit appropriate subsets of information, and many studies have addressed the role of attention in the facilitation and inhibition of cognitive processes (e.g., Ghatan, Hsieh, Peterson, Stone-Elander, Ingvar, 1998). Disruption in inhibitory processes is apparent in behaviors such as collectionism, in which individuals pathologically collect random objects. Here, individuals' inability to inhibit environmentally driven behavior results in a notable lack of autonomy (see Lhermitte et al.,

1986). Likewise, those suffering from disorders such as OCD and Tourette syndrome display severe disruption of impulse control: They are unable to inhibit successfully their thoughts, speech, or movements.

It is well documented that the process of thought suppression can be problematic to us all (Wegner, 1992; Wegner & Schneider, 1989). For example, we may have trouble suppressing thoughts of food when on a diet. However, some individuals experience severe and ongoing disruption in the ability to inhibit responses appropriately. Those with lateral PFC lesions often exhibit difficulty in suppressing previously learned material (e.g., Shimamura, Jurica, Mangels, Gershberg, & Knight, 1995). As mentioned earlier, utilization disorder illustrates the inability to suppress behavior that is strongly associated with the previous presentation of a given object (see Lhermitte, 1983). Here, the individual is unable to inhibit the behavior primed by the object (e.g., hammering with a hammer) even if that behavior is not appropriate in a given context. This behavior, Stuss, Floden, Alexander, Levine, and Katz (2001) argued, can be seen as indicative of a more general dysexecutive deficit that can affect multiple cognitive tasks, such as the Stroop and antisaccadic tasks, in which reflexive (prepotent) saccades toward a peripheral stimulus are suppressed and replaced with an intentional saccade in the opposite direction (see also Guitton, Buchtel, & Douglas, 1985).

Imaging work has started to identify the neural mechanisms underlying internal inhibition or cognitive control of thoughts and behavior. In one recent study, subjects were required to suppress a particular thought, regulate all thoughts, or to think freely about any thought. The results showed that the suppression of a particular thought led to greater activation in the ACC, when contrasted with the free-thought condition. The more generalized task involving the suppression of all thoughts was associated with greater activation in the insula bilaterally and the right inferior parietal cortex when compared with the free-thought condition (Wyland et al., in press). In another study, Mitchell, Heatherton, Kelley, Wyland, and Macrae (2003) found that ACC activity could predict the suppression of intrusive thoughts. Using a paradigm that investigated the neural mechanisms underlying failures to suppress unwanted thoughts, the authors were able to identify neural activity that differentiated between subjects' future task success (i.e., suppression) and failure (i.e., intrusion of unwanted thoughts). This study was important in demonstrating the functional significance of (rather than the correlational relationship between) the ACC and suppression.

Novelty

One of the major functions of the frontal lobes is to deal with new or surprising situations effectively; it is vital that we adjust our responses appropriately to the changes we encounter in our environment, and regulate our behavior accordingly (e.g., Daffner et al., 1998). Norman and Shallice (1986) argued that the more novel a task, the more input from the SAS (frontal lobes) is needed to carry out the task. This is consistent with the finding that when a task is new, blood flow is highest in the frontal lobes, and the presentation of novel information is particularly associated with right-hemisphere activation.

Interestingly, as the task increases in familiarity, blood flow is reduced in the frontal lobes, suggesting that input is no longer required (Raichle et al., 1994; Van Horn et al., 1998). Moreover, it has been demonstrated that novelty detection systems can operate even when subjects are unaware that they are viewing a novel stimulus, for example, following a subtle shift in the nature of a familiar sequence (see Berns, Cohen, & Mintun, 1997). Such findings highlight the significance of novelty detection in everyday information processing. Unsurprisingly, novel or surprising stimuli are usually better remembered in normal subjects (the Von Restorff effect; Von Restorff, 1933). However, decreased attention to novel events is common following frontal lobe injury (Daffner, Mesulam, Holcomb, et al., 2000; Knight, 1997; Luria, 1973).

Event-related potentials (ERPs), as measured by electroencephalograph (EEG), are ideally suited to the study of novelty processing. The good, temporal resolution allows the investigation of changes in brain function over time and with respect to context. In their review of novelty processing, Friedman, Cycowicz, and Gaeta (2001) suggested that the processing of novel events is best understood in terms of *detection* and *evaluation*. The orienting response (an involuntary shift in attention to new, unexpected, or unpredictable stimuli) can be associated with particular patterns of neural activity. It has been suggested that the detection of novel events is associated with mismatch negativity (MMN), which is thought to reflect an automatic response to stimulus deviance. However, the evaluation of those events, important for subsequent action, is associated with the later P3a response (a frontally oriented positive ERP component), which is thought to reflect the engagement of the frontal lobes in response to deviant events (e.g., Schröger, Giard, & Wolff, 2000; see Friedman et al., 2001, for a full review).

If the P3a response is implicated in novelty evaluation, this could go some way toward explaining why patients with frontal lobe damage often show difficulty solving novel problems (e.g., Duncan & Owen, 2000; Godefroy & Rousseaux, 1997) and do not show the typical memorial enhancement for novel events or stimuli. EEG studies have shown that unexpected novel stimuli do not elicit the usual electrophysiological response to the presentation of novel stimuli in persons with frontal lobe damage (e.g., Knight, 1984; Knight & Scabini, 1998). Using ERP recordings, Daffner and colleagues (2000) showed that persons with frontal lobe damage exhibit a reduced amplitude in the novelty P3a response and a reduction in the time they spend viewing novel stimuli compared to matched controls. They suggest that frontal lobe damage disrupts the novelty P3a response, therefore resulting in a reduction in attention paid to novel stimuli; perhaps the signal indicating that a novel event requires extra attention is disrupted in persons with frontal lobe damage.

In a more recent study, Daffner and colleagues (2003) investigated the role of both the PFC and the posterior parietal lobe in novelty processing. They compared responses to novel target stimuli among patients with focal lesions either to the PFC or to the posterior parietal lobe, and assessed the relative contributions of both regions to novelty processing. Using a task in which participants actively directed attention to novel events, Daffner and colleagues found that damage to the PFC resulted in greater disruption in attention to novel stimuli than to other targets. This was reflected in a marked reduction in the novelty P3 response, and a reduction in the amount of time spent viewing the novel stimuli. Those with damage to the parietal lobes, on the other hand, showed a marked reduction in both novelty and target P3 amplitude. These individuals showed a greater disruption in the processing of target than of novel stimuli.

Daffner and colleagues (2003) concluded that the PFC is not limited to *involuntary* shifts in attention to (or the detection of) novel events, as previously suggested (e.g., Knight & Scabini, 1998), with the parietal lobes capable of performing the same kind of function (e.g., Corbetta & Shulman, 2002). Rather, Daffner and colleagues proposed a cerebral novelty network, whereby the PFC determines the allocation of attentional resources to novel events, and the posterior parietal lobe is implicated in the dynamic process of updating an internal model of the environment to incorporate the novel event. They suggested that such a view is consistent with ideas of supervisory attentional control

(Shallice, 1988): "One of the most important functions of this system is the allocation and coordination of attentional processes, which includes determining the extent to which resources are devoted to selected stimuli, inhibiting further allocation of resources to irrelevant stimuli, and modulating the mental effort devoted to processing stimuli" (Daffner et al., 2003, p. 306).

Issues surrounding novelty processing have important implications for self-regulation and social interaction. We cannot deal with new or surprising situations and regulate our behavior accordingly, if we are not even aware that events are new or surprising. Self-regulation may be severely disrupted when allocation of attention to novel events is either severely diminished or exaggerated, for example, in those with posttraumatic stress disorder (e.g., Kimble, Kaloupek, Kaufman & Deldin, 2000). The processes outlined here allow us the extra time or attentional allocation needed to deal with new or unexpected events, a prerequisite for interaction within a complex social world, and the regulation of appropriate responses.

Decision Making and Choice

We have addressed the need to deal with new or surprising events to regulate our everyday behavior effectively. It is also essential that we are able to reduce ambiguity and to make meaningful decisions to smooth the path for our social relationships and daily interactions. As mentioned earlier in the chapter, persons with damage to the VPFC often experience problems with decision making and show impairments in risk-taking or gambling tasks. Individuals with early dementia also seem to lose their ability to make everyday decisions and choices.

A recent study by Tranel, Bechara, and Denburg (2002) suggests that right ventromedial PFC is particulary important in terms of decision making, as well as other aspects of social conduct and emotional processing. In their sample of patients with lesions to either the left or the right medial PFC, the authors reported that individuals with lesions on the right showed extreme disturbances in social behavior, deficits in decision making, and difficulty holding a job. By comparison, those with lesions to the left did not show such marked deficits, were generally employed, and displayed more normal social and emotional processing.

As outlined earlier, individuals with damage to the VPFC are often unable to make decisions; although they know what they should do, they find themselves incapable of actually doing it (e.g., Damasio, 1996; Eslinger & Damasio, 1985). As Bechara (2003) pointed out, this is also a common characteristic of addiction. Studies have shown that substance-dependent individuals also show dysfunction in the VPFC, and Bechara maintained that our understanding of the neural mechanisms of decision making is crucial to the understanding of disorders of self-regulation such as addiction, pathological gambling, and other compulsive or "uncontrolled" behaviors.

So what neural circuits are involved in making decisions or choosing one course of action over another? Moreover, are different types of choices subserved by different regions within the PFC? Some researchers using healthy subjects have attempted to address this question. Using positron emission tomography (PET), Frith, Friston, Liddle, and Frackowiak (1991) investigated motor responses associated with both routine and willed acts. Using both auditory (spoken words) and somatosensory (touch) cues as instructions, they required participants to make a series of "routine" or "willed" responses in one of two modalities (either by speaking a word or by lifting a finger). The routine responses were fully specified by the stimulus (e.g., repeat word, or lift first finger). On the other hand, the willed acts required an open-ended response; that is, the participants had to make a choice (generate a word beginning with the letter F, or move fingers at will in a random sequence). Frith and colleagues found that the willed acts were associated with increased activity in the DLPFC (Brodmann area 46) and the ACC. They concluded that the DLPFC is involved in internal response generation, and the ACC is implicated in response selection and attention.

Although extremely important in highlighting the distinction between willed and directed acts, one possible limitation of this study is that the DLPFC activation associated with the open-ended responses may be equally attributable to the instruction given to be "random" in the willed conditions. A potential difficulty with such an instruction is that working memory is needed to produce "random" motor or verbal responses (e.g., the generation of novel words beginning with a certain letter), because the subject may try and hold his or her previous responses in mind, in order not to produce the same response over and over again (see Spence & Frith, 1999). As mentioned previously, working memory has also been shown to be associated with activity in the DLPFC; therefore, it is hard to determine whether DLPFC activation can be attributed to the response selection or to the working memory component of the task.

In a recent attempt to study choice within a paradigm that controlled for working memory demands, Turk and colleagues (2003) employed a task that varied both the amount of choice available to the subject (choosing a stimulus from an array of 4, when either 1, 2, or 3 of the stimuli were highlighted as being available) and how meaningful the stimuli were (faces vs. faces that were potential dates). The results showed that regions of the dorsal premotor cortex, the posterior parietal cortex bilaterally, and the medial surface of the superior frontal gyrus were associated with response selection, irrespective of the type of choice to be made. Importantly, there was no choice-related increase in activation in the DLPFC. However, more anterior portions of the medial surface of the superior frontal gyrus, inferior frontal cortex, and ACC were additionally recruited when the choice to be made was socially meaningful (i.e., when it involved choosing a date). The results suggest that these areas, rather than DLPFC, may subserve certain types of willed action.

It is clear that studies such as these do not attempt to solve philosophical issues of free will, volition, and agency, but rather help to elucidate the neural systems involved in aspects of decision making, choice, and the experience of self as an agent making these choices. Many more issues to be addressed involve the nature and consequence of the decisions or choices to be made, the context in which they are made, and temporal aspects of how subjective experience corresponds with neural activity.

SUMMARY

In summary, this review of work concerning the self-regulation of behavior is by no means comprehensive; indeed, many topics fall outside the scope of this chapter, such as the development of the PFC in children (Bunge, Dudokovic, Thomason, Vaidya, & Gabrieli, 2002), and the development of the PFC and its associated executive functions over one's lifetime (e.g., Nielson, Langenecker, & Garavan, 2002). Moreover, issues of self-regulation and inhibition are also clearly relevant to a wide range of clinical disorders, such as OCD, Tourette syndrome, autism, schizophrenia, and attention deficit disorder (e.g., Bush et al., 1999; Frith, 1992; Sheppard, Bradshaw, Purcell, & Pantelis, 1999; Stuss et al., 1992). Rather, the purpose of this chapter is to highlight some key neural mechanisms involved in self-regulation and executive control. It is clear that the process of self-regulation comprises a complex interplay between anatomical, neurochemical, cognitive, and social factors. An exploration of how brain function and anatomy, combined with our existing cognitive and social theory, has become increasingly important to our understanding of "self" and how we attempt to regulate our thoughts and behavior. Accordingly, we have gained a more comprehensive insight into the failures of mental control that are, to a greater or lesser degree, common to us all.

ACKNOWLEDGMENTS

Preparation of this chapter was supported in part by Grant No. BCS 0072861 from the National Science Foundation to Todd F. Heatherton. We thank Arie van der Lugt for his helpful comments.

REFERENCES

Anderson, S. W., Bechera, A., Damasio, H., Tranel, D., & Damasio, A. R. (1999). Impairments in social and moral behavior related to early damage in human prefrontal cortex. *Nature Neuroscience, 2*(11), 1032–1037.

Awh, E., & Gehring, W. (1999). The anterior cingulate cortex lends a hand in response selection. *Nature Neuroscience, 2,* 853–854.

Baddeley, A. D. (1986). *Working memory.* Oxford, UK: Clarendon Press.

Baddeley, A. (1996). Exploring the central executive. *Quarterly Journal of Experimental Psychology, 49,* 5–28.

Baddeley, A., & Wilson, B. (1988). Frontal amnesia and the dysexecutive syndrome. *Brain and Cognition, 7,* 212–230.

Badgaiyan, R., & Posner, M. (1998). Mapping the cingulate cortex in response selection and monitering. *Neuroimage, 7,* 255–260.

Bechara, A. (2003). Risky business: Emotion, decision-making, and addiction. *Journal of Gambling Studies, 19,* 23–51.

Bechara, A., Damasio, A. R., Damasio, H., & Anderson, S. W. (1994). Insensitivity to future consequences following damage to human prefrontal cortex. *Cognition, 50,* 7–15.

Berns, G. S., Cohen, J. D., & Mintun, M. A. (1997). Brain regions responsive to novelty in the absence of awareness. *Science, 276,* 1272–1275.

Blair, R., & Cipolotti, L. (2000). Impaired social response reversal: A case of acquired sociopathy. *Brain, 123,* 1122–1141.

Blumer, D., & Benson, D. (1975). Personality changes with frontal and temporal lesions. In D. F. Benson & F. Blumer (Eds.), *Psychiatric aspects of neurologic disease.* New York: Grune & Stratton.

Botvinick, M., Nystrom, L., Fissell, K., Carter, C., & Cohen, J. (1999). Conflict monitoring versus selection for action in anterior cingulate cortex. *Nature, 402,* 179–181.

Brazzelli, B., Columbo, N., Della Sala, S., & Spinner, H. (1994). Spared and impaired cognitive abilities after bilateral frontal lode damage. *Cortex, 30,* 27–51.

Bunge, S. A., Dudukovic, N. M., Thomason, M. E., Vaidya, C. J., & Gabrieli, J. D. (2002). Immature frontal lobe contributions to cognitive control in children: Evidence from fMRI. *Neuron, 33,* 301–311.

Bush, G., Frazier, J. A., Rauch, S. L., Seidman, L. J., Whalen, P. J., Jenike, M. A., Rosen, B. R., & Biederman, J. (1999). Anterior cingulate cortex dysfunction in attention-deficit/hyperactivity disorder revealed by fMRI and the counting stroop. *Biological Psychiatry, 45,* 1542–1552.

Bush, G., Luu, P., & Posner, M. (2000). Cognitive and emotional influences in anterior cingulate cortex. *Trends in Cognitive Science, 4,* 215–222.

Bush, G., Vogt, B. A., Holmes, J., Dale, A. M., Greve, D., Jenike, J., & Rosen, B. R. (2002). Dorsal anterior cingulate cortex: A role in reward-based decision making. *Proceedings of the National Academy of Sciences of the United States of America*, 99, 507–512.

Bush, G., Whalen, P. J., Rosen, B. R., Jenike, M. A., McInerney, S. C., & Rauch, S. L. (1998). The counting stroop: An interference task specialized for functional neuroimaging—validation studywith functional MRI. *Human Brain Mapping*, 6, 270–282.

Carter, C. S., Botvinick, M. M., & Cohen, J. D. (1999). The contribution of the anterior cingulate cortex to executive processes in cognition. *Reviews in the Neurosciences*, 10(1), 49–57.

Carter, C. S., Braver, T. S., Barch, D. M., Botvinick, M. M., Noll, D., Cohen, J. D. (1998). Anterior cingulate Cortex, error detection and the on-line monitoring of performance. *Science*, 280, 747–749.

Carter, C. S., MacDonald, A. M., III, Botvinick, M., Ross, L. L., Stenger, V. A., Noll, D., & Cohen, J. D. (2000). Parsing executive processes: Strategic versus evaluative functions of the anterior cingulate cortex. *Proceedings of the National Academy of Sciences*, 97(4), 1944–1948.

Chao, L. L., & Knight, R. T. (1998). Contribution of human prefrontal cortex to delay performance. *Journal of Cognitive Neuroscience*, 10, 167–177.

Chow, T. W., & Cummings, J. L. (1999). Frontal–subcortical circuits. In B. L. Miller & J. L. Cummings (Eds.), *The human frontal lobes: Functions and disorders* (pp. 3–26). New York: Guilford Press.

Cohen, J., Botvinick, M., & Carter, C. (2000). Anterior cingulate and prefrontal cortex: Who's in control? *Nature Neuroscience*, 3, 421–423.

Cooper, R., & Shallice, T. (2000). Contention scheduling and the control of routine activities. *Cognitive Neurosychology*, 17, 297–338.

Corbetta, M., Miezin, F. M., Dobmeyer, S., Shulman, G. L., & Petersen, S. E. (1991). Selective and divided attention during visual discriminations of shape, color, and speed: Functional anatomy by positron emission tomography. *Journal of Neuroscience*, 11(8), 2383–2402.

Corbetta, M., & Shulman, G. (2002). Control of goal-directed and stimulus-driven attention in the brain. *Neuroscience*, 3, 201–215.

Daffner, K., Mesulam, M., Holcomb, P., Calvo, V., Diler, A., Chaabrerie, A., Kikinis, R., Jolesz, F., Rentz, D., & Scinto, L. (2000). Disruption of attention to novel events after frontal lobe injury in humans. *Neurology, Neurosurgery, and Psychiatry*, 68, 18–24.

Daffner, K., Mesulam, M., Scinto, L., Acar, D., Calvo, V., Faust, R., Chabrerie, A., Kennedy, B., & Holcomb, P. (2000). The central role of prefrontal cortex in directing attention to novel events. *Brain*, 123, 927–939.

Daffner, K. R., Mesulam M. M., Scinto, L. F. M., Cohen, L.G., Kennedy, B. P., West, W. C., & Holcomb, P. J. (1998). Regulation of attention to novel stimuli by frontal lobes—an event-related potential study. *Neuroreport*, 9, 787–791.

Daffner, K. R., Scinto, L. F. M., Weitzman, A. M., Faust, R., Rentz, D. M., Budson, A. E., & Holcomb, P. J. (2003). Frontal and parietal components of a cerebral network mediating voluntary attention to novel events. *Journal of Cognitive Neuroscience*, 15, 294–313.

Damasio, A. R. (1994). *Descartes' error: Emotion, reason and the human brain.* New York: Putnam.

Damasio, A. R. (1996). The somatic marker hypothesis and the possible functions of the prefrontal cortex. *Philosophical Transactions of the Royal Society of London: Series B. Biological*, 351(1346), 1413–1420.

Damasio, A. R., Tranel, D., & Damasio, H. (1990). Individuals with sociopathic behavior caused by frontal damage fail to respond automatically to social stimuli. *Behavioral Brain Research*, 41, 81–94.

Damasio, A. R., Tranel, D., & Damasio, H. (1991). Somatic markers and the guidance of behavior: theory and preliminary testing. In H. S. Levin, H. M. Eisenberg, & A. L. Benton (Eds.), *Frontal lobe function and dysfunction* (pp. 217–229). New York: Oxford Universtiy Press.

Damasio, A. R., & Van Hoesen, G. W. (1983). Emotional disturbances associated with focal lesions of the limbic frontal lobe. In K. M. Heilman & P. Satz (Eds.), *Neuropsychology of human emotion* (pp. 85–110). New York: Guilford Press.

Della Sala, S., Marchetti, C., & Spinnler, H. (1991). Right-sided anarchic (alien) hand: A longitudinal study. *Neuropsychologia, 29*(11), 1113–1127.

D'Esposito, M., Detre, J. A., Alsop, D. C., Shin, R. K., Atlas, S., & Grossman, M. (1995). The neural basis of the central executive system of working memory. *Nature, 378,* 279–281.

D'Esposito, M., & Postle, B. R. (1999). The dependence of span and delayed-response performance on prefrontal cortex. *Neuropsychologia, 37,* 1303–1315.

Devinsky, O., Morrell, M. J., & Vogt, B. A. (1995). Contributions of anterior cingulate cortex to behaviour. *Brain, 118,* 279–306.

Dimitrov, M., Granetz, J., Peterson, M., Hollnagel, C., Alexander, G., & Grafman, J. (1999). Associative learning impairments in patients with frontal lobe damage. *Brain and Cognition, 41,* 213–230.

Dolan, R. J. (1999). On the neurology of morals. *Nature Neuroscience, 2*(11), 927–929.

Dronkers, N. F., Redfern, B. B., & Knight, R. T. (2000). The neural architecture of language disorders. In M. Gazzaniga (Ed.), *The new cognitive neurosciences* (pp. 949–958). Cambridge, MA: MIT Press.

Duncan, J., & Owen, A. M. (2000). Common regions of the human frontal lobe recruited by diverse cognitive demands. *Trends in Neuroscience, 10,* 475–483.

Elliott, R., & Dolan, R. J. (1998). Neural response during preference and memory judgments for subliminally presented stimuli: A functional neuroimaging study. *Journal of Neuroscience, 18,* 4697–4704.

Elliott, R., Dolan, R. J., & Frith, C. D. (2000). Dissociable functions in the medial and lateral orbitofrontal cortex: Evidence from human neuroimaging studies. *Cerebral Cortex, 10,* 308–317.

Engle, R. W., Conway, A. R. A., Tuholski, S. W., & Shisler, R. J. (1995). A resource account of inhibition. *Psychological Science, 6*(2), 122–125.

Eslinger, P. J. (2002). The anatomic basis of utilisation behaviour: A shift from frontal-parietal to intra-frontal mechanisms. *Cortex, 38,* 273–276.

Eslinger, P. J., & Damasio, A. R. (1985). Severe disturbance of higher cognition after bilateral frontal lobe ablation: Patient EVR. *Neurology, 35,* 1731–1741.

Freeman, W., & Watts, W. (1950). *Psychosurgery* (2nd ed.). Springfield, MA: Thanas.

Friedman, D., Cycowicz, Y. M., & Gaeta, H. (2001). The novelty P3: An event-related brain potential (ERP) sign of the brain's evaluation of novelty. *Neuroscience and Biobehavioral Reviews, 25,* 355–373.

Frith, C. D. (1992). *The cognitive neuropsychology of schizophrenia.* Hove, UK: Erlbaum.

Frith, C., Friston, K., Liddle, P., & Frackowiak, R. (1991). Willed action and the prefrontal cortex in man: A study with PET. *Proceedings of the Royal Society London, 244,* 241–246.

Fuster, J. M. (1997). *The prefrontal cortex: Anatomy, physiology, and neurophysiology of the frontal lobe.* Philadelphia: Lippincott-Raven.

Fuster, J. M., & Alexander, G. E. (1970). Delayed response deficit by cryogenic depression of frontal cortex. *Brain Research, 20,* 85–90.

Fuster, J. M., Brodner, M., & Kroger, J. K. (2000). Cross-modal and cross-temporal associations in neurons of frontal cortex. *Nature, 405,* 347–351.

Gehring, W., & Knight, R. (2000). Prefrontal cingulate interactions in action monitoring. *Nature Neuroscience, 3,* 516–520.

Gehring, W. J., & Fencsik, D. E. (2001). Functions of the medial frontal cortex in the processing of conflict and errors. *Journal of Neuroscience, 21,* 9430–9437.

Ghatan, P., Hsieh, J., Peterson, K., Stone-Elander, S., & Ingvar, M. (1998). Coexistence of attention based facilitation and inhibition in the human cortex. *NeuroImage, 7,* 23–29.

Godefroy, O., & Rousseaux, M. (1997). Novel decision making in patients with prefrontal or posterior brain damage. *Neurology, 49,* 695–701.

Goldberg, E. (2001). *The executive brain: frontal lobes and the civilized mind.* New York: Oxford University Press.

Goldberg, E., Bilder, R., Hughes, J. E., Antin, S. P., & Mattis, S. (1989). A reticulo-frontal disconnection syndrome. *Cortex, 25,* 687–695.

Goldman-Rakic, P. S. (1987). Circuitry of the prefrontal cortex and the regulation of behavior by representational knowledge. In F. Plum & V. Mountcastle (Eds.), *Handbook of physiology* (pp. 373–417). Bethesda, MD: American Physiological Society.

Goldstein, K. (1944). Mental changes due to frontal lobe damage. *Journal of Psychology, 17,* 187–208.

Grafman, J., & Litvan, I. (1999). Importance of deficits in executive functions. *Lancet (England), 354,* 1921–1923.

Grafman, J., Schwab, K., Warden, D., Pridgen, A., Brown, H. R., & Salazar, A. M. (1996). Frontal lobe injuries, violence, and aggression: A report of the Vietnam Head Injury Study. *Neurology, 46*(5), 1231–8.

Guitton, D., Buchtel, H. A., & Douglas, R. M. (1985). Frontal lobe lesions in man cause difficulties in suppressing reflexive glances and in generating goal-directed saccades. *Experimental Brain Research, 58,* 455–472.

Habib, M., & Poncet, M. (1988). Loss of vitality, of interest and of affect (athymhormia syndrome) in lacunar lesions of the corpus striatum. *Revue Neurologique (Paris), 144*(10), 571–577.

Harlow, J. M. (1868). Recovery from the passage of an iron bar through the head. *Publications of the Massachusetts Medical Society, 2*(3), 327–246.

Hart, T., Schwartz, M. F., & Mayer, N. (1999). Executive function: Some current theories and their applications. In N. R. Varney & R. J. Roberts (Eds.), *The evaluation and treatment of mild traumatic brain injury* (pp. 133–148). Mahwah, NJ: Erlbaum.

Hurt, R. W., & Ballantine, H. T., Jr. (1974). Stereotactic anterior cingulate lesions for persistent pain: A report on 60 cases. *Clinical Neurosurgery, 21,* 334–351.

Jastrowitz, M. (1888). Beitrage sur Localisation im Grosshirn und uber deren praktische Verwerthung [Contributions to the localization in the cortex and their applications]. *Deutsche Medidinische Wochenschrift, 14,* 81–83, 108–112, 125–128, 151–153, 172–175, 188–192, 209–211.

Johannes, S., Wieringa, B. M., Nager, D. R., Dengler, R., Emrich, H. M., Münte, T. F., & Dietrich, D. E. (2001). Discrepant target detection and action monitoring in obsessive-compulsive disorder. *Psychiatry Research—Neuroimaging, 108,* 101–110.

Kaufer, D. I., & Lewis, D. A. (1999). Frontal lobe anatomy and cortical connectivity. In B. L. Miller & J. L. Cummings (Eds.), *The human frontal lobes: functions and disorders* (pp. 27–44). New York: Guilford Press.

Kiehl, K. A., Liddle, P. F., & Hopfinger, J. B. (2000). Error processing and the anterior cingulate: An event-related fMRI study. *Psychophysiology, 37*(2), 216–223.

Kimble, M., Kaloupek, D., Kaufman, M., & Deldin, P. (2000). Stimulus novelty differentially affects attentional allocation in PTSD. *Biological Psychiatry, 47,* 880–890.

Knight, R. T. (1984). Decreased response to novel stimuli after prefrontal lesions in man. *Electroencephalography and Clinical Neurophysiology, 59,* 9–20.

Knight, R. T. (1997). Distributed cortical network for visual attention. *Journal of Cognitive Neuroscience, 9,* 75–91.

Knight, R. T., & Grabowecky, M. (2000). Prefrontal cortex, time and consciousness. In M. Gazzaniga (Ed.), *The new cognitive neurosciences* (pp. 1319–1339). Canbridge, MA: MIT Press.

Knight, R. T., & Scabini, D. (1998). Anatomic bases of event-related potentials and their relationship to novelty detection in humans. *Journal of Clinical Neurophysiology, 15*(1), 3–13.

Knutson, B., Westdorp, A., Kaiser, E., & Hommer, D. (2000). FMRI visualisation of brain activity during a monetary incentive delay task. *Neuroimage, 12,* 20–27.

Laplane, D. (1990). Loss of psychic self-activation. *Revista del Neurologia, 146,* 397–404.

Lezak, M. (1983). *Neuropsychological assessment*. New York: Oxford University Press.

Levine, B., Freedman, M., Dawson, D., Black, S., & Stuss, D. (1999). Ventral frontal contribution to self-regulation: Convergence of episodic memory and inhibition. *Neurocase, 5*, 263–275.

Levine, B., Stuss., D. T., Milberg, W. P., Alexander, M. P., Schwartz, M., & Macdonald, R. (1998). The effects of focal and diffuse brain damage on strategy application: Evidence from focal lesions, traumatic brain injury, and normal aging. *Journal of the International Neuropsychological Society, 4*, 247–264.

Lhermitte, F. (1983). Utilization behaviour and its relation to lesions of the frontal lobes. *Brain, 106*, 237–256.

Lhermitte, F., Pillon, B., & Serdaru, M. (1986). Human anatomy and the frontal lobes. Part I: Imitation and utilization behavior: A neuropsychological study of 75 patients. *Annals of Neurology, 19*, 326–334.

Liddle, P. F., Kiehl, K. A., & Smith, A. M. (2001). Event-related fMRI study of response inhibition. *Human Brain Mapping, 12*(2), 100–109.

Luria, A. R. (1966). *Higher cortical functions in man*. New York: Basic Books.

Luria, A. R. (1973). *The working brain: An introduction to neuropsychology*. New York: Basic Books.

MacDonald, A. W., Cohen, J. D., Stenger, V. A., & Carter, C. S. (2000). Dissociating the role of the dorsolateral prefrontal cortex and anterior cingulate cortex in cognitive control. *Science, 288*, 1835–1838.

McDonald, A.W., Cohen, J. D., Stenger, V. A., & Carter, C. S. (2000). Dissociating the role of the dorsolateral prefrontal and anterior cingulate cortex in cognitive control. *Science, 288*, 1835–1838.

May, C. P., Hasher, L., & Kane, M. J. (1999). The role of interference in memory span. *Memory and Cognition, 27*, 759–767.

Menon, V., Adleman, N. E., White, C. D., Glover, G. H., & Reiss, A. L. (2001). Error-related brain activation during a Go/No Go response inhibition task. *Human Brain Mapping, 12*(3), 131–143.

Miller, E. K., & Cohen, J. D. (2001). An integrative theory of prefrontal function. *Annual Review of Neuroscience, 24*, 167–202.

Milner, B. (1982). Some cognitive effects of frontal-lobe lesions in man. *Philosophical Transactions of the Royal Society of London B Biological Science, 298*(1089), 211–26

Milner, B., & Petrides, M. (1984). Behavioural effects of frontal-lobe lesions in man. *Trends in Neurosciences, 7*, 403–407.

Mitchell, J. P., Heatherton, T. F., Kelley, W. M., Wyland, C. L., & Macrae, C. N. (2003). *Controlling the contents of consciousness: The neural substrates of thought suppression*. Manuscript under review.

Mitchell, J., Macrae, C., & Gilchrist, I. (2001). Working memory and the suppression of reflexive saccades. *Journal of Cognitive Neuroscience, 14*, 1–9.

Nauta, W. J. H. (1973). *Connections of the frontal lobe with the limbic system*. In L. V. Laitinen & K. E. Livingstone (Eds.), *Surgical approaches to psychiatry* (pp. 303–14). Baltimore: University Park Press.

Nielson, K. A., Langenecker, S. A., & Garavan, H. (2002). Differences in the functional neuroanatomy of inhibitory control across the adult lifespan. *Psychology and Aging, 17*(1), 56–71.

Nobler, M. S., Sackeim, H. A., Prohovnik, I., Moeller, J. R., Mukherjee, S., Schnur, D. B., Prudic, J., & Devanand, D. P. (1994). Regional cerebral blood flow in mood disorders: III. Treatment and clinical response. *Archives of General Psychiatry, 51*, 884–897.

Norman, D. A. (1981). Categorization of action slips. *Psychological Review, 88*, 1–15.

Norman, D. A., & Shallice, T. (1986). Attention to action: Willed and automatic control of behavior. In R. J. Davidson, G. E. Schwartz, & D. Shapiro (Eds.), *Consciousness and self-regulation: Advances in research and theory* (Vol. 4, pp. 1–18). New York: Plenum Press.

Pandya, D. N., & Barnes, C. L. (1987). Architecture and connections of the frontal lobe. In E. Perecman (Ed.), *The frontal lobes revisited* (pp. 41–72). New York: Erlbaum.

Paulus, M. P., Hozack, N., Frank, L., & Brown, G. G. (2002). Error rate and outcome predictability affect neural activation in prefrontal cortex and anterior cingulate during decision making. *Neuroimage, 15,* 836–846.

Paus, T. (2001). Primate anterior cingulate cortex: Where motor control, drive and cognition interface. *Nature Reviews Neuroscience, 2,* 417–424.

Petit, L., Courtney, S. M., Ungerleider, L. G., & Haxby, J. V. (1998). Sustained activity in the medial wall during working memory delays. *Journal of Neuroscience, 18*(22), 9429–9437.

Posner, M. I., & DiGirolamo, G. J. (1998). Executive attention: Conflict, target detection, and cognitive control. In R. Parasuraman (Ed.), *The attentive brain* (pp. 401–424). London: Bradford.

Posner, M. I., Petersen, S. E., Fox, P. T., & Raichle, M. E. (1988). Localization of cognitive operations in the human brain. *Science, 240,* 1627–1631.

Posner, M. I., & Rothbart, M. K. (1998). Attention, self regulation and consciousness. *Philosophical Transactions of the Royal Society of London B, 353,* 1915–1927.

Raichle, M. E., Fiez, J. A., Videen, T. O., MacLeod, A. M., Pardo, J. V., Fox, P. T., & Petersen, S. E. (1994). Practice-related changes in human brain functional anatomy during non-motor learning. *Cerebral Cortex, 4,* 8–26.

Ramachandran, V. S., & Blakeslee, S. B. (1998). *Phantoms in the brain.* London: Fourth Estate.

Reason, J. (1979). *Actions not as planned: The price of automization.* In G. Underwood & R. Stevens (Eds.), *Aspects of consciousness* (pp. 67–89). London: Academic Press.

Reason, J. T., & Mycielska, K. (1982). *Absentminded?: The psychology of mental lapses and everyday errors.* Englewood Cliffs, NJ: Prentice-Hall.

Ringholz, G. M. (2000). Diagnosis and treatment of vascular dementia. *Topics in Stroke Rehabilitation, 7*(3), 38–46.

Roberts, R. J., Hager, L. D., & Heron, C. (1994). Prefrontal cognitive processes: Working memory and inhibition in the antisaccade task. *Journal of Experimental Psychology: General, 123,* 374–393.

Rogers, R. D., Everitt, B. J., Baldacchino, A., Blackshaw, A. J., Swainson, R., Wynne, K., Baker, N. B., Hunter, J., Carthy, T., Booker, E., London, M., Deakin, J. F. W., Sahakian, B. J., & Robbins, T. W. (1999). Dissociable deficits in the decision-making cognition of chronic amphetamine abusers, opiate abusers, patients with focal damage to prefrontal cortex, and tryptophan-depleted normal volunteers: Evidence for monoaminergic mechanisms. *Neuropsychopharmacology, 20*(4), 322–339.

Rolls, E. T. (2000). The orbitofrontal cortex and reward. *Cerebral Cortex, 10,* 284–294.

Rolls, E. T., Hornak, J., Wade, D., & McGrath, J. (1994). Emotion-related learning in patients with social and emotional changes associated with frontal lobe damage. *Journal of Neurology, Neurosurgery and Psychiatry, 57,* 1518–1524.

Ruff, C., Woodward, T., Larens, K., & Liddle, P. (2001). The role of the anterior cingulate cortex in conflict processing: Evidence from reverse Stroop interference. *Neuroimage, 14*(5), 1150–1158.

Schröger, E., Giard, M. H., & Wolff, C. (2000). Auditory distraction: Event-related potential and behavioral indicies. *Clinical Neurophysiology, 111,* 1450–60.

Schwartz, M.F., Montgomery, M. W., Fitzpatrick-DeSalme, E. J., Ochipa, C., Coslett, H. B., & Mayer, N. H. (1995). Analysis of a disorder of everyday action. *Cognitive Neuropsychology, 12,* 863–892.

Shallice, T. (1982). Specific impairments of planning. *Philosophical Transactions of the Royal Society of London, Series B, Biological Sciences, 298,* 199–209.

Shallice, T. (1988). *From neuropsychology to mental structure.* Cambridge, UK: Cambridge University Press.

Shallice, T., & Burgess, P. (1991). Higher-order cognitive impairments and frontal lobe lesions in man. In H. S. Levin, H. M. Eisenberg, & A. L. Benton (Eds.), *Frontal lobe function and dysfunction* (pp. 125–138). New York: Oxford University Press.

Shallice, T., & Burgess, P. (1996). The domain of supervisory processes and temporal organization of behaviour. *Philosophical Transactions of the Royal Society of London, 351,* 1405–1412.

Shallice, T., Burgess, P., Schon, F., & Baxter, D. (1989). The origins of utilization behaviour. *Brain, 112,* 1587–1598.

Sheppard, D. M., Bradshaw, J. L., Purcell, R., & Pantelis, C. (1999). Tourette's and comorbid syndromes: Obsessive compulsive and attention deficit hyperactivity disorder: A common etiology? *Clinical Psychological Review, 19*(5), 531–552.

Shidara, M., & Richmond, B. J. (2002). Anterio cingulate: Single neuronal signals related to degree of reward expectancy. *Science, 296,* 1709–1711.

Shimamura, A. P., Jurica, P. J., Mangels, J. A., Gershberg, F. B., & Knight, R. T. (1995). Susceptibility to memory interference effects following frontal lobe damage: Findings from tests of paired-associate learning. *Journal of Cognitive Neuroscience, 7,* 144–152.

Spence, S. A., & Frith, C. D. (1999). Towards a functional anatomy of volition. *Journal of Consciousness Studies, 6,* 11–29.

Stone, V. E., Baron-Cohen, S., & Knight, R. T. (1998). Does frontal lobe damage produce theory of mind impairment? *Journal of Cognitive Neuroscience, 10*(5), 640–656.

Stuss, D., Floden, D., Alexander, M., Levine, B., & Katz, D. (2001). Stroop performance in focal lesion patients: Dissociation of processes and frontal lobe lesion location. *Neuropsychologia, 39,* 771–786.

Stuss, D., Gow, C., & Hetherington, C. (1992). "No longer Gage": Frontal lobe dysfunction and emotional changes. *Journal of Consulting and Clinical Psychology, 60,* 349–359.

Stuss, D., & Levine, B. (2002). Adult clinical neuropsychology: Lessons from the studies of frontal lobes. *Annual Review of Psychology, 53,* 401–433.

Stuss, D. T. (1991). Self, awareness, and the frontal lobes: A neuropsychological perspective. In J. Strauss & G. R. Goethals (Eds.), *The self: Interdisciplinary approaches* (pp. 255–278). New York: Springer-Verlag.

Stuss, D. T. (1992). Biological and psychological development of executive functions. *Brain and Cognition, 20,* 8–23.

Stuss, D. T., & Alexander, M. P. (2000). The anatomical basis of affective behavior, emotion and self-awareness: A specific role of the right frontal lobe. In G. Hatano, N. Okada, & H. Tanabe (Eds.), *Affective minds: The 13th Toyota Conference* (pp. 13–25). Shizuoka, Japan: Elsevier Science.

Stuss, D. T., Alexander, M. P., Lieberman, A., & Levine, H. (1978). An extraordinary form of confabulation. *Neurology, 28,* 1166–1172.

Stuss, D. T., & Benson, D. F. (1984). Neuropsychological studies of the frontal lobes. *Psychological Bulletin, 95,* 3–28.

Stuss, D. T., & Benson, D. F. (1986). *The frontal lobes.* New York: Raven Press.

Stuss, D. T., & Gow, C. A. (1992). Frontal dysfunction after traumatic brain injury. *Neuropsychiatry, Neuropsychology, and Behavioral Neurology, 5,* 272–282.

Stuss, D. T., Picton, T. W., & Alexander, M. P. (2001). Consciousness, self-awareness and the frontal lobes. In S. P. Salloway & P. F. Malloy (Eds.), *The frontal lobes and neuropsychiatric illness* (pp. 101–109). Washington, DC: American Psychiatric Publishing.

Tamminga, C. A., Thaker, G. K., Buchanan, R., Kirkpatrick, B., Alphs, L. D., Chase, T. N., & Carpenter, W. T. (1992). Limbic system abnormalities identified in schizophrenia using positron emission tomography with fluorodeoxyglucose and neocortical alterations with deficit syndrome. *Archives of General Psychiatry, 49,* 522–530.

Tranel, D., Bechara, A., & Denburg, N. L. (2002). Asymmetric functional roles of right and left ventromedial prefrontal cortices in social conduct, decision-making, and emotional processing. *Cortex, 38,* 589–612.

Tranel, D., & Damasio, H. (1994). Neuroanatomical correlates of electrodermal skin conductance responses. *Psychophysiology, 31,* 427–438.

Turk, D. J., Banfield, J. F., Walling, B. R., Heatherton, T. F., Grafton, S. T., Handy, T. C.,

Gazzaniga, M. S., & Macrae, C. N. (2003). *From color plates to dinner dates: The neural substrates of consequential and inconsequential choice.* Manuscript in preparation.

Van Horn, J. D., Gold, J. M., Esposito, G., Ostrem, J L., Mattay, V., Weinberger, D., R., & Berman, K. F. (1998). Changing patterns of brain activation during maze learning. *Brain Research, 793*(1–2), 29–38.

Volkow, N. D., & Fowler, J. S. (2000). Addiction, a disease of compulsion and drive: Involvement of the orbitofrontal cortex. *Cerebral Cortex, 10,* 318–325.

Von Restorff, H. (1933). Uber die Wirkung von Bereischsbildungen im spurenfeld. *Psychlogische Forschung, 18,* 299–342.

Walsch, K. W. (1978). *Neuropsychology: A clinical approach.* Edinburgh: Churchill Livingston.

Wegner, D. M. (1992). You can't always think what you want: Problems in the suppression of unwanted thoughts. In M. Zanna (Ed.), *Advances in experimental social psychology* (Vol. 25, pp. 193–225). San Diego, CA: Academic Press.

Wegner, D. M., & Schneider, D. J. (1989). Mental control: The war of the ghosts in the machine. In J. S. Uleman & J. A. Bargh (Eds.), *Unintended thought* (pp. 287–305). New York: Guilford Press.

Wyland, C. L., Kelley, W. M., Macrae, C. N., Gordon, H. L., & Heatherton, T. F. (in press). Neural correlates of thought suppression. *Neuropsychologia.*

5

Self-Regulatory Strength

Brandon J. Schmeichel
Roy F. Baumeister

The social and economic costs of self-regulation failure are enormous. Unsafe sex, AIDS, drug abuse, unethical business practices, obesity, and violence all contain elements of self-destructive behavior and self-regulatory failure. When people capitulate to their basest instincts, they create not only costly consequences for themselves in the form of poorer health, prison sentences, and conflicted interpersonal relationships, but also major disruptions in the fabric of society, for example, by consuming tax dollars, time, and social capital.

Given the prevalence and costs of self-regulatory failures, more and better self-regulation is clearly desirable, so why does self-regulation fail so often? What is the nature of the willpower used to control the self? When is it required and why is it not more successful in preventing self-regulatory failure? One likely explanation is that each person has a limited stock of willpower, and when that stock is depleted, self-control ceases to be effective.

One prominent model of self-regulation relates to a feedback loop in the form of a test–operate–test–exit (TOTE) system (see Carver, Chapter 2, this volume; Carver & Scheier, 1981, 1998; based on Powers, 1973). In the initial "test" phase, a person determines his or her current standing on a dimension (e.g., current emotional state) and compares the current state to the desired state (e.g., preferred emotional state). If a discrepancy is detected, the "operate" phase is initiated. This phase involves actions intended to move the self toward the desired end state. Progress toward the goal is monitored by further "test" phases. When the desired end state has been achieved (i.e., a good mood has been restored), the "test" phase will reveal no discrepancy between current and desired states, so the TOTE process is terminated, constituting the "exit" phase of the feedback loop.

Each step in the TOTE system is important for self-regulation and suggests a different cause of self-regulatory failure. For example, faulty monitoring of current and desired self-states may cause self-regulatory failure, because one is not clear about either the desired end state or one's current state (e.g., Kirschenbaum, 1987). However, the crucial "operate" phase, which involves self-initiated action to resolve discrepancies in current and desired states, has received less research attention than the other components of the TOTE system. One may have a perfectly clear idea that a good mood is preferred to a current bad mood, yet without sufficient ability to alter cognitive, behavioral, or emotional responses to approach the desired state, a good mood will remain elusive. This sort of self-regulatory failure is due to faulty self-regulatory operations.

The self-regulatory strength model was first suggested by Baumeister, Heatherton, and Tice (1994) and elaborated in subsequent work (see Baumeister, 2002a, 2002b; Baumeister & Heatherton, 1996; Baumeister, Muraven, & Tice, 2000; Muraven & Baumeister, 2000). It proposes that faulty self-regulatory operations implicated in self-regulation failure result from a lack of self-regulatory resources. The core of the self-regulatory strength model is that the ability to regulate responses actively (that is, to "operate" so as to move the self closer to a desired state) relies on a limited self-regulatory resource. When regulatory resources have been depleted, self-regulation failure is more likely. Regulatory resources are required to resolve self-regulatory challenges successfully, and the expenditure and resulting depletion of regulatory resources are a cause of self-regulation failure.

UNDERSTANDING THE EXECUTIVE FUNCTION

Our review focuses on the executive functions of the self, with specific emphasis on self-control and self-regulation. These volitional and active capabilities may be among the most important functions of the self (Baumeister, 1998). People are capable of transcending instinctual urges and stimulus–response conditioning, unlike other members of the animal kingdom. The ability to alter and control one's own behavior expands the range of human response options and outcomes dramatically.

The executive functions have been defined and researched primarily by cognitive psychologists, neuropsychologists, and clinicians. Broadly speaking, executive functions foster self-directed, intentional behavior. Some of these abilities include planning and problem solving (Ward & Allport, 1997), switching from one task to another (Allport, Styles, & Hseih, 1994; Phillips, Bull, Adams, & Fraser, 2002), directing mental attention (Baddeley, 1996; Wegner, 1994), resisting interference (Denckla, 1996), troubleshooting (Norman & Shallice, 1986), and performing novel tasks (Shiffrin & Schneider, 1977). Response inhibition, strategy generation and application, and flexible action are also facilitated by the executive functions (Denckla, 1996).

Executive functioning, as normally studied in cognitive psychology and neuropsychology, focuses almost exclusively on high-level cognitive processing. However, other forms of self-control that extend the information-processing focus of executive functioning have been the object of recent research attention. Self-regulated behavior such as inhibiting impulses, active choice making, persisting in the face of failure, and controlling emotions also require the self's executive function.

The extensive range of abilities engendered by executive functioning may suggest that virtually all thought and behavior require the active, controlled self. People frequently plan for the future, resist temptation, and otherwise attempt to regulate their own behavior. However, the list of behaviors that require little or no conscious control continues to grow. Evaluating novel stimuli (Duckworth, Bargh, Garcia, & Chaiken, 2002), retrieving information from long-term memory (Hasher & Zacks, 1979), nonconscious goal striving (Bargh, Gollwitzer, Lee-Chai, Barndollar, & Trotschel, 2001), and related phenomena rely on automatic processes, and conscious control by the self is un-necessary.

The automaticity of many behaviors sets important limits on the regulatory and ex-ecutive functions of the self. Regulatory resources are only required in actions that de-mand active self-control, so automatic behavior does not rely on regulatory resources. Even when self-regulatory resources have been depleted, automatic responses such as effi-cient retrieval from memory and nonconscious goal-directed behavior should function appropriately. Only self-regulated performance is affected when regulatory resources are low.

Self-regulation and executive functioning are common in everyday life and encom-pass more than flexible information processing. The self-regulatory strength model ex-plains that regulatory resources are used in all manner of active choice making, executive functioning, and self-regulation. Emotion regulation, impulse control, and interpersonal interaction are also among the unique human abilities that require the self's regulatory re-sources. However, automatic response patterns do not require active guidance by the self. The model of self-regulatory strength presented in this chapter is one attempt to locate the self in self-regulation and executive functioning.

DEFINITIONS

Since William James distinguished between the "I" and the "me," most self theorists have likewise considered the self as a combination of the knower and the known. This focus on the self as a knower has tended to downplay or overlook the self as a doer. The present consideration of the self's executive functions emphasizes the "doing" aspect of the self. The executive functions are construed as the active, conscious, and intentional core of the self, responsible for planning, initiating, and revising ongoing cognition and behavior. As such, the self's executive functions encompass self-control and self-regulatory abilities. Some theorists have suggested that the executive functions evolved to allow self-regula-tion, thereby giving the executive functions a central role in adaptive self-regulatory behavior (Barkley, 2001; Baumeister, 1998).

Self-regulation involves the self acting on itself to alter its own responses. Strictly speaking, the self does not regulate itself as a whole. Emotions and thoughts are not the self, but are felt and thought (and possibly controlled) by the self. Regulation of the self's responses is usually initiated with the goal of achieving a desired outcome, such as im-proving one's mood or avoiding an undesirable outcome.

Self-regulation and self-control are highly related and, like most authors, we use the terms interchangeably. For those who make a distinction, "self-regulation" is the broader term and may refer to both conscious and nonconscious alteration of responses by the self. Self-control typically implies a more deliberate and conscious process of altering the self's responses. "Self-control" is sometimes used specifically to refer to inhibition of un-wanted impulses. This review focuses mostly on self-regulation and, more broadly, the executive functions of the self.

SELF-REGULATORY STRENGTH

"Self-regulatory strength" refers to the internal resources available to inhibit, override, or alter responses that may arise as a result of physiological processes, habit, learning, or the press of the situation. Crucially, self-regulatory strength relies on a limited and depletable resource. When self-regulatory resources have been expended, a state of ego depletion results, and self-regulation failure is more likely. For example, attempting to control a quivering voice during a public speaking engagement may cause ego depletion, making it more difficult to restrain trips to the complimentary candy dish once the talk is over.

The self-regulatory resource is required for all manner of active self-regulation and executive functioning. Thus, not only emotion regulation (Larsen & Prizmic, Chapter 3, this volume) and impulse control require regulatory resources, but executive functions, such as making active choices, switching tasks, and solving complex problems, are also powered by regulatory resources. The domain-independent nature of these resources suggests an important relationship among varied forms of self-regulation and executive functioning: Any particular self-regulation attempt will be impaired by prior, seemingly unrelated forms of regulation and executive functioning. Suppressing a forbidden thought may impair subsequent attempts to control emotions. Inhibiting an impulse to eat sweets may impair one's facility in making a difficult choice. According to the self-regulatory strength model, depleting regulatory resources in virtually any way will make subsequent self-regulation and executive functioning more prone to failure, regardless of the specific form of the regulatory challenge.

The self-regulatory strength model differs from models of attention as a limited resource, because the strength model predicts a subsequent, not a concurrent, decrement in self-regulation. Attention models typically explain cognitive deficits, such as in dual-task processing and cognitive load situations, by positing a limited attentional resource that can focus on only a limited number of tasks at one time. When the attentional system is overloaded, current task performance suffers, but when the distraction is removed, attention returns to its full capacity. In contrast, the self-regulatory resource takes time and rest to be replenished, so the effects of ego depletion will persist even after the task that drains those resources is ended.

The difference between the resource model of attention and the resource model of self-regulation can easily be seen in the research paradigms. Studies on the limits of attention ask people to do two or more things at once. Self-regulatory depletion studies, in contrast, usually have people perform tasks one after the other, and they reveal (as we cover in more detail shortly) that performance on the latter tasks is poorer because of the resources expended on the earlier tasks. Limited attention is only relevant to simultaneous tasks. For present purposes, the important point is only that the resource involved in self-regulation is distinct from attention, because it does not follow the same patterns.

We have labeled this view of self-regulation the "strength" model, because self-regulation operates like strength: High at first, strength diminishes as the muscles are exerted, and only after some rest is strength restored to its initial power. Other implications of the analogy to strength are that people seek to conserve self-regulation once it begins to be depleted, and it can be gradually increased by exercise.

The pattern of results observed in the two-task paradigm suggests that ego depletion extends over time, so subsequent self-regulation suffers. Expending limited regulatory resources on the first task impairs performance on a subsequent task, even when the two tasks are seemingly unrelated, because the same resource is necessary for both tasks. Thus, the strength model focuses on self-regulation over time, which is crucial to many forms of self-control, including weight loss, test preparation, and fiscal responsibility. To be successful, each requires choice making and self-regulation on a moment-to-moment, day-to-day basis.

Other theories of self-regulation are plausible. In particular, a priori, it is possible that self-regulation operates as an information-processing schema instead of a strength. According to the schema view, self-regulation is essentially a matter of cognitive processing that uses information about the self and the environment (including task demands) to calculate the optimal course of action, and behavior follows directly from those calculations.

Still another possible theory of self-regulation considers it to be a skill (instead of a strength or a cognitive process). This view has been favored by developmental psychologists, who treat self-regulation as one among many skills that children gradually acquire as they grow up. If self-regulation is a general skill, then a person who performs well at one self-regulatory act is likely to perform well at another.

These three views of self-regulation predict different effects of an initial regulatory act on a subsequent regulatory attempt. According to the schema view, an initial self-regulatory attempt should prime the self-regulatory schema, so performance on a subsequent regulatory attempt should improve because of the activated schema. By analogy, a computer that has already loaded its word-processing program will be faster at doing a new word-processing task than if it had not loaded that program or perhaps was busy doing numerical data analysis.

Meanwhile, the self-regulation-as-skill view suggests that an initial self-regulatory attempt will have little effect on subsequent self-regulation except for minor benefits due to learning and practice, because skilled performance tends to be constant across trials. (Skill will show a very gradual improvement over many trials but remains essentially the same from one trial to the next.)

In contrast, the self-regulation-as-strength view predicts that an initial regulatory attempt will result in ego depletion, with adverse consequences for further behavior that relies on limited regulatory resources. Therefore, self-regulation would deteriorate over successive attempts. In the next section, we describe studies attempting to distinguish among these three competing models and their predictions.

SELF-REGULATORY STRENGTH: EMPIRICAL EVIDENCE

The initial ego depletion studies pitted the skill, schema, and strength views against each other and found strong support for the self-regulatory strength model. The inhibition of prepotent impulses, or impulse control, is a fundamental capability of the self's executive functions. Baumeister, Bratslavsky, Muraven, and Tice (1998) showed that resisting temptation impaired subsequent self-regulated persistence on an apparently unrelated task. Participants sat near a batch of chocolate-chip cookies and chocolate candies. The cookies had been freshly baked in the laboratory, and participants had been instructed to forgo eating for at least 3 hours prior to the experiment to ensure that they would be sufficiently tempted by the cookies. Participants in the ego-depletion condition were not allowed to eat the tasty cookies; instead, they had to eat radishes. Performance by participants in this group on a subsequent regulatory task was inferior to two different control conditions, in which participants were allowed to eat the sweet-tasting cookie treats, and the other in which participants performed the experiment with no food present. Specifically, participants that were not allowed to eat the tempting cookies gave up more quickly on an unsolvable geometric figure-tracing task compared to both the cookie-eating and no-food control groups. Thus, apparently, resisting the temptation to eat the cookies and chocolate depleted some inner resource, leaving participants less able to persist in the face of failure on the difficult puzzles. These results supported the predictions of the strength model and contradicted those of the schema and skill models.

The experiments reported in Baumeister and colleagues (1998) also demonstrated that acts of self-regulation could impair subsequent volition in some sphere other than self-control. Participants in Study 2 were taught an easy task that required them to read a text and cross out all instances of the letter *e*. After successfully performing this task, participants were asked to perform the task with additional rules, such as not crossing out any *e* that was adjacent or two letters removed from another vowel. These rules require people to override (repeatedly) their newly acquired habit of crossing out every *e*, thereby making this new task a self-regulatory challenge. In contrast, control participants solved three-digit multiplication problems, which are difficult and mentally taxing but do not involve self-regulation, insofar as these can be performed by simply following well-learned procedures rather than having to override incipient responses.

After both groups had performed their respective tasks, behavioral passivity was measured. People were shown a film clip of a boring movie and given control over how long they would sit and watch it. For half of the participants, continuing to view the movie was a passive option, whereas quitting was an active option: They were told that the movie would continue until they pressed the button in front of them, whereupon it would stop. For other participants, quitting was the passive option, whereas continuing required the active response. These people had to keep pressing the button to see more of the movie, and the film would stop if they did nothing. Participants in the ego-depletion condition favored the passive response, whether this response resulted in stopping the film or continued viewing; that is, ego depletion led to longer viewing of the boring movie when participants actively had to stop the movie, but depletion led to shorter viewing of the boring movie when only a passive action was required to stop the movie. Ego depletion increased subsequent passivity, consistent with the self-regulatory strength model.

Wallace and Baumeister (2002) showed that ego-depletion effects were not influenced by self-attributions or self-efficacy. They considered that performance on a second regulatory act might fail, because an initial self-regulatory task caused people to view themselves as poor at self-control. This prediction was derived from notions of self-attributions or self-efficacy (see Bandura, 1977; Bem, 1965). Lack of self-efficacy, in turn, could cause people to perform more poorly on subsequent self-regulatory tasks, because they did not feel sufficiently able to perform the second task. To pit this alternate account against the resource depletion model, Wallace and Baumeister had participants perform a resource-depleting version of the Stroop task. Some participants were then given explicit success or failure feedback regarding Stroop performance to ensure feelings of efficacy and inefficacy, respectively. Subsequent persistence at an ostensibly unrelated task was measured to assess the effects of success or failure feedback and resource depletion on further self-control. The results supported the resource-depletion view and argued against the self-perception and self-efficacy explanations. Again, participants in the ego-depletion conditions performed more poorly on a subsequent test of self-control than nondepleted participants. Performance feedback did not alter the effect of ego depletion on persistence. The success and failure feedback manipulations had no effect on the second self-control act. Even participants who rated their performance on the initial Stroop task quite favorably performed poorly at the subsequent regulatory task. Presumably, these participants had high feelings of self-efficacy, but these feelings did not diminish the ego-depletion effects.

Ego depletion has also been shown to impair physical endurance, persistence, and emotion regulation (Muraven, Tice, & Baumeister, 1998). In a first study, some participants were asked to control their emotions while viewing a sad film clip, whereas others were instructed to watch the clip naturally. Participants were then given a handgrip device and were asked to squeeze it for as long as they could. The handgrip task required self-regulation in the form of coping with physical discomfort and resisting the inclination to give up and relax one's hand muscles. People who had tried to alter their emotional reactions while watching the film clip exhibited poorer physical stamina compared to those who watched the film without trying to control their feelings, suggesting that the regulatory resources required for physical stamina had been depleted by the prior efforts at emotion control.

Another study in this series showed that controlling thoughts also impairs subsequent persistence in the face of failure, consistent with the depletion model (Muraven et al., 1998). As an initial task, some participants were asked not to think about a white bear (Wegner, Schneider, Carter, & White, 1987). Regulating the content of ongoing thoughts is a difficult and cognitively costly pursuit (Wegner, 1994). In a control condition, participants were simply asked to list their thoughts and were not instructed to control their thoughts in any way. Persistence on a series of unsolvable anagrams was measured subsequent to the thought-listing and thought-control tasks. As predicted by the ego-depletion model, participants who had depleted their regulatory resources by suppressing a forbidden thought persisted less at the difficult anagram task. These participants apparently could not marshal the resources to maintain persistence at a difficult task requiring cognitive stamina.

A related study by Muraven and colleagues (1998) demonstrated that controlling thoughts impaired subsequent attempts to control emotions. Participants in the ego-depletion condition suppressed a forbidden thought, whereas other participants only listed their thoughts. After the initial task, all participants watched a funny video clip and were instructed to suppress any laughter or signs of amusement in response to the clip. Participants that had previously been asked to suppress a forbidden thought were less able to stifle outward signs of amusement. Once again, the depleted participants were unable to muster the regulatory resources required to control their emotional expressions. This study showed that controlling thoughts may have a deleterious effect on subsequent efforts to control emotions, explicitly linking two heretofore distinct types of self-regulation.

The results of the studies reported in Muraven and colleagues (1998) indicate that the resources of the active self are limited and depletable. Furthermore, the same resource appears to be used in a variety of tasks that require self-control, including emotion regulation, physical stamina, thought control, and persistence in the face of failure. When volitional resources have been taxed, all manner of controlled self-regulatory acts may suffer.

CHOICE MAKING AND SELF-REGULATORY STRENGTH

The self's executive function may also be involved in making choices. Certainly, some choices are very simple to make and may be facilitated by preferences that have already been established, even preferences of which the person may not be aware (e.g., Nisbett & Wilson, 1977). Such choices are automatic and, therefore, do not require regulatory strength. However, some choices are novel and may therefore require the self to play a decisive and controlling role. According to the self-regulatory strength model, choices that require the active self should deplete regulatory resources, leaving people relatively unable to perform subsequent acts that also require self-control.

In a first study of the hypothesis that active choice making depletes self-regulatory resources, participants were asked to make a series of choices (Vohs, Twenge, Baumeister,

Schmeichel, & Tice, 2003). Participants made pairwise choices among products such as candy bars (e.g., Snickers or Twix), scented candles (vanilla or grape) and T-shirts of different colors (black or white). In a control condition, participants simply indicated the frequency with which they used such products. All participants then performed the cold pressor task, which requires people to immerse their hands in ice water for as long as possible. Forcing oneself to persist on this task requires overcoming the strong desire to withdraw one's hand from the aversive ice water. Consistent with the depletion hypothesis, participants who had made a series of choices persisted less at the cold pressor task than did control-condition participants.

In a separate study by the same researchers, participants that had made a series of choices were unable to force themselves to consume a healthy but bad-tasting drink compared to participants who did not make a series of choices. Because persisting at the cold pressor task and forcing oneself to drink a bad-tasting liquid required self-control and the inhibition of impulses contrary to the requirements of the task, performance on these tasks was impaired by resource depletion as a result of active choice making. Once again, ego depletion impaired executive functioning. The act of making a series of choices presumably made high demands on the self's regulatory resources, so these resources were not available to participants for the performance of the subsequent tasks.

Converging evidence that active choice making causes ego depletion was reported by Baumeister and colleagues (1998). They reported a study that used a variant of a classic cognitive dissonance manipulation, wherein some participants made a proattitudinal choice, others made a counterattitudinal choice, and still others were given no choice, but were assigned to perform a counterattitudinal behavior. The counterattitudinal choice condition is the only one in which cognitive dissonance should arise. From the self-regulatory-strength perspective, however, active choice making depletes regulatory resources, so the actual content of the choice (whether consistent with or counter to one's attitudes) should make little difference in regulatory resource expenditure, and subsequent self-regulation should be impaired in both cases. However, because assignment to a counterattitudinal condition required no choice on the part of participants, this group should show no ego-depletion effects. Subsequent persistence on unsolvable puzzles confirmed the ego-depletion account. Participants who had been assigned to a counterattitudinal position persisted the longest at the frustrating task, whereas both proattitudinal and counterattitudinal choice makers persisted the least, and there were no discernible differences in the persistence of these latter two groups. The self-regulatory strength needed to force oneself to keep trying in the face of failure was apparently the same strength used to make responsible decisions about one's own behavior.

SELF-REGULATORY RESOURCES
AND INTELLIGENT RESPONDING

The research reviewed so far has detailed ego-depletion effects on persistence in the face of failure, emotion regulation, physical endurance, and decision making. More recent research has demonstrated that ego depletion impairs high-level cognitive operations as well.

Many cognitive processes occur automatically, without active direction by the self. In contrast, other forms of cognition require self-regulation precisely because automatic operations are not sufficient. For example, solutions to difficult logic problems do not present themselves immediately. When people are faced with such challenges, the inclination to let attention wander, to think impulsively, or simply to quit and do something more en-joyable requires self-regulatory resources. Furthermore, generating possible solutions and otherwise thinking through such a problem may require self-regulated thought control.

If high-level cognitive tasks do in fact require self-regulation for successful perfor-mance, then ego depletion should result in poorer performance on them. In contrast, ego depletion should have little or no effect on tasks that do not require the self's executive function to expend its regulatory resources, such as tasks that can be done with little at-tention, or those that are highly routinized and automatic. Furthermore, these more auto-matic tasks should not cause subsequent resource depletion, and performing them should have little effect on subsequent self-regulation. Of course, there are exceptions to this claim, such as when extended persistence on even highly routinized and mindless tasks must be maintained despite impulses to quit, arising from fatigue, boredom, or stress. For example, it is easy to press a button 10 times in response to a prompt, but having to press that button 10,000 times might drain regulatory resources. In the main, however, auto-matic behavior should not be affected by, and should not cause, ego depletion.

Recent studies have shown that ego depletion makes people perform less intelligently on complex cognitive tasks but does not impact basic forms of information processing (Schmeichel, Vohs, & Baumeister, 2003). In a first study of the relationship between ego depletion and intelligent performance, some participants were asked to control carefully their attention while watching a video depicting a woman being interviewed. Specifically, these participants were asked to ignore extraneous stimuli (text) that appeared at the bot-tom of the viewing screen. They were also told to redirect their attention to the main ac-tion on the screen, if they found themselves attending to the extraneous stimuli. In the control condition, participants were given no attention-control directions, and no men-tion was made of the extraneous stimuli on the screen. Therefore, these participants were free to direct their attention to any aspect of the video clip that they wanted. After the video clip, all participants completed problems from the Analytical subtest of the Gradu-ate Record Examination (GRE). Participants who had been instructed to control their at-tention during the video clip performed worse on the GRE problems. Compared to par-ticipants in the no-depletion control group, attention-control participants attempted fewer problems in the time allotted for GRE test performance, answered fewer problems correctly, and achieved a lower proportion of correct responses on the items they did at-tempt to solve. This pattern of results is indicative of a broad impairment of higher order cognitive capacity. Presumably, good performance on the GRE test required self-regula-tory resources that had been depleted by the prior self-regulatory task.

However, not all cognitive tasks should be impaired by ego depletion. Simple infor-mation-processing activities, such as retrieving knowledge from memory, or perceiving and categorizing stimulus information, should be immune to regulatory resource deple-tion effects; that is, ego depletion should only impair activities that require active, con-trolled processing, whereas more basic and automatic forms of thought should remain in-tact.

Recent research has supported the view that ego depletion impairs higher order cog-nition, whereas basic information processing remains unaffected (Schmeichel et al., 2003). Participants completed two types of cognitive tasks. One task required higher or-der, controlled cognition, and the other required simple information retrieval from mem-ory and the application of basic computational rules. At the beginning of the study, some participants were directed to suppress their emotional reactions to an upsetting film clip. In the control condition, participants were directed to view the clip normally and react naturally. After viewing the clip, all participants performed two cognitive tests. The first test (General Mental Abilities Test [GMAT]; Janda, 1996) was a measure of basic information processing and contained sections on general knowledge, vocabulary, and basic algebra. The second test (Cognitive Estimation Test [CET]; Shallice & Evans, 1978), a measure of higher order cognitive processing, requires participants to reason their way to sensible answers, because no clear answer is readily available for any of the questions (e.g., "How many seeds are there in a watermelon?").

Consistent with the self-regulatory strength model, ego depletion due to prior emotion control led to worse performance on the test of higher order cognition (i.e., the CET). Furthermore, depleted and nondepleted participants performed equally well on the test of more basic information processing (i.e., the GMAT). Depleted participants provided a greater number of wildly inaccurate estimates on the CET than did control-condition participants, reflecting their relative inability to control sufficiently the content of their thoughts. These results suggest that the regulatory resources required to generate acceptable cognitive estimates (e.g., by generating anchor values and adjusting those anchors appropriately) were lacking because of prior ego depletion.

Ego depletion impaired controlled cognition, while leaving basic cognitive abilities intact in a third study, which used a different ego-depletion manipulation and different cognitive tests than used in prior studies. Here, we selected two tasks that clearly differed in the amount of controlled processing required for successful performance. Our measure of basic information processing was memory for nonsense syllables. Participants studied a short list of nonsense syllables and were asked to recall as many of them as possible a short while later. The measure of higher order cognition was the Reading Comprehension subtest of the GRE. As predicted, participants that had been asked to control their attention while watching a video clip performed worse on the subsequent GRE test than did participants who watched the clip naturally. However, performance on the nonsense syllable recall task was not affected by ego depletion. These results replicated the previous studies and strongly attested to the hypotheses that ego depletion impairs higher order cognition but has little or no effect on basic information processing. Depletion impairs only activities that require the self to act as a volitional, active agent.

Conceptually similar work by Kruglanski and colleagues (Webster, Richter, & Kruglanski, 1996) has demonstrated effects similar to ego depletion. After performing a lengthy final examination, students were asked to consider some information about hypothetical job applicants to form impressions of the applicants. Students experiencing mental fatigue (or ego depletion, in our terminology) due to the long final exam were more likely to base their impressions of others on early, limited information. They formed their impressions quickly, considering only a portion of the available information. A comparison group of students that had not just finished a lengthy exam were not prone to "seizing and freezing" on the limited information; therefore, they based their impressions of the target persons on broader samples of information. It is probable that the nonfatigued participants had more regulatory resources at their disposal, and could freely expend those resources and avoid leaping to conclusions based on thin slices of information. Thus, these participants opted to consider a greater amount of information to form more accurate impressions than their depleted counterparts. The depleted students presumably formed incomplete or inaccurate impressions of the target individuals because they were prone to rely on incomplete, unelaborated information. These results are consistent with the self-regulatory strength model, in that depleted students appeared to lack the resources necessary for controlled cognitive processing.

SELF-REGULATORY EXERTION AND TIME EXPERIENCE

Recent work has begun to explore some of the subjective consequences of ego depletion by focusing on the experience of time passage. A series of studies by Vohs and Schmeichel (2003) demonstrated that regulating the self is associated with an elongated perception of time. For example, when participants controlled their emotions while watching a film clip, they estimated that the clip lasted longer than did participants who watched the clip without actively controlling their emotions (Studies 1 and 2). In another study, extended-duration perceptions mediated the link between initial self-regulatory exertion and subsequent regulatory ability. When participants had controlled their emotional expressions, they experienced elongated time passage and also gave up more quickly on a subsequent self-regulated task (replicating the typical depletion effect). Finally, distorted time perception due to self-regulation extended to a subsequent and different self-regulated act. After suppressing a forbidden thought, participants performed a breath-holding task. Depleted participants estimated that they had held their breath for a longer duration than they actually did, and their breath-holding ability was actually worse than that of participants who had not initially suppressed a forbidden thought. In summary, self-regulatory exertion was associated with the perception that much time had passed, and this elongated experience of time extended into a subsequent, and quite different, self-regulatory endeavor.

Vohs and Schmeichel (2003) suggested that active self-regulation fosters an extended-now state, wherein time passage is elongated. When people experience an extended-now, current thoughts and feelings become more salient, making continued self-regulation more difficult. Ego depletion and the extended-now state appear to go hand in hand: Depleted participants give overly long estimates of the duration of self-regulated behavior, and they give up more quickly at subsequent persistence tasks as a result.

SELF-REGULATORY STRENGTH
IN ALCOHOL CONSUMPTION AND DIETING

Recent research by Muraven, Collins, and Nienhaus (2002) has applied the self-control strength model to alcohol consumption and its restraint in a sample of male social drinkers. After being informed that they would be taking a test of driving skills later in the experiment, with the opportunity to earn a reward for good performance, some participants were asked to suppress a forbidden thought provided by the experimenter. Other participants worked on simple arithmetic problems that required little or no self-regulatory resources. After completing their respective tasks, participants were given the opportunity to taste-test and rate the qualities of different alcoholic beverages (beers). In this manner, participants were encouraged to consume as much beer as they desired (in a 20-minute session) but also were provided a reason to regulate their alcohol intake, so as to perform well on the subsequent driving test.

Participants who had suppressed a forbidden thought subsequently drank more beer and had higher blood-alcohol content at the end of the experiment than did participants who performed the simple math problems. The effect of resource depletion on alcohol consumption was particularly striking among participants with high trait levels of preoccupation with alcohol. Participants who tended to have a high level of preoccupation with alcohol were particularly likely to consume alcohol following the resource-depletion manipulation. This research provides an important link to "real-world" applications of the self-control strength model. (See Hull and Sloane, Chapter 24, this volume, for an extended discussion of self-regulation and alcohol consumption.)

Research by Vohs and Heatherton (2000) applied ego depletion to dieting. Dieters' self-regulatory resources were depleted by exposure to a situation that was either strongly depleting (i.e., sitting next to a bowl of candies) or weakly depleting (i.e., sitting far from a bowl of candies). Among those who were strongly depleted, dieters ate more ice cream (Study 1) and persisted less on a demanding cognitive task (Study 2). Nondieters, conversely, were not depleted by the situational manipulation of candy, and so did not eat more ice cream or fail to persist at the difficult task. These studies emphasize the role of chronic differences among people that may render them particularly vulnerable to resource depletion in regulation-relevant situations; that is, resisting the tempting candies is depleting only for people who have the goal of inhibiting caloric intake (i.e., dieters). Presumably, nondieters found the candies less tempting and less demanding of self-regulatory resources, because they were not actively trying to inhibit caloric intake. (See Herman & Polivy, Chapter 25, this volume.)

BOOSTING SELF-REGULATORY STRENGTH
AND PREVENTING DEPLETION

The research detailing self-regulatory failure following ego depletion suggests that self-regulatory resources are used in a variety of behaviors. These depletion patterns raise an important question: How might self-regulatory resources be strengthened, allowing people to meet challenges and improve the likelihood of successful self-regulation?

If self-regulatory strength acts like a muscle, then temporary resource fatigue (ego depletion) should be a consequence of exertion. Over time, however, repeated exertion should lead to a stronger muscle, or a deeper well of resources on which to draw. Thus, one consequence of repeated self-regulation should be greater self-regulatory strength.

Muraven, Baumeister, and Tice (1999) examined this hypothesis in a longitudinal study of repeated self-regulatory practice on further self-control. Participants were assigned various self-regulatory exercises to perform for a 2-week period. One group was to try to improve posture by, for example, sitting and standing up straight; another group was told to engage in affect regulation as often as possible. Both before and after the 2 weeks of exercise, participants underwent laboratory measures of self-regulation and depletion. By comparing performance before and after the exercise period, the researchers concluded that the 2 weeks of exercise did lead to improvements in self-control, at least relative to a control group that did not practice exercising regulatory resources during the intervening 2 weeks. These results tentatively suggest that the first benefit of exercising self-control is a greater capacity to resist the debilitating effects of ego depletion. However, the overall significance of the finding was partly due to the fact that the control group performed worse at the postpractice measure of depletion. More and better research regarding the long-term benefits of exercising the self-regulatory resource may help to confirm this important implication of the self-regulatory strength model.

Other work is needed to explore how the self-regulatory resource may be replenished when it is temporarily depleted. Although systematic studies are lacking, circumstantial evidence indicates that sleep and other forms of rest help restore it. In particular, self-control appears to get progressively worse the longer a person goes without sleep, even in the course of a normal day, which suggests that sleep serves a valuable function of replenishing a resource that is expended gradually throughout the day. One study found that guided meditation helped to offset the impact of ego depletion and to restore the self's functions (Smith, 2002).

Further work is under way to explore the hypotheses that ego depletion can be counteracted by self-affirmation exercises (i.e., thinking favorable thoughts about the self) or by positive emotional experiences. Preliminary data suggest that these procedures do have some power to restore the self's capacity for self-control. If these findings continue to be supported, they may shed some light on the nature of the resource that is depleted and how it functions.

CONCLUSIONS

Self-regulation is one of the most important functions of the psyche. The research program covered in this chapter suggests that it operates on the basis of a limited resource that resembles a strength or energy. It becomes depleted when it is expended in acts of self-regulation or other executive function activity. The same resource is used for many, quite different kinds of self-regulation, and it is also used for making choices, for responding actively instead of passively, and for other executive functions. This resource promises to shed light on the neglected but highly important aspect of the self as being, instead of just a knower and a known, also a doer.

REFERENCES

Allport, D. A., Styles, E. A., & Hseih, S. (1994). Shifting intentional set: Exploring the dynamic control of tasks. In C. Umilta & M. Moscovitch (Eds.), *Attention and performance XV: Conscious and nonconscious information processing* (pp. 421–452). Cambridge, MA: MIT Press.

Baddeley, A. (1996). Exploring the central executive. *Quarterly Journal of Experimental Psychology, 49A*, 5–28.

Bandura, A. (1977). Self-efficacy: Toward a unifying theory of behavior change. *Psychological Review, 84*, 191–215.

Bargh, J. A., Gollwitzer, P. M., Lee-Chai, A., Barndollar, K., & Trotschel, R. (2001). The automated will: Nonconscious activation and pursuit of behavioral goals. *Journal of Personality and Social Psychology, 81*, 1014–1027.

Barkley, R. A. (2001). The executive functions and self-regulation: An evolutionary neuropsychological perspective. *Neuropsychology Review, 11*, 1–29.

Baumeister, R. F. (1998). The self. In D. T. Gilbert, S. T. Fiske, & G. Lindzey (Eds.), *Handbook of social psychology* (4th ed., pp. 680–740). New York: McGraw-Hill.

Baumeister, R. F. (2002a). Ego depletion and self-control failure: An energy model of the self's executive function. *Self and Identity, 1*, 129–136.

Baumeister, R. F. (2002b). Yielding to temptation: Self-control failure, impulsive purchasing, and consumer behavior. *Journal of Consumer Research, 28*, 670–676.

Baumeister, R. F., Bratslavsky, E., Muraven, M., & Tice, D. M. (1998). Ego depletion: Is the active self a limited resource? *Journal of Personality and Social Psychology, 74*, 1252–1265.

Baumeister, R. F., & Heatherton, T. F. (1996). Self-regulation failure: An overview. *Psychological Inquiry, 7*, 1–15.

Baumeister, R. F., Heatherton, T. F., & Tice, D. M. (1994). *Losing control: How and why people fail at self-regulation*. San Diego, CA: Academic Press.

Baumeister, R. F., Muraven, M., & Tice, D. M. (2000). Ego depletion: A resource model of volition, self-regulation, and controlled processing. *Social Cognition, 18*, 130–150.

Bem, D. J. (1965). An experimental analysis of self-persuasion. *Journal of Experimental Social Psychology*, *1*, 199–218.

Carver, C. S., & Scheier, M. F. (1981). *Attention and self-regulation: A control theory approach to human behavior*. New York: Springer-Verlag.

Carver, C. S., & Scheier, M. F. (1998). *On the self-regulation of behavior*. New York: Cambridge University Press.

Denckla, M. B. (1996). A theory and model of executive functioning: A neuropsychological perspective. In G. R. Lyon & N. A. Krasnegor (Eds.), *Attention, memory, and executive function* (pp. 263–277). Baltimore: Brookes.

Duckworth, K. L., Bargh, J. A., Garcia, M., & Chaiken, S. (2002). The automatic evaluation of novel stimuli. *Psychological Science*, *13*, 513–519.

Hasher, L., & Zacks, R. T. (1979). Automatic and effortful processes in memory. *Journal of Experimental Psychology*, *108*, 356–388.

Janda, L. H. (1996). *The psychologist's book of self-tests*. New York: Berkley.

Kirschenbaum, D. S. (1987). Self-regulatory failure: A review with clinical implications. *Clinical Psychology Review*, *7*, 77–104.

Muraven, M., & Baumeister, R. F. (2000). Self-regulation and depletion of limited resources: Does self-control resemble a muscle? *Psychological Bulletin*, *126*, 247–259.

Muraven, M., Baumeister, R. F., & Tice, D. M. (1999). Longitudinal improvement of self-regulation through practice: Building self-control through repeated exercise. *Journal of Social Psychology*, *139*, 446–457.

Muraven, M., Collins, R. L., & Nienhaus, K. (2002). Self-control and alcohol restraint: An initial application of the self-control strength model. *Psychology of Addictive Behaviors*, *16*, 113–120.

Muraven, M., Tice, D. M., & Baumeister, R. F. (1998). Self-control as limited resource: Regulatory depletion patterns. *Journal of Personality and Social Psychology*, *74*, 774–789.

Nisbett, R., & Wilson, T. D. (1977). Telling more than we can know: Verbal reports on mental processes. *Psychological Review*, *84*, 231–259.

Norman, D., & Shallice, T. (1986). Attention to action: Willed and automatic control of behavior. In R. J. Davidson, G. E. Schwartz, & D. Shapiro (Eds.), *Consciousness and self-regulation* (pp. 1–18). New York: Plenum Press.

Phillips, L. H., Bull, R., Adams, E., & Fraser, L. (2002). Positive mood and executive function: Evidence from Stroop and fluency tasks. *Emotion*, *2*, 21–32.

Powers, W. T. (1973). *Behavior: The control of perception*. Chicago: Aldine.

Schmeichel, B. J., Vohs, K. D., & Baumeister, R. F. (2003). Intellectual performance and ego depletion: Role of the self in logical reasoning and other information processing. *Journal of Personality and Social Psychology*, *85*, 33–46.

Shallice, T., & Evans, M. E. (1978). The involvement of the frontal lobes in cognitive estimation. *Cortex*, *14*, 294–303.

Shiffrin, R. M., & Schneider, W. (1977). Controlled and automatic human information processing: II. Perceptual learning, automatic attending and a general theory. *Psychological Review*, *84*, 127–190.

Smith, R. S. (2002). *Effects of relaxation on self-regulatory depletion*. Unpublished doctoral dissertation, Case Western Reserve University, Cleveland, OH.

Vohs, K. D., & Heatherton, T. F. (2000). Self-regulatory failure: A resource-depletion approach. *Psychological Science*, *11*, 249–254.

Vohs, K. D., & Schmeichel, B. J. (2003). Self-regulation and the extended now: Controlling the self alters the subjective experience of time. *Journal of Personality and Social Psychology*, *85*, 217–230.

Vohs, K. D., Twenge, J. M., Baumeister, R. F., Schmeichel, B. J., & Tice, D. M. (2003). *Decision fatigue: Making multiple personal decisions depletes the self's resources*. Unpublished manuscript, University of Utah, Salt Lake City.

Wallace, H. M., & Baumeister, R. F. (2002). The effects of success versus failure feedback on further self-control. *Self and Identity*, *1*, 35–42.

Webster, D. M., Richter, L., & Kruglanski, A. W. (1996). On leaping to conclusions when feeling tired: Mental fatigue effects on impressional primacy. *Journal of Experimental Social Psychology*, *32*, 181–195.

Wegner, D. M. (1994). Ironic processes of mental control. *Psychological Review*, *101*, 34–52.

Wegner, D. M., Schneider, D. J., Carter, S. R., & White, T. L. (1987). Paradoxical effects of thought suppression. *Journal of Personality and Social Psychology*, *53*, 5–13.

6

Willpower in a Cognitive–Affective Processing System

The Dynamics of Delay of Gratification

WALTER MISCHEL
OZLEM AYDUK

INTRODUCTION

The concept of *effortful control* in self-regulation or, in everyday language, "willpower," has survived a century of historical vicissitudes within psychology. Beginning with William James (1890) who made it central for the field's agenda, to its banishment as unscientific at the height of behaviorism, to its resurgence within contemporary psychology in an explosion of work on "self-regulation," the concept's popularity has waxed and waned. Currently, this now vigorously pursued and intensively researched—but still elusive—construct is more center stage than ever. It is difficult to find a conference in social, personality, or developmental psychology in which self-regulation and self-control—and a host of related executive and agentic functions (e.g., planning, future-orientation, goal-directed behavior, effortful control, proactive behavior)—are not major agenda items. As such, it remains a challenge for psychological research and theory on willpower to articulate a framework for studying and making sense of the diverse phenomena that the term encompasses. This chapter is intended as a step toward meeting that challenge. With this goal in mind, we begin by asking: What does the construct encompass? There are two related sides to the answer.

Individual Differences

As is intuitively obvious, there are widely observed individual differences in willpower. Historically in Western cultures these have been conceptualized as reflections of a stable broad trait that characterizes the person consistently across situations and over time. In this vein, the ancient Greeks used the term "akrasia" (a deficiency of the will) to distinguish between people who successfully regulated their impulses and temptations from those who did not. And in modern versions such global trait constructs as conscientiousness (Bem & Allen, 1974; McCrae & Costa, 1999) and ego resilience and ego control (Block & Block, 1980) are commonly used by researchers to explain how and why people differ in terms of their overall levels of self-regulatory ability. These trait approaches offer valuable information concerning the stability and correlates of people's self-regulatory abilities, but provide limited information about the specific processes that underlie such competencies and that enable or constrain them.

Self-Regulatory Processes

Consequently one must explicate the conditions and mechanisms that make willpower possible and that underlie the observed individual differences. Fortunately, in a rapidly accelerating trajectory, self-regulation research and theory are analyzing and illuminating many of the relevant processes influencing diverse aspects of willpower and "human agency" (e.g., Mischel & Morf, 2003; Mischel, Shoda, & Smith, 2003). For more than three decades the field has been bursting with important findings on the nature of human self-regulation, creating fresh challenges and offering exciting prospects, while at the same time still struggling with classic problems in trying to figure out the basic nature of willpower and its essential ingredients (Carver & Scheier, 1982; Gollwitzer & Bargh, 1996; Higgins, 1996; Higgins & Kruglanski, 1996; Kuhl, 1985; Mischel, Cantor, & Feldman, 1996; Mischel & Morf, 2003; Morf & Mischel, 2002).

Our overarching goal in this chapter is to outline a theoretical framework for understanding self-regulatory efforts that takes into account individual differences as well as the processes that underlie them and enable the individual to exercise willpower in the course of goal pursuit. We begin with the premise that self-regulatory processes do not operate in isolation. Rather, we assume that they are more fruitfully viewed as intrinsic aspects of the larger mental and emotional processing systems that characterize the individual. Accordingly, our specific goals in this chapter are to:

- Describe the larger processing system.
- Identify the key components of the self-regulatory system and highlight their cognitive-affective processing dynamics, drawing from research on delay of gratification illustratively.
- Illustrate how the components of the system interact with each other as well as other sub-systems in the generation of observed individual differences in self-regulation.
- Examine the implications for predicting and enhancing the individuals' ways of coping with relevant life challenges that require self-regulation.

BASIC FEATURES
OF THE SELF-REGULATORY PROCESSING SYSTEM

The explosion of work on self-regulation has led to a host of informative findings about its diverse forms, determinants, and implications. Cumulatively, they suggest an emerging consensus among process-oriented researchers concerning key ingredients for a conceptual framework that demystifies the essentials of willpower and provides a road map for its further scientific analysis. We attempt that framework here in the hope that it will have heuristic value for future research and theory development. First, we outline basic features for a self-regulatory processing system that seems to be widely assumed—albeit often only implicitly—within a broadly social cognitive-affective theoretical framework (Kunda, 1999). The view of the self-regulatory processing system presented here is closely related to Mischel and Ayduk's (2002) analysis, to the conception of the "Self as a Psycho-Social Dynamic Processing System" developed recently by Mischel and Morf (2003), to the Cognitive Affective Processing System (CAPS) presented earlier by Mischel and Shoda (1995, 1998, 1999; Shoda & Mischel, 1998), and to the Metcalfe and Mischel (1999) hot/cool model, and draws extensively on these sources. We draw on the self-system model because the very terms "willpower," "effortful control" and "self-regulation" imply an agentic self—a self-system that actively, and effortfully does the regulating. We draw on the CAPS model because self-regulation needs to be understood as an integral component within the larger cognitive-affective processing system and its sub-systems in which these processes function. And we draw on Mischel and Ayduk (2002) and Metcalfe and Mischel (1999) to illustrate key mechanisms in delay of gratification.

The Connectionist Metaphor for a Self-Regulatory Processing System

The largest challenge that faces theorists interested in constructing a scientific model, either of the self-system, self-regulation, or a broader personality processing system, is how to do so without re-invoking the "homunculus"—the little actor or "doer" in the head of the person who becomes the agent of all that follows (e.g., Kuhl, 1996). While we do not pretend to have solved this age-old problem, we try to assuage the fear of the homunculus by using connectionist models and parallel distributed processing systems as our metaphor (e.g., Baumann & Kuhl, 2002; Graziano & Tobin, 2001; Mischel & Shoda, 1995; Morf & Rhodewalt, 2001; Nowak, Vallacher, Tesser, & Borkowski, 2000; Read & Miller, 2002; Shah & Kruglanski, 2002; Shoda, LeeTiernen, & Mischel, 2002; Shoda & Mischel, 1998; Van Mechelen & Kiers, 1999). In the discussion that follows we borrow from these contributions and the connectionist metaphor. We begin with a brief summary of the key characteristics of these models.

Such models are promising metaphors because of two features. First, they are able to take account of multiple concurrent processes without invoking a single central control, thus helping to reduce the homunculus danger (Rumelhart & McClelland, 1986). As discussed by Mischel and Morf (2003), the agency is in the organization of the network, and so there is no need to invoke an internal controller. Second, connectionist models can account for a system that is biased. They do so in the sense that the patterns of activation in such a system are constrained and guided—and thus biased—by the existing network—a network that reflects the individual's unique biological, psychosocial, developmental, and life experiences. Examples of such biases are abundant and are seen every time an individual reacts predictably (e.g., with withdrawal and self-silencing or hostility and aggression) when particular threats (e.g., partner's rejection and hostility) are encountered (Ayduk, Downey, Testa, Yen, & Shoda, 1999; Ayduk, May, Downey, & Higgins, 2003; Morf & Rhodewalt, 1993; Zayas, Shoda, & Ayduk, 2002). The particular model that guides us most in this chapter, and in much of the research from which we draw, is the Cognitive-Affective Processing System or CAPS (Mischel & Shoda, 1995), which was designed as a broad processing framework for analyzing individual differences and basic processes such as self-regulation, self-control, and proactive, agentic (self-directed and future-oriented) behavior over time.

Processing Characteristics, Units, and Dynamics of the Self-Regulatory System

If we assume that self-regulatory behavior is generated by an organized, dynamic, cognitive-affective processing system like CAPS, one has to consider the nature of the units in the system, their relationship and organization, and the dynamics of their functioning. Using the connectionist, network-like metaphor, the first assumption is that in this type of processing system the mental representations consist of cognitions and affects (emotional states), abbreviated as CAUs or *cognitive–affective units*. These CAUs are interconnected within a stable network (much like a neural network, again as a metaphor) that constrains and guides their activation with pathways of activation and de-activation.

Substantively, the types of CAUs on which related theory and work has focused are based on psychological variables shown to be important in decades of past research, as proposed initially by Mischel (1973). These *person variables* include such mental–emotional representations as personal appraisals or construals (encodings) of the situation; beliefs, and expectancies (e.g., self-efficacy and outcome expectations); personal values and goals; affects (e.g., anxiety, shame, pride, eagerness); as well as evaluative self-standards, which are activated in specific situations. Particularly important for effortful control are the individual's available and accessible self-regulatory competencies. These include cognitive-attention strategies and scripts for generating diverse types of social behavior that are essential for sustained, goal-directed effort in the pursuit of difficult goals whose attainment requires impulse control and delay of gratification (Mischel & Ayduk, 2002; Mischel et al., 1996). In terms of the connectionist metaphor, the CAUs are themselves composed of activation patterns among much lower-level units (Mischel & Shoda, 1995, 1998; Shoda & Mischel, 1998). CAUs operate at multiple levels within the system and its sub-systems. These levels interact and are in part automatic and in part more deliberative, in part cognitive, and in part affective (Metcalfe & Mischel, 1999).

As in CAPS, individual differences in self-regulation are assumed to reflect both differences in the *ease of accessibility* of different CAUs (e.g., trust and efficacy expectations, self-regulatory competencies, appraisals of situations as challenging or threatening), and differences in the *stable organization* of the relationships among the CAUs. Thus, it is assumed that the CAUs are organized into distinctive idiographic networks. Each network is unique, although individuals can be grouped into types and sub-types. These types may differ both on the basis of similarities in their chronic levels of accessibility (e.g., some have higher anxious expectations for rejection, or lower fears of failure, than others) and on the basis of their organization, as will be illustrated in subsequent sections.

Figure 6.1 summarizes this model. A CAPS network is illustrated by the large circle, which consists of interconnected CAUs (shown by smaller circles). The darker the circle for a CAU the more accessible it is. The inter-connections among the CAUs may be excitatory (solid lines) or inhibitory (broken lines), and the strength of these connections differs as indicated by the darkness of the links.

Within this model, the relatively stable patterns of activation are the processing dynamics of the self-regulatory system. Situational features are encoded by CAUs, which in turn, activate a subset of mediating units that are connected to other units through a stable activation network. These situational features may be events and social stimuli that are either encountered, self-initiated (e.g., thoughts and affects activated by thinking, planning, or ruminating), or created by internal states (e.g., when hungry, or craving

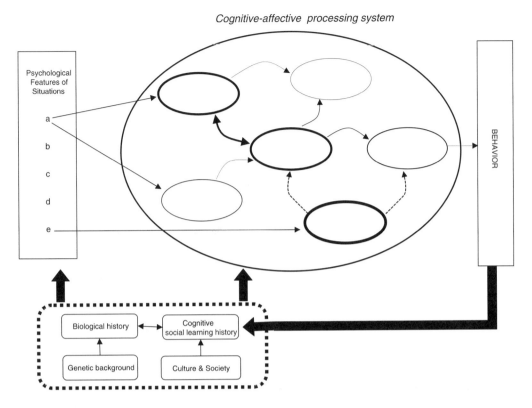

FIGURE 6.1. Illustrative self-regulatory dynamics in a cognitive–affective processing system (CAPS). Self-regulation in a CAPS network is illustrated by the large circle, and the smaller circles within it represent the cognitive–affective units (CAUs). The darker a circle, the more accessible that thought or affect is. The CAUs are inter-connected either through excitatory (solid lines) or inhibitory (broken lines); the darkness of a line indicates the strength of the association between any two CAUs. As illustrated, situational features are encoded by CAUs, which in turn activate a subset of mediating units that are inter-connected through a stable activation network. The dynamics of this network guide and constrain the individual's behavior in relation to particular situation features. The multiple influences on the CAPS network are indicated at the bottom. The system acts upon itself through a feedback loop: The behaviors that are generated influence one's subsequent experience and the social learning history, influencing the system's further development and modifying the situations encountered and generated over time.

drugs, or in other arousal states). These diverse influences may activate a contextualized construction or reconstruction process within the particular situation, rather than eliciting a retrieval of pre-existing responses or entities from storage. This reconstruction process occurs for example when the strength of the excitatory association between two CAUs is modified by a particular situation that activates one while strongly inhibiting the other. In this manner, the system becomes able to generate somewhat novel behavioral expressions; nevertheless, the preexisting dynamics of this network guide and constrain the reactions of the individual to particular features of situations. Thus the person and the situation interact reciprocally in a mutual influence process.

Development of the Self-Regulatory System

As illustrated in Figure 6.1, the CAPS network and the situational features that elicit its different aspects are assumed to develop as a function of biological and genetic predispositions as well as through the influences of the person's culture, society and idiographic social-cognitive learning history (Mischel & Shoda, 1999). Individual differences in the host of biochemical–genetic–somatic factors that influence self-regulation are conceptualized as *pre*-dispositions in this framework. The emphasis is on the "pre" to underline that these are biological precursors that may manifest themselves both directly and indirectly at multiple levels within the system and in diverse and complex forms (Grigorenko, 2002; Mischel & Shoda, 1999). These biological pre-dispositions (i.e., temperament) bias the system's development in particular directions. Nevertheless, their influences are constantly modulated by the affordances presented by the cultural, social and interpersonal contexts within which the child is situated. In particular, infant temperament and quality of parental care interact in meaningful ways in the development of effective self-regulatory mechanisms (e.g., Calkins & Fox, 2002; Kochanska, 1997). For example, children's "difficult" temperament is related to increased cortisol levels—a physiological marker of dysregulation—in the face of stress, but only in the context of poor and unresponsive adult caring (Gunnar, Larson, Hertsgaard, Harris, & Brodersen, 1992; see Gunnar & Donzella, 2002, for review).

Thus, many factors interact to influence the genesis of the person's distinctive organization, and they reflect both genetic endowment and biological history, and their interactions with social learning and developmental experiences in the course of socialization within a particular culture. Noteworthy is that the system does not merely react to the situations encountered in its course of life-long development. It also acts upon itself through a feedback loop, both by generating its own internal situations (e.g., in anticipated and planned events, in fantasy, in self-reflection), and through the behaviors that the system generates in interaction with the social world (see Figure 6.1). These behaviors (e.g., impulsive reactions, failures to carry out intentions, effective control efforts and goal pursuit) further influence the individual's social-cognitive experiences and evolving social learning history, and modify the subsequent situations encountered and generated. This way, development of the self-regulatory system becomes a life-long process of adaptation both through assimilating new stimuli into the existing CAPS network and by accommodating the network itself in response to novel or different encounters.

In the rest of this chapter, the model depicted in Figure 6.1 will be fleshed out and illustrated with research findings on delay of gratification (see Mischel, Shoda, & Rodriguez, 1989, for review) and related phenomena of willpower that exemplify its different aspects. The focus on delay of gratification reflects the fact that this program of research has data from four decades of experimental and longitudinal work that speaks both to individual differences and to basic processes that enable—or undermine—willpower or effortful self-regulation.

MOTIVATIONAL PROCESSES IN THE DECISION TO "WILL"

More than a century after James (1890) distinguished the wish or *motivation* to exert willpower in goal pursuit, and the *ability* to do so effectively, a distinction between regulatory motivation and regulatory competence is still useful because often people have one of these but not the other. This was illustrated by a recent president of the United States whose impressive abilities to self-regulate in some contexts were seen often in his skillful handling of political and foreign affairs, yet he was either unable or insufficiently motivated to apply them to himself when it came to his personal affairs to the point of impeachment (see Ayduk & Mischel, 2002, for further discussion).

First we consider the role of motivation for effortful self-regulation in the framework of the present model. The individual's response to any given situation in which effortful self-regulation may be an option begins with the encoding process in which the subjective meaning of the situation, including its self-relevance and personal importance, are appraised. The appraisal itself activates a cascade of other cognitive–affective representations within the system—expectations and beliefs, affective reactions, values and goals. These CAUs operate at multiple levels as indicated above, and interacting in a coherent organization. To illustrate, take the hungry dieter confronted with a temptingly exquisite slice of chocolate fudge cake. The motivational strength to forgo the temptation may depend on such factors as whether the person construes the cake as "unhealthy and fattening—a "threat to health and fitness" or as a great treat" to which one is entitled at the end of a long hard day. Likewise, is the affect that is triggered primarily a strong desire or an anxious concern? And what expectations about the outcome are likely to occur if the cake is eaten, and if it is bypassed? How high are the person's expectations that self-control now will pay off in better health and appearance later? How much does the person value the long-term super-ordinate goals that are served by eating healthy and being fit? Do self-regulatory behaviors like dieting serve a higher goal that is central to the self, such as being a worthy self-respecting person, or are they merely a part of a casually tried fashionable diet of the day?

Questions like these have been considered in studies of the motivational processes in self-regulation and, specifically, in the context of cross-cultural delay of gratification choice experiments that assessed people's preference patterns for larger but delayed versus smaller or less valued but immediately available rewards beginning in the 1950s (Mischel, 1961a, 1974b). Taken collectively, the findings indicated the important roles of (1) trust and control expectations about actually obtaining the delayed outcomes, and (2) the subjective relative values of the immediately available versus the temporally delayed pay-offs (Mischel, 1961b, 1974b). These person variables significantly predict whether people form the intention and make the initial decision to exert self control and, in these examples, try to delay immediate gratification for the sake of more valued but delayed rewards. To the extent that individuals trust that the delayed rewards will materialize if they put the necessary effort into it and believe that they have control over the allocation of resources they are more likely to perceive the benefits to be greater than the costs associated with delay of gratification. Perhaps as important as these expectations in determining goal commitment in delay choice is the subjective value of the delayed reward(s). Unsurprisingly, the smaller the magnitude of the delayed rewards, and the longer their temporal delay, the less people value them and are willing to wait for them in the self-delay of gratification task (Mischel & Metzner, 1962).

The motivation to delay immediate gratification for the sake of distal goals that are contingent on the individual's own efforts also depends on the activation of beliefs that one can fulfill the necessary requirements—that is, *self-efficacy beliefs* (Bandura, 1986; Mischel et al., 1996)—on which the attainment of the distal reward is contingent. For example, when self-efficacy beliefs were experimentally manipulated by giving false success/failure feedback on an unrelated performance task, participants who were given false positive feedback chose to work for the preferred but delayed contingent reward more often than the participants who were given false negative feedback (Mischel & Staub,

1965). Thus how well the participants felt that they could perform the task determined whether or not they *chose* to try for the more difficult but preferred reward. The findings on choice or preferences for delayed versus immediate gratification are consistent with the role that control expectancies and self-efficacy beliefs play in other self-regulatory contexts as well. For example, high self-efficacy beliefs lead to greater motivation to engage in health promoting behavior (Hooker & Kaus, 1992; Kaplan, Atkins, & Reinsch, 1984) and adjustment to stressful health events and procedures (Major et al., 1990).

Similarly, positive control expectancies motivate people to try to persist in the face of challenge and also improve the way they construe and behave in response to negative situations. For example, people who suffer from psychological and/or physical distress but nevertheless believe that they are capable of influencing the outcomes of their situations adjust better in response to discomfort (Averill, 1973; Miller, 1979; Rodin, 1987; Taylor, Lichtman, & Wood, 1984; Thompson, 1981) and report feeling less anxiety and distress in relation to the pain associated with their conditions (Kanfer & Seidner, 1973; Szpiler & Epstein, 1976). Conversely, people who perceive themselves as having little control over the situations they find themselves in often feel powerless and choose not to engage in adaptive forms of self-regulatory behavior (Dweck, 1986; Seligman, 1975).

In summary, findings from studies on the motivation and choice to delay gratification (i.e., goal commitment) suggest that an expectancy-subjective value mechanism underlies the initial assessments that people make regarding this decision. It is a subjective calculation of whether the value and feasibility of attaining a delayed reward relative to the value of the immediately available one is high enough to warrant their choice to wait or work to attain it. In the connectionist, network-like metaphor for the self-regulatory processing system model, self-efficacy beliefs, positive outcome and control expectations, and the subjective value of the rewards, are the CAUs that influence these decisions and intentions to commit oneself to a difficult self-regulatory goal.

FROM GOOD INTENTIONS TO WILLPOWER: OVERCOMING STIMULUS CONTROL WITH SELF-CONTROL

Goal commitment is a necessary but not a sufficient condition for goal attainment. Well-intentioned New Year's resolutions—to adhere to that diet, to forgo tobacco, to become more attentive and caring toward a partner, to persist with regular breast self-examinations—are a first step, but unless implemented by effective self-regulatory mechanisms to sustain effortful control they easily fade away when the time comes to actually exercise the will. The failure of well-motivated good intentions is documented in decades of research on the power of *stimulus control*, beginning with work on classical conditioning at the start of the last century, to the prolific studies inspired by Skinner's work on operant conditioning (e.g., Skinner, 1938) during the dominance of behaviorism, to the current resurgence of interest showing the importance and pervasiveness of *automaticity* by Bargh and colleagues (e.g., Bargh, 1997; Chartrand & Bargh, 2002). Collectively, this impressive line of research has made plain the pervasive power of the situation for eliciting prepotent responses almost reflexively without higher-order mediation and consciousness. Indeed the incisive and persuasive work of Bargh and colleagues has been so compelling that one begins to sense that the cognitive revolution is now in trouble in social and personality psychology, and in need of new defenders ready to make the case again for the power of cognitive processes against a new form of mechanistic behaviorism that may be re-emerging (see Ferguson & Bargh, 2000). The challenge to these defenders of cognition and purposeful self-regulation is to specify the processes and conditions that people can use to make them less susceptible to succumbing to the pressures and influences of the momentary situation as they attempt to pursue their long-term commitments and goals.

The next questions we address are: what are those processes and conditions in which individuals may overcome stimulus control and the pressures and temptations of the moment for the sake of more valued but delayed, or blocked, goals and outcomes? What makes it possible for some people to give up their addictions, to resist the temptations that threaten their cherished values and goals, to persist in the effort, to maintain their relationship, to overcome the more selfish motivation and take account of other people—in short, to exert "willpower"? And why do others seem to remain the victims of their own vulnerabilities and biographies?

Theoretically, in the CAPS model of self-regulation, effective pursuit of delayed rewards and difficult to attain long-term goals depends on the availability and accessibility of certain types of cognitive-attention strategies that are essential for overcoming stimulus control. Again the question has to be answered: what strategies and processes make that possible? How do they work and how can they be harnessed in the service of more constructive and effective self-regulation? Absent the availability and accessibility of such strategies, efforts to sustain delay of gratification and self-control are likely to be short-lived and the power of the immediate situation is likely to prevail and elicit the prepotent response—eat the cake, smoke the cigarette grab the money, succumb to the temptation. In contrast, in effective goal pursuit, these strategies become activated and utilized when the person tries to forgo impulsive, automatic reactions in response to immediate situational pressures and temptations for the sake of more valued but temporally delayed goals.

The Delay of Gratification Paradigm

Insights into the conditions and processes that enable effortful control have come from research in the preschool delay paradigm (Mischel, 1974a; Mischel & Baker, 1975; Mischel & Ebbesen, 1970; Mischel, Ebbesen, & Zeiss, 1972; Mischel & Moore, 1973). In this procedure, young children wait for two cookies (or other little treats) that they want and have chosen to get and which they prefer to a smaller treat, such as one cookie. They then are faced with a dilemma: they are told that the experimenter needs to leave for a while and that they can continue to wait for the larger reward until the experimenter comes back on his/her own, or they are free to ring a little bell to summon the adult at any time and immediately get the smaller treat at the expense of getting the larger preferred reward. In short, the situation creates a strong conflict between the temptation to stop the delay and take the immediately available smaller reward or to continue waiting for their original, larger, more preferred choice, albeit not knowing how long the wait will be. After children understand the situation, they are left alone in the room until they signal the experimenter. The child of course has a continuous free choice, and can resolve the conflict about whether or not to stop waiting at any time by ringing the bell, which immediately brings back the adult. If the child continues to wait, the adult returns spontaneously (after a maximum of 20 minutes).

This simple and seemingly trivial situation has turned out to be not only compelling for the young child but also surprisingly diagnostic, making it possible to significantly predict conceptually relevant and consequential long-term outcomes from the number of seconds children wait at age 4 years to diverse indices of self-regulation in goal pursuit and social–emotional cognitive competencies decades later in adulthood (e.g., Ayduk et al., 2000; Mischel et al., 1989). To illustrate, the number of seconds children can wait in certain diagnostic situations (i.e., when no regulatory strategies are provided by the experimenter and children have to access their own competencies) is significantly predictive of higher Scholastic Aptitude Test (SAT) scores and better social-cognitive, personal, and interpersonal competencies years later (Mischel, Shoda, & Peake, 1988; Shoda, Mischel, & Peake, 1990). These links between seconds of preschool delay time and adaptive life outcomes in diverse social and cognitive domains remain stable, persisting into adulthood, as discussed in later sections. Given the existence and psychological importance of the individual differences tapped in this situation it becomes important to understand what is happening psychologically that makes some children ring soon and others wait for what seems an eternity. What determines who will be under the stimulus control elicited by immediate temptations and who will be able to resist those pressures and sustain the choice to persist for the delayed rewards? We next consider the cognitive-attention control strategies that help and hurt such efforts and examine how they may play out in the proposed self-regulatory system.

Temporal Discounting

The delay of gratification paradigm for the analysis of willpower taps a phenomenon that makes effortful control especially difficult in situations when it is often most needed. It is a factor that undermines the person's motivation to keep important long-term goals in mind when faced with short-term gratifications that are immediately present. This pervasive phenomenon, found in animal species from rats to humans, is *temporal discounting* (Ainslie, 2001; Loewenstein, Read, & Baumeister, 2003; Rachlin, 2000; Trope & Liberman, 2003). Well-known to economists and philosophers as well as to psychologists, this tendency refers to the systematic discounting of the subjective value of a reward, outcome, or goal as the anticipated time delay before its expected occurrence increases. Temporal discounting is seen clearly in delay of gratification studies in the finding that the perceived subjective value of the delayed reward(s) in young children, and hence their motivation to choose to delay, decreases systematically as the length of the expected delay interval increases (Mischel, 1966, 1974b; Mischel & Metzner, 1962) as mentioned earlier. Similar findings with respect to the effect of time delays on the discounting of subjective value have long been widely documented and recognized as of central importance for understanding problems that range from the psychiatric and medical to the areas of behavioral medicine and behavioral economics (Ainslie, 2001; Loewenstein et al., 2003; Morf & Mischel, 2002; Petry, 2002; Rachlin, 2000; Wulfert, Block, Ana, Rodriguez, & Colsman, 2002). The hot/cool analysis of willpower, described next, was developed in large part to try to understand the basic mechanisms that may underlie the phenomena tapped by the delay paradigm.

Hot/Cool Systems within CAPS

Following the connectionist and parallel distributed processing neural network metaphor, two closely interacting systems—a cognitive "cool" system and an emotional "hot" system—have been proposed as components of the broader CAPS system. The interactions between these two systems are basic in the dynamics of self-regulation in general and of delay of gratification in particular and underlie the person's ability—or inability—to sustain effortful control in pursuit of delayed goals (Metcalfe & Mischel, 1999).

Briefly, the cool system is an emotionally neutral, "know" system: it is cognitive, complex, slow, and contemplative. Attuned to the informational, cognitive, and spatial aspects of stimuli, the cool system consists of a network of informational, *cool nodes* that are elaborately interconnected to each other, and generate rational, reflective, and strategic behavior. Although the specific biological roots of this system are still being explored, the cool system seems to be associated with hippocampal and frontal lobe processing (Lieberman, Gaunt, Gilbert, & Trope, 2002; Metcalfe & Mischel, 1999).

In contrast, the hot system is a "go" system. It enables quick, emotional processing: simple and fast, and thus useful for survival from an evolutionary perspective by allowing rapid flight or fight reactions, as well as necessary appetitive approach responses. The hot system consists of relatively few representations, or *hot spots* (e.g., unconditioned stimuli), which elicit virtually reflexive avoidance and approach reactions when activated by trigger stimuli. This hot system develops early in life and is the most dominant in the young infant. It is an essentially automatic system, governed by virtually reflexive stimulus–response reactions, which, unless interrupted, preclude effortful control. Although other theorists (e.g., Epstein, 1994; Lieberman, 2003) have employed somewhat different terms to describe similar sets of opponent self-regulatory processes, there is reasonable consensus that what Metcalfe and Mischel (1999) call the hot system is more affect-based relative to the cool system and generates simple, impulsive, and quick approach–avoidance responses in the presence of eliciting stimuli. The impulsive behavioral products of this system provide ample documentation for the power of stimulus control, and the formidable constraints that many hot (*affect-arousing*) situations place on a person's ability to exert willpower or volitional control. Currently, neural models of information processing suggest that the amygdala—a small, almond-shaped region in the forebrain thought to enable fight-or-flight responses—may be the seat of hot system processing (Gray, 1987; LeDoux, 1996; Metcalfe & Jacobs, 1996), but again the exact loci and circuitry remain to be mapped with increasing precision.

Consistent with a parallel-processing neural network metaphor, the hot/cool analysis assumes that cognition and affect operate in continuous interaction with one another, and emphasizes the close connections of the two sub-systems in generating phenomenological experiences as well as behavioral responses. Specifically, in the model hot spots and cool nodes that have the same external referents are directly connected to one another, and thus link the two systems (Metcalfe & Jacobs, 1996; Metcalfe & Mischel, 1999). Hot spots can be evoked by activation of corresponding cool nodes; alternately, hot representations can be cooled through inter-system connections to the corresponding cool nodes. Effortful control and willpower become possible to the extent that the cooling strategies generated by the cognitive cool system circumvents hot system activation through such inter-system connections that link hot spots to cool nodes. Thus, consequential for self-control are the conditions under which hot spots do not have access to corresponding cool representations, because these conditions are the ones that undermine or prevent cool system regulation of hot impulses.

Effects of System Maturation

Two assumptions are made about the determinants of the balance between hot and cool systems. First, this balance depends critically on the person's developmental phase. The hot system is well developed at birth, whereas the cool system develops with age. Consequently early in development the baby is primarily responsive to the pushes and pulls of hot stimuli in the external world as many of the hot spots do not have corresponding cool nodes that can regulate and inhibit hot system processing. This assumption is in line with developmental differences in the maturation rates of the biological centers for these two systems. With age and maturity, however, the cool system becomes elaborated as many more cool nodes develop and become connected to one another, thereby greatly increasing the network of cool system associations and thus the number of cool nodes corresponding to the hot spots.

Empirical evidence from the delay of gratification studies supports these expectations. Whereas delay of gratification in the paradigm described seems almost impossible—and even incomprehensible—for most children younger than 4 years of age (Mischel, l974b; Mischel & Mischel, 1983), by age 12 almost 60% of children in some studies were able to wait to criterion (25 minutes maximum; Ayduk et al., 2000, Study 2). Furthermore, the child's spontaneous use of cooling strategies such as purposeful self-distraction is positively related to both age and verbal intelligence (Rodriguez, Mischel, & Shoda, l989). By the time most children reach the age of 6 years, they are less susceptible to stimulus control from mere exposure to the desired objects facing them. As the cool system develops it becomes increasingly possible for the child spontaneously to generate diverse cognitive and attention deployment cooling strategies (e.g., self-distraction, inventing mental games to make the delay less aversive), and thus to be less controlled by whatever is salient in the immediate field of attention (Rodriguez, Mischel, & Shoda, 1989).

Effects of Stress Level

Second, the hot/cool balance depends on the stress level, which in turn depends both on the stress induced by the appraisal of the specific situation and the chronic level characteristic for the person. The theory assumes that whereas at low to moderate levels of stress cool system activation may be enhanced, at high levels it becomes attenuated and even shuts off. In contrast, the hot system becomes activated to the degree that stress is increased (Metcalfe & Jacobs, 1996; Metcalfe & Mischel, 1999). The stress level of the system reflects both individual differences in the person's chronic level of stress and the stress induced within the particular situation. Consistent with the view that high stress levels tend to attenuate the activation of the cool system, delay of gratification becomes more difficult when children experience additional psychological stress (e.g., by thinking about unhappy things that happened to them), but it becomes easier when stress is decreased, for example by priming them to "think fun" (Mischel et al., 1972). It is an ironic aspect of willpower and human nature that the cool system is most difficult to access when it is most needed.

The reader who remembers Freud's conception of the id as characterized by irrational, impulsive urges for immediate wish-fulfillment, and its battles with the rational, logical executive ego, will not fail to note their similarity to the hot and cool systems as conceptualized in contemporary thinking (e.g., Epstein, 1994; Metcalfe & Mischel, 1999). The key difference is that what has been learned from research on this topic over the course of the past century now allows us to specify more clearly the cognitive and emotional processes that underlie these two systems and their interactions to enable effective self-regulation. We consider these specific processes next, drawing on experiments conducted using the delay of gratification paradigm.

The hot/cool analysis of the dynamics of willpower summarized above was based in part on empirical evidence from the long-term research program on delay of gratification by Mischel and colleagues (e.g., see Mischel, 1974b; Mischel & Ayduk, 2002; Mischel et al., 1989, for reviews). This research provides a framework for systematically conceptualizing the processes that undermine or support the successful exertion of willpower in diverse contexts, and provides an account that seems to fit the available data reasonably well. We next consider those data and examine how they speak to the predictions and post-dictions suggested by the hot/cool analysis.

PROCESSING DYNAMICS IN DELAY OF GRATIFICATION

Mental Representation of Goals/Rewards

The experiments on mechanisms enabling delay of gratification were motivated originally by the following question, posed more than 30 years ago: how does the mental representation of deferred rewards or goals influence the person's ability to continue to wait or work for them? The question needed to be asked at that time, when behaviorism was still at its height, and because although rewards had been assigned huge power as the determinants of behavior, virtually nothing was known about how people's mental representations of them operated and influenced goal-directed behavior. Few theories or even hypotheses were available to guide the search for answers. A notable exception was Freud (1911/1959) whose writing about the transition from primary (id-based) to secondary (ego-based) processes famously theorized that the ability to endure delay of gratification begins to develop when the young child can construct a "hallucinatory wish-fulfilling image" of the wished-for but delayed object. In Freud's view, this mental image or representation of the object of desire (e.g., the maternal breast) makes it possible for the child to "bind time" and come to sustain delay of gratification volitionally.

If so, Mischel and colleagues reasoned, sustained delay behavior in goal pursuit ought to be facilitated by cues that make the delayed rewards more salient and thus more available for mental representation. Similar expectations came from a second, unexpected source, in the research on learning with animals. Struggling with the question of how a rat manages to keep running to get its rewards later at the end of all those complicated mazes, learning psychologists theorized that behavior toward a goal may be maintained by "fractional anticipatory goal responses" (Hull, 1931). While eschewing the language of cognition, the concept implied some kind of partial representation of the goal as a necessary condition for maintaining the animal's goal pursuit, for example, as the animal in a learning task tries to find its way back to the food at the end of a maze. In this sense, extrapolating to the young child, anticipation and self-instructions through which the delayed rewards are made salient should sustain delay behavior in pursuit of those rewards because it makes them easier to keep in mind and anticipate the gratification of having them. In short, collectively these views from utterly different literatures suggested that focusing attention on the delayed rewards should facilitate delay of gratification.

To explore this hypothesis and to approximate the presence versus absence of mental representations of the delayed rewards, a series of experiments varied whether or not the reward objects in the choice were available for attention while the children tried to keep waiting for them (Mischel & Ebbesen, 1970). For example, in one condition, both the delayed and immediately available rewards were exposed, whereas in another condition both the delayed and immediate rewards were concealed from children's attention. In the remaining two groups, either the delayed or the immediate rewards were exposed while the other rewards were concealed. Rather than enhancing children's delay time as was initially hypothesized by both psychodynamic and learning theories, having rewards available for attention in any combination (i.e., whether both were available or just one) dramatically reduced children's wait time.

When first obtained, these results were the opposite of what was predicted, but in retrospect, when viewed from a hot/cool systems framework, they are exactly as expected. Presumably availability of the rewards for attention increases their salience, making their consummatory, "hot" representations more accessible. This in turn, intensifies the conflict between the stimulus pull of the immediate situation (i.e., to ring the bell and get the small reward) and the desirability of the future goal (i.e., getting the larger, preferred reward), thereby increasing the child's level of frustration or stress. Under such hot system activation, it is harder to resist stimulus control, and most children reverse their initial preference, ring the bell, and settle for the less desired outcome. When the rewards are obscured from sight, however, the conflict and the frustration inherent in the delay situation is diminished, making "willpower" much less difficult, and enabling children to wait longer (Mischel, 1974b). Theoretically, when attention is not focused on the tempting reward stimuli, corresponding hot nodes are less likely to become activated, making sustained delay of gratification less effortful.

By the same rationale, moving attention away from the rewards altogether as in the use of distraction strategies even when the rewards are physically present in the environment should also prevent hot system activation and make the delay situation less difficult to endure for the child. In testing this idea, Mischel and colleagues (1972) provided children experimentally with external or internal distracters. In some conditions preschoolers were given a little toy to play with; in others they were primed with self-distracting pleasant thoughts (e.g., thinking about Mommy pushing them on a swing), or they were not given any distracters while they faced the rewards. Such self-distraction made it much easier for the children to wait (regardless of whether the distracters were external or internal), and they did so readily even though the rewards were available for attention and staring them in the face. The successful dieter who resists the desserts on the tray will not be surprised by these results.

But whereas these results showed the effects of attention to the exposed actual rewards, they still left open the more basic question: what is the effect of their internal *mental* representation? Might it be possible to represent the same stimulus in alternate ways? Foreshadowing the hot/cool formal theory by more than 30 years, a distinction had been made in the research literature between the motivational (the consummatory, arousing, action-oriented, or motivating "go" features) and the informational (cognitive cue) functions of a stimulus (Berlyne, 1960; Estes, 1972). Drawing on this distinction, Mischel and Moore (1973) reasoned that the actual rewards, or their mental representations by the child as real, puts the child's attention on the hot, arousing, consummatory features of the rewards (whether the immediately available or the delayed ones), and hence elicits the motivational effects (the "go" response: ring the bell, get the treat now). In contrast, a focus on the more cool, abstract, cue features of the rewards might have the effect of reminding the child of the delayed consequences without activating the consummatory trigger reaction, typically elicited by a focus on the motivating hot features. For example, the mental representation of the rewards as pictures emphasizes their cognitive, informational features rather than their consummatory features. Therefore, Mischel and Moore speculated that this kind of cool focus may reduce the conflict between wanting to wait and wanting to ring the bell by shifting attention away from arousing features of the stimulus and on to their informative meaning.

Hot/Cool Representations

Methodologically, the challenge was how to find operations for activating a mental representation at a time when the cognitive revolution was still in its infancy and even the concept of mental representations was still regarded suspiciously. To move beyond the effects of the actual stimulus and try to approximate their mental representations, a first step was to present the rewards in the form of *images*—literally, life-size pictures (formally, "iconic representations") of the immediate and delayed rewards presented from a slide projector on a screen facing the child. These pictorial representations were pitted against the presence of the real rewards themselves during the delay period. As predicted, the results were the opposite of those found when the real rewards were exposed: exposure to the pictures of the images of the rewards significantly increased children's waiting time whereas exposure to the actual rewards decreased delay (Mischel & Moore, 1973).

Again in retrospect, these findings are consistent with those expected from the hot/cool system analysis. The slide-presented images of the desired objects (in contrast to the actual objects) are more likely to activate cool nodes that correspond to inherently hot stimuli and attenuate the hot system. Recall that the cool nodes are conceptualized as representing informational, cognitive, and spatial aspects of stimuli. A pictorial depiction of the rewards, of a little stick of pretzel of the sort used in the studies, for example, is likely to activate a cool representation, in sharp contrast to the effects of facing the actual temptations.

Mischel and colleagues speculated that what is true for pictorial representations also should apply to diverse other forms of cognitive, cool appraisals of the "objects of desire" that might activate corresponding cool nodes for the rewards in the delay of gratification paradigm. Consequently, if the actual rewards could be construed in such a way that they psychologically become cool, for example by thinking of them as pictures rather than real, it should help the child to reduce the frustration of the delay situation cognitively rather than being at the mercy of external situational cues.

To examine this prediction, children were faced with actual rewards but this time were cued in advance by the experimenters to pretend that they were pictures by essentially "putting a frame around them in your head" (Moore, Mischel, & Zeiss, 1976). In a second condition, the children were shown pictures of the rewards but this time asked to imagine them as though they were real. Children were able to delay almost 18 minutes when they pretended that the rewards facing them were not real, but pictures. In contrast, they were able to wait for less than 6 minutes if they pretended that the real rewards, rather than the pictures, were in front of them. Theoretically, in the former group, the children were able to exert willpower by mentally activating cool nodes that corresponded to the hot stimulus in front of them (i.e., by cognitively transforming a real treat into "just a picture"). In post-tests that asked about why they waited so long, as one child put it "you can't eat a picture."

The transformations of hot, motivating representations into cool, informative ones to facilitate willpower in the delay situation also were demonstrated by Mischel and Baker (1975). In this study, children in one condition were cued with cool, informational or hot, consummatory representations of the rewards during the delay task. For example, children who were waiting for marshmallows were cued to think of them as "white, puffy clouds." Those waiting for pretzels were told to think of them as "little, brown logs." In a second hot ideation condition, the instructions cued children to think about the marshmallows as "yummy, and chewy" and the pretzels as "salty and crunchy." As expected, when children thought about the rewards in hot terms, they were able to wait only for 5 minutes, whereas when they thought about them in cool terms, delay time increased to 13 minutes.

Summary: Attention Control in the Delay Process

Taking these findings collectively, it became clear that delay of gratification depends not on whether or not attention is focused on the objects of desire, but rather on just how they are mentally represented. A focus on their hot features may momentarily increase motivation, but unless it is rapidly cooled by a focus on their cool, informative features (e.g., as reminders of what will be obtained later if the contingency is fulfilled) it is likely to become excessively arousing and trigger the "go" response.

While most of the delay of gratification experiments have involved passive waiting in order to obtain the preferred outcomes, the same mechanisms of attention deployment seem to apply when goal attainment is contingent on the person's work and performance. This was demonstrated recently in experiments in which children were required to complete a work task instead of passively waiting for the experimenter to return in order to get the larger but delayed rewards. Attention focused on the rewards undermined delay of gratification in both working and waiting situations, thus extending the generalizability of the attention control mechanisms that enable such effortful control (Peake, Hebl, & Mischel, 2002).

Flexible Attention Deployment and Discriminative Facility

Studies conducting fine-grain analyses of second by second attention deployment during efforts at sustained delay of gratification suggest that self-regulation depends not just on cooling strategies but on *flexible attention deployment* in the process (Peake et al., 2002). For example, Peake and colleagues' (2002) study on delay in working situations showed that delay ability was facilitated most when attention intermittently shifted to the rewards, as if the children tried to enhance their motivation to remain by reminding themselves about the rewards, but then quickly shifted away to prevent arousal from becoming excessive. Such flexibility in attention deployment is consistent with the view that it is the balanced interactions between the hot and cool systems that sustain delay of gratification and effortful control, as they exert their motivating and cooling effects in tandem (see also Rodriguez, Mischel, & Shoda, 1989).

Evidence that flexible attention deployment is important for effective self-regulation also is consistent with findings showing the role of *discriminative facility* in self-regulation. Discriminative facility refers to the individual's ability to perceive the subtly different demands and opportunities of different kinds of situations, and to flexibly adjust coping strategies accordingly. A good deal of research now documents that discriminative facility is basic for adaptive social and emotional coping in diverse contexts (Cantor & Kihlstrom, 1987; Cheng, Chiu, Hong, & Cheung, 2001; Chiu, Hong, Mischel, & Shoda, 1995; Mendoza-Denton, Ayduk, Mischel, Shoda, & Testa, 2001; Shoda, Mischel, & Wright, 1993).

The types of cooling strategies in these studies with preschoolers are of course only illustrative of the many adaptive ways to maintain long-term goal pursuit and to overcome stimulus control with agentic self-control. The important point is that diverse, creative cooling strategies can be constructed by the cool system, if it can be accessed before automatic impulsive action is triggered by the hot system that preempts the person from thinking rationally and creatively. In formal terms, goal pursuit in delay of gratification depends both on the activation of motivational processes as discussed earlier in this chapter, and on the accessibility and activation of the necessary cooling strategies. It depends on the network of organization connecting the motivational processes that lead to choice and goal commitment, to the activation and generation of cooling strategies. When these strategies are accessed they serve to reduce the hot stimulus pull and the frustration aroused in the situation, so that hopeful wishing can be transformed into effective willing.

Automaticity: Taking the Effort out of Effortful Control

In order for these adaptive control efforts in the hot system/cool system interactions to be maintained over time and accessed rapidly when they are urgently needed, they have to be converted from conscious, slow and effortful to automatic activation, in this sense taking the effort out of "effortful self-control." The conversion process that enables the person to go from good intentions to effective action and goal attainment has been most extensively addressed by Gollwitzer and colleagues in their research on *implementation plans* (see Gollwitzer, 1999; Patterson & Mischel, 1975). Individuals can avoid succumbing to stimulus control by planning out and rehearsing their "implementation intentions" for difficult goal pursuit. These plans specify in detail the various steps needed to protect the person from the obstacles, frustrations, and temptations likely to be encountered, keeping in mind and in awareness the demands of the current goal that is being pursued (Gollwitzer, 1999).

When planned and rehearsed, implementation intentions help self-control because goal-directed action is initiated relatively automatically when the relevant trigger cues become situationally salient. Implementation intentions help self-regulation across a wide range of regulatory tasks such as action initiation (e.g., I will start writing the paper the day after Thanksgiving), inhibition of unwanted habitual responses (e.g., when the dessert menu is served, I will not order the chocolate cake), and resistance to temptation (e.g., whenever the distraction arises, I will ignore it). In short, Gollwitzer's work indicates that some effortful, deliberative process of linking action plans to specific situational triggers (the "ifs") is needed in the initial phases of automatization. But after this link has been established and rehearsed, effective self-regulatory behavior and cool system strategies can be activated and generated much more readily, even under stressful or cognitively busy situations, without conscious effort. That is, if the specified situational cue remains highly activated, the planned behavior will run off automatically when the actual cue is encountered (Gollwitzer, 1999).

Stability and Meaningfulness of Individual Differences in Self-Regulatory Competencies

There is increasing evidence for the long-term stability and predictive value of individual differences in the self-regulatory competencies assessed in the delay of gratification paradigm early in life. As noted earlier, the number of seconds that preschoolers at age 4 years delayed gratification in the diagnostic condition of the delay paradigm described earlier significantly predicted such outcomes as their SAT scores and ratings of their social–emotional and cognitive competencies in adolescence (Mischel, Shoda, & Peake, 1988; Shoda et al., 1990). Likewise, in further follow-up studies preschool delay times predicted such outcomes as the attained educational level and use of cocaine-crack when the participants are about 27 years old (Ayduk et al., 2000).

Recently, the early antecedents of the ability to delay gratification in preschool, which are visible already in the toddler's behavior, also have been explored. They are meaningfully expressed in the ways in which the toddler deals with the delay of gratification demands produced by brief maternal separation in attachment studies using the Strange Situation (Sethi, Mischel, Aber, Shoda, & Rodriguez, 2000). Thus the same cooling attention control mechanisms demonstrated to be effective in preschool children appear to be visible in the toddler at 18 months and have been linked to delay behavior at age 4 years (Sethi et al., 2000). Further, these mechanisms also have been shown to apply in diverse populations in middle school years, and to have meaningful correlates supporting their validity as predictors of diverse adaptive social, cognitive, and emotional outcomes (Ayduk et al., 2000; Rodriguez, Mischel, & Shoda, 1989).

Individual differences in the types of self-regulatory behavior tapped in the delay paradigm may be related to distinct patterns of neural and biological reactivity as well as to aspects of temperament visible in early childhood (e.g., Derryberry, 2002; Derryberry & Rothbart, 1997; Rothbart, Derryberry, & Posner, 1994). For example, a number of studies have shown that the reactivity of the neural circuitry embedded in the limbic system, which underlies people's appetitive and defensive motivational systems, can be modulated by an executive attention control system that is sensitive to effortful intentions (Derryberry & Reed, 2002; Eisenberg, Fabes, Guthrie, & Reiser, 2000). This executive system, believed to be located in the anterior cingulate, appears to be related to the regulation of motivational impulses through "attention flexibility" and is assumed to contribute to the development of the ability to delay gratification, among a variety of other important developmental processes (Derryberry & Rothbart, 1997). It is tempting to speculate that the effective, flexible attention control that seems basic for the ability to delay gratification in goal pursuit also should be related to the neural circuitry that underlies the anterior attention system. To our knowledge, however, no empirical study to date has directly tested this assumptions and it seems important to explore those potential connections.

COOLING STRATEGIES IN EMOTION REGULATION: DEALING WITH DIVERSE AVERSIVE HOT SITUATIONS

The strategies that help people deal with the control of appetitive impulses as in the delay situation also apply to emotional self-regulation for dealing with aversive hot situations and dilemmas, including those produced by one's own vulnerabilities and negative emotions (e.g., fears of abandonment and rejection) in diverse interpersonal contexts. Experimental research reported years ago that an attitude of detachment helps people react more calmly when exposed to gory scenes portraying bloody accidents and death (Koriat, Melkman, Averill, & Lazarus, 1972) or when expecting electric shock (Holmes & Houston, 1974). Since then, experiments have helped to specify further the processes that allow people to regulate their negative emotions. In a typical study to probe the underlying processes in emotion regulation, Gross (1998) brings participants into the laboratory and informs them that they will be watching a movie. The film they will see shows detailed close up views of severe burn victims or of an arm amputation. Participants then are divided into different groups and given different instructions prior to viewing the film. For example, in one condition (called "cognitive reappraisal"), they are asked to use a cooling strategy, and to try to think about the movie in a detached unemotional way, objectively, focusing attention on the technical details of the event, not feeling anything personally (e.g., pretend that you're a teacher in medical school).

In terms of the present model, this is a cognitive cooling strategy, similar to the preschoolers' trying to think about the real treats facing them as if they were "just pictures" or by focusing on their cool rather than hot qualities. As predicted, Gross's results supported the value of the cooling strategy. Cooling enabled adaptive regulation of negative emotions better than either a control condition (in which participants are simply asked to watch the movie), or a suppression condition in which they were asked to try to hide their emotional reactions to the film as they watched it so that anyone seeing them would not know that they were feeling anything at all. The cooling strategy by means of cognitive reappraisal was a much more adaptive way to regulate negative emotions, as seen in measures of the intensity of people's negative experiences as well as in their levels of physiological autonomic nervous system arousal and distress. Thus individuals who are cued to think about the movie in a way that cools the emotional content experienced fewer feelings of disgust and less physiological activation (evidenced by less blood vessel constriction) when compared to those who attempted to completely hide and suppress their emotional responses to the film faces (Gross, 1998; see also Richards & Gross, 1999, 2000).

A word of clarification is due however about the distinction between our conceptualization self-distraction as an effective self-regulatory strategy and emotional suppression as viewed by Gross and thought suppression as discussed by Wegner (1994). Self-distraction of the kind we propose involves strategically moving attention away from hot information while actively attending to cool aspects of the situation in a way that creates "psychological distance." In this sense, it is different both from thought suppression where one simply tries to avoid thinking about an unwanted thought and emotional suppression where the individual is merely asked to not reveal his/her affective reactions without an alternative stimulus on which attention can be purposefully focused. Indeed, research on thought suppression indicates that when people are provided with focused distraction strategies (i.e., are given an alternative thought to focus on every time the to-be-suppressed idea comes to mind) they are buffered against the typical rebound effect (Wegner, Schneider, Carter, & White, 1987).

A good deal of related research further supports the conclusion that self-distraction, when possible, can be an excellent way to reduce unavoidable stresses like unpleasant medical examinations (Miller, 1987) and coping with severe life crises (Bonanno, 2001; Bonanno, Keltner, Holen, & Horowitz, 1995; Taylor & Brown, 1988). Self-distraction (e.g., watching travel slides or recalling pleasant memories) increases tolerance of experimentally-induced physical pain (e.g., Berntzen, 1987; Chaves & Barber, 1974). Similarly, distracting and relaxation-inducing activities such as listening to music reduce anxiety in the face of uncontrollable shocks (Miller, 1979), help people cope with the daily pain of rheumatoid arthritis (Affleck, Urrows, Tennen, & Higgins, 1992) and even with severe life crises (e.g., Taylor & Brown, 1988). Minimization of negative affect and instead being engaged in everyday tasks following the death of a spouse predicted minimal grief symptoms more than a year after the loss (Bonanno et al., 1995).

Cooling strategies as illustrated by re-construal mechanisms can also help one to transform potentially stressful situations to make them less aversive. For example, if surgical patients are encouraged to re-construe their hospital stay as a vacation to relax a while from the stresses of daily life, they show better postoperative adjustment (Langer, Janis, & Wolfer, 1975), just as chronically ill patients who reinterpret their conditions more positively also show better adjustment (Carver, Pozo, Harris, & Noriega, 1993). In sum, when stress and pain are inevitable, the adage to look for the silver lining and to "accentuate the positive" seems wise.

IMPLICATIONS OF EFFORTFUL CONTROL FOR COPING WITH PERSONAL VULNERABILITIES AND INTERPERSONAL DIFFICULTIES

Most of the delay of gratification studies have focused on conflicts between immediately available smaller rewards and delayed larger outcomes in essentially simple "less now" versus "more later" dilemmas. Similar psychological processes, however, underlie the subtler interpersonal conflicts that threaten to undermine many human relationships both in the work place and in intimate relations. Good intentions to maintain harmony and to work cooperatively toward common goals all too often are sabotaged by the explosion of anger, hostility, and jealousy within the daily tensions of life. It is in the heat of the moment that the need to inhibit hot, automatic—potentially destructive—reactions becomes most difficult in interpersonal relationships, particularly when those relationships are of high importance to the self.

These situations often create conflicts between the tendency to make immediate, self-centered responses, as opposed to focusing on the long-term consequences and implications for the partner and the preservation of the relationship itself (e.g., Arriaga & Rusbult, 1998). In the present model of self-regulation, a constructive approach to such conflicts requires cooling hot system activation by accessing cooling strategies that allow the long-term goals to be pursued, so that " . . . immediate, self-interested preferences are replaced by preferences that take into account broader concerns, including considerations to some degree that transcend the immediate situation" (Arriaga & Rusbult, 1998, p. 928). Basically, to attain interpersonal accommodation requires delay of gratification—making and sustaining a choice between immediate but smaller self-interest and a delayed but larger interest (larger in the sense that it is good both for the self and for the relationship).

Supporting this analysis, evidence suggests that cooling attention control processes that underlie delay ability also help in the regulation of defensive reactions in interpersonal contexts. To illustrate, we explored the hypothesis that delay ability serves as a protective buffer against the interpersonal vulnerability of *rejection sensitivity* or RS. Viewed from a CAPS perspective, RS is a chronic processing disposition characterized by anxious expectations of rejection (Downey & Feldman, 1996) and a readiness to encode even ambiguous events in interpersonal situations (e.g., partner momentarily seems inattentive) as indicators of rejection that rapidly trigger automatic hot reactions (e.g., hostility–anger, withdrawal–depression, self-silencing (Ayduk et al., 1999, 2002, 2003). Probably rooted in prior rejection experiences, these dynamics are readily activated when high RS people encounter interpersonal situations in which rejection is a possibility, triggering in them a sense of threat and foreboding. In such a state, the person's defensive, fight-or-flight system is activated, and attention narrows on detection of threat-related cues, which in turn makes the high RS person ready to perceive the threatening outcome—and to engage in behaviors (e.g., anger, hostility, exit threats) likely to ultimately confirm their worst fears by wrecking the relationship (Downey, Freitas, Michaelis, & Khouri, 1998). Repeated rejection and disillusionment with relationships tend to erode self-worth, and low self-esteem is a common characteristic of people high in RS.

In short, RS may predispose vulnerable individuals to react in automatic and reflexive impulsive hot ways, rather than engage in reflective, goal-oriented, or instrumental responses in interpersonal interactions. According to our self-regulatory processing model, however, whether this characteristic pattern unfolds or not should depend on the availability of self-regulatory competencies. To the extent that high RS individuals are capable of accessing the strategies that enable them to attenuate negative arousal, they may be able to inhibit some of their destructive behavioral patterns.

These theoretically expected processing dynamics are depicted in Figure 6.2. Panel A shows a high RS network in which potential trigger features (e.g., partner seems bored and distracted) activate anxious rejection expectations and are encoded as rejection which quickly activates hot thoughts ("she doesn't love me anymore") and negative affect. Attention control and cooling strategies are relatively inaccessible and/or have weak inhibitory links to the RS dynamics, allowing this vulnerability to have an unmediated effect on eliciting destructive behavior. In contrast, Panel B depicts a high RS network where attention control and cooling strategies are highly accessible and de-activate the RS dynamics via strong inhibitory links so that the event is not encoded as rejection, and hot thoughts and feelings are inhibited. Consequently the individual's dispositional vulnerability—the tendency to behave in a destructive manner—is attenuated and the negative consequences of this disposition are circumvented.

To explore these expectations empirically, in one set of studies self-regulatory ability was assessed by measuring the child's waiting time in the delay of gratification situation at age 4 years (Ayduk et al., 2000, Study 1). This longitudinal study showed that among vulnerable (high RS) individuals, the number of seconds participants were able to wait as preschoolers in the delay situation predicted their adult resiliency against the potentially destructive effects of RS. That is, high RS adults who had high delay ability in preschool had more positive functioning (high self-esteem, self-worth, and coping ability) compared with similarly high RS adults who were not able to delay in preschool. Furthermore, high RS participants showed higher levels of cocaine-crack use and lower levels of education than those low in RS, only if they were unable to delay gratification in preschool. That is, high RS people who had high preschool delay ability had relatively lower levels of drug use and higher education levels, and in these respects were similar to low RS participants.

A similar pattern of results was found in a second study with middle school children from a different cohort and from a very different socio-economic and ethnic population (Ayduk et al., 2000, Study 2). Namely, whereas high RS children with low delay ability were more aggressive toward their peers and thus had less positive peer relationships than children low in RS, high RS children who were able to delay longer were even less aggressive and more liked by their peers than low RS children. Consistent with the moderating role of delay ability in the RS dynamics, a cross-sectional study of preadolescents boys with behavioral problems characterized by heightened hostile reactivity to potential interpersonal threats also showed that the spontaneous use of cooling strategies in the delay task (that is, looking away from the rewards and self-distraction) predicted reduced verbal and physical aggression (Rodriguez, Mischel, Shoda, & Wright, 1989).

In a more direct experimental test of the effect of hot and cool systems on hostile reactivity to rejection, college students imagined an autobiographical rejection experience focusing either on their physiological and emotional reactions during the experience (hot ideation) or contextual features of the physical setting where this experience happened (cool ideation). In a subsequent lexical decision task, hostility and anger words were less accessible to those individuals primed with cool ideation than those primed with hot ideation. More important, this was true for both high RS and low RS participants. The same

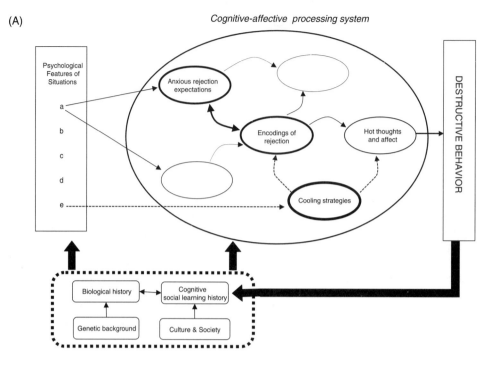

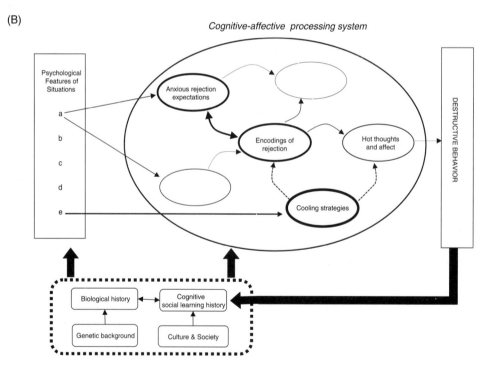

FIGURE 6.2. Interactions between attention control and rejection sensitivity (RS) in the CAPS network. (A) A high-RS network where attention control and cooling strategies are relatively inaccessible and/or weakly connected, through inhibitory links, to the RS dynamics, allowing them to have an unmediated effect on eliciting destructive behavior. (B) A high-RS network where attention control and cooling strategies are highly accessible and connect to the RS dynamics via strong inhibitory links, attenuating the individual's tendency to behave in a destructive manner.

pattern of anger reduction in the cool condition was found in people's self-report measures of angry mood and in the level of angry affect expressed in their descriptions of the rejection experience (Ayduk, Mischel, & Downey, 2002).

In sum, these correlational and experimental findings, taken collectively, suggest that how high RS translates into behavior over the course of development depends on the accessibility of self-regulatory competencies like those tapped by the delay of gratification paradigm. In the present model the extent to which an individual is likely to engage in the destructive interpersonal behavior to which the RS vulnerability readily leads depends on the connection—or lack of connection—between the activation of the RS dynamic and the activation of the relevant attention control strategies. If these two subsystems are inter-connected within the network's organization, the cooling strategies can modulate the hot reactivity of the RS dynamic, as illustrated by Figure 6.2, and the individual may be protected against the maladaptive behavioral consequences of this vulnerability.

What is true for the RS vulnerability also may apply to diverse other dispositional vulnerabilities. A growing body of research is examining similar interaction patterns between self-regulation competencies and other personality variables for diverse set of behavioral outcomes. To illustrate, Derryberry and Reed (2002) report that attention control (measured by a self-report measure of flexible shifting and focusing of attention) helps regulate attention biases of high anxious individuals in processing threat-related information. Whereas anxious individuals with poor attention control show a bias to focus on threat-related cues, anxious participants with good attention control are better able to shift their attention away from threat information, showing the buffering effects of attention control on trait anxiety. Consistently, Eisenberg and colleagues find that dispositional negative emotionality and attention control predict children's social functioning both additively and multiplicatively (see Eisenberg, Fabes, Guthrie, & Reiser, 2002, for review). More specifically, children high in negative emotionality and low in attention control seem to be at greatest risk for difficulties with peers, and externalizing as well as internalizing problems, while high regulation seems to buffer against the effect of negative emotionality on problem behaviors.

CONCLUDING REMARKS

We have argued that in the CAPS model of self-regulation, willpower requires the joint operation of regulatory motivation and competencies. Whereas strength of desire, and goal commitment, are necessary first steps in order to be able to sustain those intentions to completion, often under hot, frustrating, temptation-filled conditions, the individual has to rapidly access and flexibly utilize certain cognitive-attention deployment strategies whose key ingredients we have attempted to articulate. Furthermore, the interaction between motivation and competencies is not a one-time serial process, nor is there only one choice to be made (e.g., when the individual decides whether or not to delay gratification in the first place). Rather the process of sustaining effortful control plays out over time, as choices shift when the experience proves to be more difficult than initially anticipated, and as the power of the situation exerts its effect. In a connectionist, dynamic view of self-regulation, motivational and cognitive-attention control processes operate simultaneously and in a mutually recursive manner: the strength and commitment to one's long-term goals, and their importance within the goal hierarchies of the total system, affect how much effort may be expended in utilizing available self-regulatory skills. At the same time, utilization of attention control mechanisms and the subsequent inhibition of hot system processing helps one to stay committed to the initial goal by making all the relevant CAUs—self-efficacy beliefs, control expectancies, value of the goal and so on—highly salient and accessible.

To reiterate, for the effortful control processes necessary to maintain willpower to be accessed rapidly when they are urgently needed, and maintained over time, they have to be converted from conscious, slow and effortful to automatic activation, in this sense taking the effort out of "effortful self-control." Fortunately, as reviewed earlier in this chapter, the processes that enable this conversion (e.g., through planning and rehearsal) have become increasingly clear (see Gollwitzer, 1999; Patterson & Mischel, 1975).

We also want to re-emphasize that effective self-regulation and adaptive coping depend on the particulars of the continuous interactions between the motivating effects of the emotional, hot system and the strategic competencies enabled by the cognitive, cool system, not on the predominance of either system with the shut down of the other. It is true that in many situations in which the person wants to exercise self-control and finds it most difficult to do so, the hot system is activated by the situational pressures of the moment (the tempting pastry tray is in one's face) and cooling strategies may be urgently needed—at least some of the time. But it would be a misreading to think that adaptive goal pursuit is served by shutting down the hot system altogether and having the cool system prevail.

At the level of brain research, the work of Damasio and colleagues documents in detail the importance of both systems and their continuous interactions (e.g., Bechara, Damasio, Damasio, & Lee, 1999). For example, their somatic marker hypothesis suggests that both the ventromedial prefrontal cortex (VMF; a "cool system" structure in our conceptualization) and the amygdala (locus of the "hot" system) are essential parts of a neural circuitry that is necessary for advantageous decision making. In the "gambling tasks" in these studies, subjects choose between decks of cards that yield either immediate or delayed gratification (i.e., high immediate gain but larger future loss vs. lower immediate gain but a smaller future loss). Although we cannot elaborate the details here, briefly these studies show how both the patients with damage to the VMF and those with damage to the amygdala make disadvantageous decisions in the gambling game (i.e., choose immediate gratification), but this is the consequence of different kinds of impairments. Patients with amygdala damage cannot effectively experience somatic (emotional states) either after winning or losing money, and never develop conditioned affective reactions (i.e., increased skin conductance reflecting high arousal); subsequently, the potential impact of this kind of somatic information on decision making is precluded. VMF patients on the other hand, show somatic states in response to reward and punishment but they cannot integrate all of this information in an effective and coherent manner; thus, the somatic states (although experienced) cannot be used as feedback in subsequent decision making. These studies make it clear that patients who have impairment in what we call the hot system, as opposed to those with damage in the cool system, both encounter serious problems with delay behavior: clearly we need both systems and their interactions to make the choice to delay gratification for a larger yet distal good and to sustain effort toward its attainment.

Years ago, a distinguished humanist, Lionel Trilling (1943) also addressed both the gains and losses that either the absence or the excess of willpower can yield. After noting the place of passion in life and "the strange paradoxes of being human," he emphasized that "the will is not everything," and spoke of the "panic and emptiness which make their onset when the will is tired from its own excess" (p. 139). Excessively postponing gratification can become a stifling, joyless choice, but an absence of will leaves people the victims of their biographies. Often the choice to delay or not is difficult, yet in the absence of the competencies needed to sustain delay and to exercise the will when there is a wish to do so, the choice itself is lost.

In this chapter we have tried to show that while many of the ingredients of willpower, and particularly the processing dynamics that enable regulatory competence and delay of gratification, have long been mysterious, some of the essentials now are becoming clear. Self-regulatory ability assessed in the delay of gratification paradigm reflects stable individual differences in regulatory strength that are visible early in life and cut across different domains of behavior (e.g., eating, attachment, aggression). Much is also known about the basic attention control mechanisms that underlie and govern this self-regulatory competence. These control rules help to demystify willpower and point to the processes that enable it. Further, the implications of regulatory ability—or its lack—for the self are straightforward, influencing self-concepts and self-esteem, interpersonal strategies (e.g., aggression), coping, and the ability to buffer or protect the self against the maladaptive consequences of chronic personal vulnerabilities such as rejection sensitivity.

An urgent question remains unanswered: can self-regulation and the ability to delay gratification be taught? We already know that attention control strategies are experimentally modifiable (Ayduk et al., 2002; Mischel et al., 1989). Also, modeling effective control strategies can have positive consequences, generalizing to behavior outside of the lab in the short run for at least a period of a month or so (Bandura & Mischel, 1965). What we do not know yet is whether—and how—socialization, education, and therapy can effectively be utilized to help individuals gain the necessary attention control competencies to make willpower more accessible when they need and want it. For both theoretical and practical reasons it is time to pursue this question. We hope the answers will turn out to be affirmative—and not too long delayed.

ACKNOWLEDGMENTS

The preparation of this chapter was supported by Grant No. MH39349 from the National Institute of Mental Health. We would like to thank Ethan Kross for his constructive comments on several drafts of this chapter.

REFERENCES

Ainslie, G. (2001). *Breakdown of will*. Cambridge, UK: Cambridge University Press.

Affleck, G., Urrows, S., Tennen, H., & Higgins, P. (1992). Daily coping with pain from rheumatoid arthritis: Patterns and correlates. *Pain, 51,* 221–229.

Arriaga, X. B., & Rusbult, C. E. (1998). Standing in my partner's shoes: Partner perspective taking and reactions to accommodative dilemmas. *Personality and Social Psychology Bulletin, 24,* 927–948.

Averill, J. R. (1973). Personal control over aversive stimuli and its relationship to stress. *Psychological Bulletin, 80,* 286–315.

Ayduk, O., Downey, G., Testa, A., Yen, Y., & Shoda, Y. (1999). Does rejection sensitivity elicit hostility in rejection sensitive women? *Social Cognition, 17,* 245–271.

Ayduk, O., May, D., Downey, G., & Higgins, T. (2003). Tactical differences in coping with rejection sensitivity: The role of prevention pride. *Personality and Social Psychology Bulletin, 29,* 435–448.

Ayduk, O., Mendoza-Denton, R., Mischel, W., Downey, G., Peake, P., & Rodriguez, M. L. (2000). Regulating the interpersonal self: Strategic self-regulation for coping with rejection sensitivity. *Journal of Personality and Social Psychology, 79,* 776–792.

Ayduk, O., & Mischel, W. (2002). When smart people behave stupidly: Inconsistencies in social and emotional intelligence. In R. J. Sternberg (Ed.), *Why smart people can be so stupid* (pp. 86–105). New Haven, CT: Yale University Press.

Ayduk, O., Mischel, W., & Downey, G. (2002). Attentional mechanisms lining rejection to hostile reactivity: The role of the "hot" vs. "cool" focus. *Psychological Science, 13,* 443–448.

Bandura, A. (1986). *Social foundations of thought and action: A social cognitive theory.* Englewood Cliffs, NJ: Prentice-Hall.

Bandura, A., & Mischel, W. (1965). Modification of self-imposed delay of reward through exposure to live and symbolic models. *Journal of Personality and Social Psychology, 2,* 698–705.

Bargh, J. A. (1997). The automaticity of everyday life. In R. S. Wyer, Jr. (Ed.), *The automaticity of everyday life: Advances in social cognition* (Vol. 10, pp. 1–61). Mahwah, NJ: Erlbaum.

Baumann, N., & Kuhl, J. (2002). Intuition, affect, and personality: Unconscious coherence judgments and self-regulation of negative affect. *Journal of Personality and Social Psychology, 83,* 1213–1223.

Bechara, A., Damasio, H., Damasio, A. R., & Lee, G. (1999). Different contributions of the human amygdala and ventromedial prefrontal cortex to decision-making. *Journal of Neuroscience, 19,* 5473–5481.

Bem, D. J., & Allen, A. (1974). On predicting some of the people some of the time: The search for cross-situational consistencies in behavior. *Psychological Review, 81,* 506–520.

Berlyne, D. (1960). *Conflict, arousal, and curiosity.* New York: McGraw-Hill.

Berntzen, D. (1987). Effects of multiple cognitive coping strategies on laboratory pain. *Cognitive Therapy and Research, 11,* 613–623.

Block, J., & Block, J. J. (1980). The role of ego-control and ego resiliency in the organization of behavior. In W. A. Collins (Ed.), *The Minnesota Symposium on Child Psychology* (Vol. 13, pp. 39–101). Hillsdale, NJ: Erlbaum.

Bonanno, G. A. (2001). Grief and emotion: A social–functional perspective. In M. S. Stroebe & R. O. Hansson (Eds.), *Handbook of bereavement research: Consequences, coping, and care* (pp. 493–515). Washington, DC: American Psychological Association.

Bonanno, G. A., Keltner, D., Holen, A., & Horowitz, M. J. (1995). When avoiding unpleasant emotions might not be such a bad thing: Verbal-autonomic response dissociation and midlife conjugal bereavement. *Journal of Personality and Social Psychology, 69,* 975–989.

Calkins, S. D., & Fox, N. A. (2002). Self-regulatory processes in early development: A multilevel approach to the study of childhood social withdrawal and aggression. *Development and Psychopathology, 14,* 477–498.

Cantor, N., & Kihlstrom, J. F. (1987). *Personality and social intelligence.* Englewood Cliffs, NJ: Prentice-Hall.

Carver, C. S., Pozo, C., Harris, S. D., & Noriega, V. (1993). How coping mediates the effect of optimism on distress: A study of women with early stage breast cancer. *Journal of Personality and Social Psychology, 65,* 375–390.

Carver, C. S., & Scheier, M. F. (1982). Control theory: A useful conceptual framework for personality—social, clinical, and health psychology. *Psychological Bulletin, 92,* 111–135.

Chartrand, T. L., & Bargh, J. A. (2002). Nonconscious motivations: Their activation, operation, and consequences. In A. Tesser & D. A. Stapel (Eds.), *Self and motivation: Emerging psychological perspectives* (pp. 13–41). Washington, DC: American Psychological Association.

Chaves, J. F., & Barber, T. X. (1974). Cognitive strategies, experimenter modeling, and expectation in the attenuation of pain. *Journal of Abnormal Psychology, 83,* 356–363.

Cheng, C., Chiu, C. Y., Hong, Y. Y., & Cheung, J. S. (2001). Discriminative facility and its role in the perceived quality of interactional experiences. *Journal of Personality, 69,* 765–786.

Chiu, C., Hong, Y., Mischel, W., & Shoda, Y. (1995). Discriminative facility in social competence:

Conditional versus dispositional encoding and monitoring-blunting of information. *Social Cognition, 13,* 49–70.

Derryberry, D. (2002). Attention and voluntary self-control. *Self and Identity, 1,* 105–111.

Derryberry, D., & Reed, M. A. (2002). Anxiety-related attentional biases and their regulation by attention control. *Journal of Abnormal Psychology, 111,* 225–236.

Derryberry, D., & Rothbart, M. (1997). Reactive and effortful processes in the organization of temperament. *Development and Psychopathology, 9,* 633–652.

Downey, G., & Feldman, S. (1996). Implications of rejection sensitivity for intimate relationships. *Journal of Personality and Social Psychology, 70,* 1327–1343.

Downey, G., Freitas, A., Michealis, B., & Khouri, H. (1998). The self-fulfilling prophecy in close relationships: Do rejection sensitive women get rejected by romantic partners? *Journal of Personality and Social Psychology, 75,* 545–560.

Dweck, C. S. (1986). Motivational processes affecting learning. *American Psychologist, 41,* 1040–1048.

Eisenberg, N., Fabes, R. A., Guthrie, I. K., & Reiser, M. (2000). Dispositional emotionality and regulation: Their role in predicting quality of social functioning. *Journal of Personality and Social Psychology, 78,* 136–157.

Eisenberg, N., Fabes, R. A., Guthrie, I. K., & Reiser, M. (2002). The role of emotionality and regulation in children's social competence and adjustment. In A. Caspi (Ed.), *Paths to successful development: Personality in the life course* (pp. 46–70). New York: Cambridge University Press.

Epstein, S. (1994). Integration of the cognitive and psychodynamic unconscious. *American Psychologist, 49,* 709–724.

Estes, W. K. (1972). Reinforcement in human behavior. *American Scientist, 60,* 723–729.

Ferguson, M. J., & Bargh, J. A. (2000). Beyond behaviorism: On the automaticity of higher mental processes. *Psychological Bulletin, 126,* 925–945.

Freud, S. (1911). Formulations regarding the two principles of mental functioning. In *Collected papers* (Vol. IV). New York: Basic Books. (Original work published 1959)

Gollwitzer, P. M. (1999). Implementation intentions: Strong effects of simple plans. *American Psychologist, 54,* 493–503.

Gollwitzer, P. M., & Bargh, J. A. (Eds.). (1996). *The psychology of action: Linking cognition and motivation to behavior.* New York: Guilford Press.

Gray, J. A. (1987). *The psychology of fear and stress* (2nd ed.). New York: McGraw-Hill.

Graziano, W. G., & Tobin, R. M. (2001). The distributed processing of narcissist: Paradox lost? *Psychological Inquiry, 12,* 219–222.

Grigorenko, E. L. (2002). In search of the genetic engram of personality. In D. Cervone & W. Mischel (Eds.), *Advances in personality science* (pp. 29–82). New York: Guilford Press.

Gross, J. J. (1998). Antecedent- and response-focused emotion regulation: Divergent consequences for experience, expression, and physiology. *Journal of Personality and Social Psychology, 74,* 224–237.

Gunnar, M. R., & Donzella, B. (2002). Self regulation of the cortisol levels in early human development. *Psychoneuroendocrinology, 27,* 199–220.

Gunnar, M., Larson, M., Hertsgaard, L., Harris, M., & Brodersen, L. (1992). The stressfulness of separation among 9-month old infants: Effects of social context variables and infant temperament. *Child Development, 63,* 290–303.

Higgins, E. T. (1996). Knowledge activation: Accessibility, applicability, and salience. In E. T. Higgins & A. W. Kruglanski (Eds.), *Social psychology: Handbook of basic principles* (pp. 133–168). New York: Guilford Press.

Higgins, E. T., & Kruglanski, A. W. (Eds.). (1996). *Social psychology: Handbook of basic principles.* New York: Guilford Press.

Holmes, D. S., & Houston, B. K. (1974). Effectiveness of situation redefinition and affective isolation in coping with stress. *Journal of Personality and Social Psychology, 29,* 212–218.

Hooker, K., & Kaus, C. R. (1992). Possible selves and health behaviors in later life. *Journal of Aging and Health*, *4*, 390–411.

Hull, C. L. (1931). Goal attraction and directing ideas conceived as habit phenomena. *Psychological Review*, *38*, 487–506.

James, W. (1890). *The principles of psychology*. New York: Holt.

Kanfer, F. H., & Seidner, M. L. (1973). Self-control: Factors enhancing tolerance of noxious stimulation. *Journal of Personality and Social Psychology*, *25*, 381–389.

Kaplan, R. M., Atkins, C. J., & Reinsch, S. (1984). Specific efficacy expectations mediate exercise compliance in parents with COPD. *Health Psychology*, *3*, 233–242.

Kochanska, G. (1997). Multiple pathways to conscience for children with different temperaments: From toddlerhood to age 5. *Developmental Psychology*, *33*, 228–240.

Koriat, A., Melkman, R., Averill, J. R., & Lazarus, R. S. (1972). The self-control of emotional reactions to a stressful film. *Journal of Personality*, *40*, 601–619.

Kuhl, J. (1985). From cognition to behavior: Perspectives for future research on action control. In J. Beckmann (Ed.), *Action control from cognition to behavior* (pp. 267–276). New York: Springer-Verlag.

Kuhl, J. (1996). Who controls whom when "I control myself"? *Psychological Inquiry*, *7*, 61–68.

Kunda, Z. (1999). *Social cognition: Making sense of people*. Cambridge, MA: MIT Press.

Langer, E. J., Janis, I. L., & Wolfer, J. A. (1975). Reduction of psychological stress in surgical patients. *Journal of Experimental Social Psychology*, *11*, 155–165.

LeDoux, J. (1996). *The emotional brain*. New York: Touchstone.

Lieberman, M. D. (2003). Reflective and reflexive judgment processes: A social cognitive neuroscience approach. In J. P. Forgas, K. Williams, & W. von Hippel (Eds.), *Social judgments: Implicit and explicit processes*. Philadelphia: Psychology Press.

Lieberman, M. D., Gaunt, R., Gilbert, D. T., & Trope, Y. (2002). Reflection and reflexion: A social cognitive neuroscience approach to attributional inference. In M. Zanna (Ed.), *Advances in experimental social psychology* (Vol. 34, pp. 199–249). New York: Academic Press.

Loewenstein, G., Read, D., & Baumeister, R. (Eds.). (2003). *Time and decision: Economic and psychological perspectives on intertemporal choice*. New York: Russell Sage Foundation.

Major, B., Cozzarelli, C., Sciacchitano, A. M., Cooper, M. L., Testa, M., & Mueller, P. M. (1990). Perceived social support, self-efficacy, and adjustment to abortion. *Journal of Personality and Social Psychology*, *59*, 452–463.

McCrae, R. R., & Costa, P. T. (1999). A five-factor theory of personality. In L. A. Pervin & O. P. John (Eds.), *Handbook of personality: Theory and research* (2nd ed., pp. 139–153). New York: Guilford Press.

Mendoza-Denton, R., Ayduk, O., Mischel, W., Shoda, Y., & Testa, A. (2001). Person × situation interactionism in self-encoding (I am . . . when . . .): Implications for affect regulation and social information processing. *Journal of Personality and Social Psychology*, *80*, 533–544.

Metcalfe, J., & Jacobs, J. W. (1996). A "hot/cool-system" view of memory under stress. *PTSD Research Quarterly*, *7*, 1–6.

Metcalfe, J., & Mischel, W. (1999). A hot/cool system analysis of delay of gratification: Dynamics of willpower. *Psychological Review*, *106*, 3–19.

Miller, S. M. (1979). Coping with impending stress: Physiological and cognitive correlates of choice. *Psychophysiology*, *16*, 572–581.

Miller, S. M. (1987). Monitoring and blunting: Validation of a questionnaire to assess styles of information seeking under threat. *Journal of Personality and Social Psychology*, *52*, 344–353.

Mischel, W. (1961a). Father-absence and delay of gratification. *Journal of Abnormal and Social Psychology*, *63*, 116–124.

Mischel, W. (1961b). Preference for delayed reinforcement and social responsibility. *Journal of Abnormal Psychology*, *62*, 1–7.

Mischel, W. (1966). Theory and research on the antecedents of self-imposed delay of reward. In B. A. Maher (Ed.), *Progress in experimental personality research* (Vol. 3, pp. 85–131). New York: Academic Press.

Mischel, W. (1973). Toward a cognitive social learning reconceptualization of personality. *Psychological Review, 80*, 252–283.

Mischel, W. (1974a). Cognitive appraisals and transformations in self-control. In B. Weiner (Ed.), *Cognitive views of human motivation* (pp. 33–49). New York: Academic Press.

Mischel, W. (1974b). Processes in delay of gratification. In L. Berkowitz (Ed.), *Advances in experimental social psychology* (Vol. 7, pp. 249–292). New York: Academic Press.

Mischel, W., & Ayduk, O. (2002). Self-regulation in a cognitive-affective personality system: Attentional control in the service of the self. *Self and Identity, 1*, 113–120.

Mischel, W., & Baker, N. (1975). Cognitive appraisals and transformations in delay behavior. *Journal of Personality and Social Psychology, 31*, 254–261.

Mischel, W., Cantor, N., & Feldman, S. (1996). Principles of self-regulation: The nature of willpower and self-control. In E. T. Higgins & A. W. Kruglanski (Eds.), *Social psychology: Handbook of basic principles* (pp. 329–360). New York: Guilford Press.

Mischel, W., & Ebbesen, E. B. (1970). Attention in delay of gratification. *Journal of Personality and Social Psychology, 16*, 239–337.

Mischel, W., Ebbesen, E. B., & Zeiss, A. R. (1972). Cognitive and attentional mechanisms in delay of gratification. *Journal of Personality and Social Psychology, 21*, 204–218.

Mischel, W., & Metzner, R. (1962). Preference for delayed reward as a function of age, intelligence, and length of delay interval. *Journal of Abnormal and Social Psychology, 64*, 425–431.

Mischel, H. N., & Mischel, W. (1983). The development of children's knowledge of self-control strategies. *Child Development, 54*, 603–619.

Mischel, W., & Moore, B. (1973). Effects of attention to symbolically-presented rewards on self-control. *Journal of Personality and Social Psychology, 28*, 172–179.

Mischel, W., & Morf, C. C. (2003). The self as a psycho-social dynamic processing system: A meta-perspective on a century of the self in psychology. In M. R. Leary & J. P. Tangney (Eds.), *Handbook of self and identity* (pp. 15–43). New York: Guilford Press.

Mischel, W., & Shoda, Y. (1995). A cognitive-affective system theory of personality: Reconceptualizing situations, dispositions, dynamics, and invariance in personality structure. *Psychological Review, 102*, 246–268.

Mischel, W., & Shoda, Y. (1998). Reconciling processing dynamics and personality dispositions. *Annual Review of Psychology, 49*, 229–258.

Mischel, W., & Shoda, Y. (1999). Integrating dispositions and processing dynamics within a unified theory of personality: The cognitive-affective personality system (CAPS). In L. A. Pervin & O. P. John (Ed.), *Handbook of personality: Theory and research* (pp. 197–218). New York: Guilford Press.

Mischel, W., Shoda, Y., & Peake, P. (1988). The nature of adolescent competencies predicted by preschool delay of gratification. *Journal of Personality and Social Psychology, 54*, 687–696.

Mischel, W., Shoda, Y., & Rodriguez, M. L. (1989). Delay of gratification in children. *Science, 244*, 933–938.

Mischel, W., Shoda, Y., & Smith, R. (2003). *Introduction to personality: Toward an integration* (7th ed.). New York: Wiley.

Mischel, W., & Staub, E. (1965). Effects of expectancy on working and waiting for larger rewards. *Journal of Personality and Social Psychology, 2*, 625–633.

Moore, B., Mischel, W., & Zeiss, A. (1976). Comparative effects of the reward stimulus and its cognitive representation in voluntary delay. *Journal of Personality and Social Psychology, 34*, 419–424.

Morf, C. C., & Mischel, W. (2002). Special issue: Self-concept, self-regulation, and psychological vulnerability. *Self and Identity, 1*, 103–199.

Morf, C. C., & Rhodewalt, F. (1993). Narcissism and self-evaluation maintenance: Explorations in object relations. *Personality and Social Psychology Bulletin, 19*, 668–676.

Morf, C. C., & Rhodewalt, F. (2001). Unraveling the paradoxes of narcissism: A dynamic self-regulatory processing model. *Psychological Inquiry, 12*, 177–196.

Nowak, A., Vallacher, R. R., Tesser, A., & Borkowski, W. (2000). Society of self: The emergence of collective properties in self-structure. *Psychological Review, 107,* 39–61.

Patterson, C. J., & Mischel, W. (1975). Plans to resist distraction. *Developmental Psychology, 11,* 369–378.

Peake, P., Hebl, M., & Mischel, W. (2002). Strategic attention deployment in waiting and working situations. *Developmental Psychology, 38,* 313–326.

Petry, N. M. (2002). Discounting of delayed rewards in substance abusers: Relationship to antisocial personality disorder. *Psychopharmacology, 162,* 425–432.

Rachlin, H. (2000). *The science of self-control.* Cambridge, MA: Harvard University Press.

Read, S. J., & Miller, L. C. (2002). Virtual personalities: A neural network model of personality. *Personality and Social Psychology Review, 6,* 357–369.

Richards, J., & Gross, J. J. (1999). Composure at any cost? The cognitive consequences of emotion suppression. *Personality and Social Psychology Bulletin, 25,* 1033–1044.

Richards, J. M., & Gross, J. J. (2000). Emotion regulation and memory: The cognitive costs of keeping one's cool. *Journal of Personality and Social Psychology, 79,* 410–424.

Rodin, J. (1987). Personal control through the life course. In R. P. Abeles (Ed.), *Life-span perspective and social psychology* (pp. 103–119). Hillsdale, NJ: Erlbaum.

Rodriguez, M. L., Mischel, W., & Shoda, Y. (1989). Cognitive person variables in the delay of gratification of older children at-risk. *Journal of Personality and Social Psychology, 57,* 358–367.

Rodriguez, M. L., Mischel, W., Shoda, Y., & Wright, J. (1989). *Delay of gratification and children's social behavior in natural settings.* Paper presented at the Eastern Psychological Association, Boston.

Rothbart, M. K., Derryberry, D., & Posner, M. (1994). A psychobiological approach to the development of temperament. In T. D. Wachs (Ed.), *Temperament: Individual differences at the interface of biology and behavior* (pp. 83–116). Washington, DC: American Psychological Association.

Rumelhart, D. E., & McClelland, J. L. (1986). *Parallel distributed processing: Explorations in the microstructure of cognition: Vol. 1. Foundations.* Cambridge, MA: MIT Press/Bradford Books.

Seligman, M. E. P. (1975). *Helplessness: On depression, development, and death.* San Francisco: Freeman.

Sethi, A., Mischel, W., Aber, J. L., Shoda, Y., & Rodriguez, M. L. (2000). The role of strategic attention deployment in development of self-regulation: Predicting preschoolers delay of gratification from mother–toddler interactions. *Developmental Psychology, 36,* 767–777.

Shah, J., & Kruglanski, A. (2002). Priming against your will: How accessible alternatives affect goal pursuit. *Journal of Experimental Social Psychology, 38,* 368–383.

Shoda, Y., LeeTiernen, S., & Mischel, W. (2002). Personality as a dynamical system: Emergence of stability and distinctiveness from intra- and interpersonal interactions. *Personality and Social Psychology Review, 6,* 316–325.

Shoda, Y., & Mischel, W. (1998). Personality as a stable cognitive-affective activation network: Characteristic patterns of behavior variation emerge from a stable personality structure. In L. C. Miller (Ed.), *Connectionist models of social reasoning and social behavior* (pp. 175–208). Mahwah, NJ: Erlbaum.

Shoda, Y., Mischel, W., & Peake, P. (1990). Predicting adolescent cognitive and self-regulatory competencies from preschool delay of gratification: Identifying diagnostic conditions. *Developmental Psychology, 26,* 978–986.

Shoda, Y., Mischel, W., & Wright, J. (1993). The role of situational demands and cognitive competencies in behavior organization and personality coherence. *Journal of Personality and Social Psychology, 65,* 1023–1035.

Skinner, B. F. (1938). *The behavior of organisms: an experimental analysis.* Oxford, UK: Appleton–Century–Crofts.

Szpiler, J. A., & Epstein, S. (1976). Availability of an avoidance response as related to autonomic arousal. *Journal of Abnormal Psychology, 85,* 73–82.

Taylor, S. E., & Brown, J. D. (1988). Illusion and well-being: A social psychological perspective on mental health. *Psychological Bulletin, 103*, 193–210.

Taylor, S. E., Lichtman, R. R., & Wood, J. V. (1984). Attributions, beliefs about control, and adjustment to breast cancer. *Journal of Personality and Social Psychology, 46*, 489–502.

Thompson, S. C. (1981). Will it hurt less if I can control it?: A complex answer to a simple question. *Psychological Bulletin, 90*, 89–101.

Trilling, L. (1943). *E. M. Forster.* New York: New Directions.

Trope, Y., & Liberman, N. (2003). Temporal construal. *Psychological Review, 110*, 403–421.

Van Mechelen, I., & Kiers, H. A. L. (1999). Individual differences in anxiety responses to stressful situations: A three-mode component analysis model. *European Journal of Personality, 13*, 409–428.

Wegner, D. M. (1994). Ironic processes of mental control. *Psychological Review, 101*, 34–52.

Wegner, D. M., Schneider, D. J., Carter, S., III, & White, T. L. (1987). Paradoxical effects of thought suppression. *Journal of Personality and Social Psychology, 53*, 5–13.

Wulfert, E., Block, J. A., Ana, E. S., Rodriguez, M. L., & Colsman, M. (2002). Delay of gratification: Impulsive choices and problem behaviors in early and late adolescence. *Journal of Personality, 70*, 533–552.

Zayas, V., Shoda, Y., & Ayduk, O. (2002). Personality in context: An interpersonal systems perspective. *Journal of Personality, 70*, 851–900.

7

Self-Regulation and Behavior Change

Disentangling Behavioral Initiation and Behavioral Maintenance

ALEXANDER J. ROTHMAN
AUSTIN S. BALDWIN
ANDREW W. HERTEL

On a day-to-day basis, people face myriad behavioral challenges. Some challenges require people to form and execute a novel response, whereas others require them to continue an ongoing pattern of behavior. At first glance, one might surmise it is easier to maintain a response to a familiar challenge than to respond to a new challenge. Given their familiarity with the situation and the contingent response, people should find that they have a better sense of what to do and what they are capable of doing. Moreover, the strength of the contingency between the response and the eliciting situation should only increase as the behavior is repeated over time. From this perspective, successfully enacting a behavior should afford future success; over time, a self-sustaining pattern of behavior (i.e., a habit) will form. Accordingly, psychologists have frequently invoked the notion of habit as the logical product of a sequence of successfully enacted behaviors (Ajzen, 2002; Ouellette & Wood, 1998; Ronis, Yates, & Kirscht, 1989). But does this account adequately capture the processes that underlie the transition from behavioral initiation to behavioral maintenance and, ultimately, to habit formation? Is it correct to assume that the decision criteria that guide behavioral decision making are invariant over time?

The premise that a successfully initiated behavior will be maintained over time can be found either implicitly or explicitly in most, if not all, models of behavioral decision making (Rothman, 2000). Yet this premise is at variance with behavioral data obtained across a range of domains. Specifically, people who have successfully initiated a new pattern of behavior more often than not fail to sustain that behavior over time, for example, diet and exercise to produce weight loss (Jeffery et al., 2000), smoking cessation (Ockene et al., 2000), substance abuse (Hunt, Barnett, & Branch, 1971; Marlatt & Gordon, 1985). Further evidence for a dissociation between the processes that underlie behavioral initiation and maintenance comes from the observation that intervention strategies that help people initiate changes in their behavior have not had a similar impact on rates of behavioral maintenance (e.g., Curry & McBride, 1994; McCaul, Glasgow, & O'Neill, 1992; Perri, Nezu, Patti, & McCann, 1989).

The observation that initial behavioral success does not ensure continued success suggests that greater attention must be given to the manner in which newly enacted behaviors evolve into a habit. Although behavioral maintenance can be operationally defined as a series of similar decisions to take action, the processes that guide people's behavioral decisions need not be invariant over time. In this chapter, we first review how investigators have traditionally conceptualized the processes that underlie the ongoing self-regulation of behavior. To date, if anything, different phases in the behavior change process have been described. Although there is value in specifying the behavioral markers that characterize people at each point in the behavior change process, these descriptions must be complemented by an understanding of the factors that regulate transitions through phases of the behavior change process. We propose that once people have chosen to initiate a new pattern of behavior, four distinct phases in the behavior change process can be identified. Furthermore, the primary determinants of the behavior shift as people transition from one phase to the next. To this end, we offer a series of working hypotheses regarding the differential influence of specific factors throughout the behavior change process. Although a rigorous assessment of these predictions is constrained by the absence of empirical findings regarding ongoing behavioral practices, we hope that the framework articulated in this chapter encourages investigators to undertake a new generation of theorizing and empirical investigations that will, in turn, afford a better specification of the factors that facilitate or inhibit behavioral maintenance.

CURRENT THEORETICAL APPROACHES TO BEHAVIORAL MAINTENANCE

Current models of health behavior, for example, the health belief model (Rosenstock, Strecher, & Becker, 1988), protection motivation theory (Maddux & Rogers, 1983), social cognitive theory (Bandura, 1986), the theory of planned behavior (Ajzen, 1991), the theory of reasoned action (Ajzen & Fishbein, 1980), and the transtheoretical model of behavior change (Prochaska, DiClemente, & Norcross, 1992), have focused on elucidating how people determine whether to adopt a given behavior.[1] The decision to adopt a new behavior is predicated on an analysis of the relative costs and benefits associated with different courses of action; the manner in which these models differ is the particular set of beliefs that is predicted to be most closely associated with a decision to take action (Salovey, Rothman, & Rodin, 1998; Weinstein, 1993). Consistent with their conceptual framework, these theoretical perspectives have primarily been used to explain why people engage in a particular unhealthy or healthy behavioral practice—for example, why women decide to get a mammogram (Aiken, West, Woodward, & Reno, 1994; Rakowski et al., 1992), or why people choose to enroll in a smoking cessation program (Norman, Conner, & Bell, 1999). Very limited consideration has been given to modeling an ongoing sequence of behaviors, such as the factors that predict why a woman gets an initial mammogram but then does or does not return to obtain a subsequent screening exam

(Rothman, Kelly, Hertel, & Salovey, 2003). For instance, the health belief model (Rosenstock et al., 1988) and protection motivation theory (Maddux & Rogers, 1983) make no direct reference to issues regarding behavioral maintenance other than to define it as a course of action sustained over a specified period of time. Thus, the factors that underlie the decision to maintain a pattern of behavior are assumed to be no different than those that govern its initiation.

The theory of reasoned action (Ajzen & Fishbein, 1980) and the theory of planned behavior (Ajzen, 1991) also make no formal distinction between decisions regarding the initiation of a behavior and those regarding the maintenance of that behavior over time. Investigators have used these approaches to examine long-term behavioral outcomes. However, the primary purpose of these investigations has been to ascertain whether people's behavioral practices become sufficiently stable, such that behavior is a function of itself and no longer contingent on a set of mediating thoughts or feelings (Ajzen, 2002; Wood, Quinn, & Kashy, 2002). In a similar manner, investigators have focused on specifying the factors that increase the likelihood that people will act on their intentions (Conner, Sheeran, Norman, & Armitage, 2000; Gollwitzer, 1999; see Gollwitzer, Fujita, & Oettingen, Chapter 11, this volume). Although helping people to articulate how they will implement their behavioral intentions, or how to form strong, accurate intentions, has been shown to increase the likelihood that people will act on their intentions, these approaches provide little guidance as to the conditions that determine whether an enacted change in behavior will be maintained.

According to social cognitive theory (Bandura, 1986), self-efficacy beliefs are a crucial determinant of both the initiation and the maintenance of a change in behavior (see also Schwarzer, 2001). Confidence in one's ability to take action serves to sustain effort and perseverance in the face of obstacles. The successful implementation of changes in behavior bolsters people's confidence, which, in turn, facilitates further action, whereas failure experiences serve to undermine personal feelings of efficacy. Although the reciprocal relation between perceived self-efficacy and behavior is well documented, this relation needs to be reconciled with the observation that successfully enacted changes in behavior are not always maintained (e.g., McCaul et al., 1992). In fact, as we discuss in a subsequent section, it may be worth reconsidering the degree to which perceived self-efficacy affects the decision to maintain a behavior over and above its influence on the decision to initiate the behavior.

Although stage models have identified maintenance as a distinct stage in the behavior change process, the primary focus of these theoretical approaches has been to recognize that people differ in their readiness to take action. Therefore, research efforts have focused on delineating the processes through which people become ready to initiate a change in their behavior (Prochaska et al., 1992; Weinstein, 1988). In the transtheoretical model of behavior change (Prochaska et al., 1992), a distinction is made between people in the action and in the maintenance stage, yet the basis for this distinction rests solely on the length of time a behavior has been adopted. Accordingly, the set of cognitive and behavioral strategies that are predicted to facilitate initial action are similarly predicted to help sustain that action over time (Prochaska & Velicer, 1997).

Taken together, the dominant theoretical approaches to the study of health behavior offer little guidance as to how the processes that govern the initiation and the maintenance of behavior change might differ. Because maintenance has been operationalized as action sustained over time, it is predicted to rely on the same set of behavioral skills and motivational concerns that facilitate the initial change in behavior. Yet this perspective remains at odds with the observation that people who successfully adopt a new pattern of behavior frequently fail to maintain that pattern of behavior over time.

In a recent article, Rothman (2000) has argued that there may be important differences in the decision criteria that guide the initiation and maintenance of behavior change, and that these differences may serve to explain why people who are able to make changes in their behavior may subsequently choose not to sustain that behavior. Behavioral decisions, by definition, involve a choice between different behavioral alternatives. What differentiates decisions concerning initiation from those concerning maintenance are the criteria on which the decision is based. Decisions regarding behavioral initiation involve a consideration of whether the potential benefits afforded by a new pattern of behavior compare favorably to one's current situation and, thus, the decision to initiate a new behavior depends on a person's holding *favorable expectations* regarding future outcomes. This premise is well-grounded in a broad tradition of research endeavors indicating that the more optimistic people are about the value of the potential outcomes afforded by the new pattern of behavior and their ability to obtain those outcomes, the more likely they are to initiate changes (for reviews, see Bandura, 1997; Salovey et al., 1998). Because the decision to initiate a new behavior is predicated on obtaining future outcomes, it can be conceptualized as an approach-based self-regulatory process in which progress toward one's goal is indicated by a reduction in the discrepancy between one's current state and a desired reference state (Carver & Scheier, 1990).

Whereas decisions regarding behavioral initiation are based on expected outcomes, decisions regarding behavioral maintenance involve a consideration of the experiences people have had engaging in the new pattern of behavior and a determination of whether those experiences are sufficiently desirable to warrant continued action. Consistent with Leventhal's self-regulatory model of illness behavior (Leventhal & Cameron, 1987; Leventhal, Nerenz, & Steele, 1984), the decision to continue a pattern of behavior reflects an ongoing assessment of the behavioral, psychological, and physiological experiences afforded by the behavior change process. According to Rothman (2000), people's assessment of these experiences is ultimately indexed by their satisfaction with the experiences afforded by the new pattern of behavior, and they will maintain a change in behavior only if they are satisfied with what they have accomplished. The feeling of satisfaction indicates that the initial decision to change the behavior was correct; furthermore, it provides justification for the continued effort people must put forth to monitor their behavior and minimize vulnerability to relapse. To the extent that people choose to maintain a behavior to preserve a favorable situation, the decision processes that underlie behavioral maintenance may be conceptualized as an avoidance-based self-regulatory process in which people strive to maintain a discrepancy between their current state and an undesired reference state (Carver & Scheier, 1990).

Because different decision criteria are proposed to guide behavioral initiation and behavioral maintenance, factors that may facilitate one behavioral outcome may not have a similar effect on the other. In particular, people's outcome expectancies, a crucial determinant of their willingness to initiate a new pattern of behavior, may have a pernicious effect on decisions regarding behavioral maintenance. Optimistic outcome expectations are likely to motivate people to make changes in their behavior and, in fact, intervention strategies often work to heighten these expectancies (King, Rothman, & Jeffery, 2002). However, these expectations may also serve as the standard against which people evaluate the outcomes afforded by the new pattern of behavior (Gollwitzer, 1996; Schwarz & Strack, 1991). How it feels to have dropped down to a 32-inch waist size will differ depending on whether one's goal had been to achieve a 34-inch or a 30-inch waist size. To the extent that people's satisfaction with the behavior depends on their experiences meeting or exceeding their expectations, the unrealistically optimistic expectations that initially inspired people to make a change in their behavior may ultimately elicit feelings of dissatisfaction and disappointment, thus undermining behavioral maintenance.

Efforts to disentangle the concerns that guide decisions regarding behavioral maintenance from those that guide behavioral initiation critically depend on a clear description of the differences between these two phases of the behavior change process. Specifically, when does the initiation phase end and the maintenance phase begin? To date, distinctions between phases of the behavior change process have focused on the specific period of time the behavior has been sustained (e.g., 6 months). Conceptualizing maintenance solely in terms of time affords little insight into the factors that may facilitate or inhibit sustained behavior change. Moreover, it would appear to suggest that there is a discrete moment in time when people shift from conceptualizing a behavior as something they are trying to initiate to something they are working to maintain.

Although Rothman (2000) discussed the potential value of distinguishing between predictors of behavioral initiation and behavioral maintenance, the manner in which people transition from one phase to the next was not well delineated. The absence of a complete description of the behavior change process hinders both theoretical and empirical efforts to specify the factors that guide people's behavioral decisions. To be effective, a conceptual framework must provide investigators with both a set of features that can be used to identify what phase a person is in and a set of determinants that uniquely predict transition between each phase (Weinstein, Rothman, & Sutton, 1998). To this end, we propose unpacking the behavior change process into a series of four phases: initial response, continued response, maintenance, and habit. These phases capture the behavioral processes that begin once someone has embarked on a course of action, transitioning out of what Prochaska and colleagues (1992) have characterized as the preparation stage. In some cases this point of transition is marked by an explicit action, such as enrolling in a formal program (e.g., an addiction treatment program) or purchasing a piece of equipment (e.g., a treadmill), whereas in other cases, it is marked solely by a public or private affirmation to engage in a particular pattern of behavior (e.g., committing to exercise 3 days a week).

The structure of the four phases identified was informed, in part, by earlier efforts to construct a consensus description of the phases that individuals pass through during treatment for major depressive disorder (Frank et al., 1991). At a general level, the four proposed phases reflect our belief that distinctions needed to be made within prior conceptualizations of both behavioral initiation and behavioral maintenance. As regards behavioral initiation, we have distinguished between the decisions that underlie a person's efforts to initiate successfully a new pattern of behavior (i.e., the initial response phase) and the efforts involved with managing the new behavior and confronting the challenges associated with developing a sense of control over one's actions (i.e., the continued response phase). As we detail later, we believe the choices that people face during this period of time are distinct from those they face when deciding whether to maintain a behavior. As regards behavioral maintenance, we have distinguished between a phase in which people choose to maintain a pattern of behavior based on a repeated assessment of the behavior's value (i.e., the maintenance phase) and a phase in which people continue to maintain the behavior, but without any consideration of a behavioral alternative (i.e., the habit phase). Below we have provided a description of the defining features of each phase, as well as a general outline of the factors believed to regulate people's ability to transition successfully to the next phase (see Table 7.1 for an overview). Of course, the conceptual value of these distinctions remains an open question, the answer to which lies not in the face validity of the descriptions, but in whether empirical evidence can be obtained to support the premise that different phases of the behavior change process are contingent on distinct sets of predictors.

UNPACKING THE BEHAVIOR CHANGE PROCESS

The first phase of the behavior change process, *initial response*, begins as soon as people embark on an effort to change their behavior and continues until they first manifest a significant change. For example, a person might enroll in a smoking cessation program and subsequently report having been smoke-free for 7 consecutive days. The successful performance of the desired behavior (e.g., being smoke-free) serves as an indication that the participant has responded favorably to the treatment or intervention. Although how the behavioral outcome is operationally defined will vary across domains, the measure should indicate that a person has reliably performed the desired behavior and, thus, the behavioral response is not due to chance. People who fail to emit the desired behavioral response (e.g., someone who is unable to remain smoke-free for 7 consecutive days) are considered nonresponsive to the treatment or intervention and, thus, fail to transition to

TABLE 7.1. The Four Phases of the Behavior Change Process

Phase	Initial response	Continued response	Maintenance	Habit
Defining feature of phase	Initial effort to change behavior (e.g., enrolling in a program)	Continued effort to establish new behavior	Sustained effort to continue newly established behavior	Self-perpetuating pattern of behavior
Primary determinants of transition to next phase[a]	Efficacy beliefs (++) Outcome expectations (+) Personality/ situation (−)	Initial rewards (+) Sustained self-efficacy beliefs (+) Sustained outcome expectations (+) Demands of the behavior change process (− −) Personality/ situation (− −)	Satisfaction with new behavior (++) Personality/ situation (−)	Prior behavior (++)
Marker of end of phase/beginning of next phase[a]	First reliable performance of the desired behavior	Consistent performance of the desired behavior and complete confidence in one's ability to perform the behavior	Consistent behavior without consideration of the value of the behavior	

Note. "++" and "− −" indicate factors that have strong facilitating and inhibiting effects on behavior change, respectively. "+" and "−" indicate factors that have moderate facilitating and inhibiting effects on behavior change, respectively.
[a] Habit, the last phase of the sequence, is expected to persist as long as the behavior is sustained.

the next phase. It is assumed that these people revert back to a consideration of whether they want to begin a new attempt to modify their behavior.

Because researchers have primarily focused their efforts on identifying predictors of initial behavior change, the factors that predict successfully completing the initial response phase are relatively well understood. Specifically, the likelihood that people will initiate a change in their behavior has been shown to be a function of both their confidence in their ability to execute the behavior and their belief that engaging in the new pattern of behavior will meaningfully improve their lives (Salovey et al., 1998). In many ways, the onset of this phase of the behavior change process is characterized by a sense of optimism and hope, because people's attention is focused primarily on the reasons that have motivated them to attempt this change. Because the ability to adopt an optimistic mindset is an important determinant of initial success (Taylor & Gollwitzer, 1995), any factor that undermines a person's ability to generate and sustain this perspective, such as a facet of one's personality (e.g., pessimism) or of one's life situation (e.g., an unsupportive partner), will, in turn, make it more difficult for the person to pass through this phase.

Once a person has reliably performed the desired behavior, the second phase of the behavioral process, *continued response*, begins. This phase is characterized by a tension between a person's ability and motivation to enact the new pattern of behavior consistently, and the challenges and unpleasant experiences that leave him or her vulnerable to lapses and relapses. It is during this period of time that people strive to gain a sense of mastery over their new behavior. The length of time people remain in this phase is likely to differ across both domains and persons. Some people may find it easy to master the new pattern of behavior, whereas others may find it a continual struggle. Similarly, some behavioral domains involve a complex series of behavioral modifications, which should lengthen this phase, whereas other domains involve a very limited set of challenges, which should shorten this phase. The point at which people transition out of this phase and enter a maintenance phase occurs when they not only perform the new pattern of behavior consistently but also do so with complete confidence in their ability to manage their behavior.

A key aspect of the continued response phase is that people have to face the reality of engaging in the new pattern of behavior, including the possibility or actuality of slips and lapses. People begin to shift their attention from their expectations regarding the behavior to their experiences with it. Although people's desire to change their behavior and confidence in their ability to implement that change continue to influence behavior, it is critical that people sustain these beliefs in the face of their experience performing the new pattern of behavior. To the extent that people find the new behavior to be unpleasant or feel that it requires a considerable amount of mental and/or physical energy, their commitment to and confidence in their behavior may weaken, thus, making it difficult for them to complete this phase of the behavior change process. Moreover, as suggested by models of relapse prevention, people's explanations for both the outcomes they experience and the behaviors they perform may affect their ability to complete this phase (Brownell, Marlatt, Lichtenstein, & Wilson, 1986).

Because people's experiences with the behavior begin to affect behavioral decision making, careful consideration must be given to the nature and the timing of the consequences afforded by a new pattern of behavior. Any favorable outcomes elicited by the behavior (e.g., compliments from others) should help sustain people's motivation to change their behavior. However, in many cases, the primary benefits afforded by the new pattern of behavior arise only after extended action. In fact, people may have greater success initiating a pattern of behavior to the extent that it is motivated by goals that afford immediate, concrete outcomes (e.g., smokers who want to quit to get rid of the smell on their clothes and belongings) compared to those that afford longer term benefits (e.g., smokers who want to quit to avoid developing cancer and heart disease; Worth et al., 2002). Because the costs associated with a behavior are often closely tied to the process of enacting the behavior (e.g., having to get up early to exercise), they tend to appear with the onset of the behavior. The heightened salience of these costs can make this phase of the behavior change process particularly difficult and unpleasant, and may elicit a set of experiences that are in sharp contrast to the optimism and hope that characterized people's initial willingness to commit to the behavior change process. Given the greater prevalence of negative information about the new behavior, any aspect of a person's personality or life situation that makes it difficult for him or her to remain optimistic about the behavior change process is likely to have the most debilitating impact during this phase. Specifically, people may find that they can initiate a behavior in the absence of social support, or even in the presence of unsupportive others, but that these conditions greatly hinder their ability to sustain their efforts over time.

People who are unable to complete the continued response phase are thought to have relapsed and returned to their prior behavioral practices. However, successfully completing this phase of the behavior change process can be taken as a sign of recovery. People have put their prior, unwanted habits behind them and are consistently engaging in a new, healthy pattern of behavior. Moreover, they are doing so with a sense that they are in control of their actions. Up until now, engaging in the new pattern of behavior reflected a struggle against pressures to relapse, but with the onset of a new phase in the behavior change process, the decision to engage in the unwanted behavior becomes more volitional. From the perspective of the theory of planned behavior (Ajzen, 1991), by the end of the continued response phase, perceptions of behavioral control should no longer moderate people's ability to translate their intentions into actions.

The *maintenance* phase is characterized by the desire to sustain this new, successful pattern of behavior. Because people who have reached this phase in the behavior change process are not struggling to perform the behavior, there is an important shift in the determinants of their behavior. Having demonstrated that they can successfully perform the behavior over an extended period of time, people feel less need to question or verify their ability to engage in the behavior. Hence, the decision to continue the behavior becomes less a function of a person's ability to perform the behavior and more a function of the behavior's perceived value. It is at this phase in the behavior change process that people complete the shift from focusing on what they expect the behavior to afford to assessing what outcomes the behavior has in fact afforded (Rothman, 2000). A sufficient amount of time has passed since the onset of the behavior, so the consequences of the new behavior are now informative. Thus, people begin to form an integrated assessment of the relative costs and benefits afforded by the behavior to determine whether the behavior is worth continuing. To the extent that the cost–benefit analysis leads people to conclude that they are satisfied with the new behavior, they will choose to sustain the behavior and preserve the gains that have accrued.

During the maintenance phase, people continue to monitor the consequences of their behavior and, thus, should be sensitive to changes in the perceived benefits and costs associated with the behavior. For example, starting to receive fewer and fewer compliments as friends and family begin to take the new behavior for granted may undermine people's evaluation of the behavior and, in turn, their interest in maintaining it. Similarly, how people think about the behavior may shift as they habituate to the pleasure associated with their new experiences. Unlike the prior two phases of the behavior change process, people can remain in the maintenance phase indefinitely. As long as people feel the need to evaluate continually their perception of the relative costs and benefits of the behavior, they will remain in this phase. Because the value of continuing the pattern of behavior is continually reassessed, it is always possible that a person will choose to end the behavior after concluding that it is no longer worthwhile. At this phase, the return of the prior, unhealthy behavior is considered a recurrence rather than a relapse; that is, it represents a new episode, or instance, of the behavior as opposed to a continuation of a prior pattern of behavior.

The transition to *habit*, the final phase in the behavior change process, occurs when people are no longer actively concerned about their ability to engage in the behavior or their evaluation of the outcomes afforded by the behavior. At this point in time, people engage in the behavior in the absence of any regular analysis of whether they should or should not continue to take action (Wood et al., 2002). In other words, the behavior sustains itself. This is not to say that people in this phase do not value the behavior; rather, that they no longer need to verify or test its value. Consistently wearing seat belts when riding in a car, which has frequently been invoked as a prototypical habit, fits nicely within this framework, because it is relatively easy for people to reach the point that they question neither their ability to use a seat belt nor its value as a safety device.

Because people in this phase act based on the assumption that their behavior is worthwhile, they should be less sensitive to fluctuations in the outcomes afforded by the behavior than are those who remain in the maintenance phase of the behavior change process. Consistent with this perspective, Ferguson and Bibby (2002) observed that the subsequent behavior of occasional but not habitual blood donors was affected by having seen people faint during blood donation. Under most circumstances, people benefit from the fact that their behavior does not depend upon the constant reaffirmation (or demonstration) of its value. However, if the behavior in question ever became inadvisable, the fact that people in the habit phase are chronically less concerned with the merits of the behavior may make them less likely to reconsider their behavior than those people who remain in the maintenance phase. It is assumed that once people have reached the habit phase, they will continue in this phase until an event of sufficient magnitude causes them to reconsider the value of their behavior. Should this occur, people would shift back into the maintenance phase, where they would determine whether the behavior in question is of sufficient value to sustain.

Although our description of the behavior change process has focused on the transition from an unhealthy to a healthy pattern of behavior, the framework can also be used to describe the processes that unfolds as people choose to initiate an unhealthy pattern of behavior (e.g., substance use). The more optimistic people are that the behavior will afford favorable outcomes, such as positive reinforcement from one's peers or a better sense of self, the more likely that they will initiate the behavior (Barton, Chassin, Presson, & Sherman, 1982; Fisher & Bauman, 1988). Moreover, the decision to continue to engage in the behavior should be predicated on satisfaction with the outcomes afforded by the unhealthy behavior. Because dissatisfaction is associated with the decision not to engage in the unhealthy behavior (i.e., the healthy or wise decision), different implications are drawn from the differential effect that optimistic expectations are thought to have on behavioral initiation and maintenance. In this case, unrealistic expectations about the benefits of an unhealthy behavior such as smoking or drinking should increase the chances that people will experiment with the behavior, but decrease the chances that they would choose to maintain the behavior. Put a different way, efforts to mitigate people's expectations about the benefits associated with a given behavior may have the unintended effect of increasing the likelihood that, should they try it, they will be satisfied with their experiences and choose to continue to engage in the behavior.

DISENTANGLING BEHAVIORAL INITIATION AND BEHAVIORAL MAINTENANCE: A METHODOLOGICAL NOTE

The premise that the primary determinants of people's behavior may shift over time has important methodological implications. First and foremost, given the principle of parsimony, the burden of proof rests with investigators who assert that the determinants of behavior vary across phases of the behavior change process. Cross-sectional comparisons of individuals at different phases can be informative, but systematic longitudinal and experimental work is needed to test predictions regarding the determinants of each transition (see Weinstein, Rothman, & Nicolich, 1998, for a comprehensive description of how to test predictions derived from stage- and continuum-based models of health behavior). Second, any systematic analysis of the behavior change process, by definition, requires a methodology that provides a rich description of the ongoing relation between people's thoughts and feelings, and their behavior. Psychologists have relied on methods that enable them to delineate the manner in which people's behavior is regulated by their psychological state, but the context for these accounts is almost always a single, often brief, interval of time. Insufficient attention has been paid to how the process unfolds over several time intervals. For example, little has been done to investigate how having engaged in a behavior affects people's thoughts and feelings, then, in turn, how those thoughts and feelings influence subsequent behavior (Rothman et al., 2003). More frequent assessment of psychological constructs would enable investigators to examine the conditions under which people are and are not able to sustain their favorable views of the behavior (a crucial determinant of successful behavior change). In contrast, behavioral epidemiologists often track individuals' behavior over extended periods of time. Yet the predominant methodologies and research designs used involve infrequent assessments, thus providing minimal information regarding people's ongoing experiences as they manage their behavior (but see Shiffman & Stone, 1998). For example, despite the extensive volume of research on weight control behavior, remarkably little is known about people's experiences as they make ongoing changes in their dietary and exercise practices (Jeffery, Kelly, Rothman, Sherwood, & Boutelle, in press; also, for a review of the self-regulation of weight loss, see Herman & Polivy, Chapter 25, this volume). Given the complementary nature of the approaches associated with these two disciplines, the development of new, interdisciplinary initiatives led jointly by psychologists and epidemiologists may provide the best opportunity to examine these issues comprehensively (King et al., 2002; Suls & Rothman, in press).

Testing predictions regarding the differential determinants of initial and long-term behavior change also necessitates that investigators capture the unique effect that a particular psychological state (e.g., self-efficacy) has on each phase of the behavior change process. To date, claims regarding the determinants of behavioral maintenance are typically based on tests of whether a psychological state (e.g., self-efficacy at baseline) can predict a distal behavioral outcome (e.g., smoking status 18 months later). Yet this analytic approach is inconclusive regarding the factors that underlie behavioral maintenance, because it cannot determine whether, in the current example, people's initial feelings of self-efficacy contribute to their willingness to maintain their behavior over and above its effect on their initial behavioral efforts. With the development of theoretical models that specify differential predictors of behavior over time, the need arises to disentangle the direct relation between a psychological state and a distal outcome from the indirect relation between these two constructs that is mediated by people's initial behavioral efforts.

The proposition that factors differentially affect behavior across phases implies that phase moderates the *relative* impact of a given construct on behavior change. However, it may prove difficult to detect these shifts in a traditional analytic test of moderation. For instance, when examined on its own, the prospective effect of self-efficacy on behavior may appear equally strong across all phases of the behavior change process. Yet when other constructs are included in the model, its predictive value may shift over time (e.g., satisfaction with the behavior may emerge as the stronger predictor of behavior during the maintenance phase). One way to discern whether a construct's impact shifts as a function of phase is to separate individuals into subgroups according to their phase, then test its relative ability to predict behavior prospectively within each subgroup.

THE IMPLICATIONS OF A FOUR-PHASE BEHAVIORAL FRAMEWORK FOR THREE SUBSTANTIVE RESEARCH PROGRAMS ON BEHAVIORAL SELF-REGULATION

Although research on behavioral decision making has not systematically examined the processes by which people move from initiating to maintaining a pattern of behavior, several substantive areas of research address issues germane to the ongoing self-regulation of behavior. For example, some investigators have focused on features of the social environment that may be differentially related to behavioral initiation and maintenance (e.g., Mermelstein, Cohen, Lichtenstein, Baer, & Kamarck, 1986), whereas others have focused on personality characteristics (e.g., Stein, Newcomb, & Bentler, 1996). Here, we consider three separate research traditions that have examined the relation between a psychological state and people's ability to regulate their behavior. Specifically, we have chosen to focus on (1) self-efficacy, (2) self-regulatory strength, and (3) intrinsic–extrinsic motivation. In reviewing these research areas, we have chosen to elucidate not only the degree to which investigators have theoretically and empirically examined their influence on behavioral initiation and behavioral maintenance but also the predictions concerning the role that each of these constructs might play within our four-phase model of the behavior change process.

Self-Efficacy and Behavior Change

The premise that people's behavior is contingent on their perceived ability to execute actions in support of the behavior (i.e., self-efficacy) has had a fundamental impact on both research and theory regarding behavior change (Bandura, 1997; see also Cervone, Mor, Orom, Shadel, & Scott, Chapter 10, this volume). In fact, self-efficacy, or variables that appear to operate as proxies for the construct, can be found in many, if not all, theories of behavior change (Salovey, et al., 1998; Weinstein, 1993). As discussed earlier in the chapter, there is strong empirical support for the thesis that people's confidence in their ability to engage in a behavior positively predicts subsequent behavior, and that successfully enacting a behavior heightens people's confidence in their behavior (Bandura, 1997). However, is it appropriate to conclude that self-efficacy is an equally valuable predictor of behavior at all points in the behavior change process?

Although investigators have consistently demonstrated that self-efficacy is a robust predictor of behavioral initiation (e.g., enrolling in a smoking cessation program; Brod & Hall, 1984), most empirical investigations have failed to consider whether it has an effect at specific points in the behavior change process. To date, the precaution adoption process model is one of the few conceptual frameworks that explicitly constrains the point in the behavior change process at which self-efficacy is identified as a valuable predictor of behavior (Weinstein, 1988). In the model, high self-efficacy is identified as a critical determinant of behavioral initiation, but only once people have committed to making a change in their behavior. Empirical support for this premise was obtained in an intervention study to promote radon testing (Weinstein, Lyon, Sandman, & Cuite, 1998). Specifically, an intervention designed to heighten confidence in the ability to test for radon gas motivated people to test, but only when targeting people who had previously decided to test. People who were undecided about whether to test benefited more from an intervention emphasizing personal risk than from one emphasizing self-efficacy.

When placed in the context of our four-phase model of behavior change, the findings obtained by Weinstein, Lyon, and colleagues (1998) are consistent with the prediction that a heightened sense of personal efficacy is necessary if people are to complete the initial response phase of the behavior change process. According to our model, confidence in one's ability to perform a behavior is also a critical determinant of success during the continued response phase. In particular, it is essential that people maintain their sense of self-efficacy as they grapple with the challenges posed by the new pattern of behavior. Although the premise that self-efficacy beliefs are closely linked to people's ability to manage lapses and the threat of relapse (e.g., relapse prevention; Marlatt & Gordon, 1985), very few investigators have attempted to specify how changes in self-efficacy during this phase affect subsequent behavioral decisions. However, Shiffman and his colleagues (2000) have reported data consistent with this framework in the area of smoking cessation. Daily shifts in smokers' confidence in their ability to quit was a significant predictor of whether a lapse progressed into a relapse, even after controlling for prior smoking behavior.

According to the proposed four-phase model of behavior change, the predictive value of self-efficacy shifts as people move from initiating to maintaining a behavior. Once people have shown that they can successfully manage their behavior, the decision to maintain that behavior is thought to have less to do with variability in people's perceptions of their ability to perform the behavior, and more to do with their willingness or desire to sustain the behavior.

Although investigators often assert that self-efficacy is a critical determinant of long-term behavior change (e.g., Bandura, 1997; Schwarzer, 2001), there is surprisingly little empirical evidence that self-efficacy has a direct effect on decisions regarding behavioral maintenance. Studies that purport to demonstrate that self-efficacy beliefs predict maintenance consistently rely on tests of the relation between an initial measure of self-efficacy and a single, distal behavioral measure (e.g., Dzewaltowski, 1989; Dzewaltowski, Noble, & Shaw, 1990; Hurley & Shea, 1992; Kavanagh, Gooley, & Wilson, 1993; McCaul, Glasgow, & Schafer, 1987). As discussed earlier, this analytical approach cannot discern whether initial levels of self-efficacy have a unique (direct) effect on longer term behavior, independent of their effect on initial behavioral efforts. Research designs that allow for the repeated assessment of both people's behavior and their confidence in the ability to perform the behavior are needed to specify more precisely the role that self-efficacy plays throughout the behavior change process. We have identified two studies that meet these requirements (Hoelscher, Lichtstein, & Rosenthal, 1986; Nicki, Remington, & MacDonald, 1984); however, neither controlled for prior behavior when assessing the prospective relationship between a measure of self-efficacy beliefs and behavior. Because people's behavior is thought to both affect and be affected by self-efficacy, it is critical that tests of self-efficacy's ability to predict future behavior control for prior behavior. To the extent that analyses of nonexperimental studies fail to control for the influence of prior behavior, they may systematically overestimate the impact of self-efficacy on behavior (Weinstein, Rothman, et al., 1998).

Although it was not designed to address these issues, efforts to identify the factors that mediated the impact of the National Institute of Mental Health Multisite HIV Prevention Trial Group (2001) may shed some light on these issues. The investigators examined the degree to which participants' beliefs 3 months after the intervention predicted consistent condom use or abstinence throughout the 12-month trial. The investigators specifically examined perceived safer sex self-efficacy, condom use skills, safer sex knowledge, and perceived consequences of using condoms. It was noteworthy that beliefs about the consequences of condom use (i.e., how it would feel to use a condom, or how a partner might react to using a condom) proved to be stronger mediators than were measures of skills and self-efficacy. This pattern of results suggests that the decision to use condoms *consistently* is less a function of people's confidence in their ability to use condoms than of the belief that condom use is associated with favorable outcomes or, at least, that it does not lead to unfavorable outcomes. Although these indicators assessed people's outcome expectations, it is plausible to assume that these expectations reflect people's initial experiences during the trial with using condoms and, thus, may serve as a proxy for people's satisfaction or valuation of the behavior. Of course, before any firm conclusions can be drawn regarding the differential impact of self-efficacy on behavior change, research using the previously described analytic framework is needed.

Self-Regulatory Strength and Behavior Change

A fundamental aspect of any effort to adopt a new pattern of behavior is the need to inhibit a prior pattern of behavior. Baumeister and his colleagues (Baumeister, Heatherton, & Tice, 1994; Muraven & Baumeister, 2000; for reviews of the self-regulatory resource model, see Schmeichel & Baumeister, Chapter 5, and Vohs & Ciarocco, Chapter 20, this volume) have argued that to override, inhibit, or alter a dominant response tendency, people must possess a sufficient degree of self-regulatory strength, which is conceptualized as a limited, but renewable, cognitive resource that is drained whenever someone attempts to regulate his or her emotions, thoughts, or behavior (Baumeister & Heatherton, 1996). Because deficits in self-regulatory strength are thought to be a primary determinant of self-regulatory failure, relapses are predicted to be more likely when people are faced with repeated demands to manage their thoughts, feelings, or behavior. Support for this premise has been obtained from a series of empirical investigations across a range of behavioral domains (Baumeister, Bratslavsky, Muraven, & Tice, 1998; Muraven, Tice, & Baumeister, 1998; Vohs & Heatherton, 2000).

When considered in the context of the four-phase model we have specified in the behavior change process, self-regulatory strength would seem to be more important in the initial response and continued response phases compared to the maintenance and habit phases. During the *initial response* phase, people are likely to have difficulty initiating a new pattern of behavior successfully, if they are in a situation that involves other significant, self-regulatory demands. In fact, from a self-regulatory strength perspective, one would predict that to the extent that people overlay additional self-regulatory demands on the behavior change process (e.g., attempting to hide the new behavior from friends or family), they will have less success completing this phase.

Given that the threat posed by lapses and relapses are predicted to occur during the continued response phase, self-regulatory strength should be an important determinant of whether people are able to complete this phase of the behavior change process. In fact, most of the empirical work concerning self-regulatory strength has involved tasks analogous to the demands of this phase. To the extent to which people feel that the new behavior requires continued effort and considerable self-regulatory resources, they may find it difficult to sustain their confidence and commitment to the behavior. Moreover, even if people have allocated sufficient resources to continue their new behavior, they may find that this results in a resource deficit and undermines their ability to respond to the needs of their family, friends, or employer. The dissatisfaction that subsequently emanates from these domains may not only heighten people's need for self-regulatory strength but also lower their evaluation of the new behavior.

Because people's behavioral practices during the maintenance and habit phases reflect more their evaluation of the behavior than their ability to perform it, the cognitive resources that were necessary to perform the new behavior consistently in the first two phases are no longer needed. This does not mean that the behavior does not continue to require effort and commitment; rather, there is a steep drop in people's needs to override or inhibit an underlying behavior. The new pattern of behavior transforms into the dominant response. In fact, the onset of the maintenance phase would appear to be the time at which people can begin to take on additional self-regulatory demands, without critically undermining the new behavior. For example, if someone needed to modify two problem behaviors, such as smoking and poor dietary habits, he or she might choose to alter dietary habits only after demonstrating the ability to refrain consistently from smoking. With the onset of the habit phase, the new pattern of behavior has evolved into a person's new dominant response tendency; thus, the demands placed on self-regulatory strength should be either extremely minimal or nonexistent (Heatherton & Vohs, 1998).

Motivation and Behavior Change

People's motivation for engaging in a pattern of behavior has traditionally been considered an important determinant of their ability to initiate and maintain a pattern of behavior. Specifically, investigators have distinguished between two classes of motivation: external and internal. External motivation refers to either extrinsic motivation that arises from the desire to gain (avoid) an externally imposed reward (punishment), or controlled motivation that arises from the desire to please others (Deci & Ryan, 1985). Internal motivation refers to either the desire to obtain internally imposed rewards (intrinsic motivation) or the motivation to engage in a behavior to satisfy one's own needs (autonomous motivation; Deci & Ryan, 1985). Investigators have traditionally asserted that people are more likely to sustain a pattern of behavior over time if it is based on intrinsic or autonomous motivation compared to extrinsic or controlled motivation. The benefit associated with an internal motivation is that a person's assessment of the behavior is more under his or her control and less contingent on outside reinforcement.

When examined within the context of our four-phase model of the behavior change process, it would appear that internal motivation may exert a more positive influence than external motivation on behavior during the maintenance phase. However, it is less clear whether behavior during the first two phases of the behavior change process are differentially affected by these two classes of motivations. During the initial response phase, participants focus on the outcomes they expect to experience. Given the focus on future outcomes, the perceived desirability of the outcome is likely to be more important than whether the rewards reflect internal or external contingencies. With the onset of the continued response phase, people whose behavior reflects intrinsic or autonomous motivational needs may find it easier to sustain their confidence in and feelings about the behavior. This should be particularly true when the costs associated with engaging in the new behavior are more salient than the associated benefits. Under these conditions, people may find it easier to sustain themselves through this unpleasant period if their actions are motivated by their own needs and desires as opposed to the needs and desires of others. However, the differential impact of these two classes of motivational concerns may be attenuated to the extent that people enjoy engaging in the new behavior. In fact, to the extent that people derive a sense of satisfaction from engaging in the new pattern of behavior, they may choose to take a greater sense of personal ownership of the task and, over time, develop a stronger sense of intrinsic motivation.

The empirical literature concerning the impact of internal and external motivation on behavior change provides some insight into the relation between these constructs and behavior change. Across several studies, the degree to which people are motivated by internal concerns has been shown to predict the successful initiation and maintenance of behavior change (e.g., Williams, Freedman, & Deci, 1998; Williams, Ryan, Rodin, Grolnick, & Deci, 1998). Evidence regarding the effect of external motivation on behavior change is somewhat ambiguous. Some studies have found it to be a negative predictor of initial behavior change (e.g., Curry, Grothaus, & McBride, 1997; Curry, Wagner, & Grothaus, 1990), whereas others have found it to be unrelated to behavioral outcomes (e.g., Curry et al., 1997; Williams, Freedman, et al., 1998; Williams, Ryan, et al., 1998). However, the structure of the research designs and/or analytic strategies employed in these studies precludes drawing any specific conclusions regarding the effect that internal and external motivation has on each unique phase of the behavior change process. In particular, it would be interesting to test whether measures of intrinsic or autonomous motivations predict behavioral maintenance over and above their effect on initial behavior change. In addition, a more detailed assessment of people's experience with the behavior change process would offer an opportunity to determine whether particular classes of behavioral experiences enable people to shift from an external to an internal motivation for behavior change.

LOOKING TOWARD THE FUTURE

Even a cursory review of the goals outlined in *Healthy People 2010* (U.S. Department of Health and Human Services, 2001) reveals the practical benefits that would arise, for both individuals and society, if people would not only initiate but also maintain changes in their behavioral practices. Even modest, sustained changes in people's lifestyles would afford substantial reductions in disease morbidity and mortality, as well as reduced health care costs. Yet efforts to promote long-term behavior change effectively are constrained by our theoretical understanding of the factors that regulate people's behavioral practices over time. Investigators need to more thoroughly specify and test the implications drawn from their theoretical models regarding ongoing behavioral practices. In order to encourage this line of work, we have delineated a series of testable predictions regarding the factors that may regulate people's ability to go from successfully initiating a new behavior to making it a habit. We hope this framework inspires investigators to undertake theoretical and empirical investigations that will ultimately enable us to specify the factors that inhibit and facilitate long-term behavior change, which, in turn, can inform the design and implementation of intervention approaches that reliably elicit healthy changes in behavioral practices.

ACKNOWLEDGMENT

Preparation of this chapter was supported in part by Grant No. NS38441 from the National Institute of Neurological Disorders and Stroke.

NOTE

1. Because health behavior is the primary domain in which conceptual and empirical attention has been given to behavioral maintenance, we have chosen to ground our discussion in this area. However, the issues addressed in this chapter should generalize to other behavioral domains.

REFERENCES

Aiken, L. S., West, S. G., Woodward, C. K., & Reno, R. R. (1994). Health beliefs and compliance with mammography screening recommendations in asymptomatic women. *Health Psychology, 13*, 122–129.

Ajzen, I. (1991). The theory of planned behavior. *Organizational Behavior and Human Decision Processes, 50*, 179–211.

Ajzen, I. (2002). Residual effects of past on later behavior: Habituation and reasoned action perspectives. *Personality and Social Psychology Review, 6*, 107–122.

Ajzen, I., & Fishbein, M. (1980). *Understanding attitudes and predicting social behavior.* Englewood Cliffs, NJ: Prentice-Hall.

Bandura, A. (1986). *Social foundations of thought and action: A social cognitive theory.* Englewood Cliffs, NJ: Prentice-Hall.

Bandura, A. (1997). *Self-efficacy: The exercise of control.* New York: Freeman.

Barton, J., Chassin, L., Presson, C. C., & Sherman, S. J. (1982). Social image factors as motivators of smoking initiation in early and middle adolescence. *Child Development, 53*, 1499–1511.

Baumeister, R. F., Bratslavsky, E., Muraven, M., & Tice, D. M. (1998). Ego depletion: Is the active self a limited resource? *Journal of Personality and Social Psychology, 74*, 1252–1265.

Baumeister, R. F., & Heatherton, T. F. (1996). Self-regulation failure: An overview. *Psychological Inquiry, 7*, 1–15.

Baumeister, R. F., Heatherton, T. F., & Tice, D. M. (1994). *Losing control: How and why people fail at self-regulation.* San Diego, CA: Academic Press.

Brod, M. I., & Hall, S. M. (1984). Joiners and non-joiners in smoking treatment: A comparison of psychosocial variables. *Addictive Behaviors, 9*, 217–221.

Brownell, K. D., Marlatt, G. A., Lichtenstein, E., & Wilson, G. T. (1986). Understanding and preventing relapse. *American Psychologist, 41*, 765–782.

Carver, C. S., & Scheier, M. F. (1990). Principles of self-regulation: Action and emotion. In E. T. Higgins & R. M. Sorrentino (Eds.), *Handbook of motivation and cognition: Vol. 2. Foundations of social behavior* (pp. 645–672). New York: Guilford Press.

Conner, M., Sheeran, P., Norman, P., & Armitage, C. J. (2000). Temporal stability as a moderator of the relationships in the theory of planned behavior. *British Journal of Social Psychology, 39*, 469–494.

Curry, S. J., Grothaus, L. C., & McBride, C. M. (1997). Reasons for quitting: Intrinsic and extrinsic motivation for smoking cessation in a population-based sample of smokers. *Addictive Behaviors, 22*, 727–739.

Curry, S. J., & McBride, C. M. (1994). Relapse prevention for smoking cessation: Review and evaluation of concepts and interventions. *Annual Review of Public Health, 15*, 345–366.

Curry, S. J., Wagner, E. H., & Grothaus, L. C. (1990). Intrinsic and extrinsic motivation for smoking cessation. *Journal of Consulting and Clinical Psychology, 58*, 310–316.

Deci, E. L., & Ryan, R. M. (1985). *Intrinsic motivation and self-determination in human behavior.* New York: Plenum Press.

Dzewaltowski, D. A. (1989). Towards a model of exercise motivation. *Journal of Sport and Exercise Psychology, 11*, 251–269.

Dzewaltowski, D. A., Noble, J. M., & Shaw, J. M. (1990). Physical activity participation: Social cognitive theory versus the theories of reasoned action and planned behavior. *Journal of Sport and Exercise Psychology, 12*, 388–405.

Ferguson, E., & Bibby, P. A. (2002). Predicting future blood donor returns: Past behavior, intentions, and observer effects. *Health Psychology, 21*, 513–518.

Fisher, L. A., & Bauman, K. E. (1988). Influence and selection in the friend–adolescent relationship: Findings from studies of adolescent smoking and drinking. *Journal of Applied Social Psychology, 18*, 289–314.

Frank, E., Prien, R. F., Jarrett, R. B., Keller, M. B., Kupfer, D. J., Lavori, P. W., et al. (1991). Conceptualization and rationale for consensus definitions of terms in major depressive disorder: Remission, recovery, relapse, and recurrence. *Archives of General Psychiatry, 48*, 851–855.

Gollwitzer, P. M. (1996). The volitional benefits of planning. In P. M. Gollwitzer & J. A. Bargh (Eds.), *The psychology of action: Linking cognition and motivation to behavior* (pp. 287–312). New York: Guilford Press.

Gollwitzer, P. M. (1999). Implementation intentions: Strong effects of simple plans. *American Psychologist, 54*, 493–503

Heatherton, T. F., & Vohs, K. D. (1998). Why is it so difficult to inhibit behavior? *Psychological Inquiry, 9*, 212–215.

Hoelscher, T. J., Lichtstein, K. L., & Rosenthal, T. L. (1986). Home relaxation practice in hypertension treatment: Objective assessment and compliance induction. *Journal of Consulting and Clinical Psychology, 54*, 217–221.

Hunt, W. A., Barnett, L. W., & Branch, L. G. (1971). Relapse rates in addiction programs. *Journal of Clinical Psychology, 27*, 455–456.

Hurley, C. C., & Shea, C. A. (1992). Self-efficacy: Strategy for enhancing diabetes self-care. *Diabetes Educator, 18*, 146–150.

Jeffery, R. W., Drewnowski, A., Epstein, L. H., Stunkard, A. J., Wilson, G. T., Wing, R. R., et al. (2000), Long-term maintenance of weight loss: Current status. *Health Psychology, 19*, 5–16.

Jeffery, R. W., Kelly, K. M., Rothman, A. J., Sherwood, N. E., & Boutelle, N. (in press). The weight loss experience: A descriptive analysis. *Annals of Behavioral Medicine.*

Kavanagh, D. J., Gooley, S., & Wilson, P. H. (1993). Prediction of adherence and control in diabetes. *Journal of Behavioral Medicine, 16*, 509–522.

King, C., Rothman, A. J., & Jeffery, R. W. (2002). The challenge study: Theory-based interventions for smoking and weight loss. *Health Education Research, 17*, 522–530.

Leventhal, H., & Cameron, L. (1987). Behavioral theories and the problem of compliance. *Patient Education and Counseling, 10*, 117–138.

Leventhal, H., Nerenz, D. R., & Steele, D. J. (1984). Illness representations and coping with health threats. In A. Baum & J. Singer (Eds.), *A handbook of psychology and health* (pp. 219–252). Hillsdale, NJ: Erlbaum.

Maddux, J. E., & Rogers, R. W. (1983). Protection motivation and self-efficacy: A revised theory of fear appeals and attitude change. *Journal of Experimental Social Psychology, 19*, 469–479.

Marlatt, G. A., & Gordon, J. R. (Eds.). (1985). *Relapse prevention: Maintenance strategies in the treatment of addictive behaviors.* New York: Guilford Press.

McCaul, K. D., Glasgow, R. E., & O'Neill, H. K. (1992). The problem of creating habits: Establishing health protective dental behaviors. *Health Psychology, 11*, 101–110.

McCaul, K. D., Glasgow, R. E., & Schafer, L. C. (1987). Diabetes regimen behaviors: Predicting adherence. *Medical Care, 25*, 868–881.

Mermelstein, R., Cohen, S., Lichtenstein, E., Baer, J. S., & Kamarck, T. (1986). Social support and smoking cessation and maintenance. *Journal of Consulting and Clinical Psychology, 54*, 447–453.

Muraven, M., & Baumeister, R. F. (2000). Self-regulation and depletion of limited resources: Does self-control resemble a muscle? *Psychological Bulletin, 126*, 247–259.

Muraven, M., Tice, D. M., & Baumeister, R. F. (1998). Self-control as limited resource: Regulatory depletion patterns. *Journal of Personality and Social Psychology, 74*, 774–789.

National Institute of Mental Health Multisite HIV Prevention Trial Group. (2001). Social-cognitive theory mediators of behavior change in the National Institute of Mental Health Multisite HIV Prevention Trial. *Health Psychology, 20*, 369–376.

Nicki, R. M., Remington, R. E., & MacDonald, G. A. (1984). Self-efficacy, nicotine-fading/self-monitoring and cigarette smoking behaviour. *Behaviour Research Therapy, 22*, 477–485.

Norman, P., Conner, M., & Bell, R. (1999). The theory of planned behavior and smoking cessation. *Health Psychology, 18*, 89–94.

Ockene, J. K., Emmons, K. M., Mermelstein, R. J., Perkins, K. A., Bonollo, D. S., Vorhees, C. C., et al. (2000). Relapse and maintenance issues for smoking cessation. *Health Psychology, 19*, 17–31.

Ouellete, J. A., & Wood, W. (1998). Habit and intention in everyday life: The multiple processes by which past behavior predicts future behavior. *Psychological Bulletin, 124*, 54–74.

Perri, M. G., Nezu, A. M., Patti, E. T., & McCann, K. L. (1989). Effect of length of treatment on weight loss. *Journal of Consulting and Clinical Psychology, 57*, 450–452.

Prochaska, J. O., DiClemente, C. C., & Norcross, J. C. (1992). In search of how people change: Applications to addictive behaviors. *American Psychologist, 47*, 1102–1114.

Prochaska, J. O., & Velicer, W. F. (1997). The transtheoretical model of health behavior change. *American Journal of Health Promotion, 12*, 38–48.

Rakowski, W., Dube, C. E., Marcus, B. H., Prochaska, J. O., Velicer, W. F., & Abrams, D. B. (1992). Assessing elements of women's decisions about mammography. *Health Psychology, 11*, 111–118.

Ronis, D. L., Yates, J. F., & Kirscht, J. P. (1989). Attitudes, decisions, and habits as determinants of behavior. In A. R. Pratkanis, S. J. Breckler, & A. G. Greenwald (Eds.), *Attitude structure and function* (pp. 213–239). Hillsdale, NJ: Erlbaum.

Rosentstock, I. M., Strecher, V. J., & Becker, M. H. (1988). Social learning theory and the health belief model. *Health Education Quarterly, 15*, 175–183.

Rothman, A. J. (2000). Toward a theory-based analysis of behavioral maintenance. *Health Psychology, 19*, 1–6.

Rothman, A. J., Kelly, K. M., Hertel, A. W., & Salovey P. (2003). Message frames and illness representations: Implications for interventions to sustain healthy behavior. In L. D. Cameron & H. Leventhal (Eds.), *The self-regulation of health and illness behaviour.* London: Routledge.

Salovey, P., Rothman, A. J., & Rodin, J. (1998). Health behavior. In D. T. Gilbert, S. T. Fiske, & G. Lindzey (Eds.), *The handbook of social psychology* (4th ed., Vol. 2, pp. 633–683). New York: McGraw-Hill.

Schwarz, N., & Strack, F. (1991). Evaluating one's life: A judgmental model of subjective well-being. In F. Strack, M. Argyle, & N. Schwarz, (Eds.), *Subjective well-being: An interdisciplinary perspective* (pp. 27–47). Oxford, UK: Pergamon.

Schwarzer, R. (2001). Social-cognitive factors in changing health related behaviors. *Current Directions in Psychological Science, 10*, 47–51.

Shiffman, S., Balabanis, M. H., Paty, J. A., Engberg, J., Gwaltney, C. J., Liu, K. S., et al. (2000). Dynamic effects of self-efficacy on smoking lapse and relapse. *Health Psychology, 19*, 315–323.

Shiffman, S., & Stone, A. A. (1998). Introduction to special section: Ecological momentary assessment in health psychology. *Health Psychology, 17,* 3–5.

Stein, J. A., Newcomb, M. D., & Bentler, P. M. (1996). Initiation and maintenance of tobacco smoking: Changing personality correlates in adolescence and young adulthood. *Journal of Applied Social Psychology, 26,* 160–187.

Suls, J., & Rothman, A. J. (in press). Evolution of the psychosocial model: Implications for the future of health psychology. *Health Psychology.*

Taylor, S. E., & Gollwitzer, P. M. (1995). Effects of mindset on positive illusions. *Journal of Personality and Social Psychology, 69,* 213–226.

U.S. Department of Health and Human Services. (2001). *Healthy people 2010: National health promotion and disease prevention objectives.* Washington, DC: U.S. Government Printing Office.

Vohs, K. D., & Heatherton, T. F. (2000). Self-regulatory failure: A resource-depletion approach. *Psychological Science, 11,* 249–254.

Weinstein, N. D. (1988). The precaution adoption process. *Health Psychology, 7,* 355–386.

Weinstein, N. D. (1993). Testing four competing theories of health-protective behavior. *Health Psychology, 12,* 324–333.

Weinstein, N. D., Lyon, J. E., Sandman, P. M., & Cuite, C. L. (1998). Experimental evidence for stages of health behavior change: The precaution adoption process model applied to home radon testing. *Health Psychology, 17,* 445–453.

Weinstein, N. D., Rothman, A. J., & Nicolich, M. (1998). Using correlational data to examine the effects of risk perceptions on precautionary behavior. *Psychology and Health, 13,* 479–501.

Weinstein, N. D., Rothman, A. J., & Sutton, S. R. (1998). Stage theories of health behavior: Conceptual and methodological issues. *Health Psychology, 17,* 290–299.

Williams, G. C., Freedman, Z. R., & Deci, E. L. (1998). Supporting autonomy to motivate patients with diabetes glucose control. *Diabetes Care, 21,* 1644–1651.

Williams, G. C., Ryan, R. M., Rodin, G. C., Grolnick, W. S., & Deci, E. L. (1998). Autonomous regulation and long-term medication adherence in adult outpatients. *Health Psychology, 17,* 269–276.

Wood, W., Quinn, J. M., & Kashy, D. A. (2002). Habits in everyday life: Thought, emotion, and action. *Journal of Personality and Social Psychology, 83,* 1281–1297.

Worth, K., Sullivan, H., Hertel, A. W., Nordgren, L., Jeffery, R. W., & Rothman, A. J. (2002, August). *Avoidance goals can be beneficial: A look at smoking cessation.* Poster session presented at the annual meeting of the American Psychological Association, Chicago.

II

Cognitive, Physiological, and Neurological Dimensions of Self-Regulation

8

Automatic Self-Regulation

GRÁINNE M. FITZSIMONS
JOHN A. BARGH

What is self-regulation, exactly? What does it involve? If one looks to classic social and motivational psychology for an answer to these questions, the answer is sure to include the ability to control and determine one's behavior consciously and intentionally. For example, Carver and Scheier's (1981) influential self-regulation model posits feedback loops such that individuals must become consciously aware of the discrepancy between the current and desired self-states, then consciously choose to engage in action to reduce that discrepancy. And for the "cool system" in Metcalfe and Mischel's (1999) self-regulation model to function, individuals must consciously and intentionally attempt to control their behavior to overcome the influences of the current environment (e.g., a dieter not eating a tasty but fat-laden dessert).

In short, conscious choices and strategies permeate psychological theories of self-regulation and goal pursuit as essential mediating variables (e.g., Bandura, 1986; Deci & Ryan, 1985; Locke & Latham, 1990). Yet considerable evidence suggests that such conscious processes are neither necessary or even typical for effective self-regulation: People manage quite well on a moment-to-moment basis, without needing to select and guide every action consciously.

Consciousness has been rather unceremoniously removed from theories of many social psychological phenomena in recent years, so perhaps it is no surprise to find that it is an unnecessary guest in models of self-regulation as well. On the other hand, self-regulation may be more complex, more dynamic, and more interactive than those other phenomena (Baumeister, 1998), so conscious, intentional processes seem more at home here than in, say, models of stereotyping and person perception. Self-regulation is indeed complex: More than willpower alone, and more than just goal pursuit, it is the capacity of individuals to guide themselves, in any way possible, toward important goal states (Baumeister, 1998; Gollwitzer, 1996). Therefore, it consists of a wide range of cognitive and motivational operations, such as acting quickly to take opportunities, ignoring distractions, acting flexibly in response to situations, overcoming obstacles, and managing conflicts between goals (see Gollwitzer & Moskowitz, 1996). These operations are essential to successful self-regulation, but accumulating evidence indicates that the role of conscious processes in these operations is considerably less than previously thought. Self-regulation, it seems, can be active, complex, dynamic—and automatic.

IN PURSUIT OF NONCONSCIOUS SELF-REGULATION

For higher order motivations to be fulfilled through self-action, goals must guide and regulate action through diverse and flexible means. For example, once a person sets a higher order goal of getting a job promotion, he or she may need to regulate many aspects of thought and behavior, such as to think about his or her boss more positively, to substitute cooperative feelings for competitive ones, to work hard to successfully complete a task, and to control the desire to snap at a coworker. We suggest that all of these acts of self-regulation—of cognition, emotion, and behavior—can occur without the need for conscious intervention or guidance. In fact, due to the apparently quite limited capacity of conscious self-regulatory abilities (Baumeister, Bratslavsky, Muraven, & Tice, 1998; Muraven, Tice, & Baumeister, 1998), much of self regulation *has* to occur nonconsciously to be successful. Because even the simplest acts of conscious self-control (instigated through experimental instructions) deplete this limited resource, it would seem that most moment-to-moment self-regulation must occur nonconsciously (i.e., without using this limited resource), if it is to be effective.

An alternative (or rather, complement) to the classic self-regulatory models that highlight the mediating role of conscious choice is the auto-motive model of self-regulation (Bargh, 1990; Bargh & Gollwitzer, 1994). According to this model, the full sequence of goal pursuit—from goal setting to the completion of the attempt to attain the goal—can proceed outside of conscious awareness and guidance. But how can goals operate to guide our behavior without our knowledge? First, in harmony with several motivation theorists (see Hull, 1931; Kruglanski, 1996; Tolman, 1932), goals are hypothesized to be mentally represented in the same way as are other cognitive constructs—that is, to correspond to internal knowledge structures containing information, such as opportunity conditions, possible means (e.g., plans) for attaining the goal, and behavioral procedures, to concretely enact those means. Second, it follows from the presumed existence of these goal representations that they are capable of being activated automatically by features of one's environment, that is, by the mere presence of situational cues strongly associated with the pursuit of those goals. Automatic activation means that no intervening conscious choice or involvement is needed for the internal representation to become active and operative. Just as other social knowledge structures, such as stereotypes and attitudes, have been shown to become automatically activated in the mere presence of highly relevant environmental features (such as racial features or the object of the attitude in question; see Fazio, 1986; Greenwald & Banaji, 1995), the auto-motive model assumes that goals, too, can develop nonconscious, automatic activation capabilities, under the same conditions.[1]

Nonconsciously operating goals enable people to control thoughts, feelings, and behavior, without the need to invoke conscious choice or control processes. Moreover, the special qualities of motivational states and self-regulatory mechanisms that make for successful conscious self-regulation also appear to hold true for automatic self-regulation (see Chartrand & Bargh, 2002) in the realms of cognition, emotion, and behavior.

Automatic Regulation of Cognition

Research has demonstrated that even relatively low-level cognitive processes, such as those involved in memory and attention, can be regulated through nonconscious means. In the first set of studies to address this issue, Chartrand and Bargh (1996) showed that automatically operating information-processing goals affect the organization of information in memory and its recall. These studies conceptually replicated classic findings from the social cognition literature that had focused on the effect of various conscious goals on information processing (Hamilton, Katz, & Leirer, 1980; Hastie & Kumar, 1979). To activate these goals nonconsciously, Chartrand and Bargh (1996) used a standard "priming" manipulation in which goal-relevant stimuli were presented in a subtle and unobtrusive manner. In this task, participants formed grammatical sentences out of series of words presented in a scrambled order (Srull & Wyer, 1979). Embedded in the words presented were words related to either the goal of impression formation (e.g., "judge," "evaluate") or the goal of memorization (e.g., "remember," "retain"). Participants then read a list of behaviors ostensibly performed by a target person. Identically replicating the earlier findings involving consciously pursued goals, participants that were primed with an impression formation goal remembered more of the target's behaviors, and organized that memory around specific personality traits to a greater extent than did those primed with a memorization goal.

In a second study, words related to impression formation goals were subliminally presented during a computerized task. In this manner, half of the participants were primed with an impression formation goal, with the other half receiving no priming. All participants then read a list of behaviors allegedly performed by a target person. Again replicating previous work on consciously held impression goals (Hastie & Kumar, 1979), participants with nonconsciously activated impression formation goals automatically formed an impression of the target person while reading his behaviors, whereas those with no primed goal did not form such an impression. These findings were the first to demonstrate that basic and essential social cognitive processes can be effectively regulated through nonconscious means.

Subsequent research has supported and extended these results regarding the influence of nonconscious goals on low-level cognitions. For example, selective remembering and forgetting—both important components of optimal memory—have recently been shown to be regulated by nonconsciously activated memory strategies (Mitchell, Macrae, Schooler, Rowe, & Milne, 2002). Participants showed preferential memory for words followed by the subliminal cue "remember" and impaired memory for words followed by the subliminal cue "forget." In further evidence of the role that nonconscious goals can play in regulating low-level cognitive processes, automatic goals have also been shown to guide selective attention (Moskowitz, 2002). Selective attention is, without doubt, a strategic self-regulatory process: Individuals focus attention on what is important (the current goal) and are thereby vigilant for goal-relevant information in the environment (Gollwitzer & Moskowitz, 1996). Guided by the idea that goals can operate strategically, yet remain outside of conscious awareness, Moskowitz (2002) found that when goals were implicitly activated, attention was selectively drawn to goal-relevant items, both in a Stroop-like task and a reaction-time task. Thus, even selective attention can be regulated by nonconsciously activated goals.

Recently, such nonconscious regulation of cognitive processes has been found to extend to working memory itself—the mental system considered to be the seat of conscious control (or "executive") processes (e.g., Neisser, 1967; Smith & Jonides, 1999). To examine the nonconscious regulation of working memory, Hassin (in press) made use of a novel working memory paradigm that shared key features with standard working memory tasks, such as the reading memory span task (Daneman & Carpenter, 1980) and the N-back task (Smith & Jonides, 1999). In this novel task, sequences of disks appear individually at various locations onscreen in sets of five, each set ending with the presentation of a central fixation point. The participants are instructed to indicate on each trial, as a disk appears, whether the disk is full (i.e., a solid color) or empty (i.e., a circle). Thus participants' explicit, conscious goal is to respond to the physical nature of each disk presented. But a minority of the disk sequences follow predetermined rules or regularities, such that the implicit detection of that rule during that sequence would speed up responses to the final disk in the sequence (note that a particular sequence is never repeated, so this can not be implicit learning). Other sequences follow a rule until the final disk (i.e., the location of the fifth disk violates that rule), so that implicit detection of that rule during the sequence would hinder (slow down) responding to the final disk. (In the remaining control sets, the locations of the disks do not follow any rules.)

The results of four experiments, in the form of the pattern of reaction times to the final disk in each series, strongly supported the implicit pickup of the location rules. Compared to control sequences, participants had faster reaction times to the final disk of rule-governed trials and slower reaction times to the final disk of rule-violating trials. This occurred even though participants were never told that any of the sets would follow rules, and were entirely unaware of the existence of such rules when questioned after the experiment; indeed, in other conditions in which participants were told about the rules and instructed to try to notice and use them, no such pattern of reaction times was obtained.

Thus, even on-line working memory processes, dealing with a novel task and unique, nonrepeated sequences of stimuli, contain nonconsciously operating components. These are the processes most closely associated with conscious, executive control operations: dealing with novel, unpredictable stimuli and novel task goals, actively keeping ordered information in memory for a period of time, and updating and integrating that information with subsequent incoming information (Miyake & Shah, 1999). Thus, even executive ("conscious") control processes themselves operate at least partly in a nonconscious manner. Evident from all of these studies is that automatic processes can play a key role in regulating and guiding cognition. Much less research has directly examined the nonconscious regulation of emotional processes, a topic to which we turn next.

Automatic Regulation of Emotion

Like most kinds of self-regulation, emotion regulation—the diverse set of processes whose proximal function is to regulate control over which emotions individuals have, when they have them, and how they are experienced and expressed (Gross, 1998)—is generally considered to belong to the domain of consciousness. When fighting back tears to avoid embarrassment in public, or trying to rein in feelings of sadness when alone, the individual is likely cognizant of the emotion regulation experience. However, emotion regulation need not be conscious; indeed, emotion researchers have speculated that the procedures in which people typically engage to manage their emotions may become automated over time (Gross, 1999; Mayer & Salovey, 1995). Habits that reduce anxiety—such as nail biting or cigarette smoking—are examples of such automatized emotion regulation strategies. Indeed, because people engage in emotion regulation so frequently (Gross, 1998), it is possible that the subprocesses have become overlearned to the point of becoming automatic—at least in the sense of being efficient, or of requiring minimal attentional capacity to be performed (see Richards & Gross, 2000).

The regulation of self-esteem may be particularly likely to occur in an automatic fashion: People are highly motivated to maintain a positive sense of self (see Baumeister, 1998, for review); thus, a situational challenge to self-esteem may elicit automatic recovery attempts on the part of the individual. Indeed, people whose self-image has been threatened engage in more automatic stereotyping, shown to facilitate the restoration of a positive sense of self (Fein & Spencer, 1997; Spencer, Fein, Wolfe, Fong, & Dunn, 1998). In the Spencer and colleagues (1998) studies, receiving negative feedback was hypothesized to automatically activate a goal to restore self-image; once people had such a goal, Spencer and colleagues hypothesized that they would respond to minority-group members by automatically using stereotypes, an action previously found to increase mood and self-image (see Fein & Spencer, 1997). In a modification of a paradigm used by Gilbert and Hixon (1991), participants who received negative feedback on an "ability" test demonstrated automatic stereotyping of minority-group members, even under conditions of high cognitive load (Spencer et al., 1998, Experiment 3). Motivation to restore their threatened egos caused participants to stereotype minority-group members, even under conditions that preclude conscious processing. Participants who had not received negative feedback, on the other hand, did not engage in automatic stereotyping. This research supports the hypothesis that people can automatically engage in behaviors that protect or restore a positive sense of self, and that these kinds of self-restoration effects can occur efficiently, not requiring much cognitive capacity.

However, research on the ego-depletion model of self-regulation has shown that at least the *conscious* regulation of emotional expression, like other forms of conscious self-regulation, requires substantial mental resources (e.g., Baumeister et al., 1998; Muraven et al., 1998). People who were told to suppress their emotional responses while watching emotional films performed more poorly on subsequent self-regulatory tasks, such as solving anagrams and squeezing a handgrip exerciser (Baumeister et al., 1998). People also have been shown to have less success at regulating their emotions when they are under cognitive load (Wegner, Erber, & Zanakos, 1993), which also suggests that conscious attempts to regulate emotions may require cognitive resources. Of course, emotion regulation is not a unitary process, but rather is one term for a set of diverse processes, some of which may require heavy cognitive resources, whereas others require very few (Richards & Gross, 2000). Importantly, no research to date has examined *nonconsciously activated* emotion regulation goals or strategies, so it is as yet unclear whether emotion regulation processes can be activated automatically, and if so, whether they would consume cognitive resources in the same manner as do conscious emotion regulation attempts (see Vohs & Ciarocco, Chapter 20, this volume). In contrast, much research has examined directly the nonconscious regulation of behavior and compared the effectiveness of nonconscious and conscious goal pursuit in the behavioral realm.

Automatic Regulation of Behavior

Social behavior is automatically regulated (i.e., adapted to the current environment) in two different ways—one motivational, the other perceptual. First, goals that direct social behavior can operate nonconsciously, just as do goals that guide cognitive processing or emotion regulation. In one recent set of experiments, social and behavioral goals that were activated through subliminal and supraliminal priming manipulations were shown to guide behavior in a purposive, though nonconscious, manner (Bargh, Gollwitzer, Lee-

Chai, Barndollar, & Trotschel, 2001). In one study, after being exposed to words related to achievement (e.g., "succeed," "master," "achieve") in a word-search puzzle, participants performed significantly better on a verbal task (purportedly part of a separate experiment), though they were unaware of the relation of the priming task to the experimental task. In another study, participants presented with words related to cooperation (e.g., "fair," "share," "cooperate") behaved more cooperatively in a commons-dilemma game than did nonprimed participants. It is important to note that in both the achievement and the cooperation situations studied, the nonconscious goal operated to guide effective behavior over extended periods of time (10–15 minutes), and in complex interaction with the ongoing stream of environmental information. Thus, these behavioral effects are not one-off, reflex actions (as in the stimulus–response chains of radical behaviorism; e.g., Skinner, 1957) but instead represent a sophisticated interplay with the current environment, involving selective attention to task-relevant information, as well as its cognitive transformation, in order to meet the task goal: In short, working memory operations (Cohen, Dunbar, & McClelland, 1990). Once again, therefore, the very mental organs strongly associated with executive or "control" processes are found to operate without conscious choice, awareness, or guidance; instead, they are themselves under the control of the nonconsciously operating goal structure (see Bargh, in press).

Importantly, participants in these studies are not only unaware of the source or cause of the given goal's activation (through priming manipulations) but also unaware of its operation. For example, immediately after playing the commons-dilemma game for five rounds, participants were asked to estimate how committed they had been during the task to the goal of cooperating with their opponent (Bargh et al., 2001, Experiment 2). For participants who had been given the conscious, explicit goal to cooperate (through experimental instructions), these goal-commitment ratings correlated positively and significantly with the actual degree to which they had cooperated during the task. But for those for whom the cooperation had been nonconsciously induced (primed), these correlations were essentially zero. Even though they had just cooperated (or not) as much as did participants in the conscious goal condition, those in the nonconscious goal condition showed no awareness of the cooperative nature of their just-completed behavior in the task.

To claim the existence of "automatic self-regulation," we must show both that the phenomenon is automatic by standard criteria and also qualifies as self-regulation. For it to be truly *automatic*, it must not require conscious, intentional intervention, neither in the selection of the goal to pursue in the situation nor in the guidance of behavior toward that goal. The experimental evidence, as we have shown, is consistent with this claim. For it to be truly *self-regulation*, it must adapt thought, emotion, or behavior to the demands of both the current situation and the individual's own goal(s) within that situation. The evidence supports this part of the claim as well, because nonconsciously operating goals operate in harmony with unpredictable, unfolding events in the environment, using and transforming the available informational input in ways that help to attain the activated goal.

NONCONSCIOUS SELF-REGULATION IN REAL LIFE

In the aforementioned studies, goals were automatically activated by the presentation of words tightly associated with the goal construct. These words are hypothesized to activate a conceptual representation of the goal, which then (due to associations within the goal structure) automatically activates motivational components of the goal. However, in the real world, of course, people do not often encounter such neatly encapsulated conceptual representations of a goal; instead, they encounter varied situations that are rich with cues as to their social and psychological meaning. We certainly want to know how automatic self-regulation operates in these more natural contexts, so it is important to study how naturalistic situational cues might lead to nonconscious goal activation. Several recent studies do just that, providing evidence that a variety of real-world situational features can directly trigger self-regulatory responses.

First, characteristics of the social environment can directly prime goals. For example, being in a position of relative power can serve to activate goals that individuals associate with having power. In an important sense, having power means having the ability to attain one's important goals, so one would expect there to be strong cognitive associations between the concept of power on the one hand, and those important goal concepts on the other (Bargh & Raymond, 1995).

Having power is, of course, associated with different kinds of goals for different people. For individuals who associate power with sex, as do men who have tendencies to act in a sexually aggressive fashion, situational features that represent power have been shown to activate sexual motivations automatically (Bargh, Raymond, Pryor, & Strack, 1995). For individuals who associate power with social-responsibility goals (i.e., to take care of those over whom one has power, to use power fairly and unselfishly), as do people who possess chronically communal relationship orientations, situational power cues automatically activate such goals and lead to socially responsible behavior (Chen, Lee-Chai, & Bargh, 2001). For those who associate power with self-interest goals, as do people who possess chronically accessible exchange-relationship orientations, situational power cues automatically activate these motives and lead to self-interested behaviors (Chen et al., 2001).

In one illustrative study, researchers primed power naturalistically by seating participants in a professor's office and manipulating whether participants sat in the professor's chair (relatively high power) or in a small guest chair on the other side of the professor's desk (relatively low power). As predicted, sitting in the professor's chair led communally oriented participants to make more socially desirable responses on the Marlowe–Crowne Social Desirability Scale (Crowne & Marlowe, 1960) and the Modern Racism Scale (McConahay, 1986), reflecting their situationally accessible motives to behave in a socially responsible fashion. Situational power priming did not affect exchange-oriented participants, who do not associate power with social responsibility goals.

People as Nonconscious Triggers of Self-Regulation

Among the most frequent (and important) features of social situations are the other people with whom one has relationships, such as family, friends, and colleagues. Seeing, interacting with, and even just thinking about a significant other have been shown automatically to activate goals that guide and regulate the self's actions in a given situation (Andersen, Reznik, & Manzella, 1996; Fitzsimons & Bargh, 2003; Shah, 2003). Significant others can have nonconscious effects on self-regulation in at least two ways. First, they can serve as triggers for the goals that the individual commonly pursues with that significant other (Andersen et al., 1996; Baldwin, 1992; Fitzsimons & Bargh, 2003). Over time, goals that an individual frequently pursues with a significant other are hypothesized to become automatically associated with the mental representation of that other person, so that when that representation is activated, so are all the goals that the individual associates with that person.

In a set of studies, just thinking about a significant other was sufficient to lead to goal-directed behavior in line with goals that individuals associated with that significant other (Fitzsimons & Bargh, 2003). For example, at the beginning of the semester, college students reported the interpersonal goals they pursued with their mothers. Approximately half of the students reported wanting to please their mothers by achieving academically. Two months later, students returned to the laboratory and completed what was described to them as a "verbal achievement task." Before beginning that task, participants completed a supraliminal priming task disguised as a memory test, in which participants either answered questions about their mothers (e.g., describe your mother's appearance), or neutral, noninterpersonal, questions (e.g., describe the path you walk to school). Priming these students with questions about their mothers presumably activated interpersonal goals that students reported pursuing with their mothers, including the goal to achieve academically to please them. Indeed, participants primed with stimuli related to their mothers outperformed control participants on the verbal achievement task; importantly, though, the priming manipulation only affected participants who had previously reported a goal to please their mothers by achieving academically.

The second route through which significant others have been shown to exert a nonconscious effect on self-regulation is by activating goals that the other person has for the self, rather than the self's goals toward the other (Moretti & Higgins, 1999; Shah, 2003). To examine this issue, Shah (2003) asked participants to nominate a significant other who would want the participant to perform well on a certain task, as well as one who would not have that goal for the participant. Subliminally priming participants with these significant others produced significant effects on their goal commitment, goal accessibility, and task performance, in line with the motivations of their significant others. These effects were moderated by the closeness and importance of the relationship between the self and the significant other, as well as by the number of different goals the self associated with the significant other (Shah, 2003).

These studies demonstrate that mental representations of the significant others in one's life contain both the goals that the self pursues toward the other, and the goals that the other has for the self. Thus, thinking of or interacting with a significant other will activate one's mental representation of that person and, therefore, these associated goals as well, and can lead to either of these kinds of automatic, goal-directed behavioral responses, without a person being necessarily aware of the source of these responses. Given the frequency with which people think about and interact with significant others, this source of nonconscious self-regulatory actions may be triggered frequently and on a daily basis.

Another route by which other people can trigger automatic effects on self-regulation is through what Aarts, Gollwitzer, and Hassin (2003) call *goal contagion*, or the process by which goal-directed activity is automatically triggered simply by observing the behaviors of another person. People have been hypothesized to automatically encode others' behavior in terms of goals (Brewer & Dupree, 1983; Read & Miller, 1989; Trzebinski, 1989). If so, these inferred goals may become activated in the minds of the observers, and upon being activated, they may also activate associated means that serve these goals (see Aarts & Dijksterhuis, 2003). In a set of studies, participants that observed another person attempting to reach a certain goal were indeed found to be more likely to pursue that goal themselves, but only when the goal was applicable to the current situation (Aarts et al., 2003). Goal contagion effects were shown to be automatic, proceeding outside of conscious awareness and control; thus, they constitute another case of an automatic but motivated process that operates to guide and regulate the self's behavior.

THE ORIGINS OF NONCONSCIOUS SELF-REGULATION

A burgeoning set of social-cognitive research has found evidence for an increasing role for automaticity in self-regulation. Goals can be activated nonconsciously by situational cues and go on to guide cognition, emotion, and behavior, all without need for conscious intervention or guidance. An as yet unanswered question is, where do these nonconscious self-regulation capabilities come from? How do they develop? Following Shiffrin and Schneider's (1977) model of the automatization of basic cognitive processes, an automatic self-regulatory process is usually assumed to result from the frequent and consistent pairing of that process with a certain situational cue. Conscious monitoring and guidance have long been considered to become less necessary for mental processes that are used frequently and consistently (see Wegner & Bargh, 1998, for review). In particular, research on skill acquisition has demonstrated that once put into motion by an explicit goal, well-practiced mental operations occur quickly and effortlessly (Newell & Rosenbloom, 1981; Smith & Lerner, 1986). The auto-motive model extends the automaticity of this process out into the environment, by arguing that goals become associated with features of situations in which the goals are typically activated and used, and can thus become automatically activated simply by the presence of those features in the environment (Bargh, 1990; Bargh & Chartrand, 1999). As reviewed earlier, empirical evidence supports the proposed link between real situational cues and goals (e.g., Bargh et al., 1995; Chen at al., 2001; Fitzsimons & Bargh, 2003; Shah, 2003).

Frequently pursued goals have been shown to be automatically associated not only with the situations in which they are commonly pursued but also with the lower order means that typically serve the goals (Aarts & Dijksterhuis, 2000). When a goal is activated, the habitual plan for achieving that goal appears to be automatically activated as well; for example, habitual bicycle riders were faster to indicate that cycling was an action than were non–bicycle riders, but only after they had been unobtrusively primed with the goal to travel. The goal to travel activated the means that usually serves that goal—for bicycle riders, that means is cycling. Thus, goals are associated not only with the situations in which they are frequently pursued but also with the habitual behaviors that frequently satisfy them.

Frequency does seem to play an important role in the automatization of goals. When people are highly committed to a certain goal, and pursue it frequently over time, the goal becomes so habitualized that it is considered to be a *chronic* motivation, guiding behavior much of the time. When such chronically operating intentions are applicable, even low-level cognitive processes such as categorization can be controlled in an automatic fashion (Moskowitz, Wasel, Gollwitzer, & Schaal, 1999). For example, when people have a chronic motive to be egalitarian, they are able to avoid making stereotypical inferences and judgments, even under time constraints that preclude consciously controlled processing.

Nonhabitual Self-Regulation

Frequent and consistent goal pursuit in stable settings is likely to lead to the reduction of conscious involvement. But are frequency and consistency always necessary for self-regulation to become automatic? Not all automatic processes have become so through repeated practice: perception–behavior effects (Dijksterhuis & Bargh, 2001) and automatic evaluation effects (Duckworth, Bargh, Garcia, & Chaiken, 2002) are both examples of automatic processes that do not seem to require practice. Furthermore, even the assumption that automatic self-regulation, like other automatic processes, stems from frequent and consistent use has to this point gone largely untested. The development of automaticity has been a seriously underresearched topic in social cognition generally (for an exception, see Smith & Lerner, 1986), and, essentially, no research speaks to how self-regulatory actions become automatized.

There is in fact evidence that considerable experience (frequency and consistency) may not be necessary for a self-regulatory strategy to become automated. Gollwitzer and colleagues have demonstrated that people can successfully use *implementation intentions* purposefully to delegate control of their behavior to the environment (Gollwitzer, 1993, 1999; Gollwitzer & Brandstätter, 1997). By designating a specific if–then contingency between an environment and a plan of action (i.e., if situation X arises, then I will perform behavior Y), individuals construct a mental association between a specific situational cue and the appropriate goal-directed behavioral response. Then, when future situational events occur, the preset behavior is enacted immediately and automatically, without conscious choice at that moment. For example, experimental participants that formed the implementation intention, "When a distraction arises, I will ignore it," were more successful at avoiding tempting distractions during a tedious task than those who simply formed a goal intention, "I will not let myself get distracted" (Gollwitzer & Schaal, 1998). Implementation intentions can guide both promotive self-regulatory behavior (i.e., behavior that makes a wanted outcome more likely), and preventive self-regulatory behavior (i.e., behavior that makes an unwanted outcome less likely).

The hypothesized automatic nature of behavior guided by implementation intentions has also been supported by experiments examining how efficient and fast such behaviors can be, and the extent to which they require conscious intent at the time of action. Behaviors guided by previously formed implementation intentions are faster to be enacted (Gollwitzer & Brandstätter, 1997), and are highly efficient, functioning well even under conditions of heavy cognitive load (Brandtstätter, Lengfelder, & Gollwitzer, 2001). Even when the critical situation is subliminally presented, people who have formed implementation intentions react faster to goal-relevant words and behave in a more goal-directed fashion than do people who did not form implementation intentions (Bayer, Moskowitz, & Gollwitzer, 2002). In short, then, when people use implementation intentions, they are setting up automatic self-regulatory behaviors, without any need for frequent and consistent practice of these behaviors (Gollwitzer, Bayer, & McCulloch, 2003).

Situational Norms as Triggers of Automatic Self-Regulation

The process of self-regulation begins with the choice or selection of a goal to pursue (Gollwitzer, 1996), and nonconscious processes can play an important role in this first stage. Merely presenting goal-relevant information—even subliminally—to perceivers is sufficient to activate goals that guide behavior automatically (e.g., Bargh et al., 2001; Chartrand & Bargh, 1996). Beyond such conceptual primes, real-world primes such as significant others (Fitzsimons & Bargh, 2003; Shah, 2003), information about relative situational power positions (Bargh et al., 1995), and other people's goal-directed behavior (Aarts et al., 2003) can all activate automatic self-regulation.

Self-regulatory behaviors can also originate directly from situational norms, and this norm–behavior link need not be consciously mediated. Indeed, much of the transmission of social norms from the environment to the individual likely occurs in a nonconscious manner. Cultural norms are thought to influence, guide, and regulate behavior, while often bypassing consciousness altogether (see Bargh, 1990; Cohen, 1997). In examining the potential mechanisms through which situational norms may automatically guide behavior, recent research has focused on the cognitive structure of situational norms, hypothesizing that norms are represented mentally as associations between situations and behaviors normatively performed in those situations (e.g., Aarts & Dijksterhuis, 2003). If so, then being exposed to a feature of a given situation can automatically trigger the self-regulatory behaviors commonly performed in that situation. Indeed, when participants anticipated visiting a library and were primed with photographs of a library setting, they talked less loudly than did participants who were not primed with photographs of a library (Aarts & Dijksterhuis, 2003). Similarly, participants primed with images from the business world behaved in a more competitive fashion than did those primed with neutral images (Kay, Bargh, & Ross, 2003). Within the minimal group paradigm, participants primed with norms of loyalty behaved in ways that benefited their ingroup more than did participants primed with norms of equality, and these priming effects were partially mediated by perceptions of situational norms (Hertel & Kerr, 2001; see also Kay & Ross, in press), even though participants reported no awareness of the link between the priming task and the subsequent tasks, or of being affected by the primes in any way.

Conforming to social norms is sometimes a very deliberate process in which an individual experiences an internal conflict before deciding to go along with the group norms. However, as the aforementioned research suggests, conformity to norms can also occur nonconsciously; people who conform often report no understanding of why they went along with the norm, or even that the norm influenced their behavior at all. In a study of automatic conformity (Epley & Gilovich, 1999), participants were primed with words related to either conformity (e.g., "conform," "comply," "mimic," "follow") or nonconformity (e.g., "rebel," "deviate," "differ," "individual") in a scrambled sentence task. Participants were then asked to rate the experiment in the presence of confederates who gave extremely positive ratings. Participants primed with conformity gave much higher ratings of the experiment than did those primed with nonconformity, indicating that the nonconscious activation of the conformity and nonconformity constructs implicitly guided participants' tendency to comply with social norms.

It is important to note that participants in these studies reported no conscious awareness that their behavior was influenced by the priming manipulations. Consequently, this research suggests that situational norms may cause self-regulatory responses that are not guided by conscious control but can instead be considered automatic responses to demands of the current environment.

Potential Limiting Conditions to Nonconscious Goal Activation

Like all automatic processes, nonconscious goals are not likely to operate in conditions under which their operation is wholly inapplicable (Higgins, 1996). A nonconsciously activated goal may primarily influence behavior when the individual possesses a preexisting need state that makes the primed goal applicable. For example, people who are subliminally primed with the concept of thirst only become more likely to choose a thirst-quenching beverage if they are already somewhat thirsty (Strahan, Spencer, & Zanna, 2002). Beyond applicability, goals must also be available (Higgins, 1996), in the sense that the individual already desires that goal or has pursued it in the past (i.e., it exists as a mental representation for the individual). As Kurt Lewin (1951) often stressed, one cannot give or induce in another person a goal that he or she does not already have. Thus, a goal cannot be nonconsciously activated, unless it already exists in the mind of the individual.

In summary, nonconscious self-regulatory responses can be set into motion by environmental features, whether they be the presence of significant others or the existence of situational norms. Typically, goals will become automatically activated by a mental association to a present situational feature that is caused by their frequent and consistent co-occurrence. However, it is also possible that automatic self-regulation may result from less habitual goal pursuit, stemming instead from highly successful self-regulation–situation pairings, or from strategic delegation of control to the environment. Once set into motion, nonconscious goals must guide the self's actions through diverse and flexible means, regulating thoughts, feelings, and behaviors, without the need for conscious intervention. As we discuss in further detail in the following section, nonconscious self-regulation shares some of the essential features of conscious self-regulation and strikes an adaptive balance of efficiency and flexibility.

COMPARING CONSCIOUS
AND NONCONSCIOUS SELF-REGULATION

Conscious self-regulation can be characterized by a set of unique motivational properties, including ignoring distractions, acting flexibly in response to situations, persisting in response to obstacles, resuming goal pursuit after disruption, and managing conflicts between goals (e.g., Gollwitzer, 1990; Gollwitzer & Moskowitz, 1996; Heckhausen, 1991; Lewin, 1926, 1951; Locke & Latham, 1990). To what extent do the same qualities apply to nonconscious self-regulation? In a set of studies designed to assess whether nonconscious goal activation produces a "full-blown" motivational state, Bargh and colleagues (2001) found evidence that nonconscious goal pursuit possesses the same key features as conscious goal pursuit. For example, successful self-regulation requires individuals to *persist* toward goal attainment in the face of obstacles to success (Gollwitzer & Moskowitz, 1996). Participants in whom a nonconscious achievement goal was activated were more likely to continue working on a verbal task, even after having been told to stop (via an intercom), in an attempt to attain an ever-higher score, even if it meant violating the experimenter's explicit instructions (Bargh et al., 2001, Experiment 4).

Consciously pursued goals are also known to increase in strength over time until they are attained (Atkinson & Birch, 1970). To look at whether nonconscious goals also increase in strength over time, Bargh and colleagues (2001, Experiment 3) compared how goal priming affected performance on a verbal task immediately versus after a delay. Supporting the similarity of nonconscious and conscious goal pursuit, achievement-primed participants outperformed control participants in the no-delay condition, and this difference was actually magnified after a 5-minute delay. Achievement-primed participants in the delay condition, as predicted, outperformed those in the no-delay condition. No participants reported any conscious awareness of pursuing the achievement goal; these findings suggest that, like conscious goals, nonconsciously activated goals do increase in strength over time until they are acted upon.[2]

Another classic feature of conscious motivational states is the tendency to resume goal pursuit after a disruption (such as an interruption) has occurred (Gollwitzer & Liu, 1995). To examine whether people pursuing nonconscious goals would also resume the activity after a disruption, Bargh and colleagues (2001, Experiment 5) exposed half of their participants to achievement primes, then led all participants to engage in an intellectual task that was interrupted by an allegedly "accidental" equipment failure after 1 minute. After these "equipment problems" were resolved, the experimenter announced that there would not be enough time to complete the study as planned; therefore, participants had a choice between returning to complete the intellectual task they had started or going on to the next task, a cartoon-rating task (judged in pilot testing to be far more attractive than the intellectual task). Participants with a nonconscious achievement goal were significantly more likely to return to complete the intellectual task than were nonprimed participants (66% vs. 32%, respectively), indicating that nonconscious goal pursuit possesses still another classic feature of conscious goal pursuit.

One crucial aspect of successful self-regulation is the ability to focus on one's current goal pursuit and inhibit other goals that may interfere with progress toward the current goal (Gollwitzer & Moskowitz, 1996; Shah & Kruglanski, 2002). Intergoal conflict arises whenever two accessible goals interfere with each other's fulfillment. To maintain focus on the current goal, participants may actively inhibit other accessible goals to give full self-regulatory resources to the goal at hand (Mischel & Ebbesen, 1970). But does this preservation of goal focus also occur for nonconscious goals? Recent research by Shah and colleagues on *goal shielding theory* has demonstrated that this inhibition of alternative goals occurs outside of conscious awareness (Shah, Friedman, & Kruglanski, 2002). When participants were subliminally primed with one of their own important goals, they responded by automatically inhibiting the activation of relevant alternative goals. Thus, active nonconscious goals also possess this capability to preserve goal focus by automatically inhibiting other, competing goals as distractions.

Although this inhibition of alternative goals is an automatic self-regulatory process, it is sensitive and flexible in its application, depending on the characteristics of the goals being pursued and inhibited, as well as on the motivations and emotions of the individual engaging in self-regulatory behavior. For example, people inhibit alternative goals more when they are highly committed to the current goal, when they feel more anxiety, and when they have a high need for closure; they inhibit alternative goals less when they feel depressed (Shah et al., 2002).

These findings further establish the important point that automatic processes are not just the negation or direct opposite of controlled processes; that is, just because controlled processes are sensitive to and flexible relative to present circumstances, for example, does not necessitate that automatic processes within the same circumstances be insensitive and inflexible. Rather, the present notion of "automatic control" suggests that successful self-regulation depends on the individual's engagement in flexible automatic processes.

Another important aspect of successful self-regulation is the ability to override temptations and pursue long-term goals: Momentarily tempting desires can cause the self to engage in behaviors that contradict important higher order, longer term goals (Fishbach, Friedman, & Kruglanski, 2003; Metcalfe & Mischel, 1999). However, note that such temptations may, over time, become automatically associated with the higher order goals with which they interfere. For example, seeing a delicious chocolate cake may remind dieters of their overriding goal to eat carefully and lose weight. If such associations do exist, then this may be an automatic form of self-regulation: The accessibility of a short-term desire may automatically activate a long-term motive, which can then regulate the self's actions.

Based on their belief that such associations reflect an adaptive self-regulatory mechanism, Fishbach and colleagues (2003) predicted that although temptations would indeed activate higher order goals, such higher order goals would actually inhibit temptations.

Unlike resource-consuming, conscious self-control operations, these facilitative and inhibitive links between temptations and higher order goals are likely to become overlearned when practiced repeatedly; thus, they require very little in terms of mental resources. Indeed, a set of studies found support for these hypotheses: The activation of temptations led to the increased accessibility of goal-relevant stimuli, whereas the activation of higher order goals inhibited the accessibility of temptation-relevant stimuli (Fishbach et al., 2003).

In summary, then, nonconscious self-regulation shares many of the essential properties that make conscious self-regulation successful. People pursuing nonconscious goals respond flexibly to situational challenges by engaging self-regulatory mechanisms: They persist toward goal progress even when obstacles arise; they increase their goal strength when their goals are unfulfilled; and they tend to resume goal pursuit after disruption. Some kinds of self-regulation appear to function mainly in an automatic fashion: Alternative goals are automatically inhibited in order to maintain focus on the goal being pursued, and temptations seem automatically to activate higher order goals with which they interfere, reminding individuals of their important goal pursuits. Thus, nonconscious self-regulation can function similarly to conscious self-regulation, but more efficiently and consistently, and may also complement conscious kinds of self-control with additional, unique mechanisms.

CONSEQUENCES OF AUTOMATIC REGULATION FOR THE SELF

When people consciously pursue goals, they inevitably engage in some kind of self-assessment procedure, following the attempt, regarding their progress toward fulfilling that goal. This "postactional" phase of goal pursuit is crucial to self-regulation, because the self needs to evaluate current progress to plan for future action (Carver & Scheier, 1981; Gollwitzer, 1990). Chartrand (2003) theorized that if nonconscious goal pursuit is to be useful for self-regulatory success, it should produce the same kinds of mood and self-evaluative consequences as does conscious self-regulation: Failure should induce a negative mood and impaired future performance in the same task domain, whereas success should induce a positive mood and enhanced future performance (Bandura, 1990).

To investigate this hypothesis, Chartrand (2003) primed some participants to induce a nonconscious achievement goal. Participants then engaged in what was presented to them as a filler task—a verbal anagram task that was either extremely difficult or extremely easy to complete. The difficulty of the task served as an implicit manipulation of success or failure at the nonconscious achievement goal; note that participants were not given any explicit goal or feedback regarding the filler task. As predicted, participants who were pursuing nonconscious achievement goals were happier (in a more positive mood) after working on the easy anagram task than on the difficult one, whereas the mood of control (no primed achievement goal) participants was entirely unaffected by success or failure at the task. Similarly, in another experiment, the filler-task-difficulty manipulation produced subsequent verbal task performance differences as well, but only for those participants with a nonconsciously operating achievement goal.

Thus, the similarity between conscious and nonconscious goal pursuit extends even to this ultimate stage of self-regulation, in which the self evaluates its performance and plans future action accordingly. One important difference between the effects of conscious and nonconscious goal pursuit on self-evaluations, however, is that after engaging consciously in goal pursuit, it is possible for people to be aware of how this has affected their mood and self evaluation; in contrast, after engaging in nonconscious goal pursuit, people cannot pinpoint the cause for any effects on the self (Cheng & Chartrand, 2003). These two qualitatively different experiences—moods with and without attributable causes—can lead to different self-regulatory effects (Chartrand, Cheng, & Tesser, 2003). For example, negative moods that result from failures at nonconsciously activated goals may invoke stronger self-enhancement responses than do negative moods that originate from failures at conscious goals (Chartrand et al., 2003). In a series of studies, Chartrand and colleagues (2003) found that participants who failed at nonconscious goals created more self-serving definitions of success and engaged in more stereotyping of minority-group members than did participants who failed at conscious goals (who engaged in these behaviors more than did control participants). When participants were given the chance to understand the reason for their negative mood, these effects dissipated, again suggesting that there are unique consequences of nonconscious goal pursuit.

CONCLUSIONS

Self-regulatory action is commonly believed to be a heavy consumer of cognitive resources. Certainly, self-control attempts can often be arduous and require the input of a great deal of effort and mental resources (e.g., Baumeister et al., 1998; Mischel, 1996). The research described in this chapter presents another form of self-regulation, one that, although not nearly as labor-intensive, is effective nonetheless in guiding the self toward attainment of important goals. Because of the (oversimplified) dichotomy created between automatic and controlled processes in many dual-process theories, however, the concept of *automatic self-control* presents a challenge to our commonly held assumptions about what it means for a self-regulatory process to be automatic or controlled. As Baumeister (1998) has said, self-regulation is "active (rather than passive) and controlled (rather than automatic)" (p. 724). From our perspective, however, self-regulation can be both active and automatic.

ACKNOWLEDGMENTS

Preparation of this chapter was supported in part by a Social Sciences and Humanities Research Council of Canada (SSHRC) fellowship to Gráinne M. Fitzsimons and by U.S. Public Health Service Grant No. MH60767 to John A. Bargh.

NOTES

1. Namely, that individuals pursue the given goal within the given situation both frequently and consistently (see Bargh & Chartrand, 1999; Shiffrin & Dumais, 1981), although research has yet to address the issue of automatic goal development.
2. There must be limits to this effect of goal strength increase over time, of course, but these are expected to follow from the same factors as for the consciously held goals studied by Atkinson and Birch (1970), for example, loss of opportunity conditions, increase in strength of a more important or pressing goal at the same time, and so on.

REFERENCES

Aarts, H., & Dijksterhuis, A. (2000). Habits as knowledge structures: Automaticity in goal-directed behavior. *Journal of Personality and Social Psychology, 78*, 53–63.

Aarts, H., & Dijksterhuis, A. (2003). The silence of the library: Environment, situational norms and social behavior. *Journal of Personality and Social Psychology, 84*, 18–28.

Aarts, H., Gollwitzer, P. M., & Hassin, R. (2003). *Goal contagion: Perceiving is for pursuing.* Manuscript submitted for publication.

Andersen, S. M., Reznik, I., & Manzella, L. M. (1996). Eliciting transient affect, motivation, and expectancies in transference: Significant-other representations and the self in social relations. *Journal of Personality and Social Psychology, 71*, 1108–1129.

Atkinson, J. W., & Birch, D. (1970). *A dynamic theory of action.* New York: Wiley.

Baldwin, M. W. (1992). Relational schemas and the processing of information. *Psychological Bulletin, 112*, 461–484.

Bandura, A. (1986). *Social foundations of thought and action: A social cognitive theory.* Englewood Cliffs, NJ: Prentice-Hall.

Bandura, A. (1990). Self-regulation of motivation through anticipatory and self-reactive mechanisms. In R. A. Dienstbier (Ed.), *Nebraska Symposium on Motivation: Perspectives on motivation* (Vol. 38, pp. 69–164). Lincoln: University of Nebraska Press.

Bargh, J. A. (1990). Auto-motives: Preconscious determinants of social interaction. In E. T. Higgins & R. M. Sorrentino (Eds.), *Handbook of motivation and cognition: Vol. 2. Foundations of social behavior* (pp. 93–130). New York: Guilford Press.

Bargh, J. A. (in press). Bypassing the will: Towards demystifying the nonconscious control of social behavior. In R. Hassin, J. Uleman, & J. Bargh (Eds.), *The new unconscious.* New York: Oxford University Press.

Bargh, J. A., & Chartrand, T. L. (1999). The unbearable automaticity of being. *American Psychologist, 54*, 462–479.

Bargh, J. A., & Gollwitzer, P. M. (1994). Environmental control over goal-directed action. *Nebraska Symposium on Motivation, 41*, 71–124.

Bargh, J. A., Gollwitzer, P. M., Lee-Chai, A., Barndollar, K., & Trotschel, R. (2001). The automated will: Nonconscious activation and pursuit of behavioral goals. *Journal of Personality and Social Psychology, 81*, 1014–1027.

Bargh, J. A., & Raymond, P. (1995). The naive misuse of power: Nonconscious sources of sexual harassment. *Journal of Social Issues, 26*, 168–185.

Bargh, J. A., Raymond, P., Pryor, J., & Strack, F. (1995). Attractiveness of the underling: An automatic power–sex association and its consequences for sexual harassment and aggression. *Journal of Personality and Social Psychology, 68*, 768–781.

Baumeister, R. F. (1998). The self. In D. T. Gilbert, S. T. Fiske, & G. Lindzey (Eds.), *Handbook of social psychology* (4th ed., pp. 680–740). New York: McGraw-Hill.

Baumeister, R. F., Bratslavsky, E., Muraven, M., & Tice, D. M. (1998). Ego depletion: Is the active self a limited resource? *Journal of Personality and Social Psychology, 74*, 1252–1265.

Bayer, U. C., Moskowitz, G. B., & Gollwitzer, P. M. (2002). *Implementation intentions and action initiation without conscious intent.* Unpublished manuscript, University of Konstanz, Germany.

Brandstätter, V., Lengfelder, A., & Gollwitzer, P. M. (2001). Implementation intentions and efficient action initiation. *Journal of Personality and Social Psychology, 81*, 946–960.

Brewer, W. F., & Dupree, D. A. (1983). Use of plan schemata in the recall and recognition of goal-directed actions. *Journal of Experimental Psychology, Learning, Memory, and Cognition, 9*, 117–129.

Carver, C. S., & Scheier, M. F. (1981). *Attention and self-regulation: A control theory approach to human behaviors.* New York: Springer.

Chartrand, T. L. (2003). *Mystery moods and perplexing performance: Consequences of succeeding or failing at a nonconscious goal.* Manuscript under review.

Chartrand, T. L., & Bargh, J. A. (1996). Automatic activation of impression formation and memorization goals: Nonconscious goal priming reproduces effects of explicit task instructions. *Journal of Personality and Social Psychology, 71,* 464–478.

Chartrand, T. L., & Bargh, J. A. (2002). Nonconscious motivations: Their activation, operation, and consequences. In A. Tesser, D. A. Stapel, & J. V. Wood (Eds.), *Self and motivation: Emerging psychological perspectives* (pp. 13–41). Washington, DC: American Psychological Association.

Chartrand, T. L., Cheng, C. M., & Tesser, A. (2003). *Consequences of failing at nonconscious goals for self-enhancement and stereotyping.* Manuscript under review.

Chen, S., Lee-Chai, A. Y., & Bargh, J. A. (2001). Relationship orientation as a moderator of the effects of social power. *Journal of Personality and Social Psychology, 80,* 173–187.

Cheng, C. M., & Chartrand, T. L. (2003). Self-monitoring without awareness: Using mimicry as a nonconscious affiliation strategy. *Journal of Personality and Social Psychology, 85,* 1170–1179.

Cohen, D. (1997). Ifs and thens in cultural psychology. In R. S. Wyer, Jr. (Ed.), *Advances in social cognition* (Vol. 10, pp. 337–342). Mahwah, NJ: Erlbaum.

Cohen, J. D., Dunbar, K., & McClelland, J. L. (1990). On the control of automatic processes: A parallel distributed processing account of the Stroop effect. *Psychological Review, 97,* 332–361.

Crowne, D. P., & Marlowe, D. (1960). A new scale of social desirability independent of psychopathology. *Journal of Consulting Psychology, 24,* 349–354.

Daneman, M., & Carpenter, P. A. (1980). Individual differences in working memory and reading. *Journal of Verbal Learning and Verbal Behavior, 19,* 450–466.

Deci, E. L., & Ryan, R. M. (1985). *Intrinsic motivation and self-determination in human behavior.* New York: Plenum Press.

Dijksterhuis, A. J., & Bargh, J. A. (2001). The perception-behavior expressway: Automatic effects of social perception on social behavior. In M. P. Zanna (Ed.), *Advances in experimental social psychology* (Vol. 33, pp. 1–40). San Diego, CA: Academic Press.

Duckworth, K. L., Bargh, J. A., Garcia, M., & Chaiken, S. (2002). The automatic evaluation of novel stimuli. *Psychological Science, 13,* 513–519.

Epley, N., & Gilovich, T. (1999). Just going along: Nonconscious priming and conformity to social pressure. *Journal of Experimental Social Psychology, 35,* 578–589.

Fazio, R. H. (1986). How do attitudes guide behavior? In R. M. Sorrentino & E. T. Higgins (Eds.), *The handbook of motivation and cognition: Foundations of social behavior* (pp. 204–243). New York: Guilford Press.

Fein, S., & Spencer, S. J. (1997). Prejudice as self-image maintenance: Affirming the self through derogating others. *Journal of Personality and Social Psychology, 73,* 31–44.

Fishbach, A., Friedman, R. S., & Kruglanski, A. W. (2003). Leading us not unto temptation: Momentary allurements elicit overriding goal activation. *Journal of Personality and Social Psychology, 84,* 296–309.

Fitzsimons, G. M., & Bargh, J. A. (2003). Thinking of you: Nonconscious pursuit of interpersonal goals associated with relationship partners. *Journal of Personality and Social Psychology, 84,* 148–164.

Gilbert, D. T., & Hixon, J. G. (1991). The trouble of thinking: Activation and application of stereotypic beliefs. *Journal of Personality and Social Psychology, 60,* 509–517.

Gollwitzer, P. M. (1990). Action phases and mindsets. In E. T. Higgins & R. M. Sorrentino (Eds.), *Handbook of motivation and cognition: Vol. 2. Foundations of social behavior* (pp. 53–92). New York: Guilford Press.

Gollwitzer, P. M. (1993). Goal achievement: The role of intentions. *European Review of Social Psychology, 4,* 141–185.

Gollwitzer, P. M. (1996). The volitional benefits of planning. In P. M. Gollwitzer & J. A. Bargh (Eds.), *The psychology of action: Linking cognition and motivation to behavior* (pp. 287–312). New York: Guilford Press.

Gollwitzer, P. M. (1999). Implementation intentions: Strong effects of simple plans. *American Psychologist, 54,* 493–503.

Gollwitzer, P. M., Bayer, U., & McCulloch, K. C. (in press). The control of the unwanted. In R. Hassin, J. Uleman, & J. A. Bargh (Eds.), *The new unconscious.* New York: Oxford University Press.

Gollwitzer, P. M., & Brandstätter, V. (1997). Implementation intentions and effective goal pursuit. *Journal of Personality and Social Psychology, 73,* 186–199.

Gollwitzer, P. M., & Liu, C. (1995). Willpower. In J. Kuhl & H. Heckhausen (Eds.), *Encyclopedia of psychology: Motivation, volition and action* (pp. 209–240). Göttingen, Germany: Hogrefe.

Gollwitzer, P. M., & Moskowitz, G. B. (1996). Goal effects on action and cognition. In E. T. Higgins & A. W. Kruglanski (Eds.), *Social psychology: Handbook of basic principles* (pp. 361–399). New York: Guilford Press.

Gollwitzer, P. M., & Schaal, B. (1998). Metacognition in action: The importance of implementation intentions. *Personality and Social Psychology Review, 2,* 124–136.

Greenwald, A. G., & Banaji, M. R. (1995). Implicit social cognition: Attitudes, self-esteem, and stereotypes. *Psychological Review, 102,* 4–27.

Gross, J. J. (1998). The emerging field of emotion regulation: An integrative review. *Review of General Psychology, 2,* 271–299.

Gross, J. J. (1999). Emotion regulation: Past, present, future. *Cognition and Emotion, 13,* 551–573.

Hamilton, D. L., Katz, L. B., & Leirer, V. O. (1980). Organizational processes in impression formation. In R. Hastie, T. M. Ostrom, E. B. Ebbesen, R. S. Wyer, Jr., D. L. Hamilton, & D. E. Carlston (Eds.), *Person memory: The cognitive basis of social perception* (pp. 121–153). Hillsdale, NJ: Erlbaum.

Hassin, R. R. (in press). Non-conscious control in implicit working memory. In R. R. Hassin, J. S. Uleman, & J. A. Bargh (Eds.), *The new unconscious.* New York: Oxford University Press.

Hastie, R., & Kumar, P. A. (1979). Person memory: Personality traits as organizing principles in memory for behaviors. *Journal of Personality and Social Psychology, 37,* 25–38.

Heckhausen, H. (1991). *Motivation and action.* New York: Springer-Verlag.

Hertel, G., & Kerr, N. L. (2001). Priming ingroup favoritism: The impact of normative scripts in the minimal group paradigm. *Journal of Experimental Social Psychology, 37,* 316–324.

Higgins, E. T. (1996). Knowledge activation: Accessibility, applicability, and salience. In E. T. Higgins & A. W. Kruglanski (Eds.), *Social psychology: Handbook of basic principles* (pp. 133–168). New York: Guilford Press.

Hull, C. (1931). Goal attraction and directing ideas conceived as habit phenomena. *Psychological Review, 38,* 487–506.

Kay, A. C., Bargh, J. A., & Ross, L. (2003). *Material priming.* Manuscript under review.

Kay, A. C., & Ross, L. (in press). The perceptual push: The interplay of implicit cues and explicit situational construals on behavioral intentions in the Prisoner's Dilemma. *Journal of Experimental Social Psychology.*

Kruglanski, A. W. (1996). Goals as knowledge structures. In P. M. Gollwitzer & J. A. Bargh (Eds.), *The psychology of action: Linking cognition and motivation to behavior* (pp. 599–618). New York: Guilford Press.

Lewin, K. (1926). Vorsatz, wille, und bedürfnis [Intention, will, and need]. *Psychologische Forschung, 7,* 330–385.

Lewin, K. (1951). *Field theory in social science.* Chicago: University of Chicago Press.

Locke, E. A., & Latham, G. P. (1990). *A theory of goal setting and task performance.* Englewood Cliffs, NJ: Prentice-Hall.

Mayer, J. D., & Salovey, P. (1995). Emotional intelligence and the construction and regulation of feelings. *Applied and Preventive Psychology, 4,* 197–208.

McConahay, J. B. (1986). Modern racism, ambivalence, and the modern racism scale. In J. R.

Dovidio & S. L. Gaertner (Eds.), *Prejudice, discrimination, and racism* (pp. 91–125). Orlando, FL: Academic Press.

Metcalfe, J., & Mischel, W. (1999). A hot/cool system analysis of delay of gratification: Dynamics of willpower. *Psychological Review, 106,* 3–19.

Mischel, W. (1996). From good intentions to willpower. In P. M. Gollwitzer & J. A. Bargh (Eds.), *The psychology of action: Linking cognition and motivation to behavior* (pp. 197–218). New York: Guilford Press.

Mischel, W., & Ebbeson, E. (1970). Attention in delay of gratification. *Journal of Personality and Social Psychology, 16,* 329–337.

Mitchell, J. P, Macrae, C. N., Schooler, J. W., Rowe, A. C., & Milne, A. B. (2002). Directed remembering: Subliminal cues alter nonconscious memory strategies. *Memory, 10,* 381–388.

Miyake, A., & Shah, P. (Eds.). (1999). *Models of working memory.* New York: Cambridge University Press.

Moretti, M. M., & Higgins, E. T. (1999). Own versus other standpoints in self-regulation: Developmental antecedents and functional consequences. *Review of General Psychology, 3,* 188–223.

Moskowitz, G. B. (2002). Preconscious effects of temporary goals on attention. *Journal of Experimental Social Psychology, 38,* 397–404.

Moskowitz, G. B., Wasel, W., Gollwitzer, P. M., & Schaal, B. (1999). Preconscious control of stereotype activation through chronic egalitarian goals. *Journal of Personality and Social Psychology, 77,* 167–184.

Muraven, M., Tice, D. M., & Baumeister, R. F. (1998). Self-control as limited resource: Regulatory depletion patterns. *Journal of Personality and Social Psychology, 74,* 774–789.

Neisser, U. (1967). *Cognitive psychology.* New York: Appleton–Century–Crofts.

Read, S. J., & Miller, L. C. (1989). Inter-personalism: Toward a goal-based theory of persons in relationships. In L. A. Pervin (Ed.), *Goal concepts in personality and social psychology* (pp. 413–472). Hillsdale, NJ: Erlbaum.

Richards, J. M., & Gross, J. J. (2000). Emotion regulation and memory: The cognitive costs of keeping one's cool. *Journal of Personality and Social Psychology, 79,* 410–424.

Shah, J. (2003). Automatic for the people: How representations of significant others implicitly affect goal pursuit. *Journal of Personality and Social Psychology, 84,* 661–681.

Shah, J. Y., Friedman, R., & Kruglanski, A. W. (2002). Forgetting all else: On the antecedents and consequences of goal shielding. *Journal of Personality and Social Psychology, 83,* 1261–1280.

Shah, J. Y., & Kruglanski, A. W. (2002). Priming against your will: How goal pursuit is affected by accessible alternatives. *Journal of Experimental Social Psychology, 38,* 368–383.

Shiffrin, R. M., & Dumais, S. T. (1981). The development of automatism. In J. Anderson (Ed.), *Cognitive skills and their acquisition* (pp. 111–140). Hillsdale, NJ: Erlbaum.

Shiffrin, R. M., & Schneider, W. (1977). Controlled and automatic human information processing: II. Perceptual learning, automatic attending, and a general theory. *Psychological Review, 84,* 127–190.

Skinner, B. F. (1957). *Verbal behavior.* New York: Appleton–Century–Crofts.

Smith, E. E., & Jonides, J. (1999). Storage and executive processes in the frontal lobes. *Science, 283,* 1657–1661.

Smith, E. R., & Lerner, M. (1986). Development of automatism of social judgments. *Journal of Personality and Social Psychology, 50,* 246–259.

Spencer, S. J., Fein, S., Wolfe, C. T., Fong, C., & Dunn, M. A. (1998). Automatic activation of stereotypes: The role of self-image threat. *Personality and Social Psychology Bulletin, 24,* 1139–1152.

Srull, T. K., & Wyer, R. S., Jr. (1979). The role of category accessibility in the interpretation of information about persons: Some determinants and implications. *Journal of Personality and Social Psychology, 37,* 1660–1672.

Strahan, E. J., Spencer, S. J., & Zanna, M. P. (2002). Subliminal priming and persuasion: Striking while the iron is hot. *Journal of Experimental Social Psychology, 38,* 556–568.

Tolman, E. C. (1932). *Purposive behavior in animals and men.* London: Century/Random House.

Trzebinski, J. (1989). The role of goal categories in the representation of social knowledge. In L. A. Pervin (Ed.), *Goal concepts in personality and social psychology* (pp. 363–411). Hillsdale, NJ: Erlbaum.

Wegner, D. M., & Bargh, J. A. (1998). Control and automaticity in social life. In D. Gilbert, S. Fiske, & G. Lindzey (Eds.), *Handbook of social psychology* (4th ed.). Boston: McGraw-Hill.

Wegner, D. M., Erber, R., & Zanakos, S. (1993). Ironic processes in the mental control of mood and mood-related thought. *Journal of Personality and Social Psychology, 65,* 1093–1104.

9

Promotion and Prevention Strategies for Self-Regulation

A Motivated Cognition Perspective

E. TORY HIGGINS
SCOTT SPIEGEL

Research on motivated cognition has typically examined how *motives to arrive at certain conclusions* affect people's *judgmental processes* (cf. Dunning, Leuenberger, & Sherman, 1995; Ford & Kruglanski, 1995; Sanitioso, Kunda, & Fong, 1990; Thompson, Roman, Moskowitz, Chaiken, & Bargh, 1994). In this chapter, we extend the study of motivated cognition in two directions. First, we examine how, in addition to motives to arrive at certain outcomes, *motives to adopt certain strategies* affect people's judgmental processes (for a more general review of cognitive effects of strategic preferences, see Higgins and Molden, 2003; Molden & Higgins, in press-b). Specifically, we examine how having a promotion or a prevention focus—as well as having "regulatory fit" (Higgins, 2000) between one's promotion or prevention focus and the manner in which one pursues a goal—can affect people's judgmental processes. Second, we examine how motives to adopt certain strategies affect people's *behavior*, which can be not only the behavioral product of their judgmental processes but can also be independent of judgment. Specifically, we examine how having a promotion or a prevention focus, and having strategic "fit" with these foci, can affect behavior.

PROMOTION AND PREVENTION STRATEGIES FOR SELF-REGULATION

Regulatory focus theory (Higgins, 1997) proposes that self-regulation operates differently when serving fundamentally different needs, such as the distinct survival needs of *nurturance* (e.g., nourishment) and *security* (e.g., protection). The theory assumes that nurturance-related regulation involves a *promotion focus*, which is a regulatory state concerned with *ideals*, advancement, aspiration, and accomplishment (more generally, the presence or absence of positive outcomes). In contrast, security-related regulation involves a *prevention focus*, which is a regulatory state concerned with *oughts*, protection, safety, and responsibility (more generally, the absence or presence of negative outcomes.) *Promotion*-focused people prefer to use *eagerness*-related means, the type of means most suited to a concern with advancement, aspiration, and accomplishment (Crowe & Higgins, 1997). In contrast, *prevention*-focused people prefer to use *vigilance*-related means, the type of means most suited to a concern with protection, safety, and responsibility (Crowe & Higgins, 1997). Thus, regulatory focus theory goes beyond the basic, widely accepted hedonic principle that people approach pleasure and avoid pain, to an examination of people's strategic choices and manner of pursuing their goals. Notably, the theory proposes that differences in judgmental processes and goal pursuit can occur depending on regulatory focus above and beyond such fundamental factors as expectancy and value of attainment.

Regulatory focus has been studied both as a temporary, situationally induced orientation and as a chronic, individual-difference variable. When studied as a situationally induced orientation, regulatory focus has been manipulated either by framing an identical set of task payoffs for success or failure as involving "gain–nongain" (promotion) or "nonloss–loss" (prevention) (e.g., Shah & Higgins, 1997; Shah, Higgins, & Friedman, 1998), or by priming ideals or oughts (Higgins, Roney, Crowe, & Hymes, 1994; Liberman, Molden, Idson, & Higgins, 2001). When studied as an individual-difference variable, regulatory focus has been assessed using the Self-Guide Strength Measure (e.g., Higgins, Shah, & Friedman, 1997; Shah & Higgins, 1997), which measures the chronic accessibility of people's ideals and oughts (Higgins, 1997).

Chronic regulatory focus has also recently been studied by using the Regulatory Focus Questionnaire (RFQ; Higgins et al., 2001), which assesses people's subjective histories of effective promotion and prevention self-regulation. The RFQ distinguishes between "promotion pride"—a subjective history of success with promotion-related eagerness that orients individuals toward using eagerness means to pursue new goals— and "prevention pride"—a subjective history of success with prevention-related vigilance that orients individuals toward using vigilance means to pursue new goals. It should be noted that the RFQ measures two types of success-related pride, namely, promotion pride and prevention pride, rather than measuring success-related pride and failure-related shame. Furthermore, both promotion pride and prevention pride are positively, reliably, and independently correlated with achievement motivation (Harlow, Friedman, & Higgins, 1997); that is, both variables involve pride in success, but through different motivational orientations involving either eagerness or vigilance.

Research on regulatory focus theory has uncovered distinct patterns of sensitivities (Brendl, Higgins, & Lem, 1995) and emotional reactions to success and failure (Higgins et al., 1997; Idson, Liberman, & Higgins, 2000; for a review, see Higgins, 2001) associated with promotion and prevention orientations. This chapter, however, reviews research that highlights the ways in which regulatory focus affects people's judgmental processes and strategic behavior (i.e., the more active components of self-regulation). In summary, we have known for some time that a promotion focus is associated with *eagerness* to find means of advancing success (i.e., ensure "hits"), whereas a prevention focus is associated with *vigilance* to reject mistakes that could produce failure (i.e., "correct rejections"). The question addressed in this chapter is, how do these strategic differences influence judgmental processes and behavior?

In attempting to answer this question, we view our work as falling within the broader context of motivated cognition (see Kruglanski, 1996; Kunda, 1990, for reviews), which emphasizes the ways in which motives to arrive at certain conclusions affect people's judgmental processes. As mentioned earlier, this chapter reviews evidence that people's judgmental processes, as well as their behavior, are affected by not only their preferred conclusions but also their preferred strategies (see also Higgins & Molden, 2003; Molden & Higgins, in press-b). Because regulatory focus is a general principle of self-regulation, examining the strategic effects of promotion and prevention orientations on judgmental processes and behavior serves not only to deepen understanding of regulatory focus effects but also to broaden our understanding of the dynamics of motivated cognition.

REGULATORY FOCUS AND JUDGMENTAL PROCESSES

Here, we consider how people's *regulatory focus* affects their *judgmental processes*. How does a promotion versus a prevention focus influence individuals' *cognitive processes* when making judgments?

Expectancy   Value Effects on Goal Commitment

Which factors increase people's motivational intensity in goal pursuit? Expectancy × value (or subjective utility) theory provides a classic answer to this question (e.g., Feather, 1982). According to this theory, both higher expectancy and higher value of goal attainment increase motivational intensity. Beyond these main effects, motivational intensity is highest when the product of expectancy and value is highest. As people's expectancy for or value of goal attainment increases, the effect of the other variable on commitment also increases. For example, the high value of a goal should affect commitment more when the expectancy of goal attainment is high, rather than low.

Whereas expectancy × value models have received some empirical support, not all studies have revealed a positive multiplicative interaction between expectancy and value on goal commitment. Shah and Higgins (1997) proposed that chronic or temporary variability in people's strategic preferences may determine how expectancy and value interact to affect goal commitment. In particular, they proposed that promotion-focused people—who pursue their goals using eager strategies that involve ensuring hits and advancement—attempt to maximize their outcomes, and are thus especially motivated by a high expectancy of goal attainment when attainment is highly valued (or vice versa). Promotion-focused people, therefore, should demonstrate the classic expectancy × value effect on goal commitment.

In contrast, prevention-focused people—who pursue their goals using vigilant strategies that involve ensuring correct rejections and safety—view their goals as *necessities* when success is highly valued. It should matter less to prevention-focused people how likely they are to achieve such goals, which must be attempted regardless of difficulty or likelihood of success. Prevention-focused people are thus expected to demonstrate a *negative* expectancy × value multiplicative effect on goal commitment, such that the effect of expectancy on commitment (while continuing to have an impact) becomes smaller as the value of goal attainment increases.

These predictions were tested in a series of studies in which participants were asked to decide whether or not to take a particular class in their major (Shah & Higgins, 1997). In one study, participants' subjective expectancies and the value of success in the class were assessed; in two other studies, expectancy and value were experimentally manipulated. In addition, two of these studies manipulated participants' regulatory focus by framing the goal either as an accomplishment or as a safety concern, whereas the third study measured participants' chronic ideal and ought strength (see Higgins et al., 1997). Across all three studies, the predicted positive interactive effects between expectancy and value were found to be stronger for participants with a stronger promotion focus. In contrast, the predicted *negative* interactive effects between expectancy and value were found to be stronger for participants with a stronger prevention focus. Thus, regulatory focus as a strategic preference was found to have a profound impact on goal commitment, whereby promotion strength increased the classic effect, and prevention strength actually *reversed* it.

Counterfactual Thinking

Within decision-making contexts, people sometimes imagine, after a failure, how things might have turned out differently had they taken or *not* taken certain actions. Such *counterfactuals* have been shown to be an important judgmental process through which people learn from the outcomes of their decisions (see Roese, 1997). *Additive* counterfactuals are thoughts about what might have happened had one taken a different action. *Subtractive* counterfactuals are thoughts about what might have happened had one *not* taken a particular action. Roese, Hur, and Pennington (1999) tested the prediction that people's regulatory focus would moderate the frequency with which they generated additive versus subtractive counterfactuals in response to a failure. Because additive counterfactuals lead people to imagine how things might have turned out differently had they not missed an opportunity for advancement, they represent an eager strategy of reversing a past error of omission. Thus, additive counterfactuals should be preferred by people with a promotion focus. In contrast, because subtractive counterfactuals lead people to imagine how things might have turned out differently had they avoided a mistake, they represent a vigilant strategy of reversing a past error of commission. Thus, subtractive counterfactuals should be preferred by people with a prevention focus.

In one study conducted by Roese and colleagues (1999), participants read hypothetical scenarios involving either promotion failures (i.e., failures to attain accomplishment-related goals) or prevention failures (i.e., failures to attain safety-related goals). For each scenario, participants were then asked to expand in writing on a counterfactual stem reading, "If only. . . . " As predicted, participants who had received promotion-framed scenarios were more likely than those who had received prevention-framed scenarios to generate additive counterfactuals, whereas the reverse was true for subtractive counterfactuals. These results were conceptually replicated when other experimenters induced a promotion or prevention focus in participants by having them think of a negative experience they had had within the past year that involved feeling either *dejected* (promotion failure) or *agitated* (prevention failure) (see Higgins et al., 1997). The experimenters then asked participants to complete "If only . . . " sentences about their experiences. As predicted, promotion-focused participants were more likely than prevention-focused participants to generate additive counterfactuals, whereas the reverse was true for subtractive counterfactuals. Thus, regulatory focus has been found to have a strong influence on which information people judge to be most important about their past experiences in considering future action.

Generation of Alternatives

An important component of judgment and decision making is the generation of alternatives. Crowe and Higgins (1997) obtained evidence that regulatory focus moderates the criteria individuals use to *sort* or *describe* objects, two examples of generating alternatives in decision making. In one task, participants sorted a number of fruits and vegetables into categories, using whichever criteria they deemed appropriate. In another task, participants presented with the names of some objects of furniture were asked to list as many characteristics of each object as they could. Prior to both tasks, the experimenter induced either a promotion or a prevention focus in participants through the task-framing technique.

Because the criteria for generating categories for fruits and vegetables, and for choosing characteristics to list about furniture, were not well specified, it was possible for strategic preferences to affect the criteria people judged to be appropriate. Specifically, it was possible for participants to (1) generate few or many criteria in sorting fruits and vegetables, (2) list few or many characteristics of the furniture, and (3) use the same or different criteria to sort fruits and vegetables (e.g., color vs. shape) and to characterize the furniture (e.g., function vs. size). Generating many criteria for sorting and characteristics for description, and using different criteria and characteristics for different classes of objects represent an eager strategy, because they maximize the opportunity for "hits" by ensuring that all of the variability within and among objects is captured. In contrast, generating few criteria for sorting and characteristics for description, and using the same criteria and characteristics for different classes of objects represent a vigilant strategy, because they increase the opportunity for "correct rejections" by ensuring that one does not make a mistake in misclassifying objects. As predicted, promotion-focused participants generated more criteria and characteristics than prevention-focused participants, and they were also more likely to use different criteria and characteristics.

Two other examples of judgment contexts in which the generation of alternatives plays a fundamental role are the categorization of social behaviors, and the generation and endorsement of hypotheses about (or explanations for) social behavior. In a series of studies on regulatory focus and the resolution of uncertainty, Molden and Higgins (in press-b) demonstrated differences in promotion and prevention-focused people's generation of alternatives to categorize a target person's behavior. In one study, participants were given a *vague* behavioral description, with many possible categories in which to ascribe the behavior. In this context, generating many alternatives for classifying the behavior represents an eager strategy, because it maximizes the opportunity for selecting the correct category. In contrast, generating few alternatives represents a vigilant strategy, because it increases the opportunity for rejecting wrong categories. As predicted, promotion-focused participants endorsed more alternative descriptions of the vague behavior than did prevention-focused participants.

The generation of alternatives also plays a fundamental role in the generation and endorsement of hypotheses about social behavior. To examine this role, Liberman and colleagues (2001) primed participants with either a promotion or a prevention focus, then had them read about the helpful behavior of a target person. Participants were then asked to select possible causes for this behavior from among a set of provided alternatives. As predicted, promotion-focused participants selected more hypotheses about the causes of the target person's behavior than did prevention-focused participants. Another measure was participants' willingness to generalize from the one instance of helpful behavior they were given to the target person's future behavior in new situations. An important component of the causal attribution process is the *discounting principle*, whereby one possible cause of some behavior, such as a person's helpful disposition, is seen as less likely to the extent that other possible causes of the behavior exist (Kelley, 1973). By this logic, promotion-focused participants—who selected more possible causes of the helpful behavior than did prevention-focused participants—should have been less likely to generalize about the target person's helpful behavior in future situations. This prediction was supported.

Appraisal Efficiency

Another example of the influence of regulatory focus on judgmental processes lies in the domain of object appraisal. A promotion focus involves a concern with the presence and absence of positive outcomes, which correspond to feeling cheerful and dejected from success and failure, respectively (Higgins et al., 1997). In contrast, a prevention focus involves a concern with the absence and presence of negative outcomes, which correspond to feeling quiescent and agitated from success and failure, respectively (Higgins et al., 1997). Given this, promotion-focused people should be more efficient in appraising themselves or other attitude objects along cheerfulness- and dejection-related dimensions than along quiescence- or agitation-related dimensions, and the reverse should be true for prevention-focused people. In support of these predictions, Shah and Higgins (2001) found that both a chronic and a situationally induced promotion focus led to faster self and object appraisal for cheerfulness and dejection emotions, whereas both a chronic and a situationally induced prevention focus led to faster self and object appraisal for quiescence and agitation emotions.

Probability Estimates

Previous research suggests that people both overestimate the likelihood of conjunctive events, in which each of several preconditions must be met for the event to take place, and underestimate the likelihood of disjunctive events, in which only one of several preconditions must be met for the event to take place (see Bazerman, 1998). Brockner, Paruchuri, Idson, and Higgins (2002) proposed regulatory focus as a moderator of people's ability to estimate accurately the probability of conjunctive and disjunctive events. Because promotion-focused people use an eager strategy of looking for hits and any possible means of advancement, they should be more sensitive to the (sufficiency) notion that only one out of several preconditions must be met for a disjunctive event to occur, and should be less likely to underestimate the probability of such an event. In contrast, because prevention-focused people use a vigilant strategy of making correct rejections and avoiding impediments, they should be more sensitive to the (necessity) notion that only one out of several preconditions need go unmet for a conjunctive event not to occur, and should be less likely to overestimate the probability of such an event.

In support of these predictions, Brockner and colleagues (2002) found that people's degree of congruence between their ideal and actual selves (Higgins, 1987; Higgins et al., 2001)—that is, the extent to which they had previously experienced success in using eager means to attain their promotion goals—was positively related to their degree of accuracy in estimating the probabilities of disjunctive events, whereas congruence between ought and actual selves was unrelated to accuracy for these events. In contrast, people's degree of congruence between their ought and actual selves (Higgins, 1987; Higgins et al., 2001)—that is, the extent to which they had previously experienced success using vigilant means to attain their prevention goals—was positively related to their degree of accuracy in estimating the probabilities of conjunctive events, whereas congruence between ideal and actual selves was unrelated to accuracy for these events.

"Risky" and "Conservative" Response Biases

As noted earlier, promotion-focused people prefer to use eager strategies in goal attainment, whereas prevention-focused people prefer to use vigilant strategies. In signal-detection terms (Tanner & Swets, 1954; Trope & Liberman, 1996), an eager strategy involves a concern with achieving "hits" and ensuring against "misses." In contrast, a vigilant strategy involves a concern with achieving "correct rejections" and ensuring against "false hits." Thus, promotion-focused people should demonstrate a "risky" response bias, whereas prevention-focused people should demonstrate a "conservative" response bias. These predictions were tested in a recognition memory study by Crowe and Higgins (1997), in which participants first viewed a series of letter strings, then were presented with a series of old and new letter strings, and were asked to respond "Yes" or "No" with respect to whether they had previously seen the letter strings. The memory task had been framed beforehand with either a promotion or a prevention focus. As predicted, promotion-focused participants demonstrated a risky bias for saying "Yes" in the recognition memory task, whereas prevention-focused participants demonstrated a conservative bias for saying "No" (see also Friedman & Förster, 2001).

Levine, Higgins, and Choi (2000) extended this research to examine whether risky or conservative strategic norms could develop within group settings over time. The authors asked three-person groups to perform a recognition memory task similar to the one used by Crowe and Higgins (1997), and had participants state their "Yes" or "No" responses aloud (so that other group members could hear them). Participants were told that their group would earn $6 if the group members answered correctly 80% or more of the time, but only $3 if they answered correctly less than 80% of the time. This contingency was framed with either a promotion or a prevention focus; specifically, promotion-focused groups were told that they would begin with $3 and had a chance to earn $3 more, whereas prevention-focused groups were told that they would begin with $6 and had a chance to lose $3.

As predicted, most of the groups (27 out of 34) converged in their recognition responses from the first to the second block of the task, as reflected by decreasing within-group variance in "Yes"–"No" responses. More importantly, among those groups that converged, promotion-focused groups converged in such a way as to reflect a greater risky bias in Block 2 than in Block 1, whereas prevention-focused groups converged in such a way as to reflect a greater conservative bias in Block 2 than in Block 1. Thus, whereas Crowe and Higgins (1997) showed that people's regulatory focus affects their judgmental processes in individual settings, Levine and colleagues (2000) showed that *group*-level preferences for one strategy over another (i.e., promotion or prevention) affect group-level judgmental processes.

In summary, the research cited in this section indicates that regulatory focus as a strategic preference can have a profound effect on various judgmental processes. From expectancy × value effects on goal commitment to counterfactual thinking, from the generation of alternatives to the evaluation of attitude objects, from probability estimates to the individual and group formation of risky and conservative response biases, having a promotion versus a prevention focus has been found to be a critical determinant of people's cognitive processes while making judgments.

REGULATORY FOCUS AND STRATEGIC BEHAVIOR

In this section, we examine how people's *regulatory focus* affects their *behavior*, which can be thought of as the behavioral product of their judgmental or decision processes. How does a promotion versus a prevention focus influence individuals' behavior in the pursuit of goals?

Initiating Goal Pursuit

An important strategic component of goal pursuit is determining when to initiate activity toward a goal—or, within some contexts, when to initiate one activity over another. It should be noted that goals can be represented as either *minimal* goals that people *must* obtain, or *maximal* goals that they *hope* to attain. Regulatory focus theory predicts that because a prevention focus reflects a tendency to view goal pursuit as a necessity, a prevention focus should engender pressure to pursue goals quickly to meet the minimum standards required by these goals. In contrast, because a promotion focus reflects a tendency to view goal pursuit as progress toward some ideal maximum goal, a promotion focus should not engender any particular pressure to pursue goals quickly.

Freitas, Liberman, Salovey, and Higgins (2002) tested these hypotheses in a series of studies on regulatory focus and speed of initiating goal pursuit. In one study, they asked chronically promotion- and prevention-focused participants when they would be likely to initiate action toward applying for a hypothetical academic fellowship. As expected, higher prevention strength predicted more immediate action initiation, whereas higher promotion strength predicted later action initiation. These results were conceptually replicated in two additional studies, in which the goal was framed as being either a promotion-related accomplishment or a prevention-related necessity. As predicted, participants recorded more immediate action initiation times for the prevention-framed than the promotion-framed goal. In a final study, participants were given a $2 "account" and then completed an anagram task in which different-colored anagrams were framed with either promotion or prevention contingencies—for example, in one condition, participants were told they would gain 10 cents for each white anagram they solved, whereas they would lose 10 cents for each tan anagram they did not solve (color and contingency information were counterbalanced). As predicted, participants solved a greater proportion of prevention- than promotion-focused anagrams during the first 10 trials of the task, and a greater proportion of promotion- than prevention-focused anagrams during the second 10 trials.

Emphasizing Speed versus Accuracy

Another important strategic component of goal pursuit is people's emphasis on speed (or quantity) of accomplishment versus accuracy (or quality) of their efforts. Regulatory focus theory predicts that because quickly covering ground maximizes the opportunity to achieve "hits," promotion-focused people should be likely to emphasize speed over accuracy. In contrast, because thoroughly scrutinizing task requirements and efforts exerted minimizes the possibility of committing errors, prevention-focused people should be likely to emphasize accuracy over speed. In a pair of studies in which promotion- and prevention-focused participants were asked to complete a series of four "connect-the-dot" pictures, Förster, Higgins, and Bianco (2003) assessed the number of dots that participants connected for each picture within the allotted time frame, which constituted a measure of speed of goal completion. They also assessed the number of dots participants missed up to the highest dot they reached for each picture, which constituted a (reverse) measure of accuracy of goal completion. As predicted, promotion-focused participants were faster (i.e., got through a greater percentage of the pictures in the allotted time), whereas prevention-focused participants were more accurate (i.e., made fewer errors in the portions of the pictures that they had completed).

Förster and colleagues (2003) also found that promotion-focused participants became faster (i.e., in getting through a greater percentage of the pictures) as they approached the end of the goal (i.e., as they moved from the first to the fourth picture). In contrast, prevention-focused participants became more accurate at goal completion (i.e., made fewer errors) as they approached the end of the goal. These latter findings reflect the "goal looms larger" effect, whereby strategic motivation increases as people get closer to goal completion (see Förster, Higgins, & Idson, 1998). In the Förster and colleagues (2003) studies, this effect translated promotion-focused people's eagerness into greater speed of task completion over time, and prevention-focused people's vigilance into greater accuracy of task completion over time.

Activity and Object Substitution

Previous research has examined conditions under which people prefer to resume an interrupted activity versus switch to a substitute activity (e.g., Atkinson, 1953; Lewin, 1935, 1951; Zeigarnik, 1938), and to keep an object in their possession versus trade it for an object of equivalent value (i.e., the "endowment effect"; e.g., Kahneman, Knetsch, & Thaler, 1990; van Dijk & van Knippennberg, 1996). Liberman, Idson, Camacho, and Higgins (1999) proposed regulatory focus as a moderator of people's tendency to substitute a new activity or object for an old one. Specifically, in a situation in which an old activity or object is satisfactory, yet a new activity or object is presented for consideration, people's focus should naturally be on the new activity or object, which creates the choice situation, rather than the old activity or object, which functions as a background condition.

In this situation, promotion-focused people's eagerness for hits should make them more open to change than prevention-focused people, and promotion-focused people should be more likely to switch to the new activity or object. These predictions were supported across five studies in which participants' regulatory focus was either measured or manipulated, and their choice of a new or an old activity or prize was assessed; that is, in all five studies, promotion-focused participants were more willing than prevention-focused participants to give up an activity they were currently working on or a prize they currently possessed for a new activity or prize.

Changing Plans

In contrast to the case of a satisfactory old activity or object, an old activity or object may be unsatisfactory. A well-known example of this is the classic "sunk costs" effect, which refers to the phenomenon of people sticking to some previous plan in which they have already invested time or money (that cannot be returned) despite now having an alternative choice whose benefits they prefer and whose costs would be no greater than sticking to the old plan (see, e.g., Arkes & Blumer, 1985). In the two different versions of sunk costs, one version (see Arkes & Blumer, 1985, Experiment 1) concerns the cost of making an error of omission (i.e., omitting a "hit"): the error of missing a more enjoyable trip to Wisconsin simply because one has already paid more for a trip to Michigan that would take place at the same time. Another version (Arkes & Blumer, 1985, Experiment 3, Question 3A) concerns the cost of making an error of commission (i.e., saying "Yes" when one should say "No"): the error of wasting additional money on an endeavor, with almost no possible benefit just because one has already spent (i.e., wasted) money on it.

Higgins and colleagues (2001) predicted that regulatory focus would moderate the likelihood of making a sunk costs error, and that the moderation would be different for the two different versions of sunk costs. In the first scenario, in which an error of omission would produce the sunk costs effect, the preference for eagerness means of promotion-focused persons should make them less likely to show this type of sunk costs effect. In the second scenario, in which an error of commission would produce the sunk costs effect, the preference for vigilance means of prevention-focused persons should make them less likely to show this type of sunk costs effect. Both of these predictions were confirmed.

Motivational Effects of Success and Failure

Receiving success versus failure feedback on early attempts at goal attainment has been found to have different effects on the motivational systems and strategic behavior of people with subjective histories of promotion- versus prevention-related success (i.e., those with high "promotion pride" vs. "prevention pride"). Because people with high promotion pride are motivated through an eager strategy of attaining hits, and success feedback conveys information that they have attained a hit, success feedback maintains their eagerness to try for more hits. On the other hand, failure feedback conveys information that they have not attained a hit, and that their previous strategy of eagerness is not sufficient, thus reducing their eagerness. In contrast, because people with high prevention pride are motivated through a vigilant strategy of avoiding losses, and failure feedback conveys information that they have *not* avoided a loss, failure feedback maintains their vigilance to try to avoid additional losses. On the other hand, success feedback conveys information that they have avoided a loss, and that their previous strategy of vigilance is no longer necessary, thus reducing their vigilance.

Idson and Higgins (2000) tested these predictions and found that, as expected, people with high promotion pride improved their performance on an anagram task over time after success feedback but showed a decline in performance after failure feedback. In contrast, people with high prevention pride improved their performance on an anagram task over time after failure feedback but showed a decline in performance after success feedback. In a similar study, Spiegel and Higgins (2001) found that promotion-focused participants performed better on the second round of an anagram task after receiving success feedback on the first round of the task compared to prevention *or* control participants, whereas prevention-focused participants performed better on the second round of the task after receiving failure feedback on the first round of the task compared to promotion or control participants.

The studies described in this section have demonstrated the major influence that regulatory focus can have on people's behavior (i.e., on the behavioral product of people's judgmental processes). Across such important strategic components of goal pursuit as initiating goal-related action, emphasizing speed versus accuracy, substituting current activities or endowed objects with new ones, changing plans, and adjusting motivational intensity in response to success versus failure feedback, regulatory focus has been clearly identified as an important factor affecting people's behavior in goal pursuit.

REGULATORY FIT AND JUDGMENTAL PROCESSES

In this section, we examine how the presence of *regulatory fit* between one's regulatory focus and strategic means affects people's *judgmental processes*. In statistical terms, we consider the "interactive effects" on judgmental processes of having a promotion versus a prevention focus on the one hand, and using eager versus vigilant means on the other hand. The type of judgmental process considered is evaluating outcomes.

Value Transfer from Regulatory Fit to Outcomes

Higgins's (2000) theory of regulatory fit proposes that when the manner of pursuing a goal suits (vs. does not suit) people's regulatory orientation, the value of the goal pursuit process increases for them. For example, within the realm of regulatory focus, *promotion*-focused people who use *eager* means should experience greater regulatory fit and, consequently, value the goal pursuit process more than promotion-focused people who use vigilant means. In contrast, *prevention*-focused people who use *vigilant* means should experience greater regulatory fit and, consequently, value the goal pursuit process more than prevention-focused people who use eager means. Moreover, because people may confuse the various sources of value associated with the process versus the outcome of their goal pursuit, it is possible that the increased value of the goal pursuit process for people with regulatory fit might lead them later to evaluate more highly the outcome of their goal pursuit.

In a series of studies on "transfer of value from fit," Higgins, Idson, Freitas, Spiegel, and Molden (2003) tested the hypothesis that regulatory focus interacts with strategic means to influence the evaluative judgment of a chosen object. Across three studies, participants were asked to choose between a coffee mug and a disposable pen. (The coffee mug was more expensive than the pen and was determined by pretesting to be preferred by participants.) Half of the participants were asked to think about what they would *gain* if they chose each object, and the other half were asked to think about what they would *lose* if they did *not* choose each object. In other words, half of the participants were asked to make their choice using an eager strategy, and the other half were asked to make their choice using a vigilant strategy. After making their choice (almost all participants chose the mug), participants were asked to indicate how much they thought the mug was worth and, in one study, were asked how much of their own money they would be willing to offer to buy the mug.

Across the three studies, promotion-focused participants gave higher price estimates and offered more money when they used the eager rather than the vigilant strategy, whereas prevention-focused participants gave higher price estimates and offered more money when they used the vigilant rather than the eager strategy. In one study in which the price of the nonchosen object (i.e., the pen) was also assessed, value from fit effects were even transferred to this nonchosen object. This latter finding rules out a dissonance- (Festinger, 1957) or self-perception-based (Bem, 1967) explanation of the findings, in that these latter theories would predict that the price of the nonchosen object in fit conditions would *decrease* rather than increase.

Value Transfer from Regulatory Fit to Doing the Task Itself

Freitas and Higgins (2002) proposed that value from regulatory fit could transfer not only to evaluations of the object of a decision process but also to evaluations of the task activity itself carried out under fit or nonfit conditions; that is, these authors tested the hypothesis that using strategic means that *feel right* while doing a task can also lead people to *feel good* about doing the task. In a series of studies, participants were asked to circle any four-sided figures they found within a larger array of shapes, and to do so using either an eager strategy ("find the helpful elements") or a vigilant strategy ("eliminate the harmful elements"). Participants were subsequently asked how much they enjoyed doing the shape-finding task. As predicted, both chronically and situationally induced promotion-focused participants enjoyed doing the task more in the eager than in the vigilant condition, whereas both chronically and situationally induced prevention-focused participants enjoyed doing the task more in the vigilant than in the eager condition.

Value Transfer from Regulatory Fit to Moral Judgments

Camacho, Higgins, and Lugar (2003) tested the hypothesis that value from regulatory fit could transfer to the very means used to attain a goal, and that, in the process, use of means that *feel right* can also lead people to believe that what they are doing *is right*. In one study, chronically or situationally induced promotion- and prevention-focused participants were asked to think about a time in the past when they had failed either because of some action they had taken or *not* taken. The authors predicted that promotion-focused participants, because of their strategic tendency to maximize hits and avoid errors of omission, would feel worse about a failure resulting from an action they had *not* taken than from an action they *had* taken. In contrast, the authors predicted that prevention-focused participants, because of their strategic tendency to maximize correct rejections and avoid errors of commission, would feel worse about a failure resulting from an action they *had* taken than from an action they had *not* taken. As predicted, promotion-focused participants felt guiltier about an error of omission than about an error of commission, whereas prevention-focused people felt guiltier about an error of commission than about an error of omission.

In two additional studies involving external judgments instead of self-judgments, Camacho and colleagues (2003) found that "feeling right" from regulatory fit can transfer to evaluations of the rightness of what someone else is planning to do or has done. Participants evaluated a conflict resolution and a public policy as being more right when the described manner of pursuing the resolution or policy goal fit their regulatory orientation (an eager manner for promotion; a vigilant manner for prevention). The conflict resolution study also showed that regardless of whether the resolution occurred in a pleasurable or painful manner at the time it happened, regulatory fit increased evaluations of the resolution being "right." The fit effect was also shown to be independent of just the positivity of the participants' mood. The public policy study demonstrated that regulatory fit can influence a direct and explicit moral evaluation of an object, even when the object itself (i.e., a new afterschool program) is not intrinsically a matter of morality. In summary, in the research described in this section, the presence of regulatory fit between one's regulatory focus and strategic means of goal pursuit has a major effect on people's judgmental processes. Across domains such as rating the value of chosen attitude objects, the enjoyability of a task performed under fit or nonfit conditions, and the morality of one's own and others' actions, the interactive effect of regulatory focus and strategic means has been clearly identified as an important factor affecting the cognitive processes underlying people's evaluations.

REGULATORY FIT AND BEHAVIOR

In this final section, we examine how the presence of regulatory fit between one's regulatory focus and strategic means affects people's *behavior*, which, again, can be thought of as the behavioral product of judgmental processes. In statistical terms, we consider the "interactive effects" on the *quality of people's performance* of a promotion versus a prevention focus on the one hand, and use of eager versus vigilant means on the other hand.

Higgins's (2000) theory of regulatory fit proposes that the increased sense of value of the goal pursuit process from regulatory fit increases people's motivational intensity during the goal pursuit. Within the realm of regulatory focus, *promotion*-focused people who use *eagerness*-related means should experience greater motivational intensity than do promotion-focused people who use vigilance-related means. In addition, *prevention*-focused people who use *vigilance*-related means should experience greater motivational intensity than do prevention-focused people who use eagerness-related means. Moreover, the increased motivational intensity resulting from fit can translate into superior goal performance.

Förster and colleagues (1998) obtained evidence for this "performance hypothesis" in a set of studies in which they either measured or manipulated participants' regulatory focus. Participants were asked to perform an arm-pressure procedure while completing a set of anagrams. Half of the participants pressed upward on the bottom of a surface, which involves arm flexion, a motor action previously shown to induce an approach/eagerness orientation (Cacioppo, Priester, & Berntson, 1993). The other half of the participants pressed downward on the top of a surface, which involves arm extension, a motor action previously shown to induce an avoidance/vigilance orientation.

Förster and colleagues (1998) found that promotion-focused participants who engaged in arm flexion found more anagrams than those who engaged in arm extension, whereas prevention-focused participants who engaged in arm extension found more anagrams than those who engaged in arm flexion. In other words, participants who experienced regulatory fit between their regulatory state (i.e., promotion or prevention) and the strategic means induced by the motor action (i.e., approach/eagerness or avoidance/vigilance) found more anagrams than did participants who did not experience regulatory fit. This fit effect was replicated in other studies by Förster and colleagues that used persistence rather than number of correct solutions as the measure of performance.

In another study testing the performance hypothesis, Shah and colleagues (1998) asked participants with a chronic promotion or prevention focus to perform an anagram task framed in either promotion or prevention terms, and also had participants perform this task using either strategic eagerness or vigilance means. The performance hypothesis was supported, in that the highest number of anagrams across all conditions was found among (1) chronic promotion-focused participants who performed a promotion-framed task using eagerness means, and (2) chronic prevention-focused participants who performed a prevention-framed task using vigilance means. In other words, the best goal performance was found for participants who experienced regulatory fit between the means they used, and both their chronic and task-induced regulatory state.

Freitas, Liberman, and Higgins (2002) further tested the performance hypothesis in a study on regulatory focus and the ability to resist distraction. The authors primed participants' regulatory focus by asking them to think either about how their promotion focus aspirations (ideals) had changed over time or about how their prevention focus responsibilities (oughts) had changed over time. They then had participants perform a series of math problems under either distracting conditions, in which vigilant means had to be emphasized, or nondistracting conditions, in which eagerness means could be emphasized. Freitas and colleagues found that prevention-focused participants outperformed promotion-focused participants when vigilant means were required, but that promotion-focused participants slightly outperformed prevention-focused participants when vigilant means were not required. Again, when the strategic means suited participants' regulatory focus, higher goal performance resulted.

Finally, Spiegel, Grant-Pillow, and Higgins (in press) tested the performance hypothesis with respect to two real-world behaviors—writing a report and changing one's diet. In one experiment, predominantly promotion- and prevention-focused participants were given the goal of writing a report about their leisure time and were assigned either eagerness- or vigilance-framed means. All participants completed the same mental simulation task of imagining when, where, and how they would write their report. However, participants assigned eagerness means focused on taking advantage of good times, places, and methods in writing their reports, and participants assigned vigilance means focused on avoidance of bad times, places, and methods in writing their reports. In support of the performance hypothesis, promotion/eagerness and prevention/vigilance participants were about 50% more likely to mail in their reports than were promotion/vigilance and prevention/eagerness participants.

In a second experiment, participants were asked to read either a promotion- or a prevention-framed health message urging them to eat more fruits and vegetables. Participants were also presented with means they should use to attain this goal, which involved imagining either the benefits of compliance or the costs of noncompliance. Again, in support of the performance hypothesis, promotion/benefits and prevention/costs participants subsequently ate about 20% more fruits and vegetables over the following week than promotion/costs and prevention/benefits participants.

In this final section, the studies we have reviewed demonstrate the substantial influence on behavior of regulatory fit between one's regulatory focus and strategic means (i.e., on the behavioral product of judgmental processes). From laboratory tasks, such as finding anagrams or solving math problems, to real-world tasks, such as writing a report or changing one's diet, the interactive effect between having a promotion versus a prevention focus and the strategic means one uses have been found to be a critical determinant of the quality of people's goal performance.

CONCLUDING REMARKS

To capitalize fully on the potential of motivated cognition research to uncover basic principles of the motivation–cognition interface, we believe it is necessary to extend such research to encompass a broader perspective than just how preferred conclusions affect people's judgmental processes. In particular, we believe it is useful to examine how preferred strategies affect people's judgmental processes and behavior. Regulatory focus theory is one theory of self-regulation that has the potential to fulfill the goals of one such broader perspective on the study of motivated cognition.

We also believe that motivated cognition, as viewed within the contexts of both preferred conclusions and preferred strategies, constitute complementary perspectives, and that it may be possible to examine the interactive effects of these different types of motivated cognition on judgmental processes and behavior. In a recent study attempting such an integration, for example, Förster, Higgins, and Strack (2000) examined how people's preferences for particular outcomes (as reflected by high or low levels of prejudice toward outgroup members) and particular strategies (as reflected by promotion and prevention orientations) interact to affect memory for information about a target outgroup member. They found that the frequently obtained pattern of greater recall of stereotype-inconsistent versus consistent information was sharply pronounced for high-prejudiced participants who used (vigilant) prevention-focused strategies to evaluate the target person. This study demonstrates that the traditional view of motivated cognition as reflecting preferences for certain outcomes is complementary to the current perspective of motivated cognition as reflecting preferences for certain strategies. Future research should examine other interactive effects between promotion and prevention strategic preferences and motivations for preferred outcomes.

REFERENCES

Arkes, H. R., & Blumer, C. (1985). The psychology of sunk cost. *Organizational Behavior and Human Decision Processes, 35,* 124–140.

Atkinson, J. W. (1953). The achievement motivation and recall of interrupted and completed tasks. *Journal of Experimental Psychology, 46,* 381–390.

Bazerman, M. (1998). *Judgment in managerial decision making* (4th ed.). New York: Wiley.

Bem, D. J. (1967). Self-perception: An alternative interpretation of cognitive dissonance phenomena. *Psychological Review, 74,* 183–200.

Brendl, C. M., Higgins, E. T., & Lem, K. M. (1995). Sensitivity to varying gains and losses: The role of self-discrepancies and event framing. *Journal of Personality and Social Psychology, 69,* 1028–1051.

Brockner, J., Paruchuri, S., Idson, L. C., & Higgins, E. T. (2002). Regulatory focus and the probability estimates of conjunctive and disjunctive events. *Organizational Behavior and Human Decision Processes, 87,* 5–24.

Cacioppo, J. T., Priester, J. R., & Berntson, G. G. (1993). Rudimentary determinants of attitudes: II. Arm flexion and extension have differential effects on attitudes. *Journal of Personality and Social Psychology, 65,* 5–17.

Camacho, C. J., Higgins, E. T., & Lugar, L. (2003). Moral value transfer from regulatory fit: "What feels right *is* right" and "what feels wrong *is* wrong." *Journal of Personality and Social Psychology, 84,* 498–510.

Crowe, E., & Higgins, E. T. (1997). Regulatory focus and strategic inclinations: Promotion and prevention in decision-making. *Organizational Behavior and Human Decision Processes, 69,* 117–132.

Dunning, D., Leuenberger, A., & Sherman, D. A. (1995). A new look at motivated inference: Are self-serving theories of success a product of motivational forces? *Journal of Personality and Social Psychology, 69,* 58–68.

Feather, N. T. (1982). Actions in relation to expected consequences: An overview of a research program. In N. T. Feather (Ed.), *Expectations and actions: Expectancy-value models in psychology* (pp. 53–95). Hillsdale, NJ: Erlbaum.

Festinger, L. (1957). *A theory of cognitive dissonance.* Evanston, IL: Row, Peterson.

Ford, T. E., & Kruglanski, A. W. (1995). Effects of epistemic motivations on the use of accessible constructs in social judgment. *Personality and Social Psychology Bulletin, 21,* 950–962.

Förster, J., Higgins, E. T., & Idson, L. C. (1998). Approach and avoidance strength during goal attainment: Regulatory focus and the "goal looms larger" effect. *Journal of Personality and Social Psychology, 75,* 1115–1131.

Förster, J., Higgins, E. T., & Strack, F. (2000). When stereotype disconfirmation is a personal threat: How prejudice and prevention focus moderate incongruency effects. *Social Cognition, 18,* 178–197.

Förster, J., Higgins, E. T., & Bianco, A. T. (2003). Speed/accuracy decisions in task performance: Built-in trade-off or separate strategic concerns? *Organizational Behavior and Human Decision Processes, 90,* 148–164.

Freitas, A. L., & Higgins, E. T. (2002). Enjoying goal-directed action: The role of regulatory fit. *Psychological Science, 13,* 1–6.

Freitas, A. L., Liberman, N., & Higgins, E. T. (2002). Regulatory fit and resisting temptation during goal pursuit. *Journal of Experimental Social Psychology, 38,* 291–298.

Freitas, A. L., Liberman, N., Salovey, P., & Higgins, E. T. (2002). When to begin?: Regulatory focus and initiating goal pursuit. *Personality and Social Psychology Bulletin, 28,* 121–130.

Friedman, R. S., & Forster, J. (2001). The effects of promotion and prevention cues on creativity. *Journal of Personality and Social Psychology, 81,* 1001–1013.

Harlow, R., Friedman, R. S., & Higgins, E. T. (1997). *The Regulatory Focus Questionnaire.* Unpublished manuscript, Columbia University.

Higgins, E. T. (1987). Self-discrepancy: A theory relating self and affect. *Psychological Review, 94,* 319–340.

Higgins, E. T. (1997). Beyond pleasure and pain. *American Psychologist, 52,* 1280–1300.

Higgins, E. T. (2000). Making a good decision: Value from fit. *American Psychologist, 55,* 1217–1230.

Higgins, E. T. (2001). Promotion and prevention experiences: Relating emotions to nonemotional motivational states. In J. P. Forgas (Ed.), *Handbook of affect and social cognition* (pp. 186–211). Mahwah, NJ: Erlbaum.

Higgins, E. T., Friedman, R. S., Harlow, R. E., Idson, L. C., Ayduk, O. N., & Taylor, A. (2001). Achievement orientations from subjective histories of success: Promotion pride versus prevention pride. *European Journal of Social Psychology, 31,* 3–23.

Higgins, E. T., Idson, L. C., Freitas, A. L., Spiegel, S., & Molden, D. C. (2003). Transfer of value from fit. *Journal of Personality and Social Psychology, 84,* 1140–1153.

Higgins, E. T., & Molden, D. C. (2003). How strategies for making judgments and decisions affect cognition: Motivated cognition revisited. In G. V. Bodenhausen & A. J. Lambert (Eds.), *Foundations of social cognition* (pp. 211–235). Mahwah, NJ: Erlbaum.

Higgins, E. T., Roney, C., Crowe, E., & Hymes, C. (1994). Ideal versus ought predilections for approach and avoidance: Distinct self-regulatory systems. *Journal of Personality and Social Psychology, 66,* 276–286.

Higgins, E. T., Shah, J., & Friedman, R. (1997). Emotional responses to goal attainment: Strength of regulatory focus as moderator. *Journal of Personality and Social Psychology, 72,* 515–525.

Idson, L. C., & Higgins, E. T. (2000). How current feedback and chronic effectiveness influence motivation: Everything to gain versus everything to lose. *European Journal of Social Psychology, 30,* 583–592.

Idson, L. C., Liberman, N., & Higgins, E. T. (2000). Distinguishing gains from non-losses and losses from non-gains: A regulatory focus perspective on hedonic intensity. *Journal of Experimental Social Psychology, 36,* 252–274.

Kahneman, D., Knetsch, J. L., & Thaler, R. (1990). Experimental tests of the endowment effect and the Coase theorem. *Journal of Political Economy, 98,* 1325–1348.

Kelley, H. H. (1973). The process of causal attribution. *American Psychologist, 28,* 107–128.

Kruglanski, A. W. (1996). Motivated social cognition: Principles of the interface. In E. T. Higgins & A. W. Kruglanski (Eds.), *Social psychology: Handbook of basic principles* (pp. 493–520). New York: Guilford Press.

Kunda, Z. (1990). The case for motivated reasoning. *Psychological Bulletin, 108,* 480–498.

Levine, J. M., Higgins, E. T., & Choi, H. S. (2000). Development of strategic norms in groups. *Organizational Behavior and Human Decision Processes, 82,* 88–101.

Lewin, K. (1935). *A dynamic theory of personality.* New York: McGraw-Hill.

Lewin, K. (1951). *Field theory in social science.* New York: Harper.

Liberman, N., Idson, L. C., Camacho, C. J., & Higgins, E. T. (1999). Promotion and prevention choices between stability and change. *Journal of Personality and Social Psychology, 77*, 1135–1145.

Liberman, N., Molden, D. C., Idson, L. C., & Higgins, E. T. (2001). Promotion and prevention focus on alternative hypotheses: Implications for attributional functions. *Journal of Personality and Social Psychology, 80*, 5–18.

Molden, D. C., & Higgins, E. T. (in press-a). Categorization under uncertainty: Resolving vagueness and ambiguity with eager versus vigilant strategies. *Social Cognition.*

Molden, D. C., & Higgins, E. T. (in press-b). Motivated thinking. In K. Holyoak & R. G. Morrison (Eds.), *Handbook of thinking and reasoning.* New York: Cambridge University Press.

Roese, N. J. (1997). Counterfactual thinking. *Psychological Bulletin, 121*, 133–148.

Roese, N. J., Hur, T., & Pennington, G. L. (1999). Counterfactual thinking and regulatory focus: Implications for action versus inaction and sufficiency versus necessity. *Journal of Personality and Social Psychology, 77*, 1109–1120.

Sanitioso, R., Kunda, Z., & Fong, G. T. (1990). Motivated recruitment of autobiographical memories. *Journal of Personality and Social Psychology, 59*, 229–241.

Shah, J., & Higgins, E. T. (1997). Expectancy × value effects: Regulatory focus as a determinant of magnitude and direction. *Journal of Personality and Social Psychology, 73*, 447–458.

Shah, J., & Higgins, E. T. (2001). Regulatory concerns and appraisal efficiency: The general impact of promotion and prevention. *Journal of Personality and Social Psychology, 80*, 693–705.

Shah, J., Higgins, E. T., & Friedman, R. (1998). Performance incentives and means: How regulatory focus influences goal attainment. *Journal of Personality and Social Psychology, 74*, 285–293.

Spiegel, S., Grant-Pillow, H., & Higgins, E. T. (in press). How regulatory fit enhances motivational strength during goal pursuit. *European Journal of Social Psychology.*

Spiegel, S., & Higgins, E. T. (2001). *Regulatory focus and means substitution in strategic task performance.* Unpublished manuscript, Columbia University.

Tanner, W. P., Jr., & Swets, J. A. (1954). A decision-making theory of visual detection. *Psychological Review, 61*, 401–409.

Thompson, E. P., Roman, R. J., Moskowitz, G. B., Chaiken, S., & Bargh, J. A. (1994). Accuracy motivation attenuates covert priming: The systematic reprocessing of social information. *Journal of Personality and Social Psychology, 66*, 474–489.

Trope, Y., & Liberman, A. (1996). Social hypothesis testing: Cognitive and motivational mechanisms. In E. T. Higgins & A. W. Kruglanski (Eds.), *Social psychology: Handbook of basic principles* (pp. 239–270). New York: Guilford Press.

Van Dijk, E., & van Knippenberg, D. (1996). Buying and selling exchange goods: Loss aversion and the endowment effect. *Journal of Economic Psychology, 17*, 517–524.

Zeigarnik, B. (1938). On finished and unfinished tasks. In W. D. Ellis (Ed.), *A source book of gestalt psychology* (pp. 300–314). New York: Harcourt, Brace & World.

10

Self-Efficacy Beliefs and the Architecture of Personality

On Knowledge, Appraisal, and Self-Regulation

DANIEL CERVONE
NILLY MOR
HEATHER OROM
WILLIAM G. SHADEL
WALTER D. SCOTT

Two defining characteristics of the beings we call human are their capacities to think about (1) not only the present but also the future, and (2) not only the world around them but themselves as actors in that world. Given this combination of attributes, a class of thoughts that inevitably crosses people's minds concerns the self's capacity to cope with prospective challenges that the world may present. It is this class of thinking that is referred to as perceived self-efficacy (Bandura, 1997, 2001) and is the focus of this chapter. We review the role of self-efficacy perceptions in people's efforts to regulate their experiences and actions.

SELF-EFFICACY WITHIN THE ARCHITECTURE OF PERSONALITY

It has been suggested that "the study of no aspect of humanity is so marked by muddled thinking and confusion of thought" (Harré, 1998, p. 2) as is the study of the self. If so, it is best to express one's ideas particularly carefully. In this chapter, our central idea is that perceived self-efficacy must be understood as one aspect of an overall architecture of personality. To curtail confusion, we begin by discussing some of the terminology we used in the previous sentence and that we employ throughout this chapter.

Theorists in personality psychology try to account for both enduring structures and dynamic processes involved in personality functioning (Pervin, Cervone, & John,

188

2004). They strive, in other words, to model the overall "architecture of personality" (Cervone, 2004). The term "personality architecture" specifically refers to the within-person design and operating characteristics of those psychological systems that underlie individual personality functioning and differences among individuals (cf. Anderson, 1983).

A recent model of the cognitive architecture of personality posits two distinctions (Cervone, 2004). One differentiates knowledge from appraisal (cf. Lazarus, 1991). Knowledge refers to enduring mental representations of a typical attribute or attributes of oneself, other persons, or the physical or social world. Appraisals, in contrast, are "continuing evaluation[s] of the significance of what is happening for one's personal well-being" (Lazarus, 1991, p. 144), where those evaluations are performed by relating features of the self to features of the world. Within this personality architecture, self-efficacy beliefs are appraisals—specifically, appraisals of one's capacity to execute actions to cope with challenges the world presents. The second distinction (Cervone, 2004), which is grounded in both psychological considerations and work in the philosophy of mind (Searle, 1998), differentiates mental propositions according to whether they represent (a) beliefs about the nature of the world, (b) goals for bringing about a state of the world, or (c) standards for evaluating the goodness or worth of an entity. Within this distinction, self-efficacy appraisals are beliefs. They are conceptually distinct from—yet empirically may be systematically related to—personal goals and standards, as we discuss below.

The knowledge/appraisal distinction is important because knowledge and appraisal mechanisms play different roles in intentional self-regulation. Knowledge structures are distal determinants that influence self-regulated action through their effects on appraisals (Cervone, 1997, 2004; cf. Lazarus, 1991). For example, if one is deciding whether to participate in a group discussion on a challenging topic, and if one possesses enduring mental representations involving knowledge that one is a "smart person" or " good with words," that knowledge may prove influential in the encounter. However, the knowledge would not be influential unless it came to mind and influenced appraisals of the encounter, especially appraisals of self-efficacy for participating in the discussion successfully. Links between enduring knowledge structures and dynamic appraisals of self-efficacy are discussed in more detail below.

Generally, we discuss "the effects of perceived self-efficacy" on a given psychological outcome. We also compare people who "have high versus low perceived self-efficacy." Both phrases are examples of useful shorthands that, however, should not be taken too literally. Regarding the former phrase, it must be understood that the entity that "effects" the psychological outcomes of interest is the whole person, not the isolated psychological variable "perceived self-efficacy." It is not an individual variable but the complex person—Stern's (1935) unitas multiplex—that has the capacity to act as a causal, self-regulating agent (Harré, 1998). Regarding the latter phrase, we caution readers against interpreting "high versus low perceived self-efficacy" as "levels of a property of a person, like their weight, which has different magnitudes in different people" (as Harré, 1998, p. 130, aptly characterized traditional treatments of self-esteem). Perceived self-efficacy refers to a class of thought, namely, people's thoughts about their capabilities for performance. In any given setting, different people may think differently about their capabilities. Investigators traditionally employ quantifiable self-report measures to index these person-to-person variations. As we will see, these measures are quite valuable. Yet one should not interpret their use as an indication that self-efficacy can be reified, with different people possessing different "amounts" of the reified entity. When we refer to persons who "have high perceived self-efficacy" in any given setting, we are merely referencing individuals whose confidence regarding the level or type of performance they can accomplish in that setting exceeds the norm.

PERCEIVED SELF-EFFICACY: DEFINITION AND ASSESSMENT

Definition

Definitions describe what an entity is and, simultaneously, what it is not. Both aspects of the definition of "perceived self-efficacy" are important. As already noted, the construct refers to people's appraisals of their capabilities to execute actions in designed settings. Perceived self-efficacy, then, is a person-in-context construct; the phenomena to which it refers are people's thoughts about their capabilities for performance within a particular encounter, or type of encounters. Perceived capabilities to perform socially skilled behaviors with members of the opposite sex (Hill, 1989), to control eating (Glynn & Ruderman, 1986; Goodrick et al., 1999), to resist peer pressure (Bandura, Barbaranelli, Caprara, & Pastorelli, 1996; Caprara et al., 1998), or to engage in safe-sex practices (Dilorio, Maibach, O'Leary, & Sanderson, 1997; Montoya, 1998) are examples of the class of thinking referred to as perceived self-efficacy.

By implication, "perceived self-efficacy" does *not* refer to a variety of other self-referential psychological phenomena with which it is sometimes confused. For example, self-efficacy appraisals differ from self-esteem. Perceived self-efficacy refers to appraisals of capabilities for performance, independent of the subjective value that one attaches to the performance of the given acts. People who feel that their job has little intrinsic merit, and thus contributes little or nothing to their sense of personal esteem, may nonetheless have a high sense of self-efficacy for executing job duties. Perceived self-efficacy also does not refer to mental representations of personal attributes apart from the contexts in which those attributes may come into play. Statements such as "I am a good person," "I am a talented athlete," or "I have poor social skills" are not seen as self-efficacy appraisals, but as aspects of self-knowledge.

Other distinctions among constructs that bear on behavioral self-regulation are of note. Bandura (1977) distinguished between self-efficacy judgments and outcome expectations; the latter refer to beliefs about rewards or punishments that may follow an act, whereas the former refer to appraisals of whether one can perform the behavior in the first place. Skinner (1996) distinguished among *agents* (the entity taking action to control events), *means* (the actions to be performed to gain control), and *ends* (desired and undesired outcomes); in this framework, self-efficacy perceptions are agent–means relations. Finally, Oettingen (1996) distinguished realistic appraisals, such as self-efficacy, from fantasies; the distinction is important, because highly optimistic fantasies may be associated with goal setting and self-regulation in a manner that is distinct from efficacy judgments (Oettingen, Pak, & Schnetter, 2001).

Assessment

Requirements for assessment follow naturally from this construct definition. To assess perceived self-efficacy, one needs to tap people's appraisals of the level or type of performance they believe they can achieve when facing designated challenges.

This generally is done via structured self-report measures (Bandura, 1977). People are asked to indicate either the level of performance they believe they can achieve on a task (level of self-efficacy) or their degree of confidence in attaining designated levels of achievement (strength of self-efficacy), or both. Investigators commonly devise self-efficacy scales that are specifically tailored to tap efficacy beliefs in the particular domain of interest. Self-efficacy scales are designed to tap people's confidence in their capabilities for performance in specified circumstances. To determine the content of test items, investigators commonly perform a task analysis that identifies particular challenges that individuals face in the those circumstances. Investigators studying perceived self-efficacy and smoking cessation, for example, might determine the social and interpersonal settings in which it is particularly difficult for individuals to resist the urge to smoke (DiClemente, Fairhurst, & Piotrowski, 1995). People researching performance in the workplace might enumerate the specific challenging tasks that employees face (Saks, 1995). After this task analysis, individuals items are designed to gauge people's level of confidence in executing the behaviors required to cope with each of the challenges. Bandura (1997) provides additional valuable guidelines for scale construction.

The well-crafted self-efficacy scale can be used to gauge not only between-person differences but also within-person variations in self-appraisal across contexts. In the "microanalytic" research strategy of self-efficacy theory (Bandura, 1977; Cervone, 1985), self-efficacy measures assess people's appraisals of their ability to cope with each of a wide variety of different challenges. This enables prediction of those intraindividual patterns of cognition and action that often define an individual's personality (Mischel & Shoda, 1995).

Structured self-report questionnaires are not the only means of assessing efficacy appraisals. Below we consider alternative assessment procedures.

PERCEIVED SELF-EFFICACY: CAUSES AND CONSEQUENCES

It is no surprise that perceptions of self-efficacy may be central to self-regulation; it is difficult to envision an organism that possesses the capacity to reflect on its capabilities for action but does not incorporate those self-reflections into its decision-making calculus. One way that self-efficacy theory takes one beyond the obvious is by providing useful analytical tools for conceptualizing causes and consequences of self-efficacy appraisals.

Bandura (1977) outlined four sources of self-efficacy information, that is, four types of psychosocial experiences that influence perceptions of efficacy for coping with encounters: (1) firsthand behavioral experience, or mastery experience; (2) observation of others' experiences, that is, vicarious information conveyed via modeling; (3) evaluation of one's own emotional and physiological states, which is important, because physical state is commonly of much relevance to one's immediately subsequent capabilities; and (4) verbal persuasion, that is, speech acts by others that may boost or lower one's own self-appraisals. Much evidence indicates that firsthand mastery experiences have the greatest influence on self-efficacy appraisals (reviewed in Bandura, 1997; Williams & Cervone, 1998).

Bandura (1997) also identified four processes through which efficacy beliefs influence behavioral outcomes. First, self-efficacy perceptions influence decisions about which activities to pursue; people commonly undertake tasks for which they judge themselves efficacious and avoid activities they judge to be beyond their capacities (e.g., Hackett & Betz, 1995). Once one undertakes an activity, a second process comes into play. Self-efficacy perceptions affect effort and task persistence. Decisions about how long to persevere are based partly on self-reflections on one's capabilities (e.g., Cervone & Peake, 1986). Third, self-efficacy contribute to affective experience. People with a high sense of efficacy experience less anxiety when facing threats (e.g., Bandura, Cioffi, Taylor, & Brouillard, 1988; Bandura, Taylor, Williams, Mefford, & Barchas, 1985). People with a low sense of self-efficacy for accomplishing important life tasks are vulnerable to depression (Bandura, Pastorelli, Barbaranelli, & Caprara, 1999; Cutrona & Troutman, 1986). Finally, efficacy beliefs influence the quality of analytical cognitive performance. People with a higher sense of self-efficacy display superior performance on cognitively complex laboratory tasks (Cervone, Jiwani, & Wood, 1991; Cervone & Wood, 1995), everyday problem-solving tasks (Artistico, Cervone, & Pezzuti, 2003), and tests of memory performance (Berry, West, & Dennehey, 1989). The impact of self-efficacy appraisals on cognitive performance is partly mediated by cognitive interference (Sarason, Pierce, & Sarason, 1996); people with a low sense of self-efficacy may dwell not only on task demands but also on their personal experiences during task performance (Elliott & Dweck, 1988).

By affecting people's acceptance of challenges, persistence despite setbacks, execution of complex cognitive strategies, and anxiety versus calmness in the face of threat, higher self-efficacy perceptions generally promote superior self-regulation and achievement. The data here are quite strong. A veritable mountain of evidence (reviewed in Bandura, 1997; Caprara & Cervone, 2000) documents the influence of self-efficacy appraisals on subsequent behavior. This includes not only correlational data but also studies that manipulate self-efficacy beliefs experimentally (e.g., Cervone, 1989; Cervone & Peake, 1986; Peake & Cervone, 1989) or that relate self-efficacy perceptions to future performance, while statistically controlling for the effects of past performance (e.g., Cervone et al., 1991). Meta-analytic reviews provide particularly valuable evidence of efficacy–behavior links. Stajkovic and Luthans (1998) synthesized 114 studies relating contextualized self-efficacy assessments to work performance and found mean correlations in the .4–.5 range (with results varying somewhat as a function of the complexity of the task being performed). This numerical result, due to a restriction of range, likely underestimates the real-world impact of efficacy self-appraisals; people with a particularly low sense of efficacy may self-select out of activities rather than merely display inferior performance once an activity has begun.

In addition to their direct effect on behavioral and emotional processes, self-efficacy perceptions are important to self-regulation because they influence other personality variables that, in turn, come into play as people strive to regulate their behavior. Goal setting is one such variable. A wealth of research in personality, social, and organizational psychology documents that performance on both achievement and interpersonal tasks is greatly influenced by the nature of the personal goals that people set for themselves (e.g., Grant & Dweck, 1999). People who set explicit, challenging goals and receive feedback on their progress generally outperform others (Locke & Latham, 1990) and commonly experience greater enjoyment of activities as well (Csikszentmihalyi, 1990). People commonly reflect on their capabilities for performance when deciding on the goals to pursue. Thus, self-efficacy perceptions influence the level and type of goal that people adopt. Individuals with a high sense of self-efficacy are more likely to adopt and remain committed to highly challenging task goals (Bandura, 1997; Cervone, 1993). The relations among self-efficacy processes and goal systems are of such importance to self-regulation that they are treated in depth later in this chapter.

Another important pathway from self-efficacy perception to personal development involves the acquisition of skills. If people who judge themselves incapable of coping avoid activities, as is often the case, then they fail to acquire knowledge and skills that they might have learned had they attempted those activities. The study of self-efficacy mechanisms in career decision making illustrates the point. Among U.S. college students, women often have a lower sense of self-efficacy for mathematics than do men; differences are found even when controlling for students' tested ability (Betz & Hackett, 1981; also see Betz, 2001). As a result, women less frequently enroll in upper-level math courses. The decision not to enroll then deprives them of the skills development that they might have experienced.

SELF-EFFICACY IN CONTEXT

Conceptual and practical considerations indicate that self-efficacy perceptions should be assessed in a contextual manner. At the level of theory, the construct "perceived self-efficacy," by definition, refers to people's perceptions of their capabilities for performance. Performances, of necessity, occur in a social or environmental context. On theoretical grounds, then, a "self-efficacy assessment" procedure tests performance capabilities in designated contexts; as Bandura (1997, p. 45) phrases it, assessments procedures that match the definition of the construct "in no case" are "dissociated from context."

Pragmatic considerations also motivate contextualism. A global approach can obscure psychological phenomena that might be understood via contextualized assessment. We consider here two illustrations of this point that serve also to illustrate the general role of self-efficacy appraisal in behavioral self-regulation. The first concerns cognitive performance among older adults. The second addresses the question of whether psychosocial interventions produce changes in self-efficacy beliefs that generalize across contexts.

Cognitive Performance among Older Adults

In a world in which people increasingly live longer, identifying factors that influence older adults' capability to maintain high levels of cognitive performance is a challenge of profound social significance. On the one hand, biologically based neuroanatomical changes that foster decreases in cognitive processing speed (Willott, 1999) may cause cognitive performance to decline with age. On the other hand, increasing age is accompanied by increasing knowledge and expertise that may compensate for processing–speed losses and thus enable resilience and high performance (Baltes, 1997; Baltes & Baltes, 1990).

Because expertise generally is grounded in contextually linked knowledge structures, age-related expertise may reveal itself primarily in specific performance contexts, such as those in which older adults invest effort to develop requisite knowledge and skills (Baltes & Lang, 1997; Baltes & Staudinger, 2000). This implies that the cognitive capabilities of older adults will not be fully revealed if, in research, such persons are asked merely to perform abstract laboratory tasks that do not represent the challenges they face in daily life. Instead, to capture the cognitive capabilities of the older adult, one may need to study everyday problem solving, that is, problem solving in which individuals solve problems that resemble those they confront outside the laboratory in their everyday lives (Willis, 1996). Such problems often are amenable to multiple solutions, and the capacity to generate multiple possible solutions is a key index of performance capabilities (e.g., Allaire & Marsiske, 2002).

Generating multiple solutions to challenging problems of everyday life requires considerable cognitive effort. To devise solutions, then, one needs not only a database of social knowledge but also a strong sense of efficacy for problem solving, because people who possess knowledge but doubt their personal efficacy may fail to exert the effort required for optimal cognitive achievement. It is here that a contextual analysis is particularly valuable. Older adults may have relatively high efficacy perceptions and performance in select domains of problem solving that are ecologically representative of challenges they face in everyday life (Berry & West, 1993; Lachman & Jelalian, 1984).

This possibility was tested in research that presented younger and older adults with alternative types of problem-solving tasks (Artistico et al., 2003). Participants were asked to generate solutions to problems that were representative of activities commonly confronted either by younger adults, older adults, or both age groups. They also attempted a traditional laboratory task, namely, the Tower of Hanoi problem. Self-efficacy appraisals for each of the four types of problems were assessed prior to task performance.

The findings revealed a strong interaction between age group and task characteristics with respect to both perceived self-efficacy and problem-solving performance (Figure 10.1). Young participants had higher efficacy beliefs and displayed superior performance

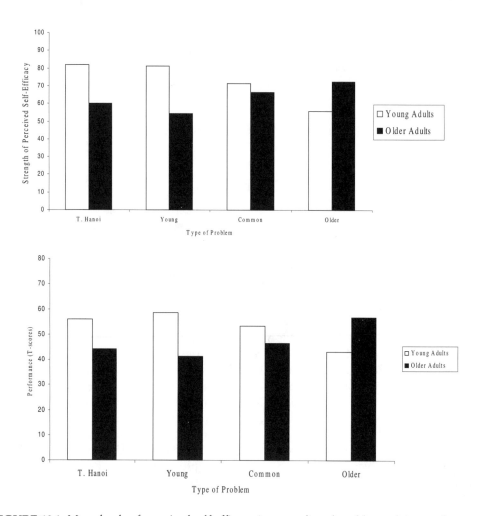

FIGURE 10.1. Mean levels of perceived self-efficacy (top panel) and problem-solving performance (bottom panel) among young and older adults on three types of everyday problems and one traditional laboratory task (see text). From Artistico et al. (2003). Copyright 2003 by the American Psychological Association. Adapted by permission.

on both the Tower of Hanoi problem and everyday problem-solving tasks that were common to both older and young adults. An even stronger difference favoring young adults was found on problems of ecological relevance to their age group. Looking merely at these three contexts (laboratory task, everyday problems of relevance to young adults, and everyday problems of relevance to both age groups), one might conclude that, as a general rule, young adults have higher self-efficacy and outperform older adults in cognitive problem solving. However, this nomothetic "rule" was completely violated in contexts of ecological relevance to the older adult (Figure 10.1). On everyday problems that were ecological relevant to their age group, older adults displayed higher self-efficacy perceptions and generated more viable solutions to the problems than did young adults (Artistico et al., 2003). Perceived self-efficacy partially or fully mediated the relations between age and performance on most problem types. The findings suggest, then, that older adults are fully capable of superior cognitive performance in particular contexts in which everyday experience has instilled in them a robust sense of problem-solving efficacy. This important result would have been overlooked if we had assessed efficacy beliefs via a global, decontextualized measurement tool.

Generalization in the Effects of Psychosocial Interventions

Another question of both theoretical and practical significance is whether the effects of a given psychosocial intervention are generalizable. Inevitably, interventions occur within a delimited context: A therapist may treat anxiety with respect to a particular class of stimuli; a social skills training program may have the resources to confront only a limited range of social and interpersonal challenges, and so on. Yet practitioners generally hope that their interventions produce widespread effects that generalize beyond the domain in which treatment is conducted (Smith, 1989). This issue can be addressed by examining psychological mechanisms that mediate behavioral change and gauging the degree to which changes in these mechanisms generalize from one domain to another. Perceived self-efficacy is one such mechanism.

There are two ways to address generalization in self-efficacy perceptions. One is to employ a generalized self-efficacy scale (e.g., Schwarzer, Babler, Kwiatek, & Shrooder, 1997; Sherer, Maddux, Mercandante, Prentice-Dunn, Jacobs, & Rogers, 1982). In this approach, the question of whether interventions produce generalized effects is operationalized by an examiniation of the intervention's influence on self-reports of whether people generally see themselves as competent, efficacious, and able to meets life's demands (e.g., Smith, 1989; Weitlauf, Smith, & Cervone, 2000). Such a strategy may indeed provide insight into the effects of interventions on self-referential beliefs. However, it has a drawback. People's self-reports of personal attributes tend to change slowly, or may fail to change despite novel life experiences (Mischel, 1968; cf. Klein & Loftus, 1993). Thus, global self-reports may fail to reveal psychological changes that would be evident if one applied a more focused assessment strategy that inquired into people's appraisals of their capabilities to deal with specific life challenges. The second strategy, then, involves contextualized measures that tap self-efficacy beliefs across each of a variety of contexts. In this contextualized, multidomain approach, generalization is gauged by determining whether an intervention changes self-efficacy beliefs in not only the domain in which the interventions occurred but also in other domains.

Building on earlier research by Ozer and Bandura (1990), Weitlauf, Cervone, Smith, and Wright (2001) examined generalization in treatment effects stemming from an intervention of significance in the lives of many women, namely, self-defense training. Women took part in a 16-hour, physical self-defense class that taught verbal and physical resistance to rape, and martial arts. Before and after self-defense training, two types of self-efficacy assessments were employed: a measure of general self-efficacy (Sherer et al., 1982) and a 32-item, situation-specific self-efficacy index that tapped perceived capabilities in a variety of specific domains, including athletics, academics, work, interpersonal encounters, and coping with life stressors of relevance to this population. Analyses of the multidomain self-efficacy questionnaire revealed that the effects of self-defense training generalized (Weitlauf et al., 2001). Self-defense training boosted efficacy beliefs in domains beyond those involving physical self-defense (e.g., interpersonal assertiveness). The generalization effects detected by our multidomain, contextualized self-efficacy measure were not replicated on the measure of general self-efficacy or self-esteem. Thus, contextualized assessment had practical benefits. An exclusive use of global self-report measures would have obscured the actual generalization effects that were detectable only when we assessed efficacy appraisals for specific challenges in specific contexts.

THE ROLE OF SELF-EFFICACY WITHIN GOAL SYSTEMS

As we have emphasized, self-efficacy perceptions do not operate in a vacuum. They are aspects of an overall architecture of knowledge structures and appraisal processes that underlie behavioral self-regulation. Another critical aspect of this architecture involves goals. Here, we present an overview of the different types of interactions among self-efficacy processes and goal systems that are indicated by contemporary theory and research on self-regulation.

In addressing this issue, it is important to recognize that the psychological phenomena referenced by the term "goals" include both enduring knowledge structures and dynamic appraisal processes. As knowledge structures, goals can be conceptualized as interlinked nodes in a semantic network (Shah & Kruglanski, 2000). Indeed, goals have been demonstrated to possess features characteristic of other knowledge structures with interlinked informational structures (Kruglanski et al., 2002), including the interconnectedness of goals and the means to attain those goals; variation in the strength of those interconnections; the transfer of properties (such as affect and beliefs) from one goal to another, or between goals and their means of attainment; the subconscious impact of goals on each other; and contextual dependence, whereby the relations between goals change across contexts (Kruglanski et al., 2002).

The term "goals" also aptly applies to dynamic appraisal processes that occur as people evaluate their relation to ongoing encounters and activities. When engaged in such activities, people formulate and reformulate aims for action, as well as strategies for achieving those aims. People devise and discard goals as they evaluate their successes and failures, and try to move from a present state to a desired future state.

Self-efficacy perceptions are linked both to enduring goal structures and to dynamic goal processes. To best understand the diverse ways in which efficacy beliefs and goals may be linked, one should recognize qualitative distinctions among aspects of goals and the ways that self-efficacy perceptions relate to these distinctions. In outlining distinctions among goals, one may focus on differences in the *content* represented by goals; in particular, some activities are pursued with the goal of accomplishing a positive outcome, whereas others are pursued to avoid a negative outcome, as many theorists have recognized (e.g., Carver & Scheier, 1998). A second distinction involves the *process* of pursuing the goals, in which processes can be construed in terms of different stages or phases of goal pursuit, such as weighing alternatives versus maximizing yield once an alternative is chosen (Gollwitzer, 1996). Content and process may interact; that is, different goal contents may be associated with greater or lesser attention being devoted to different processes of attainment. We now review the extensive work that has related goal structures and processes to self-efficacy perceptions.

Self-Efficacy Perceptions and Enduring Goal Structures

Goals differ from one other both quantitatively and qualitatively. Quantitative distinctions include difficulty level, specificity, and proximity. For example, a person may aim to complete a marathon versus a 10-kilometer race (variations in goal difficulty), volunteer at a homeless shelter versus "do something to help the homeless" (goal specificity), or read one book chapter for class each week versus reading four chapters by the end of the month (goal proximity). Variations along these goal dimensions differentially influence motivation and performance; these effects are mediated in part by self-efficacy perceptions (Bandura, 1997; Locke & Latham, 1990). For example, when people set proximal goals, they more quickly and frequently receive feedback on their progress; thus, they tend to have higher self-efficacy perceptions and in turn higher interest in, and performance of, the activities as hand (Bandura & Cervone, 1983; Stock & Cervone, 1990; see also Garland, 1985; Manderlink & Harackiewicz, 1984).

Goals also can be differentiated according to several qualitative distinctions. One such distinction is goal orientation. When pursuing a given task, different individuals may be oriented toward different types of goals; some may pursue the activity for the purpose of demonstrating or evaluating their abilities, whereas others may by trying to learn and to hone their skills (Elliott & Dweck, 1988). These two different orientations are commonly referred to as *performance* and *learning* goals (Dweck & Leggett, 1988), or similarly, as *judgment* versus *development* goal orientations (Grant & Dweck, 1999). A learning orientation, as opposed to a performance orientation, has been shown to promote self-efficacy even in the face of failure (Button, Mathieu, & Zajac, 1996) and is related to better performance (e.g., Bell & Kozlowski, 2002). Failure on performance goals induces negative self-evaluation and helplessness, and is often coupled with general beliefs about one's deficiencies (Grant & Dweck, 1999).

Another qualitative distinction differentiates between goals that involve an approach to positive outcomes and goals that entail avoidance of a negative outcome (e.g., Emmons, 1989, 1999). Avoidance goals have often been associated with negative outcomes and poor well-being (Elliott & Sheldon, 1997; Emmons & Kaiser, 1996). Self-efficacy appraisals may play a role here as well. People have been found to view avoidance goals as less clear than approach goals (i.e., as involving less clearly defined strategies and outcomes) and to have a relatively lower sense of self-efficacy for the accomplishment of avoidance goals (Mor & Cervone, 2002). Goal clarity and self-efficacy may be linked; self-efficacy perceptions may be higher when pathways to goal pursuit come to mind clearly (cf. Cervone, 1989).

Higgins (1997, 1999) has distinguished two forms of regulatory focus through which goals can be pursued: promotion and prevention. Promotion focus refers to sensitivity to positive outcomes. Individuals in a promotion focus aim to attain or to avoid loss of positive outcomes. Prevention focus, in contrast, involves an aim to avoid or to "gain the absence" of negative outcomes. Because a prevention focus involves regulation of necessary duties and obligations, expectancies play a more minor role in goal pursuit (Shah & Higgins, 1997). This raises an interesting general point about self-efficacy and goal systems: Different goals differentially engage self-efficacy processes (Bandura & Cervone, 1983); that is, they moderate the role of self-efficacy processes in the self-regulation of behavior. Efficacy appraisals play a relatively larger role when people are promotion-oriented (Shah & Higgins, 1997), and when they receive clear, easy-to-interpret feedback on performance goals (Bandura & Cervone, 1983; Cervone & Wood, 1995; Cervone et al., 1991).

Goals differ also in the extent to which the motivation for their pursuit is externally versus autonomously controlled (e.g., Ryan & Deci, 2000). People pursue autonomous goals because of a sense of personal volition and choice, whereas they pursue controlled goals because of external or internal pressure to accomplish the goal (Williams, Gagné, Ryan, & Deci, 2002). Autonomous motivation has been linked to higher task interest and enhanced persistence and performance (Deci & Ryan, 1991; Sheldon, Ryan, Rawsthorne, & Ilardi, 1997), even when people have the same level of perceived competence—a construct generally associated with autonomous motivation (Deci, 1992) that relates closely to self-efficacy, though it constitutes a more general self-evaluation. Recently, an examination of the joint role of autonomous goal pursuit and of self-efficacy revealed that although autonomous goal pursuit and self-efficacy predict both behavioral adherence to a goal and general life satisfaction, autonomous goal pursuit is a more powerful predictor of life satisfaction, whereas self-efficacy is a more potent predictor of behavioral adherence (Sene'cal, Nouwen, & White, 2000). Thus, autonomous goal pursuit may facilitate perceptions of efficacy that may in turn contribute to the self-regulation of behavior aimed toward goal attainment; however, autonomous goals may independently contribute to a general sense of satisfaction with one's life activities. In this regard, it should be remembered that self-efficacy theory is not a "unifactor" theory; instead, as we have stressed, efficacy perceptions are one of a number of personal determinants of human motivation and achievement (see Bandura, 1986, 1999).

Self-Efficacy and Nonconscious Goals

Work on perceived self-efficacy primarily has addressed the role of conscious self-reflection in self-regulation. In contrast, research on goal processes indicates that nonconscious processes also are significant. Goals can be primed and activated by environmental cues outside of awareness (e.g., Fitzsimons & Bargh, Chapter 8, this volume; Bargh & Chartrand, 1999; Bargh & Gollwitzer, 1994). Once activated, these goals can enhance performance, persistence in the face of failure, and the resumption of disrupted goal-directed behavior in the presence of alternatives (Bargh, Lee-Chai, Barndollar, Gollwitzer, & Trotschel, 2001). Thus, in these ways, nonconscious goals operate in a manner similar to that of conscious goals, despite their being relative "automatic" cognitions.

A question that arises, then, is the role of self-efficacy perceptions when goals are activated automatically by environmental stimuli (Bargh et al., 2001) rather than as a result of conscious deliberation. It must be recognized here that extant findings on automatic goal activation constitute an "existence proof"; one can create instances in which goal processes and behavioral regulation can occur outside of conscious awareness. This, however, does not imply that self-regulation occurs outside of conscious awareness in everyday settings in which people face challenging activities of personal significance. In such contexts, people naturally are prompted to dwell on the fit between their abilities and the challenges to be faced, and these conscious self-reflections on personal efficacy are key to successful self-regulation. Also, it should be noted that self-efficacy appraisal can occur rapidly, rather than through slow, deliberate cognitive processing; Lazarus

(1991) informatively explained how people may engage in rapid appraisals of their coping potential.

Self-Efficacy and Hindrance of Goal Pursuit

Self-efficacy perceptions may also hinder goal attainment. Under some circumstances, highly self-efficacious persons may be overly persistent in pursuing unattainable goals (Brandtstadter & Renner, 1990; Janoff-Bulman & Brickman, 1982) or may undertake risky endeavors that they should avoid (Haaga & Stewart, 1992; see also Baumeister & Scher, 1988). Later in life, when resources become scarce (e.g., a deterioration in health, lesser physical capacities, a shorter remaining lifespan), optimal goal pursuit involves calibration of goals to the available resources and selection of manageable goals (Freund & Baltes, 2002), whereby an inflated sense of efficacy may interfere with goal attainment.

High self-efficacy beliefs, then, are not always beneficial. Rather than asking "whether high self-efficacy beliefs are good, it is better to examine specific functional relations among self-appraisal, experience, and action. The ultimate utility of the experiences and actions that are self-regulated via efficacy beliefs, of course, may vary from one context to another.

Mood, Goals, and Standards for Performance

The previous discussion of self-regulatory processes was relatively "cold"; that is, it involved cognitive mechanisms rather than affective states. Recent work has examined the effects of affect on self-regulatory processes, with a focus on the impact of dysphoric mood (Scott & Cervone, 2002; Tillema, Scott, & Cervone, 2001).

This work has focused in particular on the relation between self-efficacy perceptions (i.e., beliefs about what one can do) and personal standards for performance (i.e., criteria that specify what one would have to achieve to be satisfied with oneself). Personal standards, of course, have long been recognized as critical to self-regulation (e.g., Lewin, Dembo, Festinger, & Sears, 1944). Correlational studies indicate that people who chronically experience dysphoric moods tend to hold relatively stringent performance standards that exceed the performances that, in their judgment, they actually can attain (Ahrens, 1987). Experimental studies indicate that affect plays a direct role in this tendency to adopt relatively perfectionistic standards. People in experimentally induced negative moods were found to display relatively high standards for performance; because negative mood did not raise efficacy beliefs, such persons exhibited the discrepancies between standards and efficacy perceptions that are typical of chronically depressed individuals (Cervone, Kopp, Schauman, & Scott, 1994).

Recent work suggests that affect-as-information processes (Schwarz & Clore, 1983, 1988) account for this result. A unique prediction of affect-as-information analyses is that mood will not influence judgment when people attribute their mood to a source unrelated to the target of judgment. The attribution to an unrelated source should cause mood no longer to serve as a source of information when evaluating the target. Scott and Cervone (2002) induced negative mood experimentally. Subsequent to this mood induction, participants completed a survey with measures of self-efficacy perceptions and personal standards for daily activities. Before completing the survey, the mood induction was made salient to some participants; that is, they were briefly reminded of the audiotaped procedure that had been used earlier to induce negative mood. In each of two studies, participants' standards for performance were similar to their self-efficacy perceptions;

that is, they felt they could achieve their minimal standards for performance—*unless* they experienced a negative mood induction, and that mood induction was not salient to them at the time of judgment (Scott & Cervone, 2002). When negative mood was made salient, participants no longer reported perfectionistic standards that exceeded their efficacy beliefs (Table 10.1), as anticipated by affect-as-information theory (Schwarz & Clore, 1983, 1988).

KNOWLEDGE STRUCTURES AND SELF-EFFICACY APPRAISAL

Investigators have devoted much attention to alternative types of experiences that influence people's perceptions of their capacity to overcoming stressful challenges, with Bandura's (1977) formulation of four main sources of efficacy information (reviewed earlier) providing a valuable guide. A delineation of types of efficacy-relevant information, however, is only one kind of question one may ask regarding determinants of self-efficacy appraisal. Another inquiry concerns internal cognitive structures that contribute to self-appraisal.

Advances in the study of social cognition (e.g., Higgins & Kruglanski, 1996) enable one to reformulate questions about the determinants of self-efficacy perceptions. This work shifts attention from a taxonomy of sources of information to the enduring elements of social and self-knowledge that develop through social interaction, and that dynamically shape people's thinking as they encounter new situations and appraise their efficacy for performance. It is particularly valuable that social cognition research has yielded a set of common principles for explaining why one versus another element of knowledge comes to mind in a given situation. Higgins (1996) describes three conditions that may determine knowledge activation. The use of knowledge to inform a given judgment depends on (1) whether the person making the judgment has the information encoded in memory (availability), (2) whether the information is relevant to the situation (applicability), and (3) the degree to which the concept is easily retrieved and used (accessibility). People may, therefore, have repertoires of chronically accessible knowledge, with relatively lower thresholds of activation, that come to mind with greater frequency and ease than other, less frequently activated concepts (Higgins & King, 1981). Extensive research has indicated that social judgments and behaviors may become automatized in instances when people's chronically accessible constructs are applicable and presumably

TABLE 10.1. Adjusted Mean Minimal Performance Standards and Evaluative Judgments for Semester GPA by Condition

Experimental condition	Minimal performance standard for semester GPA	Evaluative judgment for semester GPA
Nonsalient–negative	8.34 (2.34)	5.45 (2.91)
Salient–negative	7.16 (2.09)	6.86 (3.03)
Nonsalient–neutral	7.10 (2.73)	6.67 (3.04)

Note. Standard derivations are in parentheses. From Scott and Cervone (2002, Experiment 2). Copyright 2002 by Kluwer Academic/Plenum Press. Adapted by permission.

come to mind. Constructs that have been investigated include personality attributes (e.g., Higgins, King, & Mavin, 1982), goals (Grant & Dweck, 1999; Sanderson & Cantor, 1995), beliefs about significant others (Andersen & Chen, 2002), and beliefs about the self (Green & Sedikides, 2001; Markus, 1977; Markus, Crane, Bernstein, & Siladi, 1982).

These analyses of social and self-knowledge have been extended to the study of how chronically accessible self-schemas influence self-efficacy appraisals (Cervone, 1997, 2004; Orom & Cervone, 2002). Chronically accessible beliefs about the self may come to mind automatically in certain situations, and may lead people to make self-efficacy judgments more quickly and less effortfully than in situations in which this knowledge is unlikely to come to mind. This possibility has been explored in work that employs an idiographic assessment strategy (Cervone, 1997; Cervone, Shadel, & Jencius, 2001). Participants' beliefs about personal attributes that they consider to be strengths and weaknesses are assessed, as are their subjective beliefs about the social situations in which those attributes might come into play. In subsequent assessments, people are found to display consistently high versus low self-efficacy appraisals in situations that are subjectively linked to their self-described important strengths and weaknesses, respectively; that is, when people perceive their strengths as relevant to situations, they perceive themselves more capable than when they perceive their salient weaknesses as relevant to situations.

The idea that chronically accessible self-schemas influence self-efficacy appraisal suggests another type of prediction. In addition to displaying low versus high self-efficacy beliefs in various schema-relevant situations, people should make self-efficacy appraisals *faster* when they are contemplating a challenge relevant to schematic self-knowledge (cf. Markus, 1977). Thus, we recently have supplemented standard questionnaire assessments of self-efficacy perceptions with reaction time measures (Orom & Cervone, 2002). This study has examined not only whether people are likely to judge themselves more capable of overcoming challenges when they perceive their schematic personal strengths as relevant to challenging situations, but also whether they make these belief-relevant judgments more quickly. People judged the relevance of their salient and highly self-representative attributes to various challenging social situations. They also judged whether they could perform challenging behaviors in these situations, while the time it took to make these judgments was assessed. Finally, they rated their confidence on a 10-point self-efficacy scale typical of the literature. As predicted, people appraised their capabilities more quickly for situations perceived as relevant to an important personal strength than for situations irrelevant to the same strength or relevant to a common positive attribute not descriptive of themselves.

Results confirmed that reaction-time measures are useful for bringing to light information-processing differences between self-efficacy appraisals for schema-relevant and -irrelevant targets, which are especially notable, because these judgments are more complex than the types of decisions to which reaction times have often been applied. One possible implication is that people can take different routes to get to the same self-efficacy rating. Which route they take may depend on the accessibility of relevant information. When people are in situations that cue chronically accessible beliefs about themselves, they may make snap judgments based on automatic activation of extremely salient beliefs about themselves.

Another implication is that salient beliefs about the self that come to mind chronically can not only be sources of important interindividual differences in self-efficacy appraisal but also may underlie *within*-person coherence among thoughts and behaviors. Each person in our study (Orom & Cervone, 2002) exhibited a unique profile of situations in which he or she reported being relatively more confident in his or her capabilities. Precisely with respect to these situations, people tended to perceive that their chronically accessible personal strengths would influence their behavior, and were in turn faster to judge their capabilities. The speed with which they made efficacy appraisals in these situations appeared to be associated with activation of personal strengths. This suggests that, over time, people's chronically accessible beliefs are likely to be repeatedly activated in similar encounters, leading to consistencies in functioning across situations and emergent personality coherence.

ALTERNATIVE SELF-EFFICACY ASSESMENT TECHNIQUES: THINK-ALOUD ASSESSMENTS

In the research on self-efficacy perceptions and self-regulation that we have reviewed, efficacy perceptions have in virtually all cases been assessed via self-report questionnaires. The strength of the extant empirical results attests to the utility of this assessment technique. In closing, however, we consider an alternative assessment procedure; we do so by not only looking back, in the spirit of a handbook review, but by also looking forward to potential future developments that may capitalize on the advantages of alternative assessment procedures. The alternative that we review is think-aloud assessment methods.

Think-aloud methods and procedures have been utilized by cognitive scientists for many years (Ericsson & Simon, 1993). Clinical scientists have used think-aloud procedures in a variety of contexts to serve a variety of purposes, for example, to develop items for clinical assessments (e.g., Bystritsky, Linn, & Ware, 1990), to analyze depressive attributional styles and thought processes (Blackburn & Eunson, 1989), and to yield dependent measures responsive to diagnostic category differences (Molina, Borkovec, Peasley, & Person, 1998).

In the Articulated Thoughts in Simulated Situations paradigm (ATSS; see Davidson, Robins, & Johnson, 1983; Davidson, Vogel, & Coffman, 1997), a particular form of the think-aloud paradigm, individuals are exposed in the laboratory (usually via audiotape) to a relevant situation (e.g., a social criticism situation that elicits social anxiety; Davidson et al., 1997), and are instructed to speak aloud their thoughts and feelings at periodic intervals during exposure to the simulated situation. These responses are then coded for content and structure by trained raters, who are unaware of the circumstances of the data collection (i.e., stimuli to which the subjects had been exposed) and/or diagnostic categories (e.g., depressed vs. nondepressed) that could potentially bias their codes. The ATSS procedure offers three main advantages for cognitive assessment compared to self-report questionnaires (Davidson et al., 1997; Haaga, 1989). First, open-ended responses are collected from individuals; no predetermined set of questions is asked that might bias subject responses, and no assumptions are made about the content or structure of the individuals' cognitions. Second, the ATSS paradigm relies on assessing cognition as it occurs in response to specific, controlled situations, and does not rely on retrospective recall of how one was thinking or feeling; this procedure also controls for specific environmental factors (e.g., setting) that may bias responses. Third, the data can be reliably coded in an unbiased fashion, so as to reveal not only idiosyncratic content of the cognitions prompted by particular contextual stimuli but also differences in the underlying structure and organization of those cognitions (Cacioppo, von Hippel, & Ernst, 1997).

Research has supported the validity of the ATSS procedure. Responses coded during an ATSS experiment have reliably distinguished clinically depressed from nondepressed persons (White, Davidson, Haaga, & White, 1992) and high-anxious persons from low-anxious persons (Davidson, Feldman, & Osborn, 1984).

The ATSS procedure has been used as a novel means of assessing perceived self-efficacy. Davison and colleagues (1991) exposed undergraduates to supportive and to stressful situations, and examined their articulated thoughts in response to those situations. Self-efficacy ratings derived from articulated thoughts were associated significantly with self-reports of anxiety and behavioral observations of anxiety. Haaga and colleagues (Haaga, 1989; Haaga, Davidson, McDermut, Hillis, & Twomey, 1993; Haaga & Stewart, 1992) studied self-efficacy among smokers and ex-smokers, in the context of testing postulates of Marlatt and Gordon's (1985) cognitive social-learning model of relapse. They elicited smokers' spontaneously generated cognitions when presented with simulated high-risk situations and their responses to those cognitions; expressions of self-efficacy were drawn from their responses, as were other key constructs derived from relapse prevention theory (e.g., cognitive and behavioral coping, outcome expectancies, attributions for relapse). Analyses revealed that a greater number of positive outcome expectancies of smoking during the simulated situation prospectively predicted increased chances of relapse at 3, but not 12, months (Haaga, 1989). Moderate levels of self-efficacy to recover abstinence following a lapse were associated prospectively with increased chances of abstinence (Haaga & Stewart, 1992).

The reviewed studies coded articulated thoughts for a specific construct by counting the number of responses generated relative to that particular concept. Although this procedure is useful for quantifying the number of times a particular thought occurs, or the degree to which a particular thought dominates an individual's overall articulated thoughts response, this coding procedure does not provide information about the structure of those cognitions. This issue is a problem insofar as knowledge of this structure is important in understanding mechanisms that contribute more generally to an observed behavioral response (see Cacioppo et al., 1997). One method that has been used to infer the underlying structure of cognition from unstructured cognitive responses is the Adjusted Ratio of Clustering (ARC) score (see Cacioppo et al., 1997). If think-aloud data are collected sequentially and reliably coded into content categories, as in the ATSS procedure, the ARC score provides an index of the degree of clustering of the generated cognitive data, thus providing an index of the way the information is stored in memory. In other words, if information about a concept (in this case, self-efficacy) is stored categorically and has some degree of organization in cognitive space, then the spoken-aloud output arising from this organized cognitive structure should be similarly organized. A higher ARC score (i.e., a score that approaches 1.0) reflects a greater degree of organization of the information. Conversely, if information about a concept is stored in a disorganized fashion, then the spoken-aloud output arising from this less organized cognitive structure should be similarly less organized. A lower ARC score (i.e., approaching 0.0) should result.

An alternative index of the degree of structure and organization of cognition may be derived from latency of response during the ATSS probe (Cacioppo et al., 1997). More specifically, information that is stored in an organized fashion should take less time to access, whereas information stored in a less organized fashion should take more time to access. Thus, initial latencies to providing think-aloud responses should index the degree of organization of cognitively stored information. In terms of convergent validity, then, lower latencies to responding should be associated with higher ARC scores.

Think-aloud methods take us back to points we raised at the outset of this chapter. If self-efficacy perceptions were reified and treated as something that people have in a certain amount, "like their weight" (Harré, 1998, p. 130), then think-aloud methods would hardly make sense. Instead, from this alternative perspective, one would exclusively employ traditional measurement procedures designed to estimate an individual's self-efficacy "true score." Treating perceived self-efficacy as a dynamic appraisal process through which people evaluate their capacity to cope with shifting and sometimes unpredictable environments opens the door to novel assessment procedures and, in so doing, helps to shed light on the role of self-referential thinking processes in self-regulation.

REFERENCES

Ahrens, A. H. (1987). Theories of depression: The role of goals and the self-evaluation process. *Cognitive Therapy and Research, 11,* 665–680.

Allaire, J. C., & Marsiske, M. (2002). Well- and ill- defined measures of everyday cognition: Relationship to older adults' intellectual ability and functional status. *Psychology and Aging, 17,* 101–115.

Andersen, S. M., & Chen, S. (2002). The relational self: An interpersonal social-cognitive theory. *Psychological Review, 109,* 619–645.

Anderson, J. R. (1983). *The architecture of cognition.* Cambridge, MA: Harvard University Press.

Artistico, D., Cervone, D., & Pezzuti, L. (2003). Perceived self-efficacy and everyday problem solving among young and older adults. *Psychology and Aging, 18,* 68–79.

Baltes, P. B. (1997). On the incomplete architecture of human ontogeny: Selection, optimization, compensation as foundation of developmental theory. *American Psychologist, 52,* 366–380.

Baltes, P. B., & Baltes, M. M., (1990). *Successful aging: Perspective from the behavioral sciences.* Cambridge, UK: Cambridge University Press.

Baltes, M. M., & Lang, F. R. (1997). Everyday functioning and successful aging: The impact of resources. *Psychology and Aging, 12,* 433–443.

Baltes, P. B., & Staudinger, U. M. (2000). Wisdom: A metaheuristic (pragmatic) to orchestrate mind and virtue toward excellence. *American Psychologist, 55,* 122–136.

Bandura, A. (1977). Self-efficacy: Toward a unifying theory of behavioral change. *Psychological Review, 84,* 191–215.

Bandura, A. (1986). *Social foundations of thought and action.* Englewood Cliffs, NJ: Prentice-Hall.

Bandura, A. (1997). *Self-efficacy: The exercise of control.* New York: Freeman.

Bandura, A. (1999). Social cognitive theory of personality. In D. Cervone & Y. Shoda (Eds.), *The coherence of personality: Social-cognitive bases of consistency, variability, and organization* (pp. 185–241). New York: Guilford Press.

Bandura, A. (2001). Social cognitive theory: An agentic perspective. *Annual Review of Psychology, 52,* 1–26.

Bandura, A., Barbaranelli, C., Caprara, G. V., & Pastorelli, C. (1996). Mechanisms of moral disengagement in the exercise of moral agency. *Journal of Personality and Social Psychology, 71,* 364–374.

Bandura, A., & Cervone, D. (1983). Self-evaluative and self-efficacy mechanisms governing the motivational effects of goal systems. *Journal of Personality and Social Psychology, 45,* 1017–1028.

Bandura, A., Cioffi, D., Taylor, C. B., & Brouillard, M. E. (1988). Perceived self-efficacy in coping with cognitive stressors and opioid activation. *Journal of Personality and Social Psychology, 55,* 479–488.

Bandura, A., Pastorelli, C., Barbaranelli, C., & Caprara, G. V. (1999). Self-efficacy pathways to childhood depression. *Journal of Personality and Social Psychology, 76,* 258–269.

Bandura, A., Taylor, C. B., Williams, S. L., Mefford, I. N., & Barchas, J. D. (1985). Catecholamine secretion as a function of perceived coping self-efficacy. *Journal of Consulting and Clinical Psychology, 53,* 406–414.

Bargh, J. A., & Chartrand, T. L. (1999). The unbearable automaticity of being. *American Psychologist, 54*, 462–479.

Bargh, J. A., & Gollwitzer, P. M. (1994). Environmental control of goal-directed action: Automatic and strategic contingencies between situations and behavior. *Nebraska Symposium on Motivation, 41*, 71–124.

Bargh, J. A., Lee-Chai, A., Barndollar, K., Gollwitzer, P. M., & Trotschel, R. (2001). The automated will: Nonconscious activation and pursuit of behavioral goals. *Journal of Personality and Social Psychology, 81*, 1014–1027.

Baumeister, R. F., & Scher, S. J. (1988). Self-defeating behavior patterns among normal individuals: Review and analysis of common self-destructive tendencies. *Psychological Bulletin, 104*, 3–22.

Bell, B. S., & Kozlowski, S. W. J. (2002). Goal orientation and ability: Interactive effects on self-efficacy, performance, and knowledge. *Journal of Applied Psychology, 87*, 497–505.

Berry, J. M., & West, R. L. (1993). Cognitive self-efficacy in relation to personal mastery and goal setting across the life span. *International Journal of Behavioral Development, 16*, 351–379.

Berry, J. M., West, R. L., & Dennehey, D. M. (1989). Reliability and validity of the memory self-efficacy questionnaire. *Developmental Psychology, 25*, 701–713.

Betz, N. E. (2001). Career self-efficacy. In F. Leong & A. Barak (Eds.), *Contemporary models in vocational psychology: A volume in honor of Samuel H. Osipow* (pp. 55–77). Mahwah, NJ: Erlbaum.

Betz, N. E., & Hackett, G. (1981). The relationship of career-related self-efficacy expectations to perceived career options in college women and men. *Journal of Counseling Psychology, 23*, 399–410.

Blackburn, I., & Eunson, K. (1989). A content analysis of thoughts and emotions elicited from depressed patients during cognitive therapy. *British Journal of Medical Psychology, 62*, 23–33.

Brandtstadter, J., & Renner, G. (1990). Tenacious goal pursuit and flexible goal adjustment: Explication and age-related analysis of assimilative and accommodative strategies of coping. *Psychology and Aging, 5*, 58–67.

Button, S. B., Mathieu, J. E., & Zajac, D. M. (1996). Goal orientation in organizational research: A conceptual and empirical foundation. *Organizational Behavior and Human Decision Processes, 67*, 26–48.

Bystritsky, A., Linn, L., & Ware, J. (1990). Development of a multidimensional scale of anxiety. *Journal of Anxiety Disorders, 4*, 99–115.

Cacioppo, J., von Hippel, W., & Ernst, J. (1997). Mapping cognitive structures and processes through verbal content: The thought-listing technique. *Journal of Consulting and Clinical Psychology, 65*, 928–940.

Caprara, G. V., & Cervone, D. (2000). *Personality: Determinants, dynamics, and potentials.* New York: Cambridge University Press.

Caprara, G. V., Scabini, E., Barbaranelli, C., Pastorelli, C., Regalia, C., & Bandura, A. (1998). Impact of adolescents' perceived self-regulatory efficacy on familial communication and antisocial conduct. *European Psychologist, 3*, 125–132.

Carver, C. S., & Scheier, M. F. (1998). *On the self-regulation of behavior.* New York: Cambridge University Press.

Cervone, D. (1985). Randomization tests to determine significance levels for microanalytic congruences between self-efficacy and behavior. *Cognitive Therapy and Research, 9*, 357–365.

Cervone, D. (1989). Effects of envisioning future activities on self-efficacy judgments and motivation: An availability heuristic interpretation. *Cognitive Therapy and Research, 13*, 247–261.

Cervone, D. (1993). The role of self-referent cognitions in goal setting, motivation, and performance. In M. Rabinowitz (Ed.), *Cognitive science foundations of instruction* (pp. 57–96). Hillsdale, NJ: Erlbaum.

Cervone, D. (1997). Social-cognitive mechanisms and personality coherence: Self-knowledge, situational beliefs, and cross-situational coherence in perceived self-efficacy. *Psychological Science, 8*, 43–50.

Cervone, D. (1999). Bottom-up explanation in personality psychology: The case of cross-situational coherence. In D. Cervone & Y. Shoda (Eds.), *The coherence of personality: Social-cognitive bases of consistency, variability, and organization* (pp. 303–341). New York: Guilford Press.

Cervone, D. (in press). The architecture of personality. *Psychological Review, 111.*

Cervone, D., Jiwani, N., & Wood, R. (1991). Goal-setting and the differential influence of self-regulatory processes on complex decision-making performance. *Journal of Personality and Social Psychology, 61,* 257–266.

Cervone, D., Kopp, D. A., Schaumann, L., & Scott, W. D. (1994). Mood, self-efficacy, and performance standards: Lower moods induce higher standards for performance. *Journal of Personality and Social Psychology, 67,* 499–512.

Cervone, D., & Peake, P. K. (1986). Anchoring, efficacy, and action: The influence of judgmental heuristics on self-efficacy judgments and behavior. *Journal of Personality and Social Psychology, 50,* 492–501.

Cervone, D., Shadel, W. G., & Jencius, S. (2001). Social-cognitive theory of personality assessment. *Personality and Social Psychology Review, 5,* 33–51.

Cervone, D., & Wood, R. (1995). Goals, feedback, and the differential influence of self-regulatory processes on cognitively complex performance. *Cognitive Therapy and Research, 19,* 521–547.

Csikszentmihalyi, M. (1990). *Flow: The psychology of optimal experience.* New York: Harper & Row.

Cutrona, C. E., & Troutman, B. R. (1986). Social support, infant temperament, and parenting self-efficacy: A mediational model of postpartum depression. *Child Development, 57,* 1507–1518.

Davidson, G., Feldman, P., & Osborn, C. (1984). Articulated thoughts, irrational beliefs, and fear of negative evaluation. *Cognitive Therapy and Research, 8,* 349–362.

Davidson, G., Robins, C., & Johnson, M. (1983). Articulated Thoughts in Simulated Situations: A paradigm for studying cognition in emotion and behavior. *Cognitive Therapy and Research, 7,* 17–40.

Davidson, G., Vogel, R., & Coffman, S. (1997). Think-aloud approaches to cognitive assessment and the articulated thoughts in simulated situations paradigm. *Journal of Consulting and Clinical Psychology, 65,* 950–958.

Deci, E. L. (1992). On the nature and functions of motivation theories. *Psychological Science, 3,* 167–171.

Deci, E. L., & Ryan, R. M. (1991). A motivational approach to self: Integration in personality. In R. Dienstbier (Ed.), *Nebraska Symposium on Motivation: Vol. 38. Perspectives on motivation* (pp. 237–288). Lincoln: University of Nebraska Press.

DiClemente, C. C., Fairhurst, S. J., & Piotrowski, N. A. (1995). Self-efficacy and addictive behaviors. In J. E. Maddux (Ed.), *Self-efficacy, adaptation, and adjustment: Theory, research, and application* (pp. 109–142). New York: Plenum Press.

Dilorio, C., Maibach, E., O'Leary, A., & Sanderson, C. A. (1997). Measurement of condom use self-efficacy and outcome expectancies in a geographically diverse group of STD patients. *AIDS Education and Prevention, 9,* 1–13.

Dweck, C., & Leggett, E. (1988). A social-cognitive approach to motivation and personality. *Psychological Review, 95,* 256–273.

Elliott, A. J., & Sheldon, K. M. (1997). Avoidance achievement motivation: A personal goals analysis. *Journal of Personality and Social Psychology, 73,* 171–185.

Elliott, A. J., & Dweck, C. S. (1988). Goals: An approach to motivation and achievement. *Journal of Personality and Social Psychology, 54,* 5–12.

Emmons, R. A. (1989). The personal striving approach to personality. In L. A. Pervin (Ed.), *Goal constructs in personality and social psychology* (pp. 87–126). Hillsdale, NJ: Erlbaum.

Emmons, R. A. (1999). *The psychology of ultimate concerns: Motivation and spirituality in personality.* New York: Guilford Press.

Emmons, R. A., & Kaiser, H. A. (1996). Goal orientation and emotional well-being: Linking goals and affect through the self. In L. L. Martin & A. Tesser (Eds.), *Striving and feeling: Interactions among goals, affect, and self-regulation* (pp. 79–98). Mahwah, NJ: Erlbaum.

Ericsson, H., & Simon, H. (1993). *Protocol analysis: Verbal reports as data*. Cambridge, MA: MIT Press.

Freund, A. M., & Baltes, P. B. (2002). Life-management strategies of selection, optimization, and compensation: Measurement by self-report and construct validity. *Journal of Personality and Social Psychology, 82*, 642–662.

Garland, H. (1985). A cognitive mediation theory of task goals and human performance. *Motivation and Emotion, 9*, 345–367.

Glynn, S. M., & Ruderman, A. J. (1986). The development and validation of an eating self-efficacy scale. *Cognitive Therapy and Research, 10*, 403–420.

Gollwitzer, P. M. (1996). The volitional benefits of planning. In P. M. Gollwitzer & J. A. Bargh (Eds.), *The psychology of action: Linking cognition and motivation to behavior* (pp. 287–312). New York: Guilford Press.

Goodrick, G. K., Pendleton, V. R., Kimball, K. T., Poston, W. S. C., Reeves, R. S., & Foreyt, J. P. (1999). Binge eating severity, self-concept, dieting, self-efficacy and social support during treatment of binge eating disorder. *International Journal of Eating Disorders, 26*, 295–300.

Grant, H., & Dweck, C. S. (1999). A goal analysis of personality and personality coherence. In D. Cervone & Y. Shoda (Eds.), *The coherence of personality: Social-cognitive bases of consistency, variability, and organization* (pp. 345–371). New York: Guilford Press.

Green, J. D., & Sedikides, C. (2001). When do self-schemas shape social perception?: The role of descriptive ambiguity. *Motivation and Emotion, 25*, 67–83.

Haaga, D. A. F. (1989). Articulated thoughts and endorsement procedures for cognitive assessment in the prediction of smoking relapse. *Psychological Assessment, 1*, 112–117.

Haaga, D. A. F., Davidson, G., McDermut, W., Hillis, S., & Twomey, H. (1993). "State of mind" analysis of the articulated thoughts of ex-smokers. *Cognitive Therapy and Research, 17*, 427–439.

Haaga, D. A. F., & Stewart, B. L. (1992). Self-efficacy for recovery from a lapse after smoking cessation. *Journal of Consulting and Clinical Psychology, 60*, 24–28.

Hackett, G., & Betz, N. E. (1995). Self-efficacy and career choice. In J. Maddux (Ed.), *Self-efficacy, adaptation, and adjustment: Theory, research, and application* (pp. 249–280). New York: Plenum Press.

Harré, R. (1984). *Personal being: A theory for individual psychology*. Cambridge, MA: Harvard University Press.

Harré, R. (1998). *The singular self: An introduction to the psychology of personhood*. London: Sage.

Higgins, E. T. (1987). Self-discrepancy: A theory relating self and affect. *Psychological Review, 94*, 319–340.

Higgins, E. T. (1996). Knowledge activation: Accessibility, applicability, and salience. In E. T. Higgins & A. W. Kruglanski (Eds.), *Social psychology: Handbook of basic principles* (pp. 133–168). New York: Guilford Press.

Higgins, E. T. (1997). Beyond pleasure and pain. *American Psychologist, 52*, 1280–1300.

Higgins, E. T. (1999). Persons and situations: Unique explanatory principles or variability in general principles? In D. Cervone & Y. Shoda (Eds.), *The coherence of personality: Social-cognitive bases of consistency, variability, and organization* (pp. 61–93). New York: Guilford Press.

Higgins, E. T., & King, G. A. (1981). Accessibility of social constructs: Information-processing consequences of individual and contextual variability. In N. Cantor & J. Kihlstrom (Eds.), *Personality, cognition, and social interaction* (pp. 69–121). Hillsdale, NJ: Erlbaum.

Higgins, E. T., King, G. A., & Mavin, G. H. (1982). Individual construct accessibility and subjective impressions and recall. *Journal of Personality and Social Psychology, 43*, 35–47.

Higgins, E. T., & Kruglanski, A. W. (Eds.). (1996). *Social psychology: Handbook of basic principles*. New York: Guilford Press.

Hill, G. J. (1989). An unwillingness to act: Behavioral appropriateness, situational constraint, and self-efficacy in shyness. *Journal of Personality, 57,* 871–890.

Janoff-Bulman, R., & Brickman, P. (1982). Expectations and what people learn from failure. In N. T. Feather (Ed.), *Expectations and action: Expectancy-value models in psychology* (pp. 207–272). Hillsdale, NJ: Erlbaum.

Klein, S. B., & Loftus, J. (1993). The mental representation of trait and autobiographical knowledge about the self. In T. K. Srull & R. S. Wyer (Eds.), *Advances in social cognition* (Vol. 5, pp. 1–49). Hillsdale, NJ: Erlbaum.

Kruglanski, A. W., Shah, J. Y., Fishbach, A., Friedman, R., Chun, W. Y., & Sleeth-Keppler, D. (2002). A theory of goal-systems. In M. Zanna (Ed.), *Advances in experimental social psychology* (pp. 331–378). San Diego, CA: Academic Press.

Lachman, M. E., &, Jelalian, E. (1984). Self-efficacy and attributions for intellectual performance in young and elderly adults. *Journal of Gerontology, 39,* 577–82.

Lazarus, R. S. (1991). *Emotion and adaptation.* New York: Oxford University Press.

Lazarus, R. S., & Smith, C. A. (1988). Knowledge and appraisal in the cognition–emotion relationship. *Cognition and Emotion, 2,* 281–300.

Lewin, K., Dembo, T., Festinger, L., & Sears, P. S. (1944). Level of aspiration. In J. M. Hunt (Ed.), *Personality and the behavior disorders* (Vol. 1, pp. 333–378). New York: Ronald Press.

Locke, E. A., & Latham, G. P. (1990). *A theory of goal setting and task performance.* Englewood Cliffs, NJ: Prentice-Hall.

Manderlink, G., & Harackiewicz, J. M. (1984). Proximal versus distal goal setting and intrinsic motivation. *Journal of Personality and Social Psychology, 47,* 918–928.

Markus, H. (1977). Self-schemata and processing information about the self. *Journal of Personality and Social Psychology, 35,* 63–78.

Markus, H., Crane, M., Bernstein, S., & Siladi, M. (1982). Self-schemas and gender. *Journal of Personality and Social Psychology, 42,* 38–50.

Marlatt, G. A., & Gordon, J. (1985). *Relapse prevention: Maintenance strategies in the treatment of addictive behaviors.* New York: Guilford Press.

Mischel, W. (1968). *Personality and assessment.* New York: Wiley.

Mischel, W., & Shoda, Y. (1995). A cognitive-affective system theory of personality: Reconceptualizing situations, dispositions, dynamics, and invariance in personality structure. *Psychological Review, 102,* 246–286.

Molina, S., Borkovec, T., Peasley, C., & Person, D. (1998). Content analysis of worrisome streams of consciousness in anxious and dysphoric participants. *Cognitive Therapy and Research, 22,* 109–123.

Montoya, I. D. (1998). Social network ties, self-efficacy and condom use among women who use crack cocaine: A pilot study. *Substance Use and Misuse, 33,* 2049–2073.

Mor, N., & Cervone, D. (2002, January). *Approach and avoidance goals and subgoal mediation of the relationship between goal orientation and negative affect.* Poster presented at the annual meeting of the Society for Personality and Social Psychology, Savannah, GA.

Oettingen, G. (1996). Positive fantasy and motivation. In P. M. Gollwitzer & J. A. Bargh (Eds.), *The psychology of action: Linking cognition and motivation to behavior* (pp. 236–259). New York: Guilford Press.

Oettingen, G., Pak, H., & Schnetter, K. (2001). Self-regulation of goal-setting: Turning free fantasies about the future into binding goals. *Journal of Personality and Social Psychology, 80,* 736–753.

Orom, H., & Cervone, D. (2002, July). *The role of self-concept in self-efficacy judgments.* Poster presented at the 11th European Conference on Personality, Jena, Germany.

Ozer, E. M., & Bandura, A. (1990). Mechanisms governing empowerment effects: A self-efficacy analysis. *Journal of Personality and Social Psychology, 58,* 472–486.

Peake, P. K., & Cervone, D. (1989). Sequence anchoring and self-efficacy: Primacy effects in the consideration of possibilities. *Social Cognition, 7,* 31–50.

Pervin, L. A., Cervone, D., & John, O. P. (2004). *Personality: Theory and research* (9th ed.). New York: Wiley.

Ryan, R. M., & Deci, E. L. (2000). Self-determination theory and the facilitation of intrinsic motivation, social development, and well-being. *American Psychologist, 55,* 68–78.

Saks, A. M. (1995). Longitudinal field investigation of the moderating and mediating effects of self-efficacy on the relationship between training and newcomer adjustment. *Journal of Applied Psychology, 80,* 639–654.

Sanderson, C. A., & Cantor, N. (1995). Social dating goals in late adolescence: Implications for safer sexual activity. *Journal of Personality and Social Psychology, 68,* 1121–1134.

Sarason, I. G., Pierce, G. R., & Sarason, B. R. (1996). *Cognitive interference: Theories, methods, and findings* Mahwah, NJ: Erlbaum.

Schwarz, N., & Clore, G. L. (1983). Mood, misattribution, and judgments of well-being: Informative and directive functions of affective states. *Journal of Personality and Social Psychology, 45,* 513–523.

Schwarz, N., & Clore, G. L. (1988). How do I feel about it? Informative functions of affective states. In K. Fiedler & J. Forgas (Eds.), *Affect, cognition, and social behavior* (pp. 44–62). Toronto: Hogrefe International.

Schwarzer, R., Babler, J., Kwiatek, P., & Shrooder, K. (1997). The assessment of optimistic self-beliefs: Comparison of the German, Spanish, and Chinese versions of the General Self-Efficacy Scale. *Applied Psychology: An International Review, 46,* 69–88.

Scott, W. D., & Cervone, D. (2002). The impact of negative affect on performance standards: Evidence for an affect-as-information mechanism. *Cognitive Therapy and Research, 26,* 19–37.

Searle, J. R. (1998). *Mind, language, and society: Philosophy in the real world.* New York: Basic Books.

Sene'cal, C., Nouwen, A., & White, D. (2000). Motivation and dietary self-care in adults with diabetes: Are self-efficacy and autonomous self-regulation complementary or competing constructs? *Health Psychology, 19,* 452–457.

Shah, J. Y., & Higgins, E. T. (1997). Expectancy x value effects: Regulatory focus as a determinant of magnitude and direction. *Journal of Personality and Social Psychology, 73,* 447–458.

Shah, J. Y., & Kruglanski, A. W. (2000). Aspects of goal networks: Implication for self-regulation. In M. Boekaerts, P. R., Pintrich & M. Zeidner (Eds.), *Handbook of self-regulation* (pp. 85–110). San Diego, CA: Academic Press.

Sheldon, K. M., Ryan, R. M., Rawsthorne, L., & Ilardi, B. (1997). Trait self and true self: Cross-role variation in the Big Five traits and its relations with authenticity and subjective well-being. *Journal of Personality and Social Psychology, 73,* 1380–1393.

Sherer, M., Maddux, J. E., Mercandante, B., Prentice-Dunn, S., Jacobs, B., & Rogers, R. W. (1982). The Self-Efficacy Scale: Construction and validation. *Psychological Reports, 51,* 663–671.

Skinner, E. A. (1996). A guide to constructs of control. *Journal of Personality and Social Psychology, 71,* 549–570.

Smith, C. A., & Lazarus, R. S. (1990). Emotion and adaptation. In L. A. Pervin (Ed.), *Handbook of personality: Theory and research* (pp. 609–637). New York: Guilford Press.

Smith, R. E. (1989). Effects of coping skills training on generalized self-efficacy and locus of control. *Journal of Personality and Social Psychology, 56,* 228–233.

Stajkovic, A. D., & Luthans, F. (1998). Self-efficacy and work-related performance: A meta-analysis. *Psychological Bulletin, 124,* 240–261.

Stern, W. (1935). *Allgemeine Psychologie auf personalisticher grundlage.* Dordrecht, The Netherlands: Nijoff.

Stock, J., & Cervone, D. (1990). Proximal goal-setting and self-regulatory processes. *Cognitive Therapy and Research, 14,* 483–498.

Tillema, J., Cervone, D., & Scott, W. D. (2001). Dysphoric mood, perceived self-efficacy, and personal standards for performance: The effects of attributional cues on self-defeating patterns of cognition. *Cognitive Therapy and Research, 25,* 535–549.

Weitlauf, J., Cervone, D., Smith, R. E., & Wright, P. M. (2001). Assessing generalization in perceived self-efficacy: Multidomain and global assessments of the effects of self-defense training for women. *Personality and Social Psychology Bulletin, 27,* 1683–1691.

Weitlauf, J., Smith, R. E., & Cervone, D. (2000). Generalization of coping skills training: Influence of self-defense instruction on women's efficacy beliefs, assertiveness, and aggression, task-specific and generalized self-efficacy, aggressiveness, and personality. *Journal of Applied Psychology, 85,* 625–633.

White, J., Davidson, G. C., Haaga, D. A., & White, K. (1992). Cognitive bias in the articulated thoughts of depressed and noindepressed psychiatric patients. *Journal of Nervous and Mental Diseases, 180,* 77–81.

Williams, G. C., Gagné, M., Ryan, R. M., & Deci, E. L. (2002). Facilitating autonomous motivation for smoking cessation. *Health Psychology, 21,* 40–50.

Williams, S. L., & Cervone, D. (1998). Social cognitive theories of personality. In D. F. Barone, M. Hersen, & V. B. Van Hasselt (Eds.), *Advanced personality* (pp. 173–207). New York: Kluwer.

Willis, S. L. (1999). Everyday problem solving. In J. E. Birren & K. W. Schaie (Eds.), *Handbook of the psychology of aging* (4th ed., pp. 287–307). San Diego, CA: Academic Press.

Willot, J. F. (1999). *Neurogerontology: Aging and the nervous system.* New York: Springer.

11

Planning and the Implementation of Goals

PETER M. GOLLWITZER
KENTARO FUJITA
GABRIELE OETTINGEN

Determining the factors that promote successful goal pursuit is one of the fundamental questions studied by self-regulation and motivation researchers (Gollwitzer & Moskowitz, 1996; Oettingen & Gollwitzer, 2001). A number of theories, and supporting empirical data, suggest that the type of goal chosen and the commitment to that goal are important determinants in whether an individual carries out the behaviors necessary for goal attainment (e.g., Ajzen, 1985; Atkinson, 1957; Carver, Chapter 2, this volume; Carver & Scheier, 1998). Within these models, choosing or accepting a goal or standard is the central act of willing in the pursuit of goals. We agree with this contention but will argue in this chapter that further acts of willing should facilitate goal implementation, in particular, when goal pursuit is confronted with implemental problems (e.g., difficulties with getting started because of a lack of good opportunities; sticking to an ongoing goal pursuit in the face of distractions, temptations, and competing goal pursuits). Such acts of willing can take the form of making plans that specify when, where, and how an instrumental goal-directed response is to be implemented. More specifically, the person may take control over goal implementation by making if–then plans (i.e., from implementation intentions) that specify an anticipated critical situation and link it to an instrumental goal-directed response.

IMPLEMENTATION INTENTIONS: STRATEGIC AUTOMATICITY IN GOAL PURSUIT

Gollwitzer (1993, 1996, 1999) has proposed a distinction between goal intentions and implementation intentions. Goal intentions (goals) have the structure of "I intend to reach Z!" whereby Z may relate to a certain outcome or behavior to which the individual feels committed. Implementation intentions (plans) have the structure of "If situation X is encountered, then I will perform the goal-directed response Y!" Holding an implementation intention commits an individual to perform the specified goal-directed response once the critical situation is encountered. Both goal and implementation intentions are set in an act of willing: The former specifies the intention to meet a goal or standard; the latter refers to the intention to perform a plan. Commonly, implementation intentions are formed in the service of goal intentions, because they specify the where, when, and how of respective goal-directed responses. For instance, a possible implementation intention in the service of the goal intention to eat healthy food could link a suitable situational context (e.g., one's order is taken at a restaurant) to an appropriate behavior (e.g., asking for a low-fat meal). As a consequence, a strong mental link is established between the critical cue of the waiter taking the order and the goal-directed response of asking for a low-fat meal.

Why Implementation Intentions Are Expected to Facilitate Goal Implementation

The mental links created by implementation intentions are expected to facilitate goal attainment on the basis of psychological processes that relate to both the anticipated situation and the specified response. Because forming implementation intentions implies the selection of a critical future situation, it is assumed that the mental representation of the situation becomes highly activated and, hence, more accessible. This in turn should make it easier to detect the critical situation and readily attend to it, even when one is busy with other things. This heightened accessibility should also facilitate the recall of the critical situation. Moreover, because forming implementation intentions involves first a selection of an effective goal-directed behavior that is then linked to the selected critical situation, initiation of the intended response should become automated. Initiation should become swift and efficient, and should no longer require conscious intention once the critical situation is encountered.

Implementation Intentions: The Specified Situation

Several studies have provided support for the accessibility hypothesis by measuring how well participants' holding implementation intentions attended to, detected, and recalled the critical situation compared to participants who had only formed goal intentions (Gollwitzer, Bayer, Steller, & Bargh, 2002). One study, using a dichotic-listening paradigm, demonstrated that words describing the anticipated critical situation were highly disruptive to focused attention in implementation-intention participants compared to goal-intention participants (i.e., the shadowing performance of the attended materials decreased). In another study, using an embedded figures test (Gottschaldt, 1926), in which smaller a-figures are hidden within larger b-figures, enhanced detection of the hidden a-figures was observed with participants who had specified the a-figure in the if part of an implementation intention (i.e., had made plans on how to create a traffic sign from the a-figure). In a cued recall experiment, participants more effectively recalled the available situational opportunities to attain a set goal given that these opportunities had been specified in if–then links (i.e., in implementation intentions). Finally, Aarts, Dijksterhuis, and Midden (1999), using a lexical decision task, found that the formation of implementation intentions led to faster lexical decision times for those words that described the critical situation. Furthermore, the heightened accessibility of the critical situation (as measured by faster lexical decision responses) mediated the beneficial effects of implementation intentions on goal attainment. The latter result implies that the goal-promoting effects of implementation intentions are based on the heightened accessibility of selected critical situational cues.

Implementation Intentions: The Specified Goal-Directed Behavior

The postulated automation of action initiation (also described as strategic delegation of control to situational cues; Gollwitzer, 1993, p. 173) has been supported by the results of various experiments that tested immediacy, efficiency, and the presence–absence of conscious intent. Gollwitzer and Brandstätter (1997, Study 3) demonstrated the immediacy of action initiation in a study in which participants had been induced to form implementation intentions that specified viable opportunities for presenting counterarguments to a series of racist remarks made by a confederate. Participants with implementation intentions initiated counterarguments sooner than the participants who had formed the mere goal intention to counterargue.

The efficiency of action initiation was further explored in two experiments using a go/no-go task embedded as a secondary task in a dual-task paradigm (Brandtstätter, Lengfelder, & Gollwitzer, 2001, Studies 3 and 4). Participants formed the goal intention to press a button as fast as possible, if numbers appeared on the computer screen, but not if letters were presented. Participants in the implementation-intention condition additionally made the plan to press the response button particularly fast if the number three was presented. Implementation-intention participants showed a substantial increase in speed of responding to the number three compared to the control group, regardless of whether the simultaneously demanded primary task (a memorization task in Study 3 and a tracking task in Study 4) was either easy or difficult to perform. Apparently, the immediacy of responding induced by implementation intentions is also efficient in the sense that it does not require much in the way of cognitive resources (i.e., can be performed even when demanding dual tasks have to be performed at the same time).

Two experiments by Bayer, Moskowitz, and Gollwitzer (2002) tested whether implementation intentions lead to action initiation even in the absence of conscious intent. In these experiments, the critical situation was presented subliminally, and immediacy of initiation of the goal-directed response was assessed. Results indicated that subliminal presentation of the critical situation led to a speed-up in responding in implementation-intention but not in goal-intention participants. These effects suggest that when planned via implementation intentions, the initiation of goal-directed behavior becomes triggered by the presence of the critical situational cue, without the need for further conscious intent.

Additional process mechanisms to the stimulus perception and response initiation processes documented in the findings described earlier have been explored. For instance, furnishing goals with implementation intentions might produce an increase in goal commitment, which in turn cause heightened goal attainment. However, this hypothesis has not received any empirical support. For instance, when Brandstätter and colleagues (2001, Study 1) analyzed whether heroin addicts suffering from withdrawal benefit from forming implementation intentions to submit a newly composed curriculum vitae before the end of the day, they also measured participants' commitment to do so. Whereas the majority of the implementation-intention participants succeeded in handing in the curriculum vitae in time, none of the goal-intention participants succeeded in this task. These two groups, however, did not differ in terms of their goal commitment ("I feel committed to compose a curriculum vitae," and "I have to complete this task"), measured after the goal- and implementation-intention instructions had been administered. This finding was replicated with young adults who participated in a professional development workshop (Oettingen, Hönig, & Gollwitzer, 2000, Study 2), and analogous results were reported in research on the effects of implementation intentions on meeting health-promotion and disease-prevention goals (e.g., Orbell, Hodgkins, & Sheeran, 1997).

Implementation Intentions and Their Effects on Wanted Behavior

Given that implementation intentions facilitate attending to, detecting, and recalling viable opportunities to act toward goal attainment and, in addition, automate action initiation in the presence of such opportunities, people who form implementation intentions should show higher goal-attainment rates compared to people who do not furnish their goal intentions with implementation intentions. This hypothesis is supported by the results of a host of studies examining the attainment of various types of goal intentions (a recent meta-analysis by Gollwitzer & Sheeran, 2003, lists more than 80 studies demonstrating implementation-intention effects).

Types of Goals

Gollwitzer and Brandstätter (1997) analyzed the attainment of a goal intention that had to be acted on at an inconvenient time (e.g., writing a report about Christmas Eve during the subsequent Christmas holiday). Other studies have examined the effects of implementation intentions on goal-attainment rates with goal intentions that are somewhat unpleasant to perform. for instance, the goal intentions to perform health-protecting and -enhancing behaviors, such as regular breast examinations (Orbell et al., 1997), cervical cancer screening (Sheeran & Orbell, 2000), resumption of functional activity after joint replacement surgery (Orbell & Sheeran, 2000), and engaging in physical exercise (Milne, Orbell, & Sheeran, 2002), were all more frequently acted on when people had furnished these goals with implementation intentions. Moreover, implementation intentions were found to facilitate the attainment of goal intentions when it is easy to forget to act on them (e.g., regular intake of vitamin pills, Sheeran & Orbell, 1999; the signing of work sheets with the elderly, Chasteen, Park, & Schwarz, 2001).

Potential Moderators

The strength of the beneficial effects of implementation intentions depends on the presence or absence of several moderators. First, implementation-intention effects are more apparent the more difficult it is to initiate the goal-directed behavior. For instance, implementation intentions were more effective in completing difficult compared to easy goals (Gollwitzer & Brandstätter, 1997, Study 1). Moreover, forming implementation intentions was more beneficial to patients with frontal lobe damage, who typically have problems with executive control, than to college students (Lengfelder & Gollwitzer, 2001, Study 2).

Second, implementation intentions do not work when the respective goal intention is weak. Orbell and colleagues (1997) reported that the beneficial effects of implementation intentions on compliance in performing a breast examination were observed only in those women who strongly intended to perform breast self-examination (i.e., possessed a strong goal commitment). Similarly, results of another study (Gollwitzer, Bayer, et al., 2002, Study 3) suggest that the beneficial effects of implementation intentions on a person's recall of specified situations can no longer be observed when the respective goal intention has been abandoned (i.e., the research participants were told that the assigned goal intention need no longer be reached, because it had been performed by some other person).

Third, implementation-intention effects require the activation of the respective superordinate goal intention (Bayer, Jaudas, & Gollwitzer, 2002; Sheeran, Webb, & Gollwitzer, 2002). One study (Bayer, Jaudas, et al., 2002), which used a task-switch paradigm, manipulated whether the assigned task goal was related or unrelated to the stimulus specified in the if part of the implementation intention. Implementation-intention effects were only observed when the task goal pertained to the formed implementation intention.

Fourth, the strength of the implementation intention also matters. In one study, Gollwitzer, Bayer, and colleagues (2002, Study 3) varied the strength of the commitment to the implementation intention by telling the participants (after an extensive personality testing session) that they were the kind of people who would benefit from either strictly adhering to their plans (i.e., high commitment) or staying flexible (i.e., low commitment). The latter group showed weaker implementation-intention effects (i.e., cued recall performance for selected opportunities) than the former.

Finally, the strength of the mental link between the if and the then parts of an implementation intention should also affect how beneficial the formed implementation intentions turn out to be. For example, if a person takes much time and concentration encoding the if–then plan, or keeps repeating a formed if–then plan by using inner speech, stronger mental links should emerge, which in turn should produce stronger implementation-intention effects.

Implementation Intentions and the Control of the Unwanted Influences on an Ongoing Goal Pursuit

Research on implementation intentions has mostly focused on the self-regulatory issue of getting started with goals that one wants to achieve. However, once initiated, a goal pursuit still needs to be brought to a successful ending. People need to protect an ongoing goal from being thwarted by their attention to attractive distractions or their falling prey to conflicting bad habits (e.g., the goal of being fair may conflict with the habit of stereotyping and prejudging certain groups of people). Two major strategies in which implementation intentions can be used to control the "unwanted," potentially hampering the successful pursuit of wanted goals, include (1) directing one's implementation intentions toward the suppression of anticipated unwanted responses, and (2) blocking all kinds of (even nonanticipated) unwanted influences from inside or outside by directing one's implementation intentions toward spelling out the wanted ongoing goal pursuit.

Responding to Critical Situations with the Suppression of Anticipated Unwanted Responses

If, for instance, people want to avoid being unfriendly to a friend who is known to make outrageous requests, they can protect themselves from showing the unwanted unfriendly response by forming suppression-oriented implementation intentions, which can take different formats. A person might focus on reducing the intensity of the unwanted response by intending not to show the unwanted response: "And if my friend approaches me with an outrageous request, then I will not respond in an unfriendly manner!" But he or she may also try to reduce the intensity of the unwanted response by specifying the initiation of the respective antagonistic response: "And if my friend approaches me with an outrageous request, then I will respond in a friendly manner!" Finally, suppression-oriented implementation intentions may focus a person away from the critical situation: "And if my friend approaches me with an outrageous request, then I'll ignore it!"

Two lines of experiments analyzed the effects of suppression-oriented implementation intentions. The first looked at the control of unwanted spontaneous attending to tempting distractions (Gollwitzer & Schaal, 1998). Participants had to perform a boring task (i.e., perform a series of simple arithmetic tasks), while being bombarded with attractive, distractive stimuli (e.g., video clips of award-winning commercials). Whereas control participants were asked to form a mere goal intention ("I will not let myself get distracted!"), experimental participants, in addition, formed one of two implementation intentions: "And if a distraction arises, then I'll ignore it!" or "And if a distraction arises, then I will increase my effort at the task at hand!" The ignore-implementation intention always helped participants to ward off the distractions (as assessed by their task performance), regardless of whether the motivation to perform the tedious task (assessed at the beginning of the task) was low or high. The increase-effort implementation intention, in contrast, was effective only when motivation to perform the tedious task was low. Apparently, when motivation is high to begin with, increase-effort implementation intentions may create overmotivation that hampers task performance. It seems appropriate, therefore, to advise motivated individuals who suffer from being distracted (e.g., ambitious students doing their homework) to resort to ignore-implementation intentions rather than to implementation intentions that focus on strengthening effort.

The second line of experiments analyzing suppression-oriented implementation intentions studied the control of the automatic activation of stereotypical beliefs and prejudicial evaluations (Gollwitzer, Achtziger, Schaal, & Hammelbeck, 2002; Gollwitzer & Schaal, 1998). In various priming studies that used short stimulus-onset asynchronies of less than 300 msec between primes (presentations of members of stigmatized groups) and targets (adjectives describing relevant stereotypical attributes or neutral positive–negative adjectives), research participants using implementation intentions inhibited the automatic activation of stereotypical beliefs and prejudicial evaluations about women, the elderly, the homeless, and soccer fans. The implementation intentions specified that they be confronted with a member of the critical group in the if part, with a "Then I won't stereotype" (or "Then I won't evaluate negatively") response, or a "Then I will ignore the group membership" response in the then part. Regardless of which format was used, both types of suppression-oriented implementation intentions were effective.

Blocking Detrimental Self-States and Adverse Situational Influences

In the research presented in the previous paragraph, implementation intentions specified a critical situation or problem in the if part, which was linked to a then part that described an attempt at suppressing the unwanted response. This type of self-regulation by implementation intentions implies that the person needs to anticipate both potential hindrances to achieving the goal and what kinds of unwanted responses these hindrances elicit. However, implementation intentions can also be used to protect oneself against the "unwanted" by taking a different approach. Instead of gearing one's implementation intentions toward anticipated potential hindrances and the unwanted responses triggered therewith, the person may form implementation intentions geared at stabilizing the goal pursuit at hand. We use, again, the example of a tired person who is approached by a friend with an outrageous request and will likely respond in an unfriendly manner: If this person has in advance stipulated in an implementation intention what he or she will converse about with the friend, the critical interaction should simply run off as planned, and the self-state of being tired should fail to affect the person's response to outrageous requests in a negative, unwanted direction. As is evident from this example, the present self-regulatory strategy should be of special value whenever the influence of detrimental self-states (e.g., being tired and irritated) on derailing one's goal-directed behavior has to be controlled. This should be true regardless of whether such self-states and/or their influence on behavior reside in the person's consciousness.

Gollwitzer and Bayer (2000) tested this hypothesis in a series of experiments in which participants were asked to make plans (i.e., form implementation intentions) or not regarding their performance on an assigned task. Prior to beginning the task, participants' self-states were manipulated, so that the task at hand became more difficult (e.g., a state of self-definitional incompleteness prior to a task that required perspective taking; Gollwitzer & Wicklund, 1985; a good mood prior to a task that required evaluation of others nonstereotypically; Bless & Fiedler, 1995; and a state of ego depletion prior to solving difficult anagrams; Baumeister, 2000; Muraven, Tice, & Baumeister, 1998). The results suggested that the induced critical self-states negatively affected task performance only for those participants who had not planned out work on the task at hand via implementation intentions (i.e., had only set themselves the goal to come up with a great performance). In other words, implementation intentions that spelled out how to perform the task at hand were effective in protecting the individual from the negative effects associated with the induced detrimental self-states.

This research provides a new perspective on the psychology of self-regulation. Commonly, effective self-regulation is understood in terms of strengthening the self, so that the self can meet the challenge of being a powerful executive agent (Baumeister, Heatherton, & Tice, 1994). Therefore, most research on goal-directed self-regulation focuses on strengthening the self in such a way that threats and irritations become less likely, or on restoring an already threatened or irritated self. It is important to recognize that all of these maneuvers focus on changing the self, so that it becomes a better executive. The findings of Gollwitzer and Bayer (2000) suggest a perspective on goal-directed self-regulation that focuses on facilitating action control without changing the self. It assumes that action control becomes easier if a person's behavior is directly controlled by situational cues, and that forming implementation intentions achieves such direct action control. As this mode of action control circumvents the self, it no longer matters whether the self is threatened or secure, agitated or calm, because the self is effectively disconnected from its influence on behavior. The research by Gollwitzer and Bayer supports this line of reasoning by demonstrating that task performance (i.e., taking the perspective of another person, judging people in a nonstereotypical manner, solving difficult anagrams) does not suffer any impairment because of the respective detrimental self-states (e.g., self-definitional incompleteness, mood, and ego depletion) if performing these tasks has been planned in advance via implementation intentions.

People's goal pursuits, however, are threatened not only by detrimental self-states but also by adverse situational contexts. Many situations have negative effects on goal attainment, unbeknownst to the person who is striving for the goal. A prime example is the social-loafing phenomenon, in which people show reduced effort in the face of work settings that produce a reduction of accountability (i.e., performance outcomes can no longer be checked at an individual level). Because people are commonly not aware of this phenomenon, they cannot form implementation intentions that specify a social-loafing situation as critical, thereby rendering an implementation intention that focuses on suppressing the social-loafing response as an unviable self-regulatory strategy. As an alternative, however, people may resort to forming implementation intentions that stipulate how the intended task is to be performed, thus effectively blocking any negative situational influences.

Supporting this contention, when Endress (2001) performed a social-loafing experiment that used a brainstorming task (i.e., participants had to find as many different uses for a common knife as possible), she observed that implementation intentions ("And if I have found one solution, then I will immediately try to find a different solution!") but not goal intentions ("I will try to find as many different solutions as possible!") protected participants from social-loafing effects. Findings reported by Trötschel and Gollwitzer (2003) also support the notion that goal pursuits planned by forming implementation intentions become invulnerable to adverse situational influences. In their experiments on the self-regulation of negotiation behavior, loss-framed negotiation settings failed to unfold their negative effects on fair and cooperative negotiation outcomes when the negotiators had in advance planned out their goal intentions to be fair and cooperative with if–then plans. Similarly, Gollwitzer (1998) reported on experiments in which competing goal intentions (i.e., goal intentions contrary to an ongoing goal pursuit) were activated outside of a person's awareness with goal-priming procedures (Bargh, 1990; Bargh, Gollwitzer, Lee-Chai, Barndollar, & Trotschel, 2001). In these studies, furnishing the ongoing goal pursuit with implementation intentions protected it from the intrusive influences of the primed competing goals.

It appears, then, that the self-regulatory strategy of planning out goal pursuit in advance via implementation intentions allows the person to reap the desired positive outcomes, without having to change the environment from an adverse to a facilitative one. This is very convenient, because such environmental change is often very cumbersome (e.g., it takes the costly interventions of mediators to change the loss frames adopted by conflicting parties into gain frames), or not under the person's control. Moreover, people are often not aware of the adverse influences of the current environment (e.g., a deindividuated work setting or a loss-framed negotiation setting), or they do not know what kind of alternative environmental setting is actually facilitative (e.g., an individualized work setting or a gain-framed negotiation setting). In these situations, the self-regulatory strategy of specifying critical situations in the if part of an implementation intention and linking them to a coping response in the then part does not qualify as a viable alternative self-regulatory strategy. Rather, people need to resort to the strategy of planning out goal pursuit in advance, via implementation intentions, thereby protecting it from adverse situational influences.

Potential Costs of Using Implementation Intentions

Given the many benefits of forming implementation intentions, a question of any possible costs arises. Three issues come to mind when we consider this possibility. First, action control by implementation intentions may be characterized by rigidity and may hurt performance that requires flexibility. Second, forming implementation intentions may be a very costly self-regulatory strategy, if it produces a high degree of ego depletion and, consequently, handicaps needed self-regulatory resources. Third, even though implementation intentions can successfully suppress unwanted thoughts, feelings, and actions in a given context, these very thoughts, feelings, and actions may rebound in a temporally subsequent, different context.

With respect to rigidity, it is still an open question whether implementation-intention participants refrain from using alternative good opportunities to act toward the goal by insisting on acting only when the critical situation specified in the if part of the implementation intention is encountered. Even though implementation-intention participants may feel that they have to stick to their plans, they may very well recognize such alternative opportunities quickly. The strategic automaticity created by implementation intentions should free cognitive capacities, thus allowing effective processing of information about alternative opportunities.

The assumption that implementation intentions delegate the control of behavior to situational cues implies that the self is not implicated when behavior is controlled via implementation intentions. As a consequence, the self should not become depleted when task performance is regulated by implementation intentions (for reviews of the ego-depletion model, see Schmeichel & Baumiester, Chapter 5, and Vohs & Ciarocco, Chapter 20, this volume). Empirical data have supported the assertion that individuals who use implementation intentions to self-regulate in one task do not show reduced self-regulatory capacity in a later task. Whether the initial self-regulating task was controlling emotions while watching a humorous movie (Gollwitzer & Bayer, 2000), or performing a Stroop task (Webb & Sheeran, 2003, Study 1), implementation intentions successfully preserved self-regulatory resources, as demonstrated by participants' greater persistence on subsequent difficult or unsolvable tasks.

To test whether suppression-oriented implementation intentions create rebound effects, Gollwitzer, Trotschel, and Sumner (2002) conducted two experiments following research paradigms developed by Macrae, Bodenhausen, Milne, and Jetten (1994). In both studies, participants first had to suppress the expression of stereotypes in a first-impression formation task that focused on a particular member of a stereotyped group (i.e., homeless people). Rebound was measured either in terms of subsequent expression of stereotypes in a task that demanded the evaluation of the group of homeless people in general (Study 1), or a lexical decision task that assessed the accessibility of homeless stereotypes (Study 2). Participants who had been assigned the mere goal of controlling stereotypical thoughts, while forming an impression of the given homeless person, were more stereotypical in their judgments of homeless people in general (Study 1) and showed a higher accessibility of homeless stereotypes (Study 2) than participants who had been asked to furnish this lofty goal with relevant if–then plans. Rather than causing rebound effects, implementation intentions appear to be effective in preventing them.

Although implementation intentions seem to achieve their effects without costs in terms of rigidity, ego depletion, or rebound, this does not mean that forming implementation intentions is a foolproof self-regulatory strategy. In everyday life, people may not succeed in forming effective implementation intentions for various reasons. For instance, a person may link a critical situation to a behavior or outcome that turns out to be outside of his or her control (e.g., if a person who has the goal to eat healthy plans to ask for a vegetarian meal, but the restaurant he frequents does not offer such meals). The same is true for implementation intentions that specify opportunities that hardly ever arise (e.g., if a person who plans to ask for a vegetarian meal, when the waiter in a restaurant takes her order, mostly cooks for herself at home) or behaviors that have zero instrumentality with respect to reaching the goal (e.g., if a person with the goal of eating healthy plans to ask for a vegetarian meal does not know that most restaurants add fatty cheese to make it tasty).

Finally, there is the question of how concretely people should specify the if and then parts of their implementation intentions. If the goal is to eat healthy, one can form an implementation intention that holds either this very behavior in the then part or a more concrete operationalization of it. The latter seems appropriate whenever a whole array of specific operationalizations is possible, because as planning in advance which type of goal-directed behavior is to be executed, once the critical situation is encountered, prevents disruptive deliberation in situ (with respect to choosing one behavior over another). An analogous argument applies to the specification of situations in the if part of an implementation intention. People should specify the situation in the if part to such a degree that a given situation no longer raises the question of whether it qualifies as the critical situation.

Summary

In this section, we have argued that forming plans that specify when, where, and how an instrumental, goal-directed response is to be implemented facilitates the control of goal-directed action. Specifically, we have suggested that making if–then plans (i.e., forming implementation intentions) that specify an anticipated critical situation and link it to an instrumental, goal-directed response is an effective self-regulatory strategy. Empirical data suggest that if–then plans facilitate goal attainment through heightened accessibility of the anticipated critical situation, making it easier to detect and attend to. The cognitive link formed between this critical situation and goal-directed response in the implementation intention also allows such preselected behavior to "run off as planned" when the critical situation is encountered. This strategic automatization of goal-directed action enables individuals to respond quickly, under cognitive load, and even without conscious intent; thus, individuals can capitalize on available goal opportunities in an effective manner.

The success of such a strategy is evident in the numerous studies that document the beneficial effects of implementation intentions in helping people meet their goals. The effectiveness of implementation intentions, however, is moderated by a number of factors. If–then plans seem to be more effective with difficult rather than easy goal pursuits, when commitment to the respective goal intention is high rather than low, the goal intention is simultaneously activated with the implementation intention, commitment to the implementation intention is high rather than low, and the mental link between the if and then parts of the plan is strong rather than weak. People should also adjust the type of implementation intention formed to the self-regulation problem at hand. Although suppression-oriented implementation intentions are viable when certain distractions, temptations, and unwanted responses are anticipated, plans that bolster the ongoing goal pursuit are needed in situations in which goal pursuit is threatened by detrimental self-states and adverse situational influences of which the individual is not aware.

Finally, we reviewed potential costs of using implementation intentions. It is not clear yet whether forming if–then plans locks individuals into a specific course of action. Whether implementation intentions allow for flexible goal pursuit (e.g., to take advantage of goal opportunities other than the one specified) is still an open question. It is clear, however, that implementation intentions do not drain self-regulatory resources (i.e., produce ego depletion), and that suppression-oriented implementation intentions are not associated with rebound. Thus, forming implementation intentions is suggested as an effective and quite cost-free self-regulatory strategy. Through a simple act of willing, linking an anticipated critical situation with a goal-directed response, individuals are able to further their goal pursuits in a pretty dramatic fashion.

IMPLEMENTAL MINDSETS:
ACTIVATION OF INSTRUMENTAL COGNITIVE PROCEDURES

The concept of implementation intentions grew out of a more comprehensive approach to goal setting and goal striving: the model of action phases (Gollwitzer, 1990; Gollwitzer & Bayer, 1999; Heckhausen & Gollwitzer, 1987). The model of action phases sees successful goal pursuit as solving a series of successive tasks: deliberating wishes (potential goals) and choosing between them, planning and initiating goal-directed actions, bringing goal pursuit to a successful end, and evaluating its outcome. The task notion implies that people can self-regulate goal pursuit by developing the respective mindsets, thus facilitating task completion (Gollwitzer, 1990). Whereas the act of choosing goals activates cognitive procedures that facilitate decision making (i.e., deliberative mindset), the act of planning activates those processes that support the implementation of goals (i.e., implemental mindset).

When participants are asked to plan the implementation of a set goal, an implemental mindset with the following attributes is expected to develop (Gollwitzer & Bayer, 1999): Participants should become closed-minded to distracting, goal-irrelevant information, while processing information related to goal implementation more effectively (e.g., information on the sequencing of actions). Moreover, to maintain commitment to a chosen goal, desirability-related information should be processed in a partial manner, favoring pros over cons, and feasibility-related information should be analyzed in a manner that favors illusory optimism. Self-perception of possessing important personal attributes (e.g., cheerfulness, smartness, social sensitivity) should be strengthened, whereas perceived vulnerability to both controllable and uncontrollable risks should be lowered (e.g., developing an addiction to prescription drugs or losing a partner to an early death, respectively). Thus, the implemental mindset facilitates goal attainment by focusing individuals on implementation-related information and prevents the waning of commitment to the chosen goal.

Cognitive Features of the Implemental Mindset

The *cognitive tuning* of the implemental mindset toward implementation-related information hypothesis has found support in thought-sampling studies. Postdecisional participants report more implementation-related thoughts (e.g., "I will get started with X and then do Y") than do predecisional participants (Heckhausen & Gollwitzer, 1987; Puca & Schmalt, 2001; Taylor & Gollwitzer, 1995, Study 3). Even stronger evidence that implemental issues are highly accessible and intensively processed in the implemental compared to the deliberative mindset has been offered by Gollwitzer, Heckhausen, and Steller (1990). They primed an implemental mindset by having participants plan the implementation of a chosen personal project (e.g., "I intend to move from home!"), whereas they activated a deliberative mindset by having participants deliberate on unresolved personal concerns (e.g., "Shall I move from home or not?"). Participants were then presented with three unfinished fairy tales and, in the guise of a creativity test, asked to complete the stories in whatever manner that they wanted. Participants who had been planning were more likely to have the protagonists in the fairy tales plan how to carry out a chosen goal rather than deliberate on the choice of a goal (and the reverse was true for participants who had been deliberating). In a second study, participants viewed slides while deliberating over a task choice, or immediately after having made such a decision and while preparing its implementation. On each slide, an image of a person was presented, along with sentences containing information about goal deliberation or goal implementation. After viewing the slides and completing a brief distracter task, participants were given a cued recall test of the presented information. Planning participants had better recall of the implementation items than the deliberation items (and the reverse was true for deliberating participants).

Experiments testing the hypothesis of *closed-mindedness* in the implemental mindset have demonstrated that implemental participants have shorter noun spans (an indicator of low processing speed; Dempster, 1985) than do deliberative participants, when the noun span test contains words irrelevant to participants' implemental or deliberative concerns (Heckhausen & Gollwitzer; 1987, Study 2). This suggests that the implemental mindset leads to slower encoding of nonrelevant information than does the deliberative mindset. Moreover, Beckmann and Gollwitzer (1987) observed that among planning individuals (compared to deliberative individuals), not only does information that is not relevant to one's goal receive less processing, but information that is directly relevant also receives enhanced processing. Finally, a third set of studies by Gollwitzer and his colleagues (reported by Gollwitzer & Bayer, 1999) used modified Müller–Lyer illusions to demonstrate that planning participants' attention is more centrally focused than that of deliberative participants; the latter also attend to peripheral information.

Empirical results have also strongly supported the hypothesis that implemental mindset participants make *biased inferences* to maintain the positive evaluation of the chosen goal, thus sustaining high goal commitment. A first line of research analyzed the biased processing of feasibility-related information. Gollwitzer and Kinney (1989) had deliberative and implemental participants perform a contingency learning task. In this task, designed by Alloy and Abramson (1979), participants were asked to estimate the degree to which they could influence the presentation of a stimulus light by a button press response. The frequency of the onset of the light was not contingent on participants' responses, because target-light onset occurred with the same frequency when participants pressed or did not press the button (i.e., noncontingent to the button press response). High perceptions of control commonly occurred when noncontingent target-light onset was frequent. Gollwitzer and Kinney (1989) observed that this illusion of control was particularly pronounced in implemental participants and less so in deliberative participants. Taylor and Gollwitzer (1995) extended these findings by analyzing participants' perceived vulnerability to controllable and uncontrollable risks, and positivity of self-perception, compared to the average college student. Again, implemental mindset participants were more positive-illusionary than deliberative mindset participants, and this occurred even when increases in positive mood were accounted for. More recently, Gagné and Lydon (2001) observed that implemental mindset individuals are more optimistic in their forecasts of the survival of their romantic relationships than are deliberative mindset individuals. Moreover, Puca (2001) tested deliberative and implemental participants' realism versus optimism in terms of either choosing test materials of different difficulty (Study 1) or predicting their own future task performance (Study 2). Implemental participants preferred more difficult tasks and overestimated their probability of success more than did deliberative participants. Implemental participants also referred less to their past performance when selecting levels of difficulty or predicting future performance than did deliberative participants.

Differences between implemental and deliberative mindset participants in the biased processing of desirability-related information have recently been provided by Harmon-Jones and Harmon-Jones (2002, Study 2). They tested the effects of mindsets on the

postdecisional spreading of choice alternatives, a classic route to postdecisional dissonance reduction (Brehm & Cohen, 1962). After participants have made a choice between
two options, the chosen option is evaluated more positively, whereas the nonchosen option is evaluated more negatively. Harmon-Jones and Harmon-Jones found that, compared to a neutral control group, the implemental mindset participants increased
postdecisional spreading of alternatives, whereas deliberative mindset participants reduced it.

Implemental Mindsets and Goal Implementation

Traditionally, implemental mindsets have been analyzed primarily in terms of their cognitive features, without direct testing of these features' effects on actual implementation of
goals. In one early exception, Pösl (1994) found that participants in the implemental
mindset were faster to initiate goal-directed behavior than those in the deliberative
mindset. The speed of action initiation, however, was moderated by how much conflict
the participants experienced (i.e., whether they had a choice to perform behavior A or B,
or needed to perform only one of these). Participants benefited from the implemental mindset only when they experienced behavioral conflict. Apparently, the closed-
mindedness associated with the implemental mindset prevented planning individuals
from deliberating on behavioral alternatives, thus facilitating action initiation when two
options were provided.

There is also recent evidence that the implemental mindset generates greater persistence in goal-directed behavior. Brandstätter and Frank (2002) found that participants in
the implemental mindset persisted longer at an unsolvable puzzle task (Study 1) and a
self-paced computer task (Study 2). Similar to the findings of Pösl (1994), the impact of
the implemental mindset on persistence was evident only in situations of behavioral conflict. When the perceived feasibility and desirability of the tasks were in opposition (i.e.,
one was high, while the other was low), participants in the implemental mindset persisted
longer than did those in the deliberative mindset. This suggests that the mindset associated with planning can benefit the individual not only by facilitating action initiation but
also by generating greater persistence in the face of obstacles. Most importantly, persistence in the implemental mindset was not found to be executed in a rigid fashion.
Brandstätter and Frank (2002, Study 3) observed that whenever a task was perceived as
impossible, or when persistence was not beneficial, individuals in the implemental
mindset disengaged much more quickly than did individuals in the deliberative mindset.
Thus, persistence instigated by the implemental mindset seems flexible and adaptive, and
not stubborn and self-defeating.

Finally, Armor and Taylor (2003) have reported on an experiment demonstrating
that an implemental mindset, compared to a deliberative mindset, facilitates better task
performance (a scavenger hunt to be performed on campus), and that this effect is mediated by the cognitive features of the implemental mindset (e.g., enhanced self-efficacy, optimistic outcome expectations, perception of the task as easy). This is the first study to
demonstrate that the postulated cognitive features of the implemental mindset facilitate
goal implementation. These results suggest that optimistic expectations associated with
the implemental mindset do indeed lead to more effective self-regulation and better outcomes. Despite being optimistic, such expectations do become fulfilled. Participants' performance predictions, however, were for an immediate, imminent task. Armor and Taylor
have suggested that the temporal distance of the predicted performance event may moderate the accuracy of judgments in the two mindsets, particularly the implemental

mindset. This assumption is supported by actual performance data collected in both the Gagné and Lydon (2001) and the Puca (2001) studies reported earlier. Whereas in the Gagné and Lydon studies, long-term relationship survival was not affected by the implemental mindset participants' optimistic predictions, in the Puca research (Study 1), immediate task performance was higher in implemental mindset compared to deliberative mindset participants. It appears, then, that whenever actual goal implementation is assessed further and further away from the induction of the implemental mindset, the positive effects of its various cognitive features on goal implementation can no longer be observed.

Summary

In this section, we have argued that becoming involved with planning the implementation of a chosen goal induces an implemental mindset that uniquely tunes a person to process information related to the implementation of goals. The activated cognitive procedures activated also guarantee that the individual stays focused (closed-minded), by disregarding irrelevant and peripheral information. Moreover, they ensure that biased inferences are made on the basis of encoded information in the direction of positive illusionary evaluations of the feasibility and desirability of the chosen goal. It is the sum total of the cognitive orientation of the implemental mindset that facilitates persistence in goal pursuit and successful goal attainment.

RESEARCH ON PLANNING THE IMPLEMENTATION OF GOALS: PROSPECTS

In all of the research reported on implementation intentions and implemental mindsets, people have been asked to plan the implementation of a set goal. But when do people start planning by themselves, without being told to do so? Many factors seem to determine whether a person starts making plans for goal implementation. The first group of factors relate to the ease of goal implementation. If a given goal has been implemented consistently and repeatedly in the past, and the respective opportunity structure of the person's environment, as well as his or her capabilities to perform the required actions, has not changed, there is no necessity to plan goal implementation. The person can rely on the direct instigation of his or her habitual ways of implementing the goal by using opportunities seized in the past. Planning becomes an issue (i.e., becomes instrumental to effective goal implementation) when the way to the goal needs to be newly developed, because no established ways exist, or needs to be reinvented, because hindrances and barriers are anticipated. These hindrances and barriers may be located inside or outside the person. For instance, a person who sets herself the goal to change her diet toward less fat intake may start to plan how to implement this goal, because she either cannot resort to established habits of meeting this goal, or because the environment (e.g., she moved to a new country) or her physical condition (e.g., she has developed an allergy to certain low-fat foods) has changed, thus making useless habits she has already developed to meet this goal.

However, there are also cognitive and motivational prerequisites to planning. On the cognitive side, the potential obstacles need to be accessible, and this is also true for potential good opportunities to act, and for possible instrumental goal-directed responses. Finally, procedures relevant to effective planning need to be in an activated state (e.g., linking opportunities to instrumental responses in an if–then structure; sorting out steps to goal attainment in a temporal sequence). Supporting this line of thought, Pham and Taylor (1999; Taylor, Pham, Rivkin, & Amor, 1998) have demonstrated that mentally simulating one's way to the goal is a strong facilitator in forming relevant plans. Recent research by Grant-Pillow, Oettingen, and Gollwitzer (2003) has focused on the activation of cognitive procedures implicated in planning. In one study, placing participants in an implemental mindset with respect to a personal goal in one domain (i.e., leisure) facilitated the formation of strong implementation intentions in other domains (i.e., strong links between the specified critical situations and selected goal-directed responses were formed for achievement, interpersonal, and health goals). In a further study, people who chronically formed such strong links were observed to progress comparatively more effectively toward set achievement goals. These findings suggest that high situational (Study 1) or chronic (Study 2) accessibility of the cognitive procedures associated with making if–then plans facilitate the formation of implementation intentions.

The mere heightened accessibility of relevant knowledge (e.g., obstacles, opportunities, instrumental responses) and procedures (e.g., linking situations to responses in an if–then format) does not yet make a planner, however. Research by Oettingen (2000; Oettingen, Pak, & Schnetter, 2001) suggests that motivation to use activated knowledge and procedures for the construction of effective plans is also necessary. In one study, all participants were asked to name an unresolved interpersonal problem (e.g., "getting to know someone I like"; "improve the relationship to my partner"), and to indicate their expectations of successfully resolving it. Then, one group of participants had to dwell on obstacles that might impede successful solution of the problem. The other group of participants first had to elaborate mentally the positive future of having successfully solved the problem, then contrast these positive thoughts with thoughts about hindrances and obstacles impeding the positive future. Participants' readiness to plan how to solve the interpersonal problem was then assessed by providing them a choice either to spell out their plans or to reflect loosely on solving the problem at hand. Participants who were confident about solving their problem, who mentally contrasted the desired future with impeding hindrances, produced more plans than did participants who dwelled only on these hindrances and obstacles. Apparently, thinking about, or even intensively dwelling on, obstacles and hindrances does not make a planner either. Perceiving obstacles as standing in the way of the desired future motivates a person to engage in planning the implementation of a desired future.

In summary, people's readiness to plan seems to be guided intricately by the interplay of many different factors. Some of these factors reside in features of the goal pursuit at hand (e.g., goal implementation requires a person to be innovative or to change habitual ways). Other factors refer to the accessibility of relevant knowledge (about opportunities, obstacles, and instrumental goal-directed responses) and procedures (temporal sequencing, if–then linking). Finally, motivational factors determine whether the individual feels a need for plans and wants to go through the pain of forming them.

REFERENCES

Aarts, H., Dijksterhuis, A., & Midden, C. (1999). To plan or not to plan?: Goal achievement or interrupting the performance of mundane behaviors. *European Journal of Social Psychology*, 29, 971–979.

Ajzen, I. (1985). From intentions to actions: A theory of planned behavior. In J. Kulh & J. Beckmann (Eds.), *Action control: From cognition to behavior* (pp. 11–39). Berlin: Springer-Verlag.

Alloy, L. B., & Abramson, L. Y. (1979). Judgement of contingency in depressed and nondepressed students: Sadder but wiser? *Journal of Experimental Psychology: General, 108,* 449–485.

Armor, D. A., & Taylor, S. E. (2003). The effects of mindset on behavior: Self-regulation in deliberative and implemental frames of mind. *Personality and Social Psychology Bulletin, 29,* 86–95.

Atkinson, J. W. (1957). Motivational determinants of risk-taking behavior. *Psychological Review, 64,* 359–372.

Bargh, J. A. (1990). Auto-motives: Preconscious determinants of social interaction. In E. T. Higgins & R. M. Sorrentino (Eds.), *Handbook of motivation and cognition: Vol. 2. Foundations of social behavior* (pp. 93–130). New York: Guilford Press.

Bargh, J. A., Gollwitzer, P. M., Lee-Chai, A., Barndollar, K., & Trotschel, R. (2001). The automated will: Nonconscious activation and pursuit of behavioral goals. *Journal of Personality and Social Psychology, 81,* 1014–1027.

Baumeister, R. F. (2000). Ego-depletion and the self's executive function. In A. Tesser, R. B. Felson, & J. M. Suls (Eds.), *Psychological perspectives on self and identity* (pp. 9–33). Washington, DC: American Psychological Association.

Baumeister, R. F., Heatherton, T. F., & Tice, D. M. (1994). *Losing control: How and why people fail at self-regulation.* San Diego, CA: Academic Press.

Bayer, U. C., Jaudas, A., & Gollwitzer, P. M. (2002, July). *Do implementation intentions facilitate switching between tasks?* Poster presented at the International Symposium on Executive Functions, Konstanz, Germany.

Bayer, U. C., Moskowitz, G. B., & Gollwitzer, P. M. (2002). *Implementation intentions and action initiation without conscious intent.* Unpublished manuscript, University of Konstanz, Germany.

Beckmann, J., & Gollwitzer, P. M. (1987). Deliberative versus implemental states of mind: The issue of impartiality in predecisional and postdecisional information processing. *Social Cognition, 5,* 259–279.

Bless, H., & Fiedler, K. (1995). Affective states and the influence of activated general knowledge. *Personality and Social Psychology Bulletin, 21,* 766–778.

Brandstätter, V., & Frank, E. (2002). Effects of deliberative and implemental mindsets on persistence in goal-directed behavior. *Personality and Social Psychology, 28,* 1366–1378.

Brandstätter, V., Lengfelder, A., & Gollwitzer, P. M. (2001). Implementation intentions and efficient action initiation. *Journal of Personality and Social Psychology, 81,* 946–960.

Brehm, J. W., & Cohen, A. R. (1962). *Explorations in cognitive dissonance.* New York: John Wiley.

Carver, C. S., & Scheier, M. F. (1998). *On the self-regulation of behavior.* New York: Cambridge University Press.

Chasteen, A. L., Park, D. C., & Schwarz, N. (2001). Implementation intentions and facilitation of prospective memory. *Psychological Science, 12,* 457–461.

Dempster, F. N. (1985). Short-term memory development in childhood and adolescence. In C. J. Brainard & M. Pressley (Eds.), *Basic processes in memory development* (pp. 209–248). New York: Springer-Verlag.

Endress, H. (2001). *Die Wirksamkeit von Vorsätzen auf Gruppenleistungen. Eine empirische Untersuchung anhand von brainstorming* [Implementation intentions and the reduction of social loafing in a brain storming task]. Unpublished master's thesis, University of Konstanz, Germany.

Gagné, F. M., & Lydon, J. E. (2001). Mindset and close relationships: When bias leads to (in)accurate predictions. *Journal of Personality and Social Psychology, 81,* 85–96.

Gollwitzer, P. M. (1990). Action phases and mindsets. In T. E. Higgins & R. M. Sorrentino (Eds.), *Handbook of motivation and cognition: Vol. 2. Foundations of social behavior* (pp. 53–92). New York: Guilford Press.

Gollwitzer, P. M. (1993). Goal achievement: The role of intentions. *European Review of Social Psychology, 4,* 141–185.

Gollwitzer, P. M. (1996). The volitional benefits of planning. In P. M. Gollwitzer & J. A. Bargh

(Eds.), *The psychology of action: Linking cognition and motivation to behavior* (pp. 287–312). New York: Guilford Press.

Gollwitzer, P. M. (1998, October). *Implicit and explicit processes in goal pursuit.* Paper presented at the Symposium, Implicit vs. Explicit Processes, at the annual meeting of the Society of Experimental Social Psychology, Atlanta, GA.

Gollwitzer, P. M. (1999). Implementation intentions: Strong effects of simple plans. *American Psychologist, 54,* 493–503.

Gollwitzer, P. M., Achtziger, A., Schaal, B., & Hammelbeck, J. P. (2002). *Intentional control of strereotypical beliefs and prejudicial feelings.* Unpublished manuscript, University of Konstanz, Germany.

Gollwitzer, P. M., & Bayer, U. (1999). Deliberative versus implemental mindsets in the control of action. In S. Chaiken & Y. Trope (Eds.), *Dual-process theories in social psychology* (pp. 403–422). New York: Guilford Press.

Gollwitzer, P. M., & Bayer, U. C. (2000, October). *Becoming a better person without changing the self.* Paper presented at the Self and Identity Preconference of the annual meeting of the Society of Experimental Social Psychology, Atlanta, GA.

Gollwitzer, P. M., Bayer, U. C., Steller, B., & Bargh, J. A. (2002). *Delegating control to the environment: Perception, attention, and memory for pre-selected behavioral cues.* Unpublished manuscript, University of Konstanz, Germany.

Gollwitzer, P. M., & Brandstätter, V. (1997). Implementation intentions and effective goal pursuit. *Journal of Personality and Social Psychology, 73,* 186–199.

Gollwitzer, P. M., Heckhausen, H., & Steller, B. (1990). Deliberative and implemental mindsets: Cognitive tuning toward congruous thoughts and information. *Journal of Personality and Social Psychology, 59,* 1119–1127.

Gollwitzer, P. M., & Kinney, R. F. (1989). Effects of deliberative and implemental mindsets on illusion of control. *Journal of Personality and Social Psychology, 56,* 531–542.

Gollwitzer, P. M., & Moskowitz, G. B. (1996). Goal effects on action and cognition. In E. T. Higgins & A. W. Kruglanski (Eds.), *Social psychology: Handbook of basic principles* (pp. 361–399). New York: Guilford Press.

Gollwitzer, P. M., & Schaal, B. (1998). Metacognition in action: The importance of implementation intentions. *Personality and Social Psychology Review, 2,* 124–136.

Gollwitzer, P. M., & Sheeran, P. (2003). *Bridging the intention-behavior gap through strategic automatization: A meta-analysis of implementation intentions.* Unpublished manuscript, University of Konstanz, Germany.

Gollwitzer, P. M., Trotschel, R., & Sumner, M. (2002). *Mental control via implementation intentions is void of rebound effects.* Unpublished manuscript, University of Konstanz, Germany.

Gollwitzer, P. M., & Wicklund, R. A. (1985). Self-symbolizing and the neglect of others' perspectives. *Journal of Personality and Social Psychology, 56,* 531–715.

Gottschaldt, K. (1926). Über den Einfluß der Erfahrung auf die Wahrnehmung von Figuren [On the effects of familiarity on the perception of figures]. *Psychologische Forschung, 8,* 261–317.

Grant-Pillow, H., Oettingen, G., & Gollwitzer, P. M. (2003). *Individual differences in the self-regulation of goal setting and goal implementation.* Unpublished manuscript, New York University, NY.

Harmon-Jones, E., & Harmon-Jones, C. (2002). Testing the action-based model of cognitive dissonance: The effect of action orientation on postdecisional attitudes. *Personality and Social Psychology Bulletin, 28,* 711–723.

Heckhausen, H., & Gollwitzer, P. M. (1987). Thought contents and cognitive functioning in motivational and volitional states of mind. *Motivation and Emotion, 11,* 101–120.

Lengfelder, A., & Gollwitzer, P. M. (2001). Reflective and reflexive action control in patients with frontal brain lesions. *Neuropsychology, 15,* 80–100.

Macrae, C. N., Bodenhausen, G. V., Milne, A. B., & Jetten, J. (1994). Out of mind but back in sight: Stereotypes on the rebound. *Journal of Personality and Social Psychology, 67,* 808–817.

Milne, S., Orbell, S., & Sheeran, P. (2002). Combining motivational and volitional interventions to promote exercise participation: Protection motivation theory and implementation intentions. *British Journal of Health Psychology, 7,* 163–184.

Muraven, M., Tice, D. M., & Baumeister, R. F. (1998). Self-control as a limited resource: Regulatory depletion pattern. *Journal of Personality and Social Psychology, 74,* 774–789.

Oettingen, G. (2000). Expectancy effects on behavior depend on self-regulatory thought. *Social Cognition, 18,* 101–129.

Oettingen, G., & Gollwitzer, P. M. (2001). Goal setting and goal striving. In A. Tesser & N. Schwarz (Eds.), *The Blackwell handbook of social psychology* (pp. 329–347). Oxford, UK: Blackwell.

Oettingen, G., Hönig, G., & Gollwitzer, P. M. (2000). Effective self-regulation of goal attainment. *International Journal of Educational Research, 33,* 705–732.

Oettingen, G., Pak, H.-J., & Schnetter, K. (2001). Self-regulation of goal setting: Turning free fantasies about the future into binding goals. *Journal of Personality and Social Psychology, 80,* 736–753.

Orbell, S., Hodgkins, S., & Sheeran, P. (1997). Implementation intentions and the theory of planned behavior. *Personality and Social Psychology Bulletin, 23,* 945–954.

Orbell, S., & Sheeran, P. (2000). Motivational and volitional processes in action initiation: A field study of the role of implementation intentions. *Journal of Applied Social Psychology, 30,* 780–797.

Pham, L. B., & Taylor, S. E. (1999). From thought to action: Effects of process- versus outcome-based mental simulation on performance. *Personality and Social Psychology Bulletin, 25,* 250–260.

Pösl, I. (1994). *Wiederaufnahme unterbrochener Handlungen: Effekte der Bewusstseinslagen des Abwägens und Planens* [Deliberative and implemental mindset effects on the resumption of disrupted activities]. Unpublished master's thesis, University of Munich, Germany.

Puca, R. M. (2001). Preferred difficulty and subjective probability in different action phases. *Motivation and Emotion, 25,* 307–326.

Puca, R. M., & Schmalt, H.-D. (2001). The influence of the achievement motive on spontaneous thoughts in pre- and postdecisional action phases. *Personality and Social Psychology Bulletin, 27,* 302–308.

Sheeran, P., & Orbell, S. (1999). Implementation intentions and repeated behavior: Augmenting the predictive validity of the theory of planned behavior. *European Journal of Social Psychology, 29,* 349–369.

Sheeran, P., & Orbell, S. (2000). Using implementation intentions to increase attendance for cervical cancer screening. *Health Psychology, 19,* 283–289.

Sheeran, P., Webb, T. L., & Gollwitzer, P. M. (2002). *The interplay between goals and implementation intentions.* Manuscript under review.

Taylor, S. E., & Gollwitzer, P. M. (1995). The effects of mindsets on positive illusions. *Journal of Personality and Social Psychology, 69,* 213–226.

Taylor, S. E., Pham, L. B., Rivkin, I. D., & Armor, D. A. (1998). Harnessing the imagination: Mental simulation, self-regulation, and coping. *American Psychologist, 53,* 429–439.

Trötschel, R., & Gollwitzer, P. M. (2003). *Implementation intentions and the control of framing effects in negotiations.* Manuscript under review.

Webb, T. L., & Sheeran, P. (2003). Can implementation intentions help to overcome ego-depletion? *Journal of Experimental Social Psychology, 39,* 279–286.

12

Thinking Makes It So

A Social Cognitive Neuroscience Approach to Emotion Regulation

KEVIN N. OCHSNER
JAMES J. GROSS

One of the most remarkable of all human skills is our ability to adapt flexibly to nearly every imaginable circumstance. This ability arises in part from our capacity to regulate emotions that are engendered by the situations we face. Drawing on an array of emotion regulatory strategies, we can accentuate the positive, remain calm in the face of danger, or productively channel anger. One particularly powerful emotion regulation strategy involves changing the way we think in order to change the way we feel.

Known as reappraisal, this capacity to cognitively control emotion was eloquently described by Auschwitz survivor, neurologist, and psychiatrist Viktor Frankl. In *Man's Search for Meaning*, Frankl wrote, "We who lived in the concentration camps can remember . . . that everything can be taken from a man but one thing: The last of his freedoms—to choose one's attitude in any given set of circumstances . . . to transform a personal tragedy into triumph, to turn one's predicament into a human achievement" (1946/1985, pp. 86, 135).

Our goal in this chapter is to develop a framework for understanding the mechanisms by which reappraisal and other emotion-regulatory strategies exert their emotion-modulatory effects. Towards that end, the chapter is divided into five parts. In the first, we briefly review common conceptions of emotion and emotion regulation. In the second and third parts, we present our social cognitive neuroscience approach, which integrates theory and method from both social psychology and cognitive neuroscience (Ochsner & Lieberman, 2001) to develop a framework for studying the capacity to control emotion cognitively. In the fourth part, we present two functional magnetic resonance imaging (fMRI) studies designed to probe the neural bases of reappraisal. In the fifth part, we consider implications for other forms of emotion regulation, individual and group differences in emotion and emotion regulation, the development of emotion regulation skills, and psychopathology.

THE NATURE OF EMOTION AND EMOTION REGULATION

Lay Conceptions

In the movie/musical *Chicago*, jazz singer Velma Kelly unexpectedly discovers her husband and her own sister making love in her dressing room. The amorous pair are later found shot to death and Velma is caught literally red-handed, with blood on her hands. Accused of murder, Velma pleads her innocence, claiming to have been so overcome with emotion upon discovering the pair that she blacked out, only to find them shot when she awakened. Of course, the audience knows the truth: Enraged by the unsuspected infidelity, Velma shot them both.

Velma's denial of responsibility for her actions reflects deeply held lay conceptions of emotion, which suggest that we occasionally encounter situations triggering passions that in turn spark actions over which we may have little regulatory control. Indeed, the tug-of-war between raw feeling and reasoned control is a theme that resonates throughout the history of Western culture. According to the Hebrew Bible, our emotion regulatory struggles began with the first human beings, Adam and Eve, who knew no sin until they succumbed to their appetites and ate an apple from the Tree of Knowledge. Their children, Cain and Abel, soon followed suit: In a fit of jealous anger, Cain killed Abel after God rejected his sacrifice but accepted one from his brother.

The age-old excuse, "The devil made me do it," finds expression in these two stories and countless others, in which the protagonist is ruled by emotion rather than being a ruler of it. Examples abound in great works of philosophy and literature, from Plato to Dostoevsky, and continue to the present day in novels, television programs, and movies such as *Chicago*. Whatever the medium, the message is clear: Within every person is an essential tension between emotional impulses and our attempts to control them.

Experimental Psychological Approaches

Although current conceptions of emotion paint a more complex picture of our emotion regulatory struggles than do lay conceptions, researchers still take as their starting point the tension between processes that generate emotions and those that regulate them. On the emotion-generation side, a consensus has emerged that emotions are biologically based responses to help an organism meet challenges and opportunities, and involve changes in subjective experience, behavior, and physiology (Levenson, 1994; Smith & Ellsworth, 1985). Emotions arise when something important to us is at stake, and classic work by Lazarus in the 1960s provided the first experimental demonstration that the way we appraise, or interpret, an emotionally evocative stimulus shapes how we respond emotionally to it (Lazarus, 1991). Subsequent work on appraisal theory has examined the way in which different specific emotions are generated by appraisals of the relevance of stimuli to different goals, and current work attempts to specify the component processes of appraisal (Scherer, Schorr, & Johnstone, 2001).

Emotion regulation occurs when an individual attempts to modify one or more aspects of an emotional response (Campos & Sternberg, 1981; Gross, 1998a, 1998b).

Studies have begun to address questions about emotion regulation including who regulates their emotions, which strategies they use, and how different emotion regulation strategies influences how we feel, think, and act. It is now clear that effective emotion regulation is essential for mental and physical health (Davidson, Putnam, & Larsen, 2000; Gross, 1998b); that emotion dysregulation lies at the heart of many psychiatric disorders, such as depression (Gross & Munoz, 1995); and that different regulatory strategies have very different consequences for emotional experience, behavior, and physiology (Gross, 1998a). For example, experimental studies of emotion regulation processes have contrasted the suppression of emotion expressive behavior and cognitive reappraisal of an event's meaning in the service of emotion downregulation (Gross, 2001). Suppression can successfully mask facial and bodily manifestations of emotion, but it does so at a cost of boosting physiological responding, and it fails to diminish the emotional experience that prompted one to suppress in the first place. By contrast, reappraisal alleviates negative emotional experience and diminishes behavioral responses, without any apparent physiological cost.

A PROCESS MODEL OF EMOTION AND EMOTION REGULATION

A major aim of our research has been the specification of cognitive and neural processes that support emotion regulation. In this section, we sketch the simple model we use to describe how control processes may influence appraisal processes. In the next section, we then use neuroscience data to flesh out and constrain this model.

In our view, the appraisal process does not proceed from perception to emotion and then stop; rather, it iterates continuously, providing updated appraisals as stimuli and events (including one's own actions and feelings) change over time (see Scherer, 1994). That being said, it is useful to consider one iteration in isolation, then examine how different types of emotion regulation might impact different points of the appraisal process. In this way, differences between, and relationships among, regulatory strategies can be understood in terms of how they modulate the appraisal cycle.

For our purposes, five types of emotion regulation strategies may be distinguished (Gross, 2001). In the first, which we refer to as *situation selection*, a person can control the appraisal process before it ever begins by actively choosing to place him- or herself in particular contexts and not others. The second type of emotion regulation strategy—*situation modification*—involves direct efforts to change the situation to modify its emotional impact. These first two emotion regulation strategies serve to modify appraisal inputs, thereby controlling the cues available to generate particular emotions. Once the particular context has been set, a third strategy may direct attention to environmental cues that promote desired emotions, while ignoring cues that promote undesired emotions. *Attentional deployment* gates particular cues into the reappraisal process, while excluding others from it. A fourth strategy, *cognitive change*, allows a person to modify the meaning of particular cues once those cues have gained access to the appraisal process. For example, in the case of reappraisal, which is one kind of cognitive change, one can alter the ongoing trajectory of an emotional response by reinterpreting the meaning of stimuli and events. The fifth strategy, *response modulation*, affects only the outputs of reappraisal process. Using this strategy, control processes can suppress or augment behavioral manifestations of one's emotional state, such as smiles, frowns, or tendencies to approach or withdraw.

In the remainder of this chapter, we focus on clarifying the neurocognitive mechanisms of one form of cognitive change, namely, cognitive reappraisal. Other chapters in this volume deal extensively with situation selection and selective attention (e.g., MacCoon, Wallace, & Newman, Chapter 22; Mischel & Ayduk, Chapter 6; Rueda, Posner, & Rothbart, Chapter 14; Rothbart, Ellis, & Posner, Chapter 18), and elsewhere we have examined one form of response modulation, expressive suppression (e.g., Gross, 1998a).

Our focus on reappraisal is motivated both by the apparent commonness of reappraisal in everyday life and research demonstrating that other alternative types of strategies may have serious shortcomings: It is not always possible to avoid or modify undesirable situations, or to ignore particular aspects of them selectively, and response suppression takes both a physical (boosting blood pressure, heart rate, and skin conductance; Gross, 1998b; Gross & Levenson, 1993) and a mental toll (impairing memory; Richards & Gross, 2000). By contrast, cognitive reappraisal strategies, which influence the appraisal process itself by changing the way an event is interpreted, are widely applicable, and can successfully influence emotional experience and expression without the physiological (e.g., boosting blood pressure; Gross, 1998b; Gross & Levenson, 1993) and mental costs (impairing memory; Richards & Gross, 2000) associated with suppressing behavioral expressions of emotion.

In the next section, we develop our model of the neurocognitive mechanisms supporting reappraisal in particular, and the cognitive control of emotion more generally.

TOWARD A FUNCTIONAL NEURAL ARCHITECTURE FOR THE COGNITIVE CONTROL OF EMOTION

Because very little research has addressed the topic directly, insights regarding the neural bases of the cognitive control of emotion must be gleaned by analogy and inference from studies of emotion-processing and "cold" forms of cognitive control, such as working memory, response selection, and reasoning.

Current cognitive neuroscience models posit that cognitive control involves interactions between regions of the prefrontal cortex (PFC) that implement control processes and subcortical and posterior cortical regions that encode and represent specific kinds of information (Knight, Staines, Swick, & Chao, 1999; Miller & Cohen, 2001; Smith & Jonides, 1999). By increasing or decreasing activation of particular representations, prefrontal regions enable an individual to attend to and maintain goal-relevant information selectively in mind and resist interference from irrelevant information (Bunge, Ochsner, Desmond, Glover, & Gabrieli, 2001; Knight et al., 1999; Miller & Cohen, 2001; Smith & Jonides, 1999).

We hypothesize that similar interactions underlie the cognitive control of emotion (Davidson & Irwin, 1999; Ochsner & Feldmann Barrett, 2001). More specifically, we hypothesize that reappraisal should modulate activation of brain systems implicated in emotional appraisal, and should depend on frontal systems implicated in cognitive control. These systems are diagrammed in Figure 12.1. In the following sections, we first discuss the neural bases of emotional appraisal, then turn to the neural bases of cognitive emotional control. Our goal here is to develop a functional architecture of the neurocognitive dynamics supporting reappraisal that we can test using functional neuroimaging, as described in the next section.

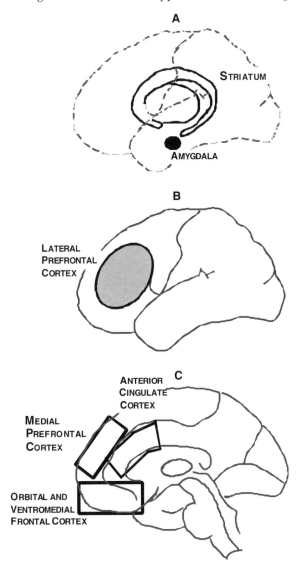

FIGURE 12.1. Schematic overview of brain systems involved in the cognitive regulation of emotion. (A) Two subcortical brain systems implicated in appraising the emotional significance of stimuli, viewed through a transparent image of the left hemisphere. The amygdala is implicated in the rapid detection and encoding of arousing stimuli, including potential threats; the striatum is implicated in the encoding and representation of sequences of thoughts and actions that lead to reinforcing outcomes, including rewards. (B) The lateral prefrontal cortex, shown here on a lateral view of the left hemisphere, has been implicated in the generation, maintenance, and strategic selection of control strategies used to regulate emotion. (C) Medial view of the right hemisphere shows two brain systems implicated in cognitive control, and one brain system implicated in emotion generation. The anterior cingulate cortex and medial prefrontal cortex are involved in the online monitoring of control strategies and drawing inferences about internal states, respectively. The orbitofrontal and the ventromedial frontal cortices are important for placing emotional responses in their appropriate social context, which may be important both for the appraisal and cognitive reappraisal of emotional responses.

What Does Reappraisal Influence?:
The Neural Bases of Emotional Appraisal

Theorists have postulated that the appraisal process involves multiple types of processing (Lazarus, 1991; LeDoux, 2000; Ochsner & Feldmann Barrett, 2001; Rolls, 2000; Smith & Kirby, 2001). Although the precise nature of component appraisal processes is not yet clear, a distinction may be made between processes that (1) evaluate rapidly the affective relevance of a stimulus, determining whether it may be potentially threatening; (2) encode sequences of actions or events that predict reward, or generally predict the occurrence of reinforcing stimuli; and (3) provide a more elaborated, context-sensitive, evaluation that may be important for decision making and representing stimulus value in awareness (Scherer et al., 2001). Different brain systems may be associated with each type of process, and it is possible that reappraisal may influence activation of each one.

Amygdalae

The amygdalae play an essential role in quickly determining whether a stimulus is affectively relevant. Both neuropsychological and neuroimaging studies demonstrate that the amygdalae are important for the preattentive detection and recognition of affectively salient stimuli (Anderson & Phelps, 2001; Morris, Ohman, & Dolan, 1999; Whalen et al., 1998), learning and generating physiological and behavioral responses to them (Bechara, Damasio, Damasio, & Lee, 1999; LeDoux, 2000), and modulating their consolidation into declarative memory (Cahill, Babinsky, Markowitsch, & McGaugh, 1995; Hamann, Ely, Grafton, & Kilts, 1999). Although the amygdalae may play a special role in fear (LeDoux, 2000), it is now clear that they respond to the arousing properties of both positive and negative stimuli (Adolphs & Tranel, 1999; Hamann et al., 1999). In keeping with their role as modulators of perception and memory, amygdala lesions do not impact the everyday experience of emotions and moods (Anderson & Phelps, 2001; Cahill et al., 1995).

Striatum

The striatum plays an essential role in learning which stimuli predict rewards and, more generally, which sequences of stimuli predict the presence or absence of reinforcing stimuli (Rolls, 2000). Imaging studies have shown differential striatal response during receipt of rewards, punishments, and pleasant sensations (Berns, McClure, Pagnoni, & Montague, 2001; Knutson, Adams, Fong, & Hommer, 2000; Knutson, Westdorp, Kaiser, & Hommer, 2001; O'Doherty, Kringelbach, Rolls, Hornak, & Andrews, 2001), as well as stimuli with acquired reinforcement value, including positive (Hamann et al., 1999) and negative photos (Canli, Desmond, Zhao, Glover, & Gabrieli, 1998; Paradiso et al., 1999), happy and sad films (Lane, Fink, Chau, & Dolan, 1997), as well as happy (Critchley et al., 2000; Morris et al., 1996), fearful (Philips et al., 1997; Schenider et al., 1997), and disgusted faces (Sprengelmeyer et al., 1996). The architecture of the striatum seems particularly suited to encode implicitly sequences of thoughts or actions that precede reinforcing stimuli, and it has been postulated that these sequences may be expressed as habits that may guide automatic behavior (Lieberman, 2000). The sensitivity of the striatum to both positive and negative stimuli may reflect its general role in encoding these predictive sequences. The ventral portion of the striatum, however, seems to play a special role in predicting the occurrence of rewarding stimuli (Knutson et al., 2001), and may be seen as a structure that allows the intuitive guidance of behavior toward rewards. Anticipation of reward activates the striatum (Knutson et al., 2001), as does viewing neutral images with positive captions (Teasdale et al., 1999), suggesting that cognitive interpretation of stimuli as positive may activate reward circuitry.

Orbitofrontal Cortex

The orbitofrontal cortex (OFC) has been implicated in appraisal processes that evaluate the emotional meaning of stimuli in context, and determine the appropriateness of possible responses to them (Lazarus, 1991; Scherer et al., 2001). The OFC is important for emotional experience and social behavior (Hornak, Rolls, & Wade, 1996; Rolls, Hornak, Wade, & McGrath, 1994; Zald & Kim, 1996), as well as the perception (Beauregard et al., 1998; Blair, Morris, Frith, Perrett, & Dolan, 1999; Paradiso et al., 1999), sensation (Francis et al., 1999), generation (Crosson et al., 1999), imagery (Shin et al., 1997), and recall (Reiman et al., 1997) of pleasant and unpleasant stimuli across sensory modalities. It has been suggested that the medial OFC (MOFC) may play a particularly important role in emotional appraisal (Elliott, Dolan, & Frith, 2000; Ongur & Price, 2000) given the high level of connectivity of the MOFC and the amygdalae (Ongur & Price, 2000). The MOFC (along with the adjacent ventromedial prefrontal cortex) may be important for representing the pleasant or unpleasant affective value of a stimulus (Davidson & Irwin, 1999; Elliott, Frith, & Dolan, 1997; Knutson et al., 2001; O'Doherty et al., 2001) in a flexible format that is sensitive to momentary changes in social and motivational contexts (Bechara, Damasio, & Damasio, 2000; Ochsner & Feldmann Barrett, 2001; Rolls, 2000). Together, the amygdala and the MOFC are thought to encode and represent differentially the affective properties of stimuli (Bechara et al., 1999; Schoenbaum, Chiba, & Gallagher, 1999).

What Implements Reappraisal?: The Neural Bases of Cognitive Reappraisal

Reappraisal involves complex strategic processing and seems unlikely to be represented by a single, unitary process. However, we hypothesize that the component processes on which reappraisal depends may involve (1) the active generation of a strategy for cognitively reframing an emotional event, as well as the maintenance of that strategy over time; (2) the mediation of interference between the newly constructed top–down interpretation of an event (as more or less emotional) and a bottom–up appraisal that may continue to generate the initial affective impulse; and (3) the reinterpretation of the meaning of internal states with respect to the stimuli that elicited them. These functions have been associated with a network of four interconnected brain structures, which, working together, support the reappraisal process.

Lateral Prefrontal Cortex

Both neuropsychological and functional imaging studies have implicated the lateral PFC in the first of these functions: Lateral prefrontal lesions impair working memory, reasoning, problem solving, and the ability to generate and organize plans of action (Barcelo & Knight, 2002; Miller & Cohen, 2001), and tasks that tap these abilities reliably activate the PFC in both fMRI (Cabeza & Nyberg, 2000; Smith & Jonides, 1999) and electrophysiological (Barcelo, Suwazono, & Knight, 2000; Nielsen-Bohlman & Knight, 1999) studies. Although lateral PFC is commonly activated in studies of emotion, its functional relationship to emotion-processing brain systems, such as the amygdalae, is unclear. Consider, for example, that during the perception, recall, or learning of affective stimuli, studies have found activation of the PFC but not the amygdalae (Canli et al., 1998; Mayberg et al., 1999; O'Doherty et al., 2001; Paradiso et al., 1999; Teasdale et al., 1999), of the amygdalae but not the PFC (e.g., Buchel, Morris, Dolan, & Friston, 1998, LaBar, Gatenby, Gore, LeDoux, & Phelps, 1998; Morris et al., 1996; 1999; Reiman et al., 1997; Taylor, Liberzon, & Koeppe, 2000), of both the PFC and amygdalae (Crosson et al., 1999; Damasio et al., 2000; Phillips et al., 1997), or activation of the PFC and deactivation of amygdalae (Critchley et al., 2000; Hariri, Bookheimer, & Mazziotta, 2000; Liberzon et al., 2000). Lateral prefrontal activations also have been associated with induced (Baker, Frith, & Dolan, 1997; Chua, Krams, Toni, Passingham, & Dolan, 1999) or endogenous moods (Davidson & Irwin, 1999). Unfortunately, it is difficult to determine the regulatory significance of these activations, because most studies have used uninstructed viewing conditions that do not take into account the possible spontaneous regulation of emotional responses in which participants tend to engage (Erber, 1996), have employed stimulus judgments unrelated to emotional appraisal or reappraisal, or have used stimuli that do not elicit strong emotional responses (such as faces). In line with our predictions, however, some have suggested that the PFC may represent emotion-related goals (Davidson & Irwin, 1999), although this hypothesis has yet to be tested systematically in the context of emotion regulation.

Anterior Cingulate Cortex

The dorsal anterior cingulate cortex (ACC) may be essential for mediating interference between top–down regulation and bottom–up appraisals that generate competing emotional response tendencies (Botvinick, Braver, Barch, Carter, & Cohen, 2001; Ochsner & Feldman Barrett, 2001). Dorsal cingulate activity consistently has been found in a variety of conditions that involve response conflict (Barch et al., 2001; Botvinick, Nystrom, Fissell, Carter, & Cohen, 1999; for reviews, see Botvinick et al., 2001; Bush, Luu, & Posner, 2000), including tasks that require overriding prepotent response tendencies (Carter et al., 2000; Peterson et al., 1999). It has been suggested that the dorsal ACC works hand in hand with the PFC during cognitive control: Whereas the PFC implements control processes, the ACC monitors the degree of response conflict or error and signals the need for control to continue (Botvinick et al., 2001; Gehring & Knight, 2000; MacDonald, Cohen, Stenger, & Carter, 2000; Miller & Cohen, 2001). Unfortunately, just as in the literature on the PFC, it is difficult to interpret the regulatory significance of dorsal ACC activation in studies of the perception (e.g., Beauregard et al., 1998; Francis et al., 1999; O'Doherty, Rolls, Francis, Bowtell, & McGlone, 2001; Teasdale et al., 1999), recall (Damasio et al., 2000), or learning (Fredrikson et al., 1998) of emotional stimuli.

Orbitofrontal Cortex

For many of the same reasons that the OFC may play an important role in the initial appraisal of emotional stimuli, evidence suggests that it may play an important role in reappraisal as well. In supporting the contextual evaluation of stimuli, the OFC may participate in updating the meaning of emotional stimuli as they change over time (Bechara et al., 2000; Ochsner & Feldmann Barrett, 2001; Rolls, 2000), which is essential to altering stimulus meaning during reappraisal. For example, orbitofrontal lesions in humans can result in the inability to select appropriate behavioral and emotional responses across varying social contexts (Bechara et al., 2000; Hornak et al., 1996; Zald & Kim, 1996), and monkeys can impair reversals of stimulus–reward mappings (Butter, 1969; Dias, Robbins, & Roberts, 1996; Iversen & Mishkin, 1970) and cause perseveration of responding to a previously rewarded stimulus for a few trials after this reversal is made (Dias et al., 1996). In humans, neuroimaging studies have shown activation of the lateral OFC when stimulus–reward mappings are changed (O'Doherty, Critchley, Deichmann, & Dolan, 2003). Some have suggested that the lateral OFC is necessary for inhibiting prepotent responses or mediating interference between conflicting responses more generally (see Ongur & Price, 2000; Roberts & Wallis, 2000), which is consistent with neuroimaging studies showing activation of lateral OFC and related areas of ventral lateral frontal cortex when participants are performing the Stroop task (Bench et al., 1993), preparing but not executing a finger movement (Krams, Rushworth, Deiber, Frackowiak, & Passingham, 1998), making a finger or speech response in the direction opposite of that indicated by a cue (Paus, Petrides, Evans, & Meyer, 1993), inhibiting an attentional shift when a stimulus appears in an invalidly cued location (Nobre, Coull, Frith, & Mesulam, 1999), changing well-learned response mappings (Taylor, Kornblum, Minoshima, Oliver, & Koeppe, 1994), or reasoning deductively or inductively (Goel, Gold, Kapur, & Houle, 1997).

Medial Prefrontal Cortex

Recent fMRI work suggests that dorsal regions of the medial prefrontal cortex (MPFC; including rostral portions of the ACC implicated in emotion; Bush et al., 2000; Lane, Fink, Chau, & Dolan, 1997) may play an important role in reappraising the relationship between internal states and external events. Medial prefrontal activation has been observed when evaluating one's own (Lane et al., 1997; Paradiso et al., 1999) or another person's (Gallagher et al., 2000; Happe et al., 1996) mental states, when judging the self-relevance of stimuli (Craik et al., 1999; Kelley et al., 2002) and during viewing of emotional films (Beauregard et al., 1998; Lane, Reiman, Ahern, Schwartz, & Davidson, 1997; Reiman et al., 1997). Importantly, activation of the MPFC when anticipating painful shock (Chua et al., 1999; Hsieh, Stone-Elander, & Ingvar, 1999) may be inversely correlated with the experience of anxiety (Simpson, Drevets, Snyder, Gusnard, & Raichle, 2001), and in rats, medial prefrontal lesions increase freezing in response to an aversive conditioned stimulus (Morgan & Ledoux, 1995), suggesting impairment of regulatory control.

TESTING OUR WORKING MODEL OF REAPPRAISAL USING FUNCTIONAL MAGNETIC RESONANCE IMAGING

To test predictions drawn from our literature review, we conducted two fMRI studies of reappraisal whose design allowed us to make direct inferences regarding the roles that cognitive- and emotion-processing systems play in the reappraisal process.

Using fMRI to Examine Reappraisal

Before describing how fMRI might be used to test our reappraisal model, it is important to emphasize two interrelated points about the use of fMRI in particular, and neuroscientific methods more generally, to address psychological questions (for a more complete discussion of these points, see Kosslyn, 1999, and Ochsner & Lieberman, 2001).

First, neuroscientific techniques should be seen as tools in a researcher's methodological toolbox that can be used to provide, along with many other tools, converging evidence concerning a question of interest. This means that neuroscientific data are not special in the sense that they provide a "magic window" on the mind that tells us what "really" is going on. No matter what technique is employed, whether neuroscientific or behavioral, researchers must draw inferences about what a given dependent measure tells us about the psychological processes under investigation, which in turn depends on considering a given result in the context of related findings.

This leads to the second point: Neuroscientific data *are* special insofar as they more directly reflect the participation in a behavior of a given neural information processing system than do purely behavioral methods that measure only the inputs to, and outputs of, such systems. As illustrated below, neuroscientific studies can tell us when and how particular information processing systems are engaged in a task, while also deepening our understanding of the functions carried out by particular brain systems.

The Neural Bases of Cognitive Reappraisal: An Initial Study

With these considerations in mind, in an initial study, we sought to use fMRI to address the general question of how reappraisal exerts its emotion modulatory effects. More specifically, we asked first, what types of cognitive processes support reappraisal, and second, what types of emotion processing does reappraisal modulate (Ochsner, Bunge, Gross, & Gabrieli, 2002)?

Using the model of reappraisal described earlier, we formulated concrete predictions about the psychological and neural processes involved in the cognitive control of emotion that could be tested using fMRI. On the one hand, reappraisal should activate prefrontal and cingulate regions implicated in cognitive control; on the other hand, reappraisal should involve modulation of one or more emotion-processing systems, such as the OFC and the amygdalae.

The logic of our approach was to use the presence or absence of activation in particular cognitive and emotion processing systems as markers of the engagement or disengagement of particular psychological processes. Thus, by determining whether and how prefrontal regions are activated during reappraisal, we could draw inferences about how systems involved in implementing cognitive control strategies enable individuals to reinterpret the meaning of an affectively charged event. Similarly, by determining whether and how emotion-processing systems are more or less activated during reappraisal, we could infer that reappraisal modulates either the low-level processes associated with the amygdala, and/or the complex contextual processes associated with the OFC.

In this study, we asked 15 female participants to view a series of negative and neutral photos for 8 sec each. Drawing on a paradigm used by Jackson, Malmstadt, Larson, and Davidson (2000), we had participants simply view the image for the first 4 sec. At the 4-sec mark, participants were cued either to reappraise the image in such a way that they no longer felt negative in response to it, or were cued, on baseline trials, to attend to their feelings and let themselves respond naturally. In a prescan session, participants received substantial prior training in reappraisal, which involved imagining less negative outcomes or dispositions for pictured individuals. For example, an image of women weeping outside a church might initially be appraised as a sad scene of women at a funeral. Reappraisal training helped participants to view the scene either as a wedding rather than a funeral or, if appraised as a funeral, to see weeping as a natural and healthy way of grieving the passing of an individual who had lived a long and fulfilling life.

Two contrasts were performed to identify brain regions involved in, and modulated by, reappraisal: In the *cognitive control contrast*, regions more active on reappraise than on attend trials should be involved in the cognitive control of emotion, which, we could infer, support the reappraisal process; in the *emotion-processing contrast*, regions more active on attend than on reappraise trials should be involved in the generation of an emotional response, which, we could infer, are modulated by reappraisal.

As shown in Figure 12.2, results were generally consistent with our expectations. The cognitive control contrast showed activation primarily in left prefrontal regions implicated in working memory and response selection. The left lateralized nature of these

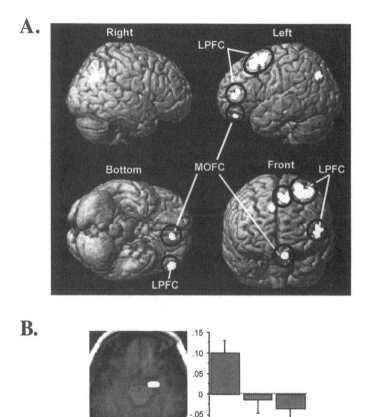

FIGURE 12.2. Lateral prefrontal and amygdala regions activated in our first study (Ochsner et al., 2002). (A) Lateral prefrontal (LPFC) and medial orbitofrontal (MOFC) regions activated or deactivated by reappraisal used to downregulate negative emotion. (B) Group averages for parameter estimates of activation across trial types in right amygdala region of interest. Activation decreased significantly ($p < .05$) on reappraise as compared to attend trials with negative photos and was not significantly different from activation on attend trials with neutral photos. Right panel shows representative region of interest for one participant.

activations is consistent with the idea that participants use verbal strategic processes to construct novel reframes of the evocative photos they viewed. The emotion-processing contrast showed modulation of the left MOFC, and in a region-of-interest analysis (see Figure 12.2), modulation of the amygdala as well. These findings are consistent with the idea that reappraisal can influence low-level emotion processes involved in the initial detection and recognition of arousing stimuli, as well as high-level emotion processes involved in the translation of arousal into a context-appropriate sense of positive or negative affect. As our working model of the neural bases of reappraisal would predict, reappraisal-related activations of the PFC correlated with concomitant modulations of the amygdalae and the OFC (see Figure 12.2), suggesting a sensitive regulatory relationship between them.

Interestingly, in the cognitive control contrast, we did not observe activation in the ACC. Sometimes the failure to observe activation in an overall group contrast occurs because a given brain region is not consistently recruited in all participants. Some participants might recruit the region a great deal, whereas others might not recruit that region at all, and when averaged together, no activation is observed. In such cases, one can correlate a performance measure with brain activation to determine whether individuals who perform well or poorly on the task recruit particular brain regions more or less. When we correlated a measure of reappraisal success with brain activation during reappraisal, only two brain regions were identified: (1) a region of parietal cortex involved in semantic analysis, and (2) a region of the right ACC, shown in Figure 12.3. Increasing activation in this region was coupled with greater reappraisal efficacy. Given the cingulate's role in monitoring and evaluating the success of cognitive control, this finding may suggest that individuals who more closely monitor the selection and application of reappraisal strategies are able to regulate their negative emotions more successfully.

The Neural Bases of Cognitive Reappraisal: Up- and Downregulation of Emotion

In the initial fMRI experiment just described, we examined the use of reappraisal only to attenuate, or downregulate, negative emotion. This seemed like a reasonable starting point, because attenuation is commonly employed to neutralize negative reactions, as when one interprets a hurtful remark as unintended and inconsequential. However, reappraisal also may be used to dampen positive reactions, such as when a researcher tries not to get carried away by an initial positive finding.

One important question is whether reappraisal that enhances rather than diminishes the emotional impact of a situation engages similar neural systems. After all, reappraisal can be used to interpret an evocative stimulus in terms that not only diminish but also increase, or enhance, its emotional impact, whether negative or positive. For example, reappraisal may be used either to augment a response that already is under way, such as when one enhances joy at a wedding, or to generate an emotional response to a stimulus that initially was appraised as neutral, such as when one imagines that an innocuous creak signals an intruder in the next room (Langston, 1994). The use of attenuation and enhancement has been shown to play an important role in subjective well-being and adaptation to stress (Diener, 1984; Folkman, 1984; Gross, 1998a; Nolen-Hoeksema & Morrow, 1991; Parrott, 1993).

In a second study, therefore, we used fMRI to compare directly the use of reappraisal to either down- or upregulate negative emotional responses. The goals of this study were twofold: First, we sought to determine whether the down- and upregulation of emotion

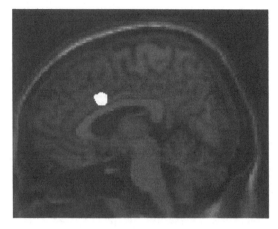

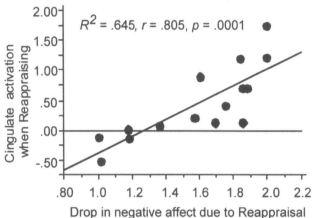

FIGURE 12.3. Left panel shows region of right anterior cingulate cortex whose level of activation across participants predicted a drop in negative affect on reappraise compared to attend trials. The right panel plots activation against drop in negative affect. Each point represents one participant's level of cingulate activation and the corresponding magnitude of affect change.

depend on similar control systems, and second, we sought to determine whether these two different uses of reappraisal might divergently modulate activation in emotion-processing systems, such as the amygdala (Ochsner et al., 2003).

Turning first to the control side of the reappraisal equation, our basic hypothesis was that changing the goal of reappraisal from the downregulation to the upregulation of emotion should not change many of the essential processes used to generate a verbal strategy for reinterpreting an event. In either case, participants would be telling stories about pictured events. In one case, the stories would make them feel better, and in others, the stories would make them feel worse about what they were viewing. But in both cases, a common set of control systems used to generate the stories should be recruited.

However, generating stories that make us feel worse or better about negative events may also recruit some distinct control systems. We hypothesized that using reappraisal to upregulate negative emotion would uniquely recruit prefrontal systems implicated in the self-generation of emotional content. For example, when viewing an image of a sick individual in the hospital, one could upregulate negative affect by generating negative descriptions of the emotions, dispositions, or outcomes experienced by that individual. This is, in fact, what we instructed participants to do. Participants could imagine that a sick individual was in great pain, had a weak constitution, and would be likely to get sicker and perhaps even die in the future. By contrast, we hypothesized that using reappraisal to downregulate negative emotion would uniquely recruit lateral OFC systems implicated in updating and altering the affective value of stimuli. When downregulating, we instructed participants once again to focus on the emotions, dispositions, or outcomes experienced by pictured individuals, but this time to imagine that things were getting better for that person. Participants could imagine that a sick individual was not in great pain, was hearty, and would be getting better in the future. The application of this neutralizing top–down reinterpretation of an otherwise negative event should require a reversal of that event's meaning.

On the emotions side of the reappraisal equation, we hypothesized that downregulating negative affect should once again decrease activation in the amygdala, but that upregulating negative affect should increase it. This prediction followed from our first study, which showed activation of the amygdala when generating a negative emotion, and attenuation of that response during reappraisal. Our reasoning was that cognitive control may modulate low-level emotion processes that encode the emotionally salient properties of a stimulus. These properties should become more or less salient as one up- or downregulates negative affect. With respect to the MOFC, which also was modulated in our initial study, we hypothesized that activation in this region should increase or decrease in concordance with the up- or downregulatory goal of reappraisal. Our reasoning was that cognitive control may modulate high-level emotion processes as one cognitively restructures the mental context in which an event's meaning is being appraised.

To test these hypotheses, we employed a variant of the experimental method employed in our initial study. This time, on each trial, participants first were cued either to increase or decrease their negative affect in response to a subsequently presented photo. In the baseline condition, participants were instructed simply to look at each photo and let themselves respond naturally. To identify regions associated with the up- or downregulation of negative emotion, we contrasted activation on increase or decrease trials with activation on baseline trials. As shown in Figure 12.4, results provided support for our hypothesis that these two uses of reappraisal should involve some common and some distinct control systems. Both up- and downregulating negative emotion engaged left lateral prefrontal control systems implicated in verbal strategic processes, such as the maintenance and manipulation of verbal information in working memory processes essential to reappraisal.

We identified regions unique to each form of reappraisal by directly comparing activation on increase and decrease trials. In keeping with predictions, upregulating negative affect uniquely recruited a region of left rostral lateral PFC previously implicated in self-generating negative words to emotional category cues (Crosson et al., 1999), whereas downregulating negative affect recruited right lateral PFC and lateral OFC regions previously implicated in inhibiting prepotent responses and altering emotional associations (Bechara et al., 2000; Dias et al., 1996; Hornak et al., 1996; O'Doherty et al., 2003; Rolls, 2000; Zald & Kim, 1996).

Two intriguing aspects of these results should be noted. First, we now observed bilateral activation of the PFC when downregulating negative emotion compared to the left-sided activation observed in our initial study. The reason for this difference is very likely due to an increase in the power in our second study: This study employed 24, compared

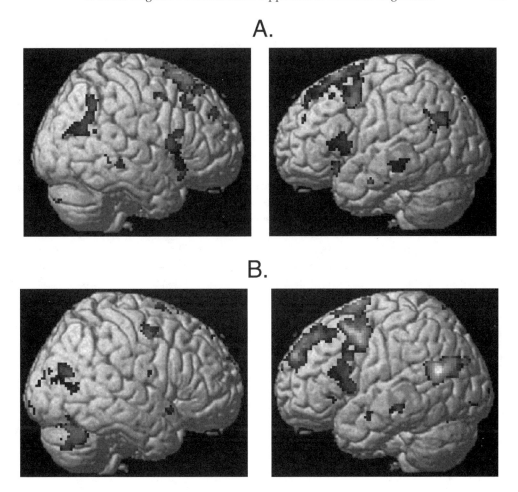

FIGURE 12.4. Prefrontal regions activated when decreasing (A) or increasing (B) negative emotion via reappraisal. (A) Lateral views of the right and left hemisphere, showing regions activated when participants cognitively decreased their negative affect. (B) Lateral views of the right and left hemisphere, showing regions activated when participants cognitively increased their negative affect. Note that activations are primarily left-sided. Note that activations are substantially bilateral. Common activation of left lateral prefrontal systems by both the cognitive increase and decrease of negative emotion suggests that these two types of reappraisal rely on a common set of verbal strategic control processes associated with these left-lateralized regions. Selective recruitment of right prefrontal regions when decreasing negative affect is consistent with the involvement of these regions in behavioral inhibition and withdrawal more generally. See text for details.

to 15, participants; used a more powerful fMRI pulse sequence to acquire data; and involved numerous procedural improvements over the initial study, designed to train participants better to reappraise stimuli preselected to be even more strongly negative. This conclusion is further supported by examining activation in our initial study at a more liberal threshold, which reveals a bilateral pattern of prefrontal activation when regulating negative emotion that is essentially identical to the pattern observed in our second study.

A second intriguing aspect of these results is the lateralization of prefrontal activations associated with up- and downregulating emotion. Davidson and colleagues

(Davidson & Irwin, 1999; Davidson et al., 2000) have marshaled evidence supporting the hypothesis that left prefrontal systems are associated with approach motivation, whereas right prefrontal systems are associated with withdrawal motivation. In this study, we observed an association between left prefrontal activation and increasing negative affect on the one hand, and right prefrontal activation and a decrease in negative affect on the other. Our results may be consistent with Davidson's hypothesis to the extent that increasing negative affect involves increasing closeness or approach to an event, whereas decreasing negative affect involves withdrawal from an event.

Also in keeping with our predictions, we found that up- or downregulating negative affect resulted in increases or decreases in amygdala activation, respectively. Furthermore, the extent to which amygdala activation increased or decreased was correlated with activation in the PFC. When upregulating negative affect, prefrontal activation correlated positively with amygdala activation, and when downregulating negative affect, prefrontal activation correlated negatively with amygdala activation. These results suggest a sensitive relationship between the PFC and the amygdala, further support the findings of our initial study, and indicate that cognitive control influences low-level emotion processes.

We did not observe modulations of the MOFC, however, which contrasts with the results of our initial study. When considered in light of procedural modifications that included changes in instructions on baseline trials, the failure to observe MOFC modulations to reappraisal may not be altogether surprising. In our initial study, participants were instructed to attend to, but not to try to change, their emotions on baseline trials. One concern we had with this instruction is that asking participants to attend to their emotional responses may have selectively amplified MOFC responses to aversive photographs on baseline trials. This concern led us to modify our baseline instructions in the second study, eliminating the instruction to attend to one's emotional state, and simply ask participants to look at a stimulus and let themselves respond naturally. Interestingly, our concern seems to have had some merit, as relatively increased activation on baseline compared to downregulation reappraisal trials was no longer observed.

Summary and Conclusions

In summary, these two studies of the neurocognitive bases of reappraisal converge to support two inferences. The first is that reappraisal depends on prefrontal systems implicated in other forms of cognitive control, such as working memory and response selection. Depending on the goal of reappraisal, to up- or downregulate negative emotion, similar and overlapping but distinct networks of prefrontal control systems will be recruited to make one feel better or worse. The second is that reappraisal modulates low-level emotion-processing systems such as the amygdala. Whether and when reappraisal modulates higher level emotion-processing systems is less clear.

Since we began this work, other investigators have begun investigating reappraisal and related forms of attentional regulation of emotion processing. Work by Beauregard and colleagues, for example, has investigated the use of reappraisal to modulate feelings of sexual arousal (2001) or sadness (Levesque et al., 2003). Their findings generally dovetail with ours: Regions of lateral PFC showed greater activation when participants reappraised, whereas emotion-processing systems, such as the amygdala, in the case of sexual arousal, or the insula, in the case of sadness, show decreased activation. As described below, an important goal for future work is to determine how different types of reappraisal strategies, and other forms of self-regulation more generally, involve the same kinds of interactions we have observed here.

IMPLICATIONS AND FUTURE DIRECTIONS

Our working model of the cognitive control of emotion necessarily simplifies matters, and much work remains to further test the model and extend it to other types of emotion regulatory phenomena. In this section, we use the model to help generate hypotheses concerning emotion and emotion regulation in a series of domains to illustrate one way in which neurocognitive analyses could develop our model and deepen our understanding of emotion regulation across levels of analysis.

Relations to Other Forms of Reappraisal and Self-Regulation

In developing our working model of the cognitive control of emotion, our goal was to create a framework for understanding not only reappraisal in the service of the downregulation of negative emotion but also other forms of reappraisal, and even other forms of self-regulation. One important next step, therefore, is to apply this framework to other kinds of reappraisal, and to other important forms of self-regulation.

In our initial fMRI studies described earlier, we examined the use of reappraisal only in the context of negative emotion. This seemed like a reasonable starting point, because reappraisal is often used to neutralize negative reactions, such as when one interprets a hurtful remark as unintended and inconsequential. However, reappraisal also may be used to manage positive or appetitive reactions, such as when a researcher tries not to get carried away by an initial positive finding, or a child attempts to delay gratification (Mischel & Ayduk, Chapter 6, this volume). One important question, therefore, is whether the findings of our initial study will generalize to the downregulation of positive emotion. It is possible, for example, that reappraisal of appetitive reactions will engage prefrontal control systems that overlap highly with those used to regulate negative reactions, but that these prefrontal systems will modulate structures specifically involved in generating appetitive reactions, such as the striatum.

How might our work on cognitive regulation of emotion relate to other important forms of self-regulation? In this volume (MacCoon et al., Chapter 22; Rothbart et al., Chapter 18; and Rueda et al., Chapter 14) all deal with mechanisms of selective attention, which is one of the five strategies for regulating emotion that we outlined in a preceding section. Work by Posner and colleagues, reviewed in Rueda and colleagues, Chapter 14, this volume, has supported the notion that cingulate and prefrontal systems are essential for supporting attention to target stimuli and ignoring irrelevant distracters, as well as sustaining maintenance of attention over time. As discussed earlier, cingulate and prefrontal control systems also figure prominently in our model of reappraisal. Cognitive neuroscience research suggests that these systems may participate in multiple forms of cognitive control, but it is not yet clear whether control systems supporting selective attention are distinct from those supporting the maintenance and manipulation of cognitive strategies that are part and parcel of reappraisal.

Some studies have addressed the way in which full or divided attention to affectively salient stimuli influences their processing by the amygdala. Amygdala responses to fearful faces seem to be unaffected by attentional manipulations (e.g., Anderson et al., 2003; Vuillumier, Armony, Driver, & Dolan, 2001; however, cf. Pessoa, Kastner, & Ungerleider, 2002). Other studies have examined the way in which processing of fearful faces is influenced by direct or indirect judgments of their affective properties. Amygdala activation has been shown to be greater when participants indirectly process affective content, for example, by judging the gender of a fearful face, compared to when participants must directly process affective content, for example by rating the degree of negative affect expressed (e.g., Critchley et al., 2000; Hariri et al., 2000; Winston, Strange, O'Doherty, & Dolan, 2002). These studies have not investigated the regulation of emotional experience or responses per se, but instead have investigated processing of social cues to emotional experience in others that may have evolutionarily conserved significance (e.g., alerting us to the presence of threats detected by conspecifics). Nonetheless, in the context of our reappraisal studies, they suggest that there may be important differences between the cognitive restructuring of emotional experience and simple inattention to, or superficial processing of, stimuli with some affective relevance.

An important goal for future research is to differentiate control systems important for reappraisal as opposed to selective attention or other forms of cognitive self-regulation, and the way in which they interact with emotion-processing systems.

Individual Differences in Emotion and Emotion Regulation

Individuals differ in both their emotional responding and their use of reappraisal. Our working model might be used to characterize and test hypotheses about the neurocognitive bases of these differences. Such investigations would be important for at least two reasons. First, studies of emotion regulation that explicitly consider these two important sources of variation among individuals may have increased power to detect the cognitive and neural mechanisms of emotion regulation. Second, differences in emotional responding and regulation also may help to account for gender differences in emotional experience and brain activation (George, Ketter, Parekh, Herscovitch, & Post, 1996; Kring & Gordon, 1998).

Individual Differences in Emotional Responding

Individual differences in emotional responding arise—at least in part—from early-appearing, biologically based differences among individuals. The dimensions of extraversion and neuroticism have been found to be associated with positive and negative emotional experience, respectively (Costa & McCrae, 1980; Eysenck, 1990; John, 1990; Meyer & Shack, 1989). Individuals who exhibit a high degree of extraversion—the tendency to be upbeat, optimistic, and to enjoy social contact—report more positive emotions in everyday life than less extraverted individuals (Costa & McCrae, 1980). Individuals who exhibit a high degree of neuroticism—the tendency to worry, to be anxious and apprehensive—report more negative emotions in everyday life than less neurotic individuals (Costa & McCrae, 1980). Experimental manipulations of emotion have likewise documented strong personality–emotion level/reactivity relations (Gross, Sutton, & Ketelaar, 1998) whose neural basis is suggested by Canli and colleagues (2001), who showed that extraversion predicts right amygdala, striatum, cingulate, and prefrontal activation to positive photos, whereas neuroticism predicts right prefrontal deactivation to negative photos. These data are consistent with the hypothesis that persons who are extraverted use prefrontal regions to enhance positive emotion, whereas persons who are neurotic fail to regulate negative emotion using these same regions. This hypothesis needs to be tested in future work.

Individual Differences in Reappraisal

Less is known about individual differences in emotion regulation than about individual or group differences in emotional responding. However, recent research has shown that individuals do differ in their typical use of reappraisal (Gross & John, 2003). Such individual differences in the use of reappraisal can be measured reliably and validly, and predict self- and peer-reports of (1) more positive emotion and (2) less negative emotion. Future work may determine whether typical use of reappraisal in the real world is related to reappraisal efficacy as measured in the functional imaging laboratory. Such analyses could reveal ways in which life experience tunes cognitive control systems to support the reappraisal process better.

Emotion Regulation across the Lifespan

Emotion regulation processes play an important role throughout the lifespan. There are indications, however, that the use of cognitive reappraisal as an emotion regulation strategy may vary across the lifespan.

Emotion Regulation in Childhood

One crucial step in the lifelong acquisition of emotion regulation skills is the development of the capacity to cognitively reappraise emotion-eliciting situations. As early as the preschool years, children understand that emotions can be caused by internal (mental), as well as external (physical), events (Harris, 1989). However, it is not until age 10 or so that children start to explain changes in their own or others' emotions by invoking mental events (Saarni, 1993). At about the same age, children report using more cognitively oriented emotion regulation strategies to change their emotions. Thus, in contrast to younger children (age 6), older children (age 10) at boarding school said that they tried to alleviate negative emotions such as sadness and homesickness by using cognitive strategies such as distraction and reappraisal (Harris & Lipian, 1989). Although little is currently known about the frequency of use of cognitive reappraisal from late childhood through adulthood, it appears that there may be an increase in the use of cognitive reappraisal not only through adolescence (Harris, 1989) but also through adulthood (Gross et al., 1997).

The emergence of reappraisal capacity around age 10 is striking given that we have found that (1) reappraisal depends on prefrontal cognitive control systems in adults; (2) that cold forms of cognitive control, such as working memory, develop between the ages of 6 and 12 years (Dempster, 1981; Swanson, 1996); (3) that the development of these control abilities is thought to depend on delayed maturation of the PFC that continues into adolescence (Casey, Giedd, & Thomas, 2000; Diamond, 2002); and (4) that amygdala responses to fear-relevant stimuli in children 10 years of age may be indistinguishable from those of adults (Baird et al., 1999; Thomas et al., 2001), suggesting adultlike functioning of at least one emotion-processing system at a time when the PFC is still maturing. Given these facts, we have hypothesized that the development of the PFC may undergird the development of cognitive reappraisal as children mature into adolescence and young adulthood. We recently have begun studies that directly address these hypothesis, using modified versions of our reappraisal paradigm described in this chapter.

Emotion Regulation in Later Life

As we age, many of our cognitive and physical abilities decline. By contrast, both field and laboratory evidence suggest that emotional well-being may actually improve with age. How can these apparently discrepant findings be reconciled? We have hypothesized that as people age, they become increasingly skilled at using effective emotion regulation strategies, such as cognitive reappraisal (Gross et al., 1997). This hypothesis derives from two related observations. On the one hand, data from experience sampling (Carstensen, Pasopathi, Mayr, & Nesselroade, 2000), longitudinal (Charles, Reynolds, & Gatz, 2001), and cross-cultural (Diener & Suh, 1998) field studies demonstrate that whereas the frequency and duration of positive emotions remain constant across adulthood, negative emotions decline in frequency and duration. And in the laboratory, older people experience induced negative emotions as intensely as younger adults (Malatesta & Kalnok, 1984). Taken together, these data suggest that the capacity to generate emotion does not decline with age. On the other hand, older adults report greater control over emotion (Gross et al., 1997), as shown by their ability to limit the escalation of negative affect in social interactions (Carstensen et al., 2000) and to express diminished physiological activation when recalling emotional autobiographical events (Levenson, 1994).

Although many factors may contribute to an improvement in emotion regulation in older adults, including a relative prioritization of affect regulatory goals (as posited by socioemotional selectivity theory; Carstensen, Isaacowitz, & Charles, 1999), at present, the contextual factors and processing mechanisms responsible are not clear. In the context of our neurocognitive model of reappraisal, we might hypothesize that older adults may be better able to attenuate negative emotions and/or enhance positive emotions, which might be tested in fMRI studies contrasting these two forms of reappraisal in the same participants. Interestingly, it is known that some of the prefrontal neural machinery supporting cognitive control declines with age (DeCarli et al., 1994; Raz et al., 1997; Reuter-Lorenz et al., 2000; Rypma & D'Esposito, 2000), which might suggest that older adults employ more efficient strategies and/or recruit additional systems to support emotion regulation not used by younger individuals (Reuter-Lorenz et al., 2000).

CONCLUSIONS

In his *Nichomachean Ethics*, Aristotle argued that emotions are useful only when they are about the right things, are expressed in the right way, arise at the right time, and last the right amount of time. This formulation points to—but does not address—a fundamental question that has intrigued scientists since Aristotle: How can individuals regulate their emotions so as to maximize their emotions' adaptive value? This question motivates our own work, as well as that of many other contributors to this volume. As demonstrated in this volume, many different answers can be provided for this question. In our chapter, we have taken a few steps toward providing an answer of a very particular kind. This answer has to do with reappraisal, and makes heavy use of neuroscientific methods and findings to identify neural information-processing systems that support reappraisal, and are in turn modulated by it. We hope that both our process model of emotion regulation and the empirical findings it has generated have helped to clarify the neural bases of emotion regulation. In particular, we hope to have shed some light on what Frankl memorably called "the last freedom," namely, the capacity to tailor how one responds emotionally to a given situation by using cognitive reappraisal.

ACKNOWLEDGMENTS

Our thanks to Elaine Robertson for assistance in preparation of the manuscript. This work was supported by the National Science Foundation, Grant No. BCS-93679, and the National Institute of Health, Grant No. MH58147.

REFERENCES

Adolphs, R., & Tranel, D. (1999). Preferences for visual stimuli following amygdala damage. *Journal of Cognitive Neuroscience*, *11*(6), 610–616.

Anderson, A. K., Christoff, K., Stappen, I., Panitz, D., Ghahremani, D. G., Glover, G., Gabrieli, J. D., & Sobel, N. (2003). Dissociated neural representations of intensity and valence in human olfaction. *Nature Neuroscience*, *6*(2), 196–202.

Anderson, A. K., & Phelps, E. A. (2001). Lesions of the human amygdala impair enhanced perception of emotionally salient events. *Nature*, *411*(6835), 305–309.

Baird, A. A., Gruber, S. A., Fein, D. A., Maas, L. C., Steingard, R. J., Renshaw, P. F., Cohen, B. M., & Yurgelun-Todd, D. A. (1999). Functional magnetic resonance imaging of facial affect recognition in children and adolescents. *Journal of the American Academy of Child and Adolescent Psychiatry*, *38*(2), 195–199.

Barcelo, F., & Knight, R. T. (2002). Both random and perseverative errors underlie WCST deficits in prefrontal patients. *Neuropsychologia*, *40*(3), 349–356.

Barcelo, F., Suwazono, S., & Knight, R. T. (2000). Prefrontal modulation of visual processing in humans. *Nature Neuroscience*, *3*(4), 399–403.

Barch, D. M., Braver, T. S., Akbudak, E., Conturo, T., Ollinger, J., & Snyder, A. (2001). Anterior cingulate cortex and response conflict: Effects of response modality and processing domain. *Cerebral Cortex*, *11*(9), 837–848.

Beauregard, M., Leroux, J. M., Bergman, S., Arzoumanian, Y., Beaudoin, G., Bourgouin, P., & Stip, E. (1998). The functional neuroanatomy of major depression: An fMRI study using an emotional activation paradigm. *Neuroreport*, *9*(14), 3253–3258.

Beauregard, M., Levesque, J., & Bourgouin, P. (2001). Neural correlates of conscious self-regulation of emotion. *Journal of Neuroscience*, *21*(18), RC165.

Bechara, A., Damasio, H., & Damasio, A. R. (2000). Emotion, decision making and the orbitofrontal cortex. *Cerebral Cortex*, *10*(3), 295–307.

Bechara, A., Damasio, H., Damasio, A. R., & Lee, G. P. (1999). Different contributions of the human amygdala and ventromedial prefrontal cortex to decision-making. *Journal of Neuroscience*, *19*(13), 5473–5481.

Bench, C. J., Frith, C. D., Grasby, P. M., Friston, K. J., Paulesu, E., Frackowiak, R. S., & Dolan, R. J. (1993). Investigations of the functional anatomy of attention using the Stroop test. *Neuropsychologia*, *31*(9), 907–922.

Berns, G. S., McClure, S. M., Pagnoni, G., & Montague, P. R. (2001). Predictability modulates human brain response to reward. *Journal of Neuroscience*, *21*(8), 2793–2798.

Blair, R. J., Morris, J. S., Frith, C. D., Perrett, D. I., & Dolan, R. J. (1999). Dissociable neural responses to facial expressions of sadness and anger. *Brain*, *122*(5), 883–893.

Botvinick, M. M., Braver, T. S., Barch, D. M., Carter, C. S., & Cohen, J. D. (2001). Conflict monitoring and cognitive control. *Psychology Review*, *108*(3), 624–652.

Botvinick, M. M., Nystrom, L. E., Fissell, K., Carter, C. S., & Cohen, J. D. (1999). Conflict monitoring versus selection-for-action in anterior cingulate cortex. *Nature*, *402*(6758), 179–181.

Buchel, C., Morris, J., Dolan, R. J., & Friston, K. J. (1998). Brain systems mediating aversive conditioning: An event-related fMRI study. *Neuron*, *20*(5), 947–957.

Bunge, S. A., Ochsner, K. N., Desmond, J. E., Glover, G. H., & Gabrieli, J. D. (2001). Prefrontal regions involved in keeping information in and out of mind. *Brain*, *124*(10), 2074–2086.

Bush, G., Luu, P., & Posner, M. I. (1999). Cognitive and emotional influences in anterior cingulate cortex. *Trends in Cognitive Sciences*, *4*(6), 215–222.

Butter, C. M. (1969). Perseveration in extinction and in discrimination reversal tasks following selective frontal ablations in *Macaca mulatta*. *Physiology and Behavior*, *4*, 163–171.

Cabeza, R., & Nyberg, L. (2000). Imaging cognition: II. An empirical review of 275 PET and fMRI studies. *Journal of Cognitive Neuroscience*, *12*(1), 1–47.

Cahill, L., Babinsky, R., Markowitsch, H. J., & McGaugh, J. L. (1995). The amygdala and emotional memory [Letter]. *Nature*, *377*(6547), 295–296.

Campos, J. J., & Sternberg, C. (1981). Perception, appraisal, and emotion: The onset of social referencing. In M. E. Lamb & L. R. Sherrod (Eds.), *Infant social cognition: Empirical and theoretical considerations* (pp. 273–314). Hillsdale, NJ: Erlbaum.

Canli, T., Desmond, J. E., Zhao, Z., Glover, G., & Gabrieli, J. D. (1998). Hemispheric asymmetry for emotional stimuli detected with fMRI. *Neuroreport, 9*(14), 3233–3239.

Canli, T., Zhao, Z., Desmond, J. E., Kang, E., Gross, J., & Gabrieli, J. D. (2001). An fMRI study of personality influences on brain reactivity to emotional stimuli. *Behavioral Neuroscience, 115*(1), 33–42.

Carstensen, L. L., Isaacowitz, D. M., & Charles, S. T. (1999). Taking time seriously: A theory of socioemotional selectivity. *American Psychologist, 54*, 165–181.

Carstensen, L. L., Pasupathi, M., Mayr, U., & Nesselroade, J. R. (2000). Emotional experience in everyday life across the adult life span. *Journal of Personality and Social Psychology, 79*, 644–655.

Carter, C. S., MacDonald, A. M., Botvinick, M., Ross, L. L., Stenger, V. A., Noll, D., & Cohen, J. D. (2000). Parsing executive processes: Strategic vs. evaluative functions of the anterior cingulate cortex. *Proceedings of the National Academy of Sciences, USA, 97*(4), 1944–1948.

Casey, B. J., Giedd, J. N., & Thomas, K. M. (2000). Structural and functional brain development and its relation to cognitive development. *Biological Psychology, 54*(1–3), 241–257.

Charles, S. T., Reynolds, C. A., & Gatz, M. (2001). Age-related differences and change in positive and negative affect over 23 years. *Journal of Personality and Social Psychology, 80*, 136–151.

Chua, P., Krams, M., Toni, I., Passingham, R., & Dolan, R. (1999). A functional anatomy of anticipatory anxiety. *Neuroimage, 9*(6), 563–571.

Costa, J. T. P., & McCrae, R. R. (1980). Influence of extraversion and neuroticism on subjective well-being: Happy and unhappy people. *Journal of Personality and Social Psychology, 38*, 668–678.

Craik, F. I. M., Moroz, T. M., Moscovitch, M., Stuss, D. T., Winocur, G., Tulving, E., et al. (1999). In search of the self: A positron emission tomography study. *Psychological Science, 10*, 26–34.

Critchley, H., Daly, E., Phillips, M., Brammer, M., Bullmore, E., Williams, S., et al. (2000). Explicit and implicit neural mechanisms for processing of social information from facial expressions: A functional magnetic resonance imaging study. *Human Brain Mapping, 9*(2), 93–105.

Crosson, B., Radonovich, K., Sadek, J. R., Gokcay, D., Bauer, R. M., Fischler, I. S., Cato, M. A., Maron, L., Auerbach, E. J., Browd, S. R., & Briggs, R. W. (1999). Left-hemisphere processing of emotional connotation during word generation. *Neuroreport, 10*(12), 2449–2455.

Damasio, A. R., Grabowski, T. J., Bechara, A., Damasio, H., Ponto, L. L., Parvizi, J., & Hichwa, R. D. (2000). Subcortical and cortical brain activity during the feeling of self-generated emotions. *Nature Neuroscience, 3*(10), 1049–1056.

Davidson, R. J., & Irwin, W. (1999). The functional neuroanatomy of emotion and affective style. *Trends in Cognitive Sciences, 3*(1), 11–21.

Davidson, R. J., Putnam, K. M., & Larson, C. L. (2000). Dysfunction in the neural circuitry of emotion regulation—a possible prelude to violence. *Science, 289*(5479), 591–594.

DeCarli, C., Murphy, D. G., Gillette, J. A., Haxby, J. V., Teichberg, D., Schapiro, M. B., & Horwitz, B. (1994). Lack of age-related differences in temporal lobe volume of very healthy adults. *American Journal of Neuroradiology, 15*, 689–696.

Dempster, F. N. (1981). Memory span: Sources of individual and developmental differences. *Psychological Bulletin, 89*(1), 63.

Diamond, A. (2002). Normal development of prefrontal cortex from birth to young adulthood: Cognitive functions, anatomy, and biochemistry. In D. T. Stuss & R. T. Knight (Eds.), *Principles of frontal lobe function* (pp. 466–503). London: Oxford University Press.

Dias, R., Robbins, T. W., & Roberts, A. C. (1996). Dissociation in prefrontal cortex of affective and attentional shifts. *Nature, 380*(6569), 69–72.

Diener, E. (1984). Subjective well-being. *Psychological Bulletin, 95*, 542–575.

Diener, E., & Suh, M. E. (1998). Subjective well-being and age: An international analysis. In B. Tucker & J. Libby (Eds.), *Annual review of gerontology and Geriatrics* (Vol. 17, pp. 304–324). New York: Springer.

Elliott, R., Dolan, R. J., & Frith, C. D. (2000). Dissociable functions in the medial and lateral orbitofrontal cortex: Evidence from human neuroimaging studies. *Cerebral Cortex*, *10*(3), 308–317.

Elliott, R., Frith, C. D., & Dolan, R. J. (1997). Differential neural response to positive and negative feedback in planning and guessing tasks. *Neuropsychologia*, *35*(10), 1395–1404.

Erber, R. (1996). The self-regulation of moods. In L. L. Martin & A. Tesser (Eds.), *Striving and feeling: Interactions among goals, affect, and self-regulation* (pp. 251–275). Mahwah, NJ: Erlbaum.

Eysenck, H. J. (1990). Biological dimensions of personality. In L. A. Pervin (Ed.), *Handbook of personality: Theory and research* (pp. 244–276). New York: Guilford Press.

Folkman, S. (1984). Personal control and stress and coping processes: A theoretical analysis. *Journal of Personality and Social Psychology*, *46*, 839–852.

Francis, S., Rolls, E. T., Bowtell, R., McGlone, F., O'Doherty, J., Browning, A., Clare, S., & Smith, E. (1999). The representation of pleasant touch in the brain and its relationship with taste and olfactory areas. *Neuroreport*, *10*(3), 453–459.

Frankl, V. I. (1985). *Man's search for meaning*. New York: Washington Square Press. (Original work published 1946)

Fredrikson, M., Furmark, T., Olsson, M. T., Fischer, H., Andersson, J., & Langstrom, B. (1998). Functional neuroanatomical correlates of electrodermal activity: A positron emission tomographic study. *Psychophysiology*, *35*(2), 179–185.

Gallagher, H. L., Happe, F., Brunswick, N., Fletcher, P. C., Frith, U., & Frith, C. D. (2000). Reading the mind in cartoons and stories: An fMRI study of "theory of mind" in verbal and nonverbal tasks. *Neuropsychologia*, *38*(1), 11–21.

Gehring, W. J., & Knight, R. T. (2000). Prefrontal–cingulate interactions in action monitoring. *Nature Neuroscience*, *3*(5), 516–520.

George, M. S., Ketter, T. A., Parekh, P. I., Herscovitch, P., & Post, R. M. (1996). Gender differences in regional cerebral blood flow during transient self-induced sadness or happiness. *Biological Psychiatry*, *40*(9), 859–871.

Goel, V., Gold, B., Kapur, S., & Houle, S. (1997). The seats of reason?: An imaging study of deductive and inductive reasoning. *Neuroreport*, *8*(5), 1305–1310.

Gross, J. J. (1998a). Antecedent- and response-focused emotion regulation: Divergent consequences for experience, expression, and physiology. *Journal of Personality and Social Psychology*, *74*(1), 224–237.

Gross, J. J. (1998b). The emerging field of emotion regulation: An integrative review. *Review of General Psychology*, *2*, 271–299.

Gross, J. J. (2001). Emotion regulation in adulthood: Timing is everything. *Current Directions in Psychological Science*, *10*(6), 214–219.

Gross, J. J., Carstensen, L. L., Pasupathi, M., Tsai, J., Skorpen, C. G., & Hsu, A. Y. (1997). Emotion and aging: Experience, expression, and control. *Psychology Aging*, *12*(4), 590–599.

Gross, J. J., & John, O. P. (2003). Individual differences in two emotion regulation processes: Implications for affect, relationships, and well-being. *Journal of Personality and Social Psychology*, *85*, 348–362.

Gross, J. J., & Levenson, R. W. (1993). Emotional suppression: Physiology, self-report, and expressive behavior. *Journal of Personality and Social Psychology*, *64*(6), 970–986.

Gross, J. J., & Munoz, R. F. (1995). Emotion regulation and mental health. *Clinical Psychology: Science and Practice*, *2*, 151–164.

Gross, J. J., Sutton, S. K., & Ketelaar, T. V. (1998). Relations between affect and personality: Support for the affect-level and affective-reactivity views. *Personality and Social Psychology Bulletin*, *24*, 279–288.

Hamann, S. B., Ely, T. D., Grafton, S. T., & Kilts, C. D. (1999). Amygdala activity related to enhanced memory for pleasant and aversive stimuli. *Nature Neuroscience*, *2*(3), 289–293.

Happe, F., Ehlers, S., Fletcher, P., Frith, U., Johansson, M., Gillberg, C., Dolan, R., Frackowiak, R., & Frith, C. (1996). "Theory of mind" in the brain. Evidence from a PET scan study of Asperger syndrome. *Neuroreport*, *8*(1), 197–201.

Hariri, A. R., Bookheimer, S. Y., & Mazziotta, J. C. (2000). Modulating emotional responses: Effects of a neocortical network on the limbic system. *Neuroreport*, *11*(1), 43–48.

Harris, P. L. (1989). *Children and emotion: The development of psychological understanding.* Cambridge, MA: Blackwell.

Harris, P. L., & Lipian, M. S. (1989). Understanding emotion and experiencing emotion. In C. Saarni & P. L. Harris (Eds.), *Children's understanding of emotion* (pp. 241–258). New York: Cambridge University Press.

Hornak, J., Rolls, E. T., & Wade, D. (1996). Face and voice expression identification in patients with emotional and behavioural changes following ventral frontal lobe damage. *Neuropsychologia*, *34*(4), 247–261.

Hsieh, J. C., Stone-Elander, S., & Ingvar, M. (1999). Anticipatory coping of pain expressed in the human anterior cingulate cortex: A positron emission tomography study. *Neuroscience Letters*, *262*(1), 61–64.

Iversen, S. D., & Mishkin, M. (1970). Perseverative interference in monkeys following selective lesions of the inferior prefrontal convexity. *Experimental Brain Research*, *11*(4), 376–386.

Jackson, D. C., Malmstadt, J. R., Larson, C. L., & Davidson, R. J. (2000). Suppression and enhancement of emotional responses to unpleasant pictures. *Psychophysiology*, *37*(4), 515–522.

John, O. P. (1990). The "Big Five" factor taxonomy: Dimensions of personality in the natural language and in questionnaires. In L. A. Pervin (Ed.), *Handbook of personality: Theory and research* (pp. 66–100). New York: Guilford Press.

Kelley, W. M., Macrae, C. N., Wyland, C. L., Caglar, S., Inati, S., & Heatherton, T. F. (2002). Finding the self?: An event-related fMRI study. *Journal of Cognitive Neuroscience*, *14*(5), 785–794.

Knight, R. T., Staines, W. R., Swick, D., & Chao, L. L. (1999). Prefrontal cortex regulates inhibition and excitation in distributed neural networks. *Acta Psychology (Amsterdam)*, *101*(2–3), 159–178.

Knutson, B., Adams, C. M., Fong, G. W., & Hommer, D. (2001). Anticipation of increasing monetary reward selectively recruits nucleus accumbens. *Journal of Neuroscience*, *21*(16), RC159.

Knutson, B., Westdorp, A., Kaiser, E., & Hommer, D. (2000). fMRI visualization of brain activity during a monetary incentive delay task. *Neuroimage*, *12*(1), 20–27.

Kosslyn, S. M. (1999). If neuroimaging is the answer, what is the question? *Philosophical Transactions of the Royal Society of London B: Biological Sciences*, *354*(1387), 1283–1294.

Krams, M., Rushworth, M. F., Deiber, M. P., Frackowiak, R. S., & Passingham, R. E. (1998). The preparation, execution and suppression of copied movements in the human brain. *Experimental Brain Research*, *120*(3), 386–398.

Kring, A. M., & Gordon, A. H. (1998). Sex differences in emotion: Expression, experience, and physiology. *Journal of Personality and Social Psychology*, *74*(3), 686–703.

LaBar, K. S., Gatenby, J. C., Gore, J. C., LeDoux, J. E., & Phelps, E. A. (1998). Human amygdala activation during conditioned fear acquisition and extinction: A mixed-trial fMRI study. *Neuron*, *20*(5), 937–945.

Lane, R. D., Fink, G. R., Chau, P. M., & Dolan, R. J. (1997). Neural activation during selective attention to subjective emotional responses. *Neuroreport*, *8*(18), 3969–3972.

Lane, R. D., Reiman, E. M., Ahern, G. L., Schwartz, G. E., & Davidson, R. J. (1997). Neuroanatomical correlates of happiness, sadness, and disgust. *American Journal of Psychiatry*, *154*(7), 926–933.

Langston, C. A. (1994). Capitalizing on and coping with daily-life events: Expressive responses to positive events. *Journal of Personality and Social Psychology*, *67*(6), 1112–1125.

Lazarus, R. S. (1991). Progress on a cognitive–motivational–relational theory of emotion. *American Psychologist*, *46*(8), 819–834.

LeDoux, J. E. (2000). Emotion circuits in the brain. *Annual Review of Neuroscience,* *23*, 155–184.

Levenson, R. W. (1994). Human emotions: A functional view. In P. Ekman & R. J. Davidson (Eds.), *The nature of emotion: Fundamental questions* (pp. 123–126). New York: Oxford University Press.

Levesque, J., Eugene, F., Joanette, Y., Paquette, V., Mensour, B., Beaudoin, G., Leroux, J. M., Bourgouin, P., & Beauregard, M. (2003). Neural circuitry underlying voluntary suppression of sadness. *Biological Psychiatry, 53*(6), 105–121.

Liberzon, I., Taylor, S. F., Fig, L. M., Decker, L. R., Koeppe, R. A., & Minoshima, S. (2000). Limbic activation and psychophysiologic responses to aversive visual stimuli: Interaction with cognitive task. *Neuropsychopharmacology, 23*(5), 508–516.

Lieberman, M. D. (2000). Intuition: A social cognitive neuroscience approach. *Psychology Bulletin, 126*(1), 109–137.

Malatesta, C., & Kalnok, M. (1984). Emotional experience in younger and older adults. *Journal of Gerontology, 39*(3), 301–308.

Mayberg, H. S., Liotti, M., Brannan, S. K., McGinnis, S., Mahurin, R. K., Jerabek, P. A., Silva, J. A., Tekell, J. L., Martin, C. C., Lancaster, J. L., & Fox, P. T. (1999). Reciprocal limbic–cortical function and negative mood: Converging PET findings in depression and normal sadness. *American Journal of Psychiatry, 156*(5), 675–682.

Meyer, G. J., & Shack, J. R. (1989). Structural convergence of mood and personality: Evidence for old and new directions. *Journal of Personality and Social Psychology, 57,* 691–706.

Miller, E. K., & Cohen, J. D. (2001). An integrative theory of prefrontal cortex function. *Annual Review of Neuroscience, 24,* 167–202.

Morgan, M. A., & LeDoux, J. E. (1995). Differential contribution of dorsal and ventral medial prefrontal cortex to the acquisition and extinction of conditioned fear in rats. *Behavioral Neuroscience, 109*(4), 681–688.

Morris, J. S., Frith, C. D., Perrett, D. I., Rowland, D., Young, A. W., Calder, A. J., & Dolan, R. J. (1996). A differential neural response in the human amygdala to fearful and happy facial expressions. *Nature, 383*(6603), 812–815.

Morris, J. S., Ohman, A., & Dolan, R. J. (1999). A subcortical pathway to the right amygdala mediating "unseen" fear. *Proceedings of the National Academy of Sciences, USA, 96*(4), 1680–1685.

Nielsen-Bohlman, L., & Knight, R. T. (1999). Prefrontal cortical involvement in visual working memory. *Cognitive Brain Research, 8*(3), 299–310.

Nobre, A. C., Coull, J. T., Frith, C. D., & Mesulam, M. M. (1999). Orbitofrontal cortex is activated during breaches of expectation in tasks of visual attention. *Nature Neuroscience, 2*(1), 11–12.

Nolen-Hoeksema, S., & Morrow, J. (1991). A prospective study of depression and distress following a natural disaster: The 1989 Loma Prieta earthquake. *Journal of Personality and Social Psychology, 61,* 105–121.

O'Doherty, J., Critchley, H., Deichmann, R., & Dolan, R. (2003). *Dissociating outcome from response switching in human orbitofrontal cortex.* Paper presented at the 10th annual meeting of the Cognitive Neuroscience Society, New York.

O'Doherty, J., Kringelbach, M. L., Rolls, E. T., Hornak, J., & Andrews, C. (2001). Abstract reward and punishment representations in the human orbitofrontal cortex. *Nature Neuroscience, 4*(1), 95–102.

O'Doherty, J., Rolls, E. T., Francis, S., Bowtell, R., & McGlone, F. (2001). Representation of pleasant and aversive taste in the human brain. *Journal of Neurophysiology, 85*(3), 1315–1321.

Ochsner, K. N., Bunge, S. A., Gross, J. J., & Gabrieli, J. D. (2002). Rethinking feelings: An FMRI study of the cognitive regulation of emotion. *Journal of Cognitive Neuroscience, 14*(8), 1215–1229.

Ochsner, K. N., & Feldman Barrett, L. (2001). A multiprocess perspective on the neuroscience of emotion. In T. J. Mayne & G. A. Bonanno (Eds.), *Emotions: Currrent issues and future directions* (pp. 38–81). New York: Guilford Press.

Ochsner, K. N., Ray, R., Cooper, J., Robertson, E., Chopra, S., Gabrieli, J. D. E., & Gross, J. J. (2003). *For better or for worse: Neural systems supporting the cognitive down- and up-regulation of negative emotion.* Manuscript submitted for publication.

Ochsner, K. N., & Lieberman, M. D. (2001). The emergence of social cognitive neuroscience. *American Psychologist, 56*(9), 717–734.

Ongur, D., & Price, J. L. (2000). The organization of networks within the orbital and medial prefrontal cortex of rats, monkeys and humans. *Cerebral Cortex*, *10*(3), 206–219.

Paradiso, S., Johnson, D. L., Andreasen, N. C., O'Leary, D. S., Watkins, G. L., Ponto, L. L., & Hichwa, R. D. (1999). Cerebral blood flow changes associated with attribution of emotional valence to pleasant, unpleasant, and neutral visual stimuli in a PET study of normal subjects. *American Journal of Psychiatry*, *156*(10), 1618–1629.

Parrott, W. G. (1993). Beyond hedonism: Motives for inhibiting good moods and for maintaining bad moods. In D. M. Wegner & J. W. Pennebaker (Eds.), *Handbook of mental control* (pp. 278–308). Englewood Cliffs, NJ: Prentice-Hall.

Paus, T., Petrides, M., Evans, A. C., & Meyer, E. (1993). Role of the human anterior cingulate cortex in the control of oculomotor, manual, and speech responses: A positron emission tomography study. *Journal of Neurophysiology*, *70*(2), 453–469.

Pessoa, L., Kastner, S., & Ungerleider, L. G. (2002). Attentional control of the processing of neural and emotional stimuli. *Cognitive Brain Research*, *15*(1), 31–45.

Peterson, B. S., Skudlarski, P., Gatenby, J. C., Zhang, H., Anderson, A. W., & Gore, J. C. (1999). An fMRI study of Stroop word–color interference: Evidence for cingulate subregions subserving multiple distributed attentional systems. *Biological Psychiatry*, *45*(10), 1237–1258.

Phillips, M. L., Young, A. W., Senior, C., Brammer, M., Andrew, C., Calder, A. J., Bullmore, E. T., Perrett, D. I., Rowland, D., Williams, S. C., Gray, J. A., & David, A. S. (1997). A specific neural substrate for perceiving facial expressions of disgust. *Nature*, *389*(6650), 495–498.

Raz, N., Gunning, F. M., Head, D., Dupuis, J. H., McQuain, J., Briggs, S. D., Loken, W. J., Thornton, A. E., & Acker, J. D. (1997). Selective aging of the human cerebral cortex observed in vivo: Differential vulnerability of the prefrontal gray matter. *Cerebral Cortex*, *7*(3), 268–282.

Reiman, E. M., Lane, R. D., Ahern, G. L., Schwartz, G. E., Davidson, R. J., Friston, K. J., Yun, L. S., & Chen, K. (1997). Neuroanatomical correlates of externally and internally generated human emotion. *American Journal of Psychiatry*, *154*(7), 918–925.

Reuter-Lorenz, P. A., Jonides, J., Smith, E. E., Hartley, A., Miller, A., Marshuetz, C., & Koeppe, R. A. (2000). Age differences in the frontal lateralization of verbal and spatial working memory revealed by PET. *Journal of Cognitive Neuroscience*, *12*(1), 174–187.

Richards, J. M., & Gross, J. J. (2000). Emotion regulation and memory: The cognitive costs of keeping one's cool. *Journal of Personality and Social Psychology*, *79*(3), 410–424.

Roberts, A. C., & Wallis, J. D. (2000). Inhibitory control and affective processing in the prefrontal cortex: Neuropsychological studies in the common marmoset. *Cerebral Cortex*, *10*(3), 252–262.

Rolls, E. T. (2000). The orbitofrontal cortex and reward. *Cerebral Cortex*, *10*(3), 284–294.

Rolls, E. T., Hornak, J., Wade, D., & McGrath, J. (1994). Emotion-related learning in patients with social and emotional changes associated with frontal lobe damage. *Journal of Neurol Neurosurg Psychiatry*, *57*(12), 1518–1524.

Rypma, B., & D'Esposito, M. (2000). Isolating the neural mechanisms of age-related changes in human working memory. *Nature Neuroscience*, *3*(5), 509–515.

Saarni, C. (1993). Socialization of emotion. In M. Lewis & J. M. Haviland (Eds.), *Handbook of emotions* (pp. 435–446). New York: Guilford Press.

Scherer, K. R. (1994). Emotion serves to decouple stimulus and response. In P. Ekman & R. J. Davidson (Eds.), *The nature of emotion: Fundamental questions* (pp. 127–130). New York: Oxford University Press.

Scherer, K. R., Schorr, A., & Johnstone, T. (Eds.). (2001). *Appraisal processes in emotion: Theory, methods, research*. New York: Oxford University Press.

Schneider, F., Grodd, W., Weiss, U., Klose, U., Mayer, K. R., Nagele, T., & Gur, R. C. (1997). Functional MRI reveals left amygdala activation during emotion. *Psychiatry Research*, *76*(2–3), 75–82.

Schoenbaum, G., Chiba, A. A., & Gallagher, M. (1999). Neural encoding in orbitofrontal cortex and basolateral amygdala during olfactory discrimination learning. *Journal of Neuroscience*, *19*(5), 1876–1884.

Shin, L. M., Kosslyn, S. M., McNally, R. J., Alpert, N. M., Thompson, W. L., Rauch, S. L., Macklin, M. L., & Pitman, R. K. (1997). Visual imagery and perception in posttraumatic stress disorder. A positron emission tomographic investigation. *Archives of General Psychiatry, 54*(3), 233–241.

Simpson, J. R., Jr., Drevets, W. C., Snyder, A. Z., Gusnard, D. A., & Raichle, M. E. (2001). Emotion-induced changes in human medial prefrontal cortex: II. During anticipatory anxiety. *Proceedings of the National Academy of Sciences, USA, 98*(2), 688–693.

Smith, C. A., & Ellsworth, P. C. (1985). Patterns of cognitive appraisal in emotion. *Journal of Personality and Social Psychology, 48*, 813–838.

Smith, C. A., & Kirby, L. D. (2001). Toward delivering on the promise of appraisal theory. In K. R. Scherer & A. Schorr (Eds.), *Appraisal processes in emotion: Theory, methods, research* (pp. 121–138). New York: Oxford University Press.

Smith, E. E., & Jonides, J. (1999). Storage and executive processes in the frontal lobes. *Science, 283*(5408), 1657–1661.

Sprengelmeyer, R., Young, A. W., Calder, A. J., Karnat, A., Lange, H., Homberg, V., Perrett, D. I., & Rowland, D. (1996). Loss of disgust: Perception of faces and emotions in Huntington's disease. *Brain, 119*(7), 1647–1665.

Swanson, H. L. (1996). Individual and age-related differences in children's working memory. *Memory and Cognition, 24*(1), 70–82.

Taylor, S. F., Kornblum, S., Minoshima, S., Oliver, L. M., & Koeppe, R. A. (1994). Changes in medial cortical blood flow with a stimulus–response compatibility task. *Neuropsychologia, 32*(2), 249–255.

Taylor, S. F., Liberzon, I., & Koeppe, R. A. (2000). The effect of graded aversive stimuli on limbic and visual activation. *Neuropsychologia, 38*(10), 1415–1425.

Teasdale, J. D., Howard, R. J., Cox, S. G., Ha, Y., Brammer, M. J., Williams, S. C., & Checkley, S. A. (1999). Functional MRI study of the cognitive generation of affect. *American Journal of Psychiatry, 156*(2), 209–215.

Thomas, K. M., Drevets, W. C., Whalen, P. J., Eccard, C. H., Dahl, R. E., Ryan, N. D., & Casey, B. J. (2001). Amygdala response to facial expressions in children and adults. *Biological Psychiatry, 49*(4), 309–316.

Vuilleumier, P., Armony, J. L., Driver, J., & Dolan, R. J. (2001). Effects of attention and emotion on face processing in the human brain: An event-related fMRI study. *Neuron, 30*(3), 829–841.

Whalen, P. J., Rauch, S. L., Etcoff, N. L., McInerney, S. C., Lee, M. B., & Jenike, M. A. (1998). Masked presentations of emotional facial expressions modulate amygdala activity without explicit knowledge. *Journal of Neuroscience, 18*(1), 411–418.

Winston, J. S., Strange, B. A., O'Doherty, J., & Dolan, R. J. (2002). Automatic and intentional brain responses during evaluation of trustworthiness of faces. *Nature Neuroscience, 5*(3), 277–283.

Zald, D. H., & Kim, S. W. (1996). Anatomy and function of the orbital frontal cortex: I. Anatomy, neurocircuitry; and obsessive-compulsive disorder. *Journal of Neuropsychiatry and Clinical Neurosciences, 8*(2), 125–138.

III

Development of Self-Regulation

13

Effortful Control

Relations with Emotion Regulation, Adjustment, and Socialization in Childhood

NANCY EISENBERG
CYNTHIA L. SMITH
ADRIENNE SADOVSKY
TRACY L. SPINRAD

Our purpose in this chapter is to discuss the construct of effortful control and review literature relevant to its importance, development, and significance for optimal development in childhood. First, we review important definitional and conceptual issues, then the literature on the emergence of effortful control in childhood. Next, we consider the issue of its role in development—for example, its associations with emotionality, compliance, delay of gratification, moral development, empathy, adjustment, social competence, and cognitive and academic performance. Finally, we consider what is known about the socialization of effortful control, especially in the family.

THE DEFINITION OF EFFORTFUL CONTROL

The term "effortful control" was first used in 1989 by Mary Rothbart in a chapter on temperament to describe a level of control that emerges in children's development. Her thinking about this construct was further developed in research and writings with collaborators studying personality and cognitive neuroscience (e.g., Ahadi, Rothbart, & Ye, 1993; Rothbart, Derryberry, & Posner, 1994). For example, Rothbart, Derryberry, and colleagues (1994) described effortful control as involving the anterior attention network in the midprefrontal cortex, which seems to play a major role in planning and controlling attention and related behavior (see Rueda, Posner, & Rothbart, Chapter 14, this volume).

Rothbart has defined effortful control as "the ability to inhibit a dominant response to perform a subdominant response" (Rothbart & Bates, 1998, p. 137) or the "efficiency of executive attention, including the ability to inhibit a dominant response and/or to activate a subdominant response, to plan, and to detect errors" (personal communication, January 26, 2002). Effortful control pertains to the ability to willfully or voluntarily inhibit, activate, or change (modulate) attention and behavior. Measures of effortful control often include indices of attentional regulation (e.g., the ability to voluntarily focus or shift attention as needed, called "attentional control") and/or behavioral regulation (e.g., the ability to inhibit behavior effortfully as appropriate, called "inhibitory control"). Investigators sometimes have included measures of the ability to activate behavior when needed (even if someone does not feel like doing so, called "activation control"; Eisenberg, Fabes, & Murphy, 1995), for example, when one needs to complete a task or respond to a signal (e.g., Ellis & Rothbart, 1999; Kochanska, Murray, & Harlan, 2000). Effortful control, as part of executive attention, is viewed as involved in the awareness of one's planned behavior (Posner & DiGirolamo, 2000) and subjective feelings of voluntary control of thoughts and feelings, and is believed to come into play when resolving conflict (e.g., in regard to discrepant information), correcting errors, and planning new actions (Posner & Rothbart, 1998; see Rueda, Posner, & Rothbart, Chapter 14, this volume).

Effortful control is viewed by Rothbart as one of the primary dimensions of temperament (Ahadi & Rothbart, 1994; Rothbart, Ahadi, Hershey, & Fisher, 2001; see Rothbart, Ellis, & Posner, Chapter 18, this volume). She has defined temperament as

> constitutionally based individual differences in emotional, motor, and attentional reactivity and self-regulation. Temperamental characteristics are seen to demonstrate consistency across situations, as well as relative stability over time.... In our characterization of temperament, reactivity and self-regulation are umbrella terms for psychological processes within the temperament domain. (Rothbart & Bates, 1998, p. 109)

The self-regulation aspect of temperament is operationalized as effortful control, whereas temperamental reactivity includes emotional reactivity and characteristics such as activity level.

THE ROLE OF EFFORTFUL CONTROL IN EMOTION REGULATION AND SOCIAL FUNCTIONING: CONCEPTUAL ISSUES

Eisenberg (2002; Eisenberg & Morris, 2002) has defined "emotion-related regulation" as the process of initiating, avoiding, inhibiting, maintaining, or modulating the occurrence, form, intensity, or duration of internal feeling states, emotion-related physiological processes, emotion-related goals, and/or behavioral concomitants of emotion, generally in the service of accomplishing one's goals. She and her colleagues (Eisenberg, Fabes, Guthrie, & Reiser, 2000; Eisenberg & Morris, 2002) have suggested that effortful control plays a central role in emotion-related regulation. For example, when people are experiencing (or are likely to experience) negative emotions, they often use attentional processes, such as distracting themselves by shifting their attention to something else or simply breaking off input from the fear-inducing stimuli (e.g., Sandler, Tein, & West, 1994). They also may use inhibitory control, for example, to mask the expression of negative emotion or to inhibit their aggressive impulses when angered. Moreover, the planning capacities linked to effortful control (or executive attention) can be viewed as contributing to attempts to cope actively with stress—that is, active coping (Sandler et al., 1994) or engagement coping (Compas, Connor-Smith, & Saltzman, 2001). In stressful situations, or when experiencing negative emotion, people also may need to force themselves to take action that will ameliorate the situation; that is, they may use activational control.

Eisenberg (2002; Eisenberg & Morris, 2002) has attempted to differentiate what she has labeled as "emotion-related regulation" from less voluntary, reactive emotion-related processes. Recall that she defines "emotion-related regulation" as involving the abilities to manage attention, motivation, and behavior voluntarily (cognitions may also be changed in an attempt to regulate emotion). She argues that this sort of regulation should be differentiated from the general construct of "control," defined in the dictionary as inhibition or restraint. Although voluntarily managed inhibition (or control) is part of emotion-related regulation (i.e., what Rothbart has labeled "inhibitory control"), inhibition often may be involuntary or so automatic that it usually is not under voluntary control. For example, the behaviorally inhibited children studied by Kagan (1998), who were wary and overly constrained in novel or stressful contexts, seemed to have difficulty modulating their inhibition. Similarly, the impulse to activate behavior and approach people or things in the environment often may be relatively nonvoluntary—for example, people may be "pulled" toward rewarding or positive situations, with little ability to inhibit themselves. Like other emotion researchers (e.g., Cole, Michel, & Teti, 1994), Eisenberg (2002; Eisenberg, Spinrad, & Morris, 2002) argues that optimal emotion-related regulation is flexible and can be modulated so that a person is not overly controlled or out of control. Regulated individuals should be able to respond in a spontaneous manner in contexts in which such reactions are acceptable, and also able to rein in their approach or avoidant tendencies, when appropriate.

The biological or temperamental systems related to less voluntary approach or inhibition have sometimes been labeled as "reactive systems" (Derryberry & Rothbart, 1997), which include impulsivity and surgent approach behavior (perhaps based on reward dominance; Gray, 1975, 1987) or, at the other extreme, very low impulsivity and high inhibition. Whereas effortful control appears to be seated primarily in the anterior cingulate gyrus (in the paleocortex; Posner & DiGirolamo, 2000), Pickering and Gray (1999) and others (Cacioppo, Gardner, & Berntson, 1999; Derryberry & Reed, 1994) have argued that approach–avoidance motivational systems related to impulsive (undercontrolled) and overly inhibited behaviors are associated with subcortical systems, such as Gray's behavioral inhibition system (BIS; which is activated in situations involving novelty and stimuli signaling punishment or frustrative nonreward) and the behavioral activation system (BAS; which involves sensitivity to cues of reward or cessation of punishment). According to Gray (Pickering & Gray, 1999), impulsive behavior is associated with high BAS and relatively low BIS functioning, whereas the BIS system inhibits behavior (e.g., due to fear of punishment). Fowles (1987), Patterson and Newman (1993), DePue and Collins (1999), and others have proposed variations of Gray's BAS/BIS systems; nonetheless, numerous researchers (such as these) discuss separate (albeit related) social withdrawal and social facilitation (or approach) systems.

Effortful control and reactive control are conceptually and statistically related (e.g., Eisenberg, Fabes, & Shepard, 1997), in part because people viewed as impulsive are likely to be especially low in effortful control. If impulsive people were not low in effortful control, they could inhibit the overt expression of their impulsive tendencies. However, a person might be prone to high impulsive (or inhibition) motivational tendencies and partly manage their overt expression with effortful control. Indeed, in Rothbart's

(Rothbart & Bates, 1998) theory of temperament, effortful control processes (i.e., regulation) serve to manage reactive (including emotional) processes (see Rothbart et al., Chapter 18, this volume).

Unfortunately, in research on regulation, it often is difficult to know whether one is assessing effortful control or reactive impulsivity or behavioral inhibition. Some measures clearly tap executive attention (e.g., Stroop-type tasks) or the child's ability to focus attention (e.g., attention focusing scale; Rothbart et al., 2001) or voluntarily inhibit behavior (stop-and-go tasks; e.g., Kochanska et al., 2000; Oosterlaan, Logan, & Sergeant, 1998; or an inhibitory control scale; Rothbart et al., 2001). However, for some tasks, reactive tendencies or effortful control (or both) may affect performance. For example, in Mischel's (e.g., Shoda, Mischel, & Peake, 1990) delay of gratification tasks, children are presented with tempting commodities (e.g., candy, pretzels) and left alone with them for some period of time. They are told that they can eat the reward without waiting or wait for a period of time, after which they will be given a larger number of rewards. Children who wait often seem to use attentional strategies, such as distracting themselves by playing with, or looking at, other objects (or perhaps singing, or a similar activity). Thus, delay of gratification likely involves both effortful attentional control and the ability to inhibit the urge to take the desirable commodity. However, the reward also may activate impulsive reactive tendencies, such that children may be pulled toward the reward with little voluntary control. Therefore, children who cannot delay may be high in impulsive tendencies, whereas those who delay their gratification may be moderate or low in impulsive tendencies. More generally, when a measure of regulation involves rewards, it may be difficult or impossible to determine whether the individual's behavior reflects effortful control or reactive tendencies. This problem should be kept in mind when we review the relevant literature on the correlates of effortful control because the measures often used to assess effortful control (or regulation) may also tap reactive tendencies.

DEVELOPMENT OF EFFORTFUL CONTROL

In tracing the development of executive attention and effortful control, Rothbart and colleagues (Derryberry & Rothbart, 1997; Posner & Rothbart, 1998; Rothbart & Bates, 1998) have differentiated between attentional systems that are largely reactive and those that appear to denote self-regulatory mechanisms (i.e., effortful processes). The former system is present very early in life and is evident in behaviors such as infants' orienting responses to novelty, early attentional persistence, duration and latency of orienting, and early state control. This early attentional system is thought to be controlled by the brain's posterior orienting systems involved in orienting to sensory stimuli.

Rothbart and colleagues have proposed that the attentional processes involved in effortful control (i.e., executive attention) develop later than the posterior attentional system. Executive attention is viewed as being involved not only in the abilities to willfully focus and shift attention as needed to adapt, but also in inhibitory control and activational control (i.e., the abilities to inhibit or activate behavior as needed, especially when one is not inclined to do so). As already noted, this second system is thought to be centered primarily in anterior cingulate gyrus.

Posner and Rothbart (1998) believe there is modest development in the anterior attentional system around the second half of the first year of life, although this system is believed to be quite immature in the child's first couple of years of life. Indeed, the capacity for effortful control is believed to increase markedly in the preschool years and may continue to develop into adulthood (Murphy, Eisenberg, Fabes, Shepard, & Guthrie, 1999; Posner & Rothbart, 1998; Williams, Ponesse, Schachar, Logan, & Tannock, 1999).

Early evidence of executive attention, which is a large part of effortful control, has been demonstrated in infancy and toddlerhood. Between 9 and 18 months of age, attention becomes more voluntary (Ruff & Rothbart, 1996) as infants learn to resolve conflicts (e.g., when processing information), correct errors, and plan new actions (Posner & Rothbart, 1998). Diamond (1991), for example, has shown that, around 12 months of age, infants develop the ability to inhibit predominant responses and are, therefore, able to control their behavior. For example, she found that 12-month-olds are able to reach for a target not in their line of sight, which shows that they are able to coordinate reach and vision, and attend to both. Also during this developmental transition, Diamond found that infants were able to inhibit predominant response tendencies, an ability believed to involve the execution of intentional behavior, planning, and the resistance of more automatic action tendencies.

According to Posner and Rothbart (1998), another transition in the development of executive attention (and inhibition of related behavior) can be seen around 30 months of age. Using a Stroop-like task that requires toddlers to switch attention and inhibit behavior accordingly, Posner and Rothbart reported that children showed significant improvement in performance by 30 months of age and performed with high accuracy by 36–38 months of age. Moreover, toddlers' ability on this sort of task, which improved from age 24 to 36 months, was positively related to parents' ratings of attention-shifting abilities at 30 and 36 months of age (Gerardi-Caulton, 2000).

The ability to inhibit behavior on command is typically not much in evidence until 24–36 months of age (Rothbart & Bates, 1998). Kochanska and colleagues (2000) developed a battery of effortful control tasks designed to measure five components of effortful control: delaying, slowing down motor activity, suppressing or initiating activity to signal, lowering the voice, and effortful attention. Kochanska and colleagues demonstrated significant improvement in children's effortful control between 22 and 33 months of age; Gerardi-Caulton (2000) found improvement on a different Stroop task in children from 24 to 36 months. Other researchers have shown that children's ability to inhibit behavior effortfully on tasks such as "Simon Says" appears to emerge at approximately 44 months and is fairly good by 4 years of age (Posner & Rothbart, 1998; Reed, Pien, & Rothbart, 1984).

Interestingly, relatively few data exist on the interindividual (i.e., correlational) stability of effortful control in the early years of life. However, Kochanska and colleagues found that effortful control observed at 22 months substantially predicted effortful control at both 33 months (Kochanska et al., 2000) and 45 months (Kochanksa & Knaack, 2002). Moreover, early focused attention has been shown to predict later effortful control (Kochanska et al., 2000). In addition, teachers' and parents' reports of aspects of effortful control have been found to be relatively stable over 4, or sometimes 6, years during childhood (especially for attention focusing and inhibitory control, but less so for attention shifting; Murphy et al., 1999). Given her longitudinal findings of stability from toddlerhood through preschool and into early school years (Kochanska & Knaack, 2002; Kochanska, Murray, & Coy, 1997), Kochanska has compared the stability of effortful control to the stability of IQ. According to Kochanska and colleagues (2000), the robust stability findings in their work indicate a trait-like quality of effortful control and support Rothbart and Bates's (1998) view of effortful control as a temperamental characteristic.

RELATIONS OF EFFORTFUL CONTROL
TO DEVELOPMENTAL OUTCOMES

Because of its purported role in emotion-related regulation and in the ability to suppress or initiate socially appropriate or desirable behaviors, effortful control is believed to play an important role in the development of a wide range of socioemotional outcomes, including negative emotionality, internalized compliance, the development of a conscience, prosocial behavior, empathy-related responding, social competence, and adjustment (see Eisenberg, Fabes, et al., 2000; Kopp, 1982; and the references below). Due to space limitations, our review is illustrative rather than exhaustive, and we include few studies with adults. However, we try to highlight the major findings and bodies of work. Moreover, we do not include studies in which measures of regulation or control clearly tapped diverse constructs, such as social competence or aspects of adjustment.

Relations to Emotionality

Researchers have been interested in whether effortful control is related to lower negative emotionality in children. In work with young children, attention shifting or focusing has been associated with a decrease in distress in infancy. For example, 4-month-old infants who demonstrated high levels of refocusing attention away from one location to another were less distressed in laboratory situations (Rothbart, Ziaie, & O'Boyle, 1992). Harman, Rothbart, and Posner (1997) found that distress displayed by 3- to 6-month-old infants in response to overstimulation decreased when infants attended to interesting visual and auditory events (which may have involved some intentional shift of attention); however, once the distraction was removed, the infants' level of distress returned to the level before the distraction. In addition, Matheny, Riese, and Wilson (1985) demonstrated that infants' focused attention to objects was concurrently related to better regulated negative affect and more positive affect at 9 months. In another investigation, 8- to 10-month-olds who were capable of longer focused attention during block play exhibited less discomfort and fewer anger reactions in response to aversive stimuli (Kochanska, Coy, Tjebkes, & Husarek, 1998).

Some findings with young children more clearly suggest that effortful attentional control is involved in the regulation of negative emotion. For example, 18-month-olds who showed relatively high distress during a frustration task were less likely than their peers to use adaptive regulation strategies, which included distracting their attention away from the source of the frustration (Calkins & Johnson, 1998). Calkins, Dedmon, Gill, Lomax, and Johnson (2002) recruited two groups of 6-month-old infants based on a composite score of their level of frustration in laboratory tasks and maternal report. Compared to the group of infants who were not easily frustrated, easily frustrated infants exhibited less focused attention during an attention task and showed less attentional regulation during frustration tasks (i.e., they were less likely to distract their attention away from the focal object). In a study with 4- to 6-year-olds, Eisenberg and colleagues (1993) found that teachers' reports of attentional effortful control were negatively related to their reports of children's negative emotionality. Thus, attentional processes appear to be linked to negative emotionality in the first years of life and contribute to infants', toddlers', and preschoolers' attempts to regulate negative emotions.

Other measures of regulation (besides attentional control) also seem to be related to children's emotionality. Gerardi-Caulton (2000) found that 30- and 36-month-olds' delay scores on a spatial conflict (Stroop-like) task were negatively related to parents' ratings of the toddlers' anger and frustration. In addition, Kochanka and colleagues (2000) found that at 22 and 33 months, toddlers who performed better on a composite measure of effortful control tasks—many of which involved inhibitory or activational control—also expressed less intense anger at the same ages during frustrating situations. Toddlers who showed higher levels of effortful control also expressed less intense joy during a positive task, but this association was found only at 33 months. Furthermore, Kochanska and Knaack (2003) noted that toddlers who were more emotionally intense (more prone to display anger and joy at 14 and 22 months of age) scored lower on a composite measure of effortful control tasks at 22, 33, and 45 months of age. Not only were there concurrent associations between emotional intensity and effortful control, but the toddlers' emotional intensity also predicted effortful control at ages 22–45 months. Kochanska and Knaack believe that executive attention may be a common developmental antecedent to both early emotional system and effortful control. Alternatively, effortful control may help children to regulate emotions, and/or children high in negative emotionality may have more difficulty than their more placid peers in developing effortful control.

The association between effortful control and negative emotionality also has been noted in middle childhood and adulthood. Adults' reports of elementary school children's effortful control (Eisenberg, Fabes, et al., 1998; Eisenberg et al., 1999) and their self-reports of effortful control or regulation of emotion (Derryberry & Rothbart, 1988; Eisenberg et al., 1994) have been linked to relatively low levels of reported negative emotionality. Moreover, delay of gratification in preschool children has predicted their ability to deal with frustration in adolescence (Mischel, Shoda, & Peake, 1988).

Relations to Delay of Gratification

Preschoolers' use of attentional regulation during delay-of-gratification tasks is related to their ability to control behavior. For example, children who are able to wait to touch an attractive toy tend to use distraction as a strategy (Raver, Blackburn, Bancroft, & Torp, 1999). Also suggestive of a link between effortful attentional processes and delay of gratification, Mischel and Baker (1972) found that providing children with strategies to divert their attention helped them to delay gratification. Furthermore, toddlers' use of effective attentional strategies to cope with maternal separation (e.g., distraction) has predicted their use of effective delay-of-gratification strategies at age 5 (Sethi, Mischel, Aber, Shoda, & Rodriguez, 2000). Thus, as mentioned previously, performance on a delay-of-gratification task may depend at least partly on differences in children's effortful control, although it also may tap impulsive (reactive) tendencies. Nonetheless, because of the role of effortful control in delay of gratification, we review some studies that assess regulation with delay-of-gratification measures.

Relations to Compliance

Many researchers interested in young children's regulation have focused on toddlers' or preschoolers' compliance. In regard to the attentional capacities, Kochanska, Tjebkes, and Forman (1998) found that early focused attention at 8–10 months was related to committed compliance, which is an index of children's internalized compliance, at 14 months. In addition, attentional regulation (defined as looking away from the mother and focusing attention on objects in the room) at 4 months during a still face procedure with mothers was positively associated with higher rates of committed compliance and lower rates of situational compliance (compliance motivated only by external forces, as opposed to internalized compliance) when the children were 36 months of age (Hill & Braungart-Rieker, 2002).

Similar relations seem to hold when effortful control has been assessed in toddlers and young children. In longitudinal studies of compliance, inhibitory effortful control, measured through a battery of effortful control tasks, has been related to observed committed compliance in toddlerhood and the preschool years (Kochanska, Coy, & Murray, 2001; Kochanska et al., 1997). The context of the compliance situation is also important: Effortful control has been found to be more strongly linked to committed compliance to requests to suppress a desired action ("don't" contexts) than to requests to initiate and sustain a mundane activity ("do" contexts; Kochanska et al., 2001) for which relations were more modest. As suggested by Kochanska, by multiple reasons, suppressing behavior may be easier for younger children than initiating and sustaining a mundane activity. Young children may have more experience in situations in which they are not allowed to do something because parents enforce prohibitions early in their children's lives; therefore, children's self-regulatory skills may develop earlier in response to prohibitions than "do" commands. Also, sustaining an undesired behavior may require more behavioral control than suppressing a prohibited behavior. Moreover, children's abilities in "don't" situations may be especially related to their ability to self-regulate emotions because many "don't" situations involve high levels of potential frustration or anger (anger at having to put toys away, or frustration at not being able to play with attractive toys).

Relations to Moral Development

Measures of effortful control or related constructs have been linked to the development of conscience, empathy-related responding, and prosocial behavior.

Conscience

In regard to the development of conscience, Kochanska and colleagues (1997) found that effortful control and conscience were positively related at each age (i.e., in concurrent analyses at toddler, preschool, and early school age), and that effortful control at all three ages predicted early conscience in school-age children. Measures of conscience in children included ratings on items reflecting dimensions of moral self (such as concern about others' wrongdoing, apology, and empathy), responses to hypothetical moral dilemmas, internalization of their mothers' rules, internalization of the experimenter's rules (not cheating at a game while the experimenter was not in the room), and internalization of the experimenter's rules in a peer context (not cheating on a game while the experimenter was not in the room but two other children were also present). Kochanska and Knaack (2003), who were able to replicate the results of Kochanska and colleagues, found that effortful control at ages 22, 33, and 45 months, as well as the composite score of effortful control across those ages, predicted a more internalized conscience at age 56 months. In this study, measures of conscience included ratings of children's moral self, internalization of their mothers' rules, and internalization of the experimenter's rules.

Few investigators have assessed the relation between conscience and effortful control in older children. However, Rothbart and colleagues (1994) found that parents' reports of children's effortful control were associated with their reports of their 7-year-old children's tendencies to experience guilt. In addition, Krueger, Caspi, Moffitt, White, and Stouthamer-Loeber (1996) found a modest relation between a behavioral measure of early adolescents' delay of gratification and parents' reports of the child showing "con-cern about what's right and what's wrong" (e.g., "He tries to be fair"; p. 122).

Empathy and Prosocial Behavior

Eisenberg and colleagues have hypothesized that individuals high in effortful regulation would be expected to experience sympathy (an other-oriented response to another's emotion or condition) rather than personal distress (i.e., a self-focused, aversive response to another's emotional state or condition) because empathic overarousal is aversive and leads to a self-focus and self-concern (rather than concern for others; see Eisenberg, Wentzel, & Harris, 1998). Consistent with this premise, relations between effortful control and empathy-related responding have been found in studies with both children and adults. For example, Guthrie and colleagues (1997) asked parents and teachers to rate 5- to 8-year-old children's effortful regulation using select items from Rothbart's Children's Behavior Questionnaire (CBQ; Rothbart et al., 2001). Guthrie and colleagues videotaped children watching an evocative film about a young girl burned during a home fire (and teased by peers for her appearance). Finally, after the film, they probed children's reactions to the film by having them rate their feelings during the film, using simple adjectives and scales. Guthrie and colleagues found that children who were rated high on effortful regulation exhibited greater facial sadness during the film than did children who were rated low in effortful control. Children's postfilm reports of sadness and sympathy to the film were also positively correlated with parents' ratings of regulation. Conversely, children low in parent-related effortful regulation were prone to experience personal distress (e.g., anxiety, tension) during the film. In another study, facial concern when viewing an empathy-inducing film was correlated with teachers' ratings of children's high attentional control (Eisenberg & Fabes, 1995). Taken together, these findings indicate children higher in effortful control were more likely than those lower in such control to exhibit sadness and sympathy in response to viewing the distressing situation.

Effortful control also has been positively related to self- or other-report measures of empathy/sympathy. Eisenberg, Fabes, Murphy, and colleagues (1996), Murphy and colleagues (1999), and Rothbart, Ahadi, and Hershey (1994) have all found links between children's effortful control (as assessed through parents' and teachers' reports; e.g., on the CBQ; Rothbart et al., 2001) and parents' reports of sympathy or children's self-reported empathy or sympathy. In some of this work, effortful control (or a composite comprised mostly of effortful control and low impulsivity) predicted sympathy over 2 or 4 years (e.g., Murphy et al., 1999). Similar concurrent relations have been noted in studies in which adults reported on their own sympathy and regulation (Eisenberg & Okun, 1996), although sometimes the association was not significant until the effects of individual differences in negative emotionality were controlled (Eisenberg et al., 1994; Okun, Shepard, & Eisenberg, 2000). In addition, effortful control has been negatively related to adults' reports of personal distress (Eisenberg et al., 1994; Eisenberg & Okun, 1996).

Consistent with the relation between effortful control and sympathy/empathy, adults' ratings of elementary school children's effortful attentional control and/or a behavioral measure assessing effortful control (and perhaps impulsivity, to some degree) have been correlated with peers' ratings of prosocial behavior in two studies (Eisenberg, Fabes, Karbon, et al., 1996; Eisenberg, Guthrie, et al., 1997), as well as with preschoolers' peer- and teacher-reported agreeableness (including niceness, sharing, and helpfulness; Cumberland et al., in press). Thus, individuals who can regulate their emotion and behavior are more likely not only to experience sympathy but also to act in morally desirable ways with others.

Social Competence and Adjustment

In general, measures that likely tap effortful control have been positively related to children's adjustment and social competence (see Vohs & Ciarocco, Chapter 20, this volume). In one of the most relevant longitudinal studies to examine this issue, at ages 3 and 5, children's lack of control—likely a combination of effortful control, low reactive control, and negative emotionality (e.g., variables such as fleeting attention, emotional lability)—was rated from their behaviors when performing a variety of tasks (e.g., Henry, Caspi, Moffitt, Harrington, & Silva, 1999). In addition, at age 3, children were classified into various personality types based, in part, on this index of lack of control (the undercontrolled group was characterized primarily by lack of control). Lack of control at age 3 or age 5 was positively associated with parents' and/or teachers' reports of externalizing (e.g., hyperactive behavior, inattention, antisocial behavior, or conduct disorder) and internalizing problems (anxiety/fearfulness) in late childhood (age 9 and/or 11) and adolescence (age 13 and/or 15), and negatively related with the number of children's strengths (e.g., parents' and teachers' ratings of caring, mature, friendly, interested, determined, well behaved, enthusiastic, creative, confident, sense of humor, popular, cooperative, helpful, good at sports, clean, active) in adolescence (Caspi, Henry, McGee, Moffitt, & Silva, 1995). At age 18, the undercontrolled individuals scored high on measures of impulsivity, danger seeking, aggression, and interpersonal alienation (Caspi & Silva, 1995). At age 21, lack of control was related to number of criminal convictions for men and women, with this relation being stronger for men (but not women) who dropped out of school (Henry et al., 1999). In addition, undercontrolled children at age 3 were more antisocial at age 21 and had poorer social relations and high levels of interpersonal conflict (Newman, Caspi, Moffitt, & Silva, 1997). They also were less likely to be employed in adolescence and had more psychiatric disorders at age 21 (Caspi, 2000; Caspi, Moffitt, Newman, & Silva, 1996). Similarly, in another study in which the measure of regulation reflected a combination of behavioral and attentional regulation and moodiness (e.g., the child is impulsive, lacks concentration, and changes mood), Pulkkinen and Hamalainen's (1995) index of weak self-control at age 14 predicted criminal offenses at age 20 and amount of criminal behavior at age 32 (see also Pulkkinen, 1982, 1987).

Although the measure of undercontrol used in the aforementioned studies likely assessed impulsivity and emotionality as well as effortful control, other investigators have obtained similar results using somewhat purer measures of effortful control. Moreover, the links between effortful control and social competence or adjustment have been noted at an early age. For example, preschoolers who used more attentional strategies (self-distraction) during a delay task were rated by their teachers as higher in social competence, and peers tended to rate them as popular and average rather than as rejected or neglected (Raver et al., 1999). Furthermore, adults' ratings of preschoolers' and kindergarteners' effortful attention shifting and focusing have been associated with children's socially appropriate behavior, boys' (but not girls') peer status, and children's constructive coping with real-life incidents involving negative emotion at preschool (Eisenberg et al., 1993, 1994). In addition, teachers' and/or mothers' reports of attentional control at this age often predicted children's social functioning and prosocial/social behavior at school 2, 4, and 6 years later (Eisenberg, Fabes, Murphy, et al., 1995; Eisenberg, Fabes, et al., 1997; Murphy, Shepard, Eisenberg, & Fabes, in press).

Effortful control and related constructs also have been linked with social competence in older samples of children. For example, Olson (1989) found that children who could delay gratification at age 4–5 years were relatively unlikely to be perceived negatively by peers concurrently and 1 year later. This relation held for inhibitory control only at age 5–6 (and there were no significant relations with positive peer nominations). Eisenberg, Guthrie, and colleagues (1997) also found an association between peer nominations for social status and teachers' and parents' reports of elementary school children's attentional control, as well as a behavioral measure of persistence (rather than cheating or being off-task). In this same study, children's adult-rated effortful attentional control and performance on a behavioral task generally were related to teachers' ratings of socially appropriate behavior (at two points in time, and especially for children prone to negative emotions; Eisenberg, Fabes, et al., 2000; Eisenberg, Guthrie, et al., 1997). In Mischel's (Mischel et al., 1988; Mischel, Shoda, & Rodriguez, 1989) longitudinal study, delay of gratification at age 4 or 5 predicted parent-reported social competence and coping with problems in adolescence. For vulnerable children (those who were sensitive to rejection), the ability to delay gratification predicted better peer relationships (lower peer rejection and aggression), higher self-worth in middle school children, and lower use of drugs in adulthood (Ayduk et al., 2000).

Consistent with the findings of Caspi (2000), low effortful control has been rather consistently linked to problems with adjustment from a relatively young age (e.g., Kyrios & Prior, 1990). For example, Calkins and Dedmon (2000) examined the differences between a group of 2-year-olds at risk for problem behaviors (i.e., who had a t score greater than 60 on the Child Behavior Checklist Externalizing Problems scale) and a group of toddlers at low risk (a t score of less than 50). When compared to low-risk children, high-risk toddlers engaged in less regulated behavior, including high rates of distraction and low attention to challenging tasks, as well as more negative affect. In addition, Kochanska and Knaack (2003) found that children's lack of effortful control (as measured by a battery of tasks at 22, 33, and 45 months) was related to increased mother-reported behavior problems at 73 months. Lemery, Essex, and Snider (2002) found that mothers' reports of children's attention focusing and inhibitory control (averaged across ratings provided when the children were 3.5 and 4.5 years of age) predicted mothers' and fathers' reports of externalizing problems and attention-deficit/hyperactivity disorder at age 5.5 years. In contrast, Eisenberg and colleagues (Eisenberg, Fabes, Murphy, Maszk, et al. 1995; Eisenberg, Fabes, et al., 1997; Murphy et al., in press) found that parents' reports of children's externalizing behavior in elementary school were only occasionally predicted by parents' (but not teachers') reports of attentional control in preschool or kindergarten. However, mothers' and fathers' reports of externalizing problems in elementary school were much more consistently predicted by mothers' (but not teachers') reports of effortful control (including attentional control, inhibitory control, and low impulsivity), either concurrently or earlier in elementary school (Eisenberg, Fabes, Murphy, Maszk, et al., 1995; Eisenberg, Fabes, et al., 1997; Murphy et al., in press). At age 9 to 12 years, children's conduct problems (child- and parent-reported) consistently were negatively related to their attention focusing (child- and parent-reported; Lengua, West, & Sandler, 1998).

In a different longitudinal study, Eisenberg, Fabes, Guthrie, and colleagues (1996) examined the relations of both adult-reported attentional effortful control (shifting and focusing) and behavior control (including adult-reported inhibitory control and low levels of reactive undercontrol, as well as a behavioral measure of regulation and low impulsivity) to school children's externalizing behaviors. At a 2-year follow-up, both types of regulation–control provided unique prediction of externalizing behavior, even when controlling for prior levels of regulation (Eisenberg, Guthrie, et al., 2000). In another sample, children with teacher- and parent-reported externalizing problems tended to be low in adult-reported attentional effortful control and inhibitory control, as well as in behavioral measures of persistence and inhibitory control (e.g., persisting on a puzzle task rather than cheating, sitting still when asked to do so). Similarly, schoolchildren's externalizing problems have been associated with low delay of gratification (Krueger, Caspi, Moffitt, White, & Stouthamer-Loeber, 1996), with the inability to inhibit behavior on signal (Oosterlaan et al., 1998; Oosterlaan & Sergeant, 1996), and with parents' reports of effortful control (Rothbart, Ahadi, & Hershey, 1994).

Other investigators have linked effortful control (or related measures) to delinquency. White and colleagues (1994) assessed preteen boys' "impulsivity" through a variety of behavioral and cognitive tasks and reports from parents, teachers, and participants. The behavioral measures tapped a range of actions subsumed under effortful control (e.g., inhibition via the Trail Making Test; attention via the Stroop task) and likely tapped effortful control as much, or more, than reactive impulsivity. What the authors labeled as "behavioral impulsivity" (e.g., observer-rated motor restlessness, teacher-rated impulsivity) was more highly related to delinquent behavior than was cognitive impulsivity (e.g., performance on the Stroop task and on the Trail Making Test, circle tracing), although both composite measures were correlated with delinquency at ages 10 and 13 (with only the former contributing unique variance to prediction; see also Lynam, 1997, for analyses predicting psychopathy with the same sample). In another study that included an assessment of cognitive and behavioral regulation–impulsivity, 6- to 16-year-old boys with externalizing problems were higher than controls on both cognitive and behavioral impulsivity–effortful control, but especially on the latter (Mezzacappa, Kindlon, & Earls, 1999). Furthermore, Olson, Schilling, and Bates (1999) found some modest negative relations between behavioral measures of inhibitory control or delay of gratification and aggressive or hyperactive behavior at ages 6 and 8 (however, sample sizes were small, so power was low; also see Olson, 1989).

Findings in regard to the relation between effortful control and internalizing problems are less consistent. Mothers' reports of preschoolers' attention-focusing and inhibitory control have been modestly negatively related with internalizing problems when the children were 5.5 years old, and these relations held even when items that overlapped between the constructs of regulation and internalizing problems were removed from the scales (Lemery et al., 2002). Young school-age children with internalizing problem have been found to be low in adult-rated attentional control (Eisenberg, Cumberland, et al., 2001); 9- to 12-year-olds' child- or parent-reported depressive symptoms have been correlated with low levels of child- and parent-reported attention focusing (Lengua et al., 1998); shyness has been linked to teachers', but not parents', reports of low effortful attentional control (Eisenberg, Shepard, Fabes, Murphy, & Guthrie, 1998). Moreover, children high in test anxiety demonstrate some difficulties in selective attention (e.g., they are biased to look at threatening words; Vasey, El-Hag, & Daleiden, 1996). However, Krueger and colleagues (1996) did not find a relation between delay of gratification and young adolescents' internalizing problems.

Nonlinear relations between attentional control and social competence also have been found. Specifically, attentional regulation has been found to interact with emotionality to predict later social behavior. Belsky, Friedman, and Hsieh (2001) concluded that observed attentional persistence moderated the relation of negative emotionality to mothers' ratings of social competence (but not problem behavior, perhaps due to the nature of the measure). In particular, high levels of negative emotionality at age 15 months predicted lower social competence at age 3, but only for toddlers classified as low in attentional persistence. Similarly, in elementary school, negative and/or general emotionality has been found to moderate the relation between effortful control and social functioning at school, such that regulation predicts the quality of social functioning at school for all children, but more so for those prone to intense emotions (Eisenberg, Fabes, Shepard, et al., 1997). Analogous interactions have been found when predicting schoolchildren's externalizing problems from measures of effortful control (sometimes combined with indexes of reactive undercontrol) and negative emotional intensity (e.g., Eisenberg, Fabes, Guthrie, et al., 1996; Eisenberg, Guthrie, et al., 2000). In addition, some initial evidence indicates that the relation between parents' reports of their children's shyness and negative emotional intensity was greater for children with low ability to shift attention (Eisenberg, Shepard, et al., 1998). Finally, because dispositional impulsivity is corrected with alcohol use (Colder & Chassin, 1997; Stice & Gonzales, 1998) and has been found to moderate the relations of positive emotionality (Colder & Chassin, 1997) and depression (Hussong & Chassin, 1994) to alcohol use and/or impairment, it seems likely that effortful control predicts substance/alcohol use and moderates the relation of emotionality to substance and alcohol abuse (see also Wills, Windle, & Cleary, 1998).

Cognitive and Academic Outcomes

It is reasonable to hypothesize that early cognitive development is fostered by the abilities to focus attention and persist at tasks. Similarly, academic achievement likely necessitates the behaviors implicit in our working definition of effortful control. For instance, one must be able to maintain attention to succeed at academic tasks and to continue working on tasks when more appealing options are available.

Consistent with these propositions, the limited available research suggests an association between effortful control and cognitive/academic performance. For example, measures of executive functioning and inhibitory control have been linked to children's understanding of the mental states of others (i.e., theory of mind; Carlson & Moses, 2001; Hughes, 1998). Moreover, Mischel and colleagues (1990) and Shoda and colleagues (1990) found that preschool-age children's ability to delay gratification during a task in which they were exposed to a reward predicted high Scholastic Aptitude Test (SAT) scores in adolescence. In adulthood, sensitivity to rejection was linked to attaining a lower level of education, but only for individuals who had been low in delay of gratification many years earlier (Ayduk et al., 2000).

Summary

Although the relevant literature is not entirely consistent, there is mounting evidence that individual differences in effortful control are linked to a variety of important developmental outcomes. It seems likely children's relative lack of ability to regulate their attention effectively puts them at risk for behavior problems, either directly or indirectly, through deficits in the ability to regulate negative emotions. Children high in effortful control tend to exhibit relatively low levels of negative emotion, high committed compliance, high social competence, high levels of conscience and prosocial responding, high academic success, and low levels of problem behaviors and delinquency or criminality (concurrently or at older ages). In contrast, researchers have found that children with low effortful control tend to be at risk for social, moral, academic, emotional, and psychological problems. Thus, it appears that effortful control contributes to the emergence of desirable patterns of behavior in the toddler and early years, and also is involved in the continued development and maintenance of positive emotional, social, and cognitive development.

THE SOCIALIZATION OF EFFORTFUL CONTROL

According to Kopp (1989), successful regulation of behavior in infants and young children can be indexed by how closely the children meet familial and social conventions. Infants and young children must have external support for regulating their behavior, and the development of self-regulation involves give-and-take between the children's needs and caregivers' behaviors (Kopp, 1989; see also Calkins, Chapter 16, this volume). Consistent with Kopp's theorizing, although effortful control likely has relatively strong hereditary and constitutional origins, the socialization practices of parents have been linked to children's abilities to regulate attention and their inhibitory control.

Socialization in the Toddler and Preschool Years

Several investigators have documented associations between parenting and young children's effortful control (or related measures). Calkins and Johnson (1998) found links between 18-month-old infants' regulatory strategies and their mothers' behavior. Toddlers who were more likely to use distraction and constructive coping during frustrating situations had mothers who were more likely to use positive guiding behaviors as opposed to more negative and directive behaviors. In a follow-up on this sample, Calkins, Smith, Gill, and Johnson (1998) found that maternal positive- and negative-caregiving strategies during mother–child interaction were related to the regulatory strategies employed by the children during emotion-eliciting tasks at 24 months of age. Mothers with more directive and controlling caregiving styles had children who used less adaptive regulatory strategies. When frustrated, these children were more likely to orient to and manipulate an object they had been prohibited from using, and were less likely to distract themselves from the denied object. Similarly, Calkins and colleagues found that the mothers of easily frustrated 6-month-olds (who used less distraction in a frustrating task and displayed less attention during attention tasks than nonfrustrated infants; Calkins et al., 2002) were less sensitive, more intrusive, and provided less physical stimulation to the infants than did mothers of nonfrustrated infants (Calkins, Gill, Dedmon, Johnson, & Lomax, 2000).

Consistent with Calkins's findings, Gilliom, Shaw, Beck, Schonberg, and Lukon (2002) found that warm and supportive (vs. hostile and punitive) parenting when children were 1½ years old predicted children's ability to shift attention from a source of frustration at age 3½. Similarly, Olson, Bates, and Bayles (1990) found that a secure attachment at age 13 months predicted boys' inhibitory and attentional control (including a number of behavioral measures and delay of gratification); observed nonpunitive, nonrestrictive parenting also predicted boys' effortful control at age 6. Those same maternal variables did not predict effortful control for girls, although maternal verbal stimulation was positively related with girls' regulation. Furthermore, Kyrios and Prior (1990), in a study using quite different measures, found that mothers' reports of the use of rewards during socialization efforts at approximately age 3 were negatively related to concurrent maternal reports of their children's temperamental persistence and soothability (believed to reflect temperamental self-regulation), and children's temperamental self-regulation mediated the relation of maternal use of rewards to later adjustment problems.

Kochanska and colleagues (2000) have obtained similar results. They found that maternal responsiveness to children at 22 months, measured by the quality of maternal responses to the toddlers' bids, predicted effortful control at both 22 and 33 months. It may be that the responsiveness supports children's autonomy, which has positive implications for their self-regulatory abilities. Conversely, mothers' use of power-assertive discipline, which reflects low sensitivity and lack of support for autonomy, was related to low levels of young children's effortful control. In turn, effortful control appeared to mediate the relation between parental use of power assertion and children's later conscience development (Kochanska & Knaack, 2003). Results from these studies indicate that children with mothers who are controlling and relatively low in positive affect and behavior may have trouble shifting and regulating attention, which could foster poorer self-regulation later or in different situations.

In addition, Kochanska and colleagues (2000) found that mothers who rated themselves higher on a socialization scale (e.g., ratings of acceptance of cultural norms, patience, and persistence) had toddlers who exhibited higher effortful control. Thus, in this study, not only were the mothers' behaviors during interactions with their children important, but mothers' own ability to follow rules and show patience was also a predictor of effortful control. Thus, it appears that toddlers may be learning some aspects of effortful control by modeling the same behavior in mothers, and/or effortful control may have a genetic component (see Goldsmith, Buss, & Lemery, 1997).

Researchers have also examined the relation between maternal behavior and children's ability to delay their behavior during delay tasks. As discussed earlier, children who are able to control their attention frequently do better at delay tasks; however, young children often need external regulation to learn how to divert their attention away from desirable objects. Putnam, Spritz, and Stifter (2002) found that toddlers who focused on something other than the prohibited item during a delay showed more restraint in regard to touching the prohibited object. However, the toddlers did not spontaneously attend to other aspects in the environment. Instead, this behavior frequently occurred in response to maternal directives to do so.

Whereas maternal directives might help children learn the skill of distraction, the quality of the maternal directives is very important. Silverman and Ippolito (1995) found that delay ability at age 2 was negatively related to mothers' use of directives in free play and takeovers during a teaching task, and positively related to feedback in a teaching task. Given these findings, and those on links between maternal behavior and attentional control, maternal directives issued in a positive manner may be necessary to help children learn to self-regulate.

In addition to the quality of the mothers' behavior, children's response to maternal behavior is important in predicting their self-regulation abilities. For example, Sethi and colleagues (2000) found an interaction between toddlers' response to maternal bids and maternal control when predicting children's ability to demonstrate delay during the late preschool years. Toddlers' response to maternal bids was defined as whether toddlers approached the mother after she made a bid (i.e., an attempt to initiate interaction), or whether toddlers explored at a distance following the bids (i.e., did not approach). The authors reasoned that it is more appropriate for toddlers with low-controlling mothers to approach after bids than not to approach (i.e., these toddlers should want to engage their mothers). In contrast, it is more appropriate for toddlers of controlling mothers to disengage after maternal bids. Furthermore, the children's pattern of behavior regulation with their mothers predicted their delay ability at a later assessment. Toddlers with more controlling mothers, who responded to maternal control by exploring away from their mothers, showed relatively longer delays, less hot focus (i.e., less of a focus on the rewards and the bell), and more cool focus (i.e., a focus away from the reward and bell). Toddlers with less controlling mothers, who approached their mothers after maternal bids, also exhibited less hot focus, more cool focus, and longer delays. This pattern of findings suggests that there is more than one socialization-related pathway to developing self-regulation. In the case of overly controlling and intrusive mothers, it may be more adaptive for toddlers to develop strategies of focusing their attention away from the maternal bids. Sethi and colleagues concluded that the link between maternal control and self-regulation (shown by longer delay capacity) may be mediated by the ability to use attention effectively. However, it also is possible that the ability to use attention underlies both the use of strategies that help toddlers to delay and toddlers' strategies for dealing with overcontrolling mothers.

Socialization in the School Years

Research on the socialization correlates of effortful control in childhood and adolescence is limited. Much of this work deals with the relations between parents' expression of emotion and children's regulation. For example, Eisenberg, Gershoff, and colleagues (2001) examined the relation between children's effortful control and mothers' reports of their positive and negative expressivity (expression of emotion) in the family, and their positive and negative emotion in an interaction with their child. Children were ages 4.5 to just turning 8 years. Children's effortful control was assessed with parents' and teachers' ratings on Rothbart's CBQ scales for attention shifting, attention focusing, and inhibitory control, and a behavioral measure of persistence rather than cheating on a rewarded puzzle task. The adult-reported ratings likely reflected mostly effortful control, whereas the puzzle task might have tapped effortful control and impulsivity. In a structural equation modeling (SEM) analysis, as well as in correlations, mothers' positive expressivity (including mother-reported and observed measures of positive emotion) was positively related to their children's effortful control, whereas mothers' negative expressivity (including the reported and observed measure) was negatively related to effortful control.

Similar measures were obtained 2 years later (Eisenberg, Valiente, et al., 2003). Mothers' reports of their own positive expression of emotion were associated with teachers' and their own reports of children's regulation in the expected directions (but not with persistence on the box task). Observed maternal positive emotion expressed with the child (negative emotion was too infrequent to use) was positively related with teachers', but not mothers', reports of children's effortful control. Observed positive expressivity at the first assessment also was correlated with persistence on the box task 2 years later. In a concurrent SEM model at the follow-up, positive maternal expressivity was positively related to effortful control. Moreover, in regression analyses (but not SEM analyses, likely due in part to weaker power in the SEM), there was evidence that this relation held over time when researchers controlled for initial levels of the variables. Unexpectedly, at the second assessment, mothers' negative expressivity was no longer negatively related to children's effortful control (except for maternal reports); indeed, it was positively related to teacher-reported effortful control. This finding is similar to that reported by Greenberg (personal communication, July 2, 2001), in which parental negative expressivity was related to teachers' reports of children's compliance at school (perhaps because compliant children are likely to be viewed as regulated by teachers).

In a similar study, in which parental expressivity was assessed only with parents' reports (primarily mothers'), parental negative expressivity, but not positive expressivity, was associated with low levels of Indonesian third graders' effortful regulation (Eisenberg, Liew, & Pidada, 2001). Moreover, mother-reported positive expressivity in the family has been related to higher levels of toddlers' self-soothing behavior, whereas mother-reported sadness was inversely related (Garner, 1995; see Garner & Power, 1996, for more mixed findings). In a study with 11- and 12-year-olds, Brody and Ge (2001) found that parental nurturance/support versus negativity—a construct that likely included more than just parental emotional expressivity—predicted children's self-control at two points in time; children's self-control was assessed with teachers' reports (e.g., their ability to plan, pay attention to tasks, finish a job without an adult watching). Furthermore, college students and adults from negatively expressive families reported less control than their peers over feelings of anger, even when the intensity of anger was controlled statistically (Burrowes & Halberstadt, 1987). Thus, although the findings are not entirely consistent (e.g., Greenberg, Lengua, Coie, & Pinderhughes, 1999), in general, positive parental expression of emotion and parental warmth have been linked to regulation indexes likely to partly (or fully) tap effortful control, whereas parental negative expression of emotion has been negatively related.

Parental discipline also has been linked to children's effortful control. Zhou, Eisenberg, Wang, and Reiser (in press) found positive relations of Chinese schoolchildren's effortful control with parents' (but not teachers') reports of authoritative parenting (e.g., involving warmth, reasoning, and democratic participation). In addition, teachers' and parents' reports of regulation were negatively related to children's effortful control. Consistent with the latter finding, parents' (usually mothers') punitive reactions or self-focused distressed reactions to children's displays of emotion have been related to low levels of schoolchildren's effortful control (including inhibitory control, attention focusing, low impulsivity, and a self-control scale; Eisenberg, Fabes, et al., 1999). Similarly, Gottman, Katz, and Hoover (1997) found that parents who were supportive in regard to encouraging the appropriate expression of emotion and coaching children about their emotions had children who were relatively high in regulation (as assessed with parents' reports of their need to help their children calm themselves when aroused and children's physiological vagal tone). Thus, in general, supportive parenting (including support for children's expressivity) seems to be positively related to the development of effortful control.

In summary, initial findings are consistent with the view that shared environment (Goldsmith, Buss, & Lemery, 1997), including the quality of parenting, may contribute to the development of effortful control. Parental supportive directives, behaviors, and expression of positive emotion have been correlated with higher levels of effortful control in children. In addition, parental attempts to scaffold children's use of effective self-regulatory strategies, and their use of positive discipline, are associated with the level of children's effortful control. Thus, although effortful control has a genetic, temperamental basis, it likely can be fostered in interactions with socializers.

CONCLUSIONS

In the past decade, it has become increasingly clear that effortful control is intimately related to social, emotional, moral, and cognitive development in childhood. Of course, because the research generally is correlational in design, it is very difficult to prove causal relations. Nonetheless, researchers have found that early measures of effortful control (or measures including effortful control) predict a broad range of important outcomes in childhood and beyond. Moreover, relations between effortful control and emotionality, adjustment, and social competence are evident across childhood and at older ages. Thus, as was noted in a National Academy of Science (NAS) committee report, *From Neurons to Neighborhoods*, "The growth of self-regulation is a cornerstone of early childhood development that cuts across all domains of behavior" (Shonkoff & Phillips, 2000, p. 3). We would add that effortful control also plays a major role in many aspects of development after early childhood.

Findings also suggest that socialization in the home may contribute to the development of effortful control. It is possible that a number of effects of parental socialization on developmental outcomes are partly mediated through their relations to effortful control. However, experimental studies in which parents are trained to interact with their children in ways likely to foster effortful control are needed to prove a causal link. This is an important task for future study. Moreover, given the critical role of effortful control in many aspects of development, it is important that behavioral scientists find ways to stimulate its development outside of the home. Although some intervention/prevention researchers have designed programs to foster emotion regulation (e.g., Greenberg, Kusche, Cook, & Quamma, 1995), much more could, and should, be done in this domain.

ACKNOWLEDGMENT

This research was supported by Grant No. 1 R01 MH60838 from the National Institute of Mental Health to Nancy Eisenberg and Richard Fabes, and by Grant No. DA05227 from the National Institute on Drug Abuse to Laurie Chassin and Nancy Eisenberg.

REFERENCES

Ahadi, S. A., & Rothbart, M. K. (1994). Temperament, development, and the Big Five. In C. F. Halverson, Jr. & G. A. Kohnstamm (Eds.), *The developing structure of temperament and personality from infancy to adulthood* (pp. 189–207). Hillsdale, NJ: Erlbaum.

Ahadi, S. A., Rothart, M. K., & Ye, R. (1993). Children's temperament in the US and China: Similarities and differences. *European Journal of Personality, 7,* 359–377.

Ayduk, O., Mendoza-Denton, R., Mischel, W., Downey, G., Peake, P. K., & Rodriguez, M. (2000). Regulating the interpersonal self: Strategic self-regulation for coping with rejection sensitivity. *Journal of Personality and Social Psychology, 79,* 776–792.

Belsky, J., Friedman, S. L., & Hsieh, K. H. (2001). Testing a core emotion-regulation prediction: Does early attentional persistence moderate the effect of infant negative emotionality on later development? *Child Development, 72,* 123–133.

Brody, G. H., & Ge, X. (2001). Linking parenting processes and self-regulation to psychological functioning and alcohol use during early adolescence. *Journal of Family Psychology, 15,* 82–93.

Burrowes, B. D., & Halberstadt, A. G. (1987). Self- and family-expressiveness styles in the experience and expression of anger. *Journal of Nonverbal Behavior, 11,* 254–268.

Cacioppo, J. T., Gardner, W. L., & Berntson, G. G. (1999). The affect system has parallel and integrative processing components: Form follows function. *Journal of Personality and Social Psychology, 76,* 839–855.

Calkins, S. D., & Dedmon, S. E. (2000). Physiological and behavioral regulation in two-year-old children with aggressive/destructive behavior problems. *Journal of Abnormal Child Psychology, 28,* 103–118.

Calkins, S. D., Dedmon, S. E., Gill, K. L., Lomax, L. E., & Johnson, L. M. (2002). Frustration in infancy: Implications for emotion regulation, physiological processes, and temperament. *Infancy, 3,* 175–197.

Calkins, S. D., Gill, K., Dedmon, S., Johnson, L., & Lomax, L. (April, 2000). *Mothers' interactions with temperamentally frustrated infants.* Poster presented at the 12th Biennial International Conference on Infant Studies, Brighton, UK.

Calkins, S. D., & Johnson, M. J. (1998). Toddler regulation of distress to frustrating events: Temperamental and maternal correlates. *Infant Behavior and Development, 21*(3), 379–395.

Calkins, S. D., Smith, C. L., Gill, K. L., & Johnson, M. C. (1998). Maternal interactive style across contexts: Relations to emotional, behavioral, and physiological regulation during toddlerhood. *Social Development, 7*(3), 350–369.

Carlson, S. M., & Moses, L. J. (2001). Individual differences in inhibitory control and children's theory of mind. *Child Development, 72,* 1032–1053.

Caspi, A. (2000). The child is the father of the man: Personality continuities from childhood to adulthood. *Journal of Personality and Social Psychology, 78,* 158–172.

Caspi, A., Henry, B., McGee, R. O., Moffitt, T. E., & Silva, P. (1995). Temperamental origins of child and adolescent behavior problems: From age three to age fifteen. *Child Development, 66,* 55–68.

Caspi, A., Moffitt, T. E., Newman, D. L., & Silva, P. A. (1996). Behavioral observations at age 3 predict psychiatric disorders: Longitudinal evidence from a birth cohort. *Archives of General Psychiatry, 53,* 1033–1039.

Caspi, A., & Silva, P. (1995). Temperamental qualities at age three predict personality traits in young adulthood: Longitudinal evidence from a birth cohort. *Child Development, 66,* 486–498.

Colder, C. R., & Chassin, L. (1997). Affectivity and impulsivity: Temperament risk for adolescent alcohol involvement. *Psychology of Addictive Behaviors, 11,* 83–97.

Cole, P. M., Michel, M. K., & Teti, L. O. (1994). The development of emotion regulation and dysregulation: A clinical perspective. In N. A. Fox (Ed.), *Monographs of the Society for Research in Child Development 59* (Serial No. 240, pp. 73–100). Chicago: University of Chicago Press.

Compas, B. E., Connor-Smith, J. K., & Saltzman, H. (2001). Coping with stress during childhood and adolescence: Problems, progress, and potential in theory and research. *Psychological Bulletin, 127,* 87–127.

Cumberland, A., Eisenberg, N., & Reiser, M. (in press). Relations of young children's agreeableness and resiliency to effortful control, impulsivity, and social competence. *Social Development.*

DePue, R. A., & Collins, P. F. (1999). Neurobiology of the structure of personality: Dopamine, facilitation of incentive motivation, and extraversion. *Behavioral and Brain Sciences, 22,* 491–599.

Derryberry, D., & Reed, M. A. (1994). Temperament and attention: Orienting toward and away from positive and negative signals. *Journal of Personality and Social Psychology, 66,* 1128–1139.

Derryberry, D., & Rothbart, M. K. (1988). Arousal, affect, and attention as components of temperament. *Journal of Personality and Social Psychology, 55,* 958–966.

Derryberry, D., & Rothbart, M. K. (1997). Reactive and effortful processes in the organization of temperament. *Development and Psychopathology, 9,* 1997, 633–652.

Diamond, A. (1991). Neuropsychological insights into the meaning of object concept development. In S. Carey & R. Gelman (Eds.), *The epigenesis of mind: Essays on biology and cognition* (pp. 67–110). Hillsdale, NJ: Erlbaum.

Eisenberg, N. (2002). Emotion-related regulation and its relation to qualify of social functioning. In W. W. Hartup & R. A. Weinberg (Eds.), *Child psychology in retrospect and prospect: In celebration of the 75th anniversary of the Institute of Child Development* (Vol. 32, pp. 133–171). Mahwah, NJ: Erlbaum.

Eisenberg, N., Cumberland, A., Spinrad, T. L., Fabes, R. A., Shepard, S. A., Reiser, M., Murphy, B. C., Losoya, S. H., & Guthrie, I. K. (2001). The relations of regulaton and emotionality to children's externalizing and internalizing problem behavior. *Child Development, 72,* 1112–1134.

Eisenberg, N., & Fabes, R. A. (1995). The relation of young children's vicarious emotional responding to social competence, regulation, and emotionality. *Cognition and Emotion*, 9, 203–229.

Eisenberg, N., Fabes, R. A., Bernzweig, J., Karbon, M., Poulin, R., & Hanish, L. (1993). The relations of emotionality and regulation to preschoolers' social skills and sociometric status. *Child Development*, 64, 1418–1438.

Eisenberg, N., Fabes, R. A., Guthrie, I., Murphy, B. C., Maszk, P., Holmgren, R., & Suh, K. (1996). The relations of regulation and emotionality to problem behavior in elementary school children. *Development and Psychopathology*, 8, 141–162.

Eisenberg, N., Fabes, R. A., Guthrie, I. K., & Reiser, M. (2000). Dispositional emotionality and regulation: Their role in predicting quality of social functioning. *Journal of Personality and Social Psychology*, 78, 136–157.

Eisenberg, N., Fabes, R. A., Karbon, M., Murphy, B. C., Wosinski, M., Polazzi, L., Carlo, G., & Juhnke, C. (1996). The relations of children's dispositional prosocial behavior to emotionality, regulation, and social functioning. *Child Development*, 67, 974–992.

Eisenberg, N., Fabes, R. A., & Murphy, B. C. (1995). Relations of shyness and low sociability to regulation and emotionality. *Journal of Personality and Social Psychology*, 68, 505–517.

Eisenberg, N., Fabes, R. A., Murphy, B., Karbon, M., Maszk, P., Smith, M., O'Boyle, C., & Suh, K. (1994). The relations of emotionality and regulation to dispositional and situational empathy-related responding. *Journal of Personality and Social Psychology*, 66, 776–797.

Eisenberg, N., Fabes, R. A., Murphy, B., Karbon, M., Smith, M., & Maszk, P. (1996). The relations of children's dispositional empathy-related responding to their emotionality, regulation, and social functioning. *Developmental Psychology*, 32, 195–209.

Eisenberg, N., Fabes, R. A., Murphy, B., Maszk, P., Smith, M., & Karbon, M. (1995). The role of emotionality and regulation in children's social functioning: A longitudinal study. *Child Development*, 66, 1360–1384.

Eisenberg, N., Fabes, R. A., Shepard, S. A., Murphy, B. C., Guthrie, I. K., Jones, S., Friedman, J., Pulin, R., & Maszk, P. (1997). Contemporaneous and longitudinal prediction of children's social functioning from regulation and emotionality. *Child Development*, 68, 642–664.

Eisenberg, N., Fabes, R. A., Shepard, S. A., Guthrie, I. K., Murphy, B. C., & Reiser, M. (1999). Parental reactions to children's negative emotions: Longitudinal relations to quality of children's social functioning. *Child Development*, 70, 513–534.

Eisenberg, N., Fabes, R. A., Shepard, S. A., Murphy, B. C., Jones, S., & Guthrie, I. K. (1998). Contemporaneous and longitudinal prediction of children's sympathy from dispositional regulation and emotionality. *Developmental Psychology*, 34, 910–924.

Eisenberg, N., Gershoff, E. T., Fabes, R. A., Shepard, S. A., Cumberland, A. J., Lososya, S. H., Guthrie, I. K., & Murphy, B. C. (2001). Mothers' emotional expressivity and children's behavior problems and social competence: Mediation through children's regulation. *Developmental Psychology*, 37, 475–490.

Eisenberg, N., Guthrie, I. K., Fabes, R. A., Resier, M., Murphy, B. C., Holmgren, R., Maszk, P., & Losoya, S. (1997). The relations of regulation and emotionality to resiliency and competent social functioning in elementary school children. *Child Development*, 68, 367–383.

Eisenberg, N., Guthrie, I. K., Fabes, R. A., Shepard, S., Losoya, S., Murphy, B. C., Jones, S., Poulin, R., & Reiser, M. (2000). Prediction of elementary school children's externalizing problem behaviors from attentional and behavioral regulation and negative emotionality. *Child Development*, 71, 1367–1382.

Eisenberg, N., Liew, J., & Pidada, S. (2001). The relations of parental emotional expressivity with the quality of Indonesian children's social functioning. *Emotion*, 1, 107–115.

Eisenberg, N., & Morris, A. S. (2002). Children's emotion-related regulation. In R. Kail (Ed.), *Advances in child development and behavior* (Vol. 30, pp. 90–229). Amsterdam: Academic Press.

Eisenberg, N., & Okun, M. A. (1996). The relations of dispositional regulation and emotionality to elders' empathy-related responding and affect while volunteering. *Journal of Personality, 64,* 157–183.

Eisenberg, N., Shepard, S. A., Fabes, R. A., Murphy, B. C., & Guthrie, I. K. (1998). Shyness and children's emotionality, regulation, and coping: Contemporaneous, longitudinal, and across-context relations. *Child Development, 69,* 767–790.

Eisenberg, N., Spinrad, T. L., & Morris, A. S. (2002). Regulation, resiliency, and quality of social functioning. *Self and Identity, 1,* 121–128.

Eisenberg, N., Valiente, C., Morris, A. S., Fabes, R. A., Cumberland, A., Reiser, M., Gershoff, E. T., Shepard, S. A., & Losoya, S. (2003). Longitudinal relations among parental emotional expressivity, children's regulation, and quality of socioemotional functioning. *Developmental Psychology, 39,* 2–19.

Eisenberg, N., Wentzel, M., & Harris, J. D. (1998). The role of emotionality and regulation in empathy-related responding. *School Psychology Review, 27,* 506–521.

Ellis, L. K., & Rothbart, M. K. (1999). *Early Adolescent Temperament Questionnaire—Revised Short Form.* Unpublished document, University of Oregon, Eugene.

Fowles, D. C. (1987). Application of a behavioral theory of motivation to the concepts of anxiety and impulsivity. *Journal of Research in Personality, 21,* 417–435.

Garner, P. W. (1995). Toddlers' emotion regulation behaviors: The roles of social context and family expressiveness. *Journal of Genetic Psychology, 156,* 417–430.

Garner, P. W., & Power, T. G. (1996). Preschoolers' emotional control in the disappointment paradigm and its relation to temperament, emotional knowledge, and family expressiveness. *Child Development, 67,* 1406–1419.

Gerardi-Caulton, G. (2000). Sensitivity to spatial conflict and the development of self-regulation in children 24–36 months of age. *Developmental Science, 3,* 397–404.

Gilliom, M., Shaw, D. S., Beck, J. E., Schonberg, M. A., & Lukon, J. L. (2002). Anger regulation in disadvantaged preschool boys: Strategies, antecedents, and the development of self-control. *Developmental Psychology, 38,* 222–235.

Goldsmith, H. H., Buss, K. A., & Lemery, K. S. (1997). Toddler and childhood temperament: Expanded content, stronger genetic evidence, new evidence for the importance of environment. *Developmental Psychology, 33,* 891–905.

Goldsmith, H. H., Buss, K. A., & Lemery, K. S. (1997). Toddler and childhood temperament: Expanded content, stronger genetic evidence, new evidence for the importance of environment. *Developmental Psychology, 33,* 891–905.

Gottman, J. M., Katz, L. F., Hooven, C. (1997). *Meta-emotion: How families communicate emotionally.* Mahwah, NJ: Erlbaum.

Gray, J. A. (1975). *Elements of a two-process theory of learning.* New York: Academic Press.

Gray, J. A. (1987). Perspectives and anxiety and impulsivity: A commentary. *Journal of Research in Personality, 21,* 493–509.

Greenberg, M. T., Kusche, C. A., Cook, E. T., & Quamma, J. P. (1995). Promoting emotional competence in school-aged children: The effects of the PATHS curriculum. *Development and Psychopathology, 7,* 117–136.

Greenberg, M. T., Lengua, L. J., Coie, J. D., & Pinderhughes, E. E. (1999). Predicting developmental outcomes at school entry using a multiple-risk model: Four American communities. *Developmental Psychology, 35,* 403–417.

Guthrie, I. K., Eisenberg, N., Fabes, R. A., Murphy, B. C., Holmgren, R., Maszk, P., & Suh, K. (1997). The relations of regulation and emotionality to children's situational empathy-related responding. *Motivation and Emotion, 21,* 87–108.

Harman, C., Rothbart, M. K., & Posner, M. I. (1997). Distress and attention interactions in early infancy. *Motivation and Emotion, 21,* 27–43.

Henry, B., Caspi, A., Moffitt, T. E., Harrington, H., & Silva, P. (1999). Staying in school protects boys with poor self-regulation in childhood from later crime: A longitudinal study. *International Journal of Behavioral Development, 23,* 1049–1073.

Hill, A. L., & Braungart-Rieker, J. M. (2002). Four-month attentional regulation and its prediction of three-year compliance. *Infancy, 3,* 261–273.

Hughes, C. (1998). Finding your marbles: Does preschoolers' strategic behavior predict later understanding of mind? *Developmental Psychology, 34,* 1326–1339.

Hussong, A. M., & Chassin, L. (1994). The stress-negative affect model of adolescent alcohol use: Disaggregating negative affect. *Journal of Studies in Alcohol, 55,* 707–718.

Kagan, J. (1998). Biology and the child. In W. Damon (Series Ed.) & N. Eisenberg (Vol. Ed.), *Handbook of child psychology: Vol. 3. Social, emotional and personality development* (pp. 177–235). New York: Wiley.

Kochanska, G., Coy, K. C., & Murray, K. T. (2001). The development of self-regulation in the first four years of life. *Child Development, 72,* 1091–1111.

Kochanska, G., Coy, K. C., Tjebkes, T. L., & Husarek, S. J. (1998). Individual differences in emotionality in infancy. *Child Development, 64,* 375–390.

Kochanska, G., & Knaack, A. (2003). Effortful control as a personality characteristic of young children: Antecedents, correlates, and consequences. *Journal of Personality, 71,* 1087–1112.

Kochanska, G., Murray, K., & Coy, K. C. (1997). Inhibitory control as a contributor to conscience in childhood: From toddler to early school age. *Child Development, 68,* 263–277.

Kochanska, G., Murray, K. L., & Harlan, E. T. (2000). Effortful control in early childhood: Continuity and change, antecedents, and implications for social development. *Developmental Psychology, 36,* 220–232.

Kochanska, G., Tjebkes, T. L., & Forman, D. R. (1998). Children's emerging regulation of conduct: Restraint, compliance, and internalization from infancy to the second year. *Child Development, 69,* 1378–1389.

Kopp, C. B. (1982). Antecedents of self-regulation: A developmental perspective. *Developmental Psychology, 18,* 199–214.

Kopp, C. B. (1989). Regulation of distress and negative emotions: A developmental view. *Developmental Psychology, 25,* 343–354.

Krueger, R. F., Caspi, A., Moffitt, T. E., White, J., & Stouthamer-Loeber, M. (1996). Delay of gratification, psychopathology, and personality: Is low self-control specific to externalizing problems? *Journal of Personality, 64,* 107–129.

Kyrios, M., & Prior, M. (1990). Temperament, stress and family factors in behavioural adjustment of 3-5-year-old children. *International Journal of Behavioral Development, 13,* 67–93.

Lemery, K. S., Essex, M. J., & Snider, N. A. (2002). Revealing the relation between temperament and behavior problem symptoms by eliminating measurement confounding: Expert ratings and factor analyses. *Child Development, 73,* 867–882.

Lengua, L. J., West, S. G., & Sandler, I. N. (1998). Temperament as a predictor of symptomatology in children: Addressing contamination of measures. *Child Development, 69,* 164–181.

Lynam, D. R. (1997). Pursuing the psychopath: Capturing the fledgling psychopath in a nomological net. *Journal of Abnormal Psychology, 106,* 425–438.

Matheny, A. P., Riese, M. L., & Wilson, R. S. (1985). Rudiments of infants' temperament: Newborn to 9 months. *Developmental Psychology, 21,* 486–494.

Mezzacappa, E., Kindlon, D., & Earls, F. (1999). Relations of age to cognitive and motivational elements of impulse control in boys with and without externalizing behavior problems. *Journal of Abnormal Child Psychology, 27,* 473–483.

Mischel, W., & Baker, N. (1972). Cognitive appraisals and transformations in delay behavior. *Journal of Personality and Social Psychology, 31,* 254–261.

Mischel, W., Shoda, Y., & Peake, P. K. (1988). The nature of adolescent competencies predicted by preschool delay of gratification. *Journal of Personality and Social Psychology, 54,* 687–696.

Mischel, W., Shoda, Y., & Rodriguez, M. L. (1989). Delay of gratification in children. *Science, 244,* 933–938.

Murphy, B. C., Eisenberg, N., Fabes, R. A., Shepard, S., & Guthrie, I. K. (1999). Consistency and change in children's emotionality and regulation: A longitudinal study. *Merrill–Palmer Quarterly, 46*, 413–444.

Murphy, B. C., Shepard, S. A., Eisenberg, N., & Fabes, R. A. (in press). Concurrent and across time prediction of young adolescents' social functioning: The role of emotionality and regulation. *Social Development.*

Newman, D. L., Caspi, A., Moffitt, T. E., & Silva, P. (1997). Antecedents of adult interpersonal functioning: Effects of individual differences in age 3 temperament. *Developmental Psychology, 33*, 206–217.

Okun, M. A., Shepard, S. A., & Eisenberg, N. (2000). The relations of emotionality and regulation to dispositional empathy-related responding among volunteers-in-training. *Personality and Individual Differences, 28*, 367–382.

Olson, S. L. (1989). Assessment of impulsivity in preschoolers: Cross-measure convergences, longitudinal stability, and relevance to social competence. *Journal of Clinical Child Psychology, 18*, 176–183.

Olson, S. L., Bates, J. E., & Bayles, K. (1990). Early antecedents of childhood impulsivity: The role of parent–child interaction, cognitive competence, and temperament. *Journal of Abnormal Child Psychology, 18*, 317–334.

Olson, S. L., Schilling, E. M., & Bates, J. E. (1999). Measurement of impulsivity: Construct coherence, longitudinal stability, and relationship with externalizing problems in middle childhood and adolescence. *Journal of Abnormal Child Psychology, 27*, 151–165.

Oosterlaan, J., Logan, G. D., & Sergeant, J. A. (1998). Response inhibition in AD/HD, CD, comorbid AD/HD + CD, anxious, and control children: A meta-analysis of studies with the stop task. *Journal of Child Psychology and Psychiatry and Allied Disciplines, 39*, 411–425.

Oosterlaan, J., & Sergeant, J. A. (1996). Inhibition in ADHD, aggressive, and anxious children: A biologically based model of child psychopathology. *Journal of Abnormal Child Psychology, 24*, 19–36.

Patterson, C. M., & Newman, J. P. (1993). Reflectivity and learning from aversive events: Toward a psychological mechanism for the syndromes of disinhibition. *Psychological Review, 100*, 716–736.

Pickering, A. D., & Gray, J. A. (1999). The neuroscience of personality. In L. A. Pervin & O. P. John (Eds.), *Handbook of personality: Theory and research* (2nd ed., pp. 277–299). New York: Guilford Press.

Posner, M. I., & DiGirolamo, G. J. (2000). Cognitive neuroscience: Origins and promise. *Psychological Bulletin, 126*, 873–889.

Posner, M. I., & Rothbart, M. K. (1998). Attention, self-regulation, and consciousness. *Transactions of the Philosophical Society of London, B*, 1915–1927.

Posner, M. I., & Rothbart, M. K. (2000). Developing mechanisms of self-regulation. *Development and Psychopathology, 12*, 427–441.

Pulkkinen, L. (1982). Self-control and continuity from childhood to late adolescence. In P. B. Baltes & O. G. Brim, Jr. (Eds.), *Life-span development and behavior* (Vol. 4, pp. 63–105). New York: Academic Press.

Pulkkinen, L. (1987). Offensive and defensive aggression in humans: A longitudinal pespective. *Aggressive Behavior, 13*, 197–212.

Pulkkinen, L., & Hamalainen, M. (1995). Low self-control as a precursor to crime and accidents in a Finnish longitudinal study. *Criminal Behaviour and Mental Health, 5*, 424–438.

Putnam, S. P., Spritz, B. L., & Stifter, C. A. (2002). Mother–child coregulation during delay of gratification at 30 months. *Infancy, 3*, 209–225.

Raver, C. C., Blackburn, E. K., Bancroft, M., & Torp, N. (1999). Relations between effective emotional self-regulation, attentional control, and low-income preschoolers' social competence with peers. *Early Education and Development, 10*, 333–350.

Reed, M., Pien, D. L., & Rothbart, M. K. (1984). Inhibitory self control in preschool children. *Merrill–Palmer Quarterly, 30*, 131–147.

Rothbart, M. K. (1989). Temperament and development. In G. A. Kohnstamm, J. E. Bates, & M. K. Rothbart (Eds.), *Temperament in childhood* (pp. 187–247). New York: Wiley.

Rothbart, M. K., Ahadi, S. A., & Hershey, K. L. (1994). Temperament and social behavior in childhood. *Merrill–Palmer Quarterly, 40*, 21–39.

Rothbart, M. K., Ahadi, S. A., Hershey, K. L., & Fisher, P. (2001). Investigations of temperament at three to seven years: The Children's Behavior Questionnaire. *Child Development, 72*, 1394–1408.

Rothbart, M. K., & Bates, J. E. (1998). Temperament. In W. Damon (Series Ed.) & N. Eisenberg (Vol. Ed.), *Handbook of child psychology: Vol. 3. Social, emotional, personality development* (pp. 105–176). New York: Wiley.

Rothbart, M. K., Derryberry, D., & Posner, M. I. (1994). A psychobiological approach to the development of temperament. In J. E. Bates & T. D. Wachs (Eds.), *Temperament: Individual differences at the interface of biology and behavior* (pp. 83–116). Washington DC: American Psychological Association.

Rothbart, M. K., Ziaie, H., & O'Boyle, C. G. (1992). Self regulation and emotion in infancy. *New Directions for Child Development, 55*, 7–23.

Ruff, H. A., & Rothbart, M. K. (1996). *Attention in early development.* New York: Oxford University Press.

Sandler, I. N., Tein, J., & West, S. G. (1994). Coping, stress, and the psychological symptoms of children of divorce: A cross-sectional and longitudinal study. *Child Development, 65*, 1744–1763.

Sethi, A., Mischel, W., Aber, J. L., Shoda, Y., & Rodriguez, M. L. (2000). The role of strategic attention deployment in development of self-regulation: Predicting preschoolers' delay of gratification from mother–toddler interactions. *Developmental Psychology, 36*, 767–777.

Shoda, Y., Mischel, W., & Peake, P. K. (1990). Predicting adolescent cognitive and self-regulatory competencies from preschool delay of gratification: Identifying diagnostic conditions. *Developmental Psychology, 26*, 978–986.

Shonkoff, J. P., Phillips, D. A. and the Committee on Integrating the Science of Early Childhood Development. (Eds.). (2000). *From neurons to neighborhoods: The science of early childhood development.* Washington, DC: National Academy of Science.

Silverman, I. W., & Ippolito, M. F. (1995). Maternal antecedents of delay ability in young children. *Journal of Applied Developmental Psychology, 16*, 569–591.

Stice, E., & Gonzales, N. (1998). Adolescent temperament moderates the relation of parenting to antisocial behavior and substance use. *Journal of Adolescent Research, 13*, 5–31.

Vasey, M. W., El-Hag, N., & Daleiden, E. L. (1996). Anxiety and the processing of emotionally threatening stimuli: Distinctive patterns of selective attention among high- and low-test-anxious children. *Child Development, 67*, 1173–1185.

White, J. L., Moffitt, T. E., Caspi, A., Bartusch, D. J., Needles, D. J., & Stouthamer-Loeber, M. (1994). Measuring impulsivity and examining its relationship to delinquency. *Journal of Abnormal Psychology, 103*, 192–205.

Wills, T. A., Windle, M., & Cleary, S. D. (1998). Temperament and novelty seeking in adolescent substance use: Convergence of dimensions of temperament with constructs from Cloninger's theory. *Journal of Personality and Social Psychology, 74*, 387–406.

Williams, B. R., Ponesse, J. S., Schachar, R. J., Logan, G. D., & Tannock, R. (1999). Development of inhibitory control across the life span. *Developmental Psychology, 35*, 205–213.

Zhou, Q. (2001). *Parental socialization of children's emotion-related regulation in the People's Republic of China.* Unpublished master's thesis, Arizona State University, Tempe.

Zhou, Q., Eisenberg, N., Wang, Y., & Reiser, M. (in press). Chinese children's effortful control and dispositional anger/frustration: Relations to parenting styles and children's social functioning. *Developmental Psychology.*

14

Attentional Control and Self-Regulation

M. ROSARIO RUEDA
MICHAEL I. POSNER
MARY K. ROTHBART

Self-regulation has been a central concept in developmental psychology and in the study of psychopathologies. According to a recent paper by Fonagy and Target (2002, p. 307), "Self-regulation is the key mediator between genetic predisposition, early experience and adult functioning." In their view, self-regulation refers to children's ability to "(1) control the reaction to stress, (2) capacity to maintain focused attention and (3) the capacity to interpret mental states in themselves and others." Self-regulation is also an obvious feature of normal socialization apparent to caregivers, teachers, and others who work with children.

A recent historical prospective and review of self-regulation (Bronson, 2000) outlined perspectives from psychoanalysis, social learning theory, Vygotsky, Piaget (including neo-Piagetians), and the information-processing tradition. Each of these approaches seeks to account for how children achieve the ability to regulate their emotions, and to an extent, their thought processes.

In this chapter, we stress recent efforts to develop a neurological basis for self-regulation based on the use of neuroimaging, studies of the assessment of attention from questionnaires (see Rothbart & Bates, 1998; Rothbart, Ellis & Posner, Chapter 18, this volume), and individual differences in performance on attention tasks that can be used to define phenotypes for genetic analysis (Fossella, Posner, Fan, Swanson, & Pfaff, 2002). Although we talk about the neural networks related to self-regulation, our goal is not to review the field, as Bronson (2000) has done, but to provide an example of one analysis based on imaging and genetic studies that may prove to be relevant to all of the theoretical perspectives cited by Bronson.

ATTENTION AS SELF-REGULATION

The study of attention has been a central topic from the start of human experimental psychology (Broadbent, 1958; Titchener, 1909). Generally, the focus has been on probing fundamental mechanisms, by training or instructions, to perform tasks that call for various attentional functions, such as remaining vigilant to external events, selecting among concurrent information, processing difficult targets, or ignoring conflicting signals.

A usually unstated idea related to these studies is that by controlling the focus of attention through instructions, one can observe the properties of mechanisms that would also be used during self-motivated performance. For example, artificial displays can be developed, in which the small movements and luminance cues thought to invoke a shift of attention are eliminated. Under these conditions, subjects are very often unaware of large and significant changes in a scene, when they occur away from the current focus of attention (Rensink, O'Regan, & Clark, 1997). The understanding that arises from these studies is that, in the natural world, where movement and luminance cues are present, these cues automatically summon attention and, thus, underlie our subjective impression of attending to the whole scene. Similarly, when cues are introduced to direct attention covertly (without any eye or head movement) to a visual location, either automatically or voluntarily (Posner, 1980), the resulting mechanisms (Corbetta & Shulman, 2002) are also thought to be active during voluntary searches of the visual world, or prior to voluntary eye movements (saccades).

Due largely to the development of neuroimaging in humans and cellular recording in nonhuman primates, an understanding of the specific neural networks that underlie these shifts of attention has emerged (Corbetta & Shulman, 2002; Desimone & Duncan, 1995). Studies using both functional magnetic resonance imaging (fMRI) and cellular recording have demonstrated that a number of brain areas, such as the superior parietal lobe and temporal parietal junction, play a key role in modulating the activity within primary and extrastriate visual systems. Thus, attention acts to control or regulate the visual input that then exercises a strong influence on behavior.

Many of the best studies of the regulatory aspect of attention involve modulation of sensory systems. However, many fMRI studies have suggested that the regulatory effects of attention are common to all or most areas of the brain (Posner & Raichle, 1994, 1998). This finding suggests that the principles studied so intensively in the regulation of sensory input by attention apply just as well to brain areas involved in the processing of the semantics of words, storing information in memory, and generating emotions such as fear and sadness.

INTEGRATION

Although discussion of neural networks in the human brain has the potential for linking knowledge of the human brain with the efforts of educators and parents to socialize their young, until recently, these goals seemed remote. Two major developments changed the prospect for such integration.

First, neuroimaging combined with electrical or magnetic recordings from outside the skull allow us to see in real time the circuits computing sensory, semantic, and emotional response to input (Dale et al., 2000; Posner & Raichle, 1994, 1998). Although some aspects of this technology had been around for a long time, only in the last decade has it become clear that a new era has arrived: our ability to create local images of human brain activity through changes in cerebral blood flow. The second event was the sequencing of the human genome (Ventner et al., 2001), making it possible to study not only the functional anatomy of brain networks but also to examine how genetic differences might lead to individual variations in the potential to use these networks to acquire and perform skills.

Ruff and Rothbart (1996) attempted to integrate the study of attention and self-regulation in their volume on early development of attention. They viewed attention as "part of the larger construction of self-regulation—the ability to modulate behavior according to the cognitive, emotional and social demands of specific situations" (p. 7). They argued further that self-regulation places emphasis on inhibitory control, strategies of problem solving, memory, and self-monitoring. In addition to their argument that attention is a part of the mechanisms of self-regulation, Ruff and Rothbart discussed how the role of individual differences in attentional efficiency plays a part in the degree of successful self-regulation.

In previous work, we have stressed important results showing that some brain networks provide control operations that facilitate or inhibit the functions of other networks, providing a neural basis for self-regulation (Posner & Rothbart, 1998, 2000). For example, different parts of the cingulate gyrus have been involved in cognitive and emotional monitoring processes. Areas of the dorsal anterior cingulate are highly interconnected with lateral frontal and parietal structures, and become very active when a task requires selection among conflicting alternatives (Botvinick, Braver, Barch, Carter, & Cohen, 2001; Bush, Luu, & Posner, 2000). More ventral areas of the cingulate, in conjunction with other limbic structures (e.g., the amygdala), provide a basis for regulation of emotion (Bush et al., 2000; Drevets & Raichle, 1998). Despite these important technical advances, it is still a major task to isolate neural networks responsible for self-regulation by neuroimaging to observe how genes and environment regulate them during development. We have been involved in this effort for some time (Posner & Rothbart, 1998, 2000) and provide in this chapter an overview of our approach and findings.

Fonagy and Target (2002) have used a psychoanalytic framework to connect self-regulation to attachment. They argue that the attachment process allows children to develop a theory of the minds of other people. This mentalizing function in turn allows the child to operate successfully within society. There is evidence that effortful control, the individual-differences variable most closely related to executive attention, is highly correlated with aspects of theory of mind in middle childhood (Carlson & Moses, 2001). Similarly, Kochanska, Murray, Jacques, Koenig, and Vandegeest (1996) have identified developmental links between effortful control and the development of conscience.

The approach in this chapter follows the framework of Ruff and Rothbart (1996) but involves a more detailed analysis of the links between self-regulation and attention, available from more recent studies. The functions associated with the executive attention network overlap with the more general notion of executive functions in childhood. These functions include working memory, planning, switching, and inhibitory control (Welch, 2001). For example, "working memory," as defined by Baddeley (1986), included both storage and executive components, the same as what we refer to as "executive attention" in this chapter. Some functions of working memory and other executive functions are self-regulatory, and are carried out by brain structures that involve the executive attention network. However, we place emphasis on the monitoring and control functions of attention, without attempting to develop a strict boundary between these and other executive functions that may not emphasize attention.

ATTENTIONAL NETWORKS

Functional neuroimaging has allowed the analysis of many cognitive tasks in terms of the brain areas they activate. Attention studies have been among the tasks most often examined in this way (Corbetta & Shulman, 2002, Driver, Eimer, & Macaluso, in press; Posner & Fan, in press). Imaging data have supported the presence of three networks related to different aspects of attention. These networks carry out the functions of alerting, orienting, and providing executive control (Posner & Fan, in press). The anatomy and transmitters involved in the three networks are summarized in Table 14.1. "Alerting" is defined as achieving and maintaining a state of high sensitivity to incoming stimuli; "orienting" is the selection of information from sensory input; and "executive control" involves the mechanisms for monitoring and resolving conflict among thoughts, feelings, and responses.

The alerting system has been associated with frontal and parietal regions of the right hemisphere. A particularly effective way to vary alertness has been to use warning signals prior to presentation of targets. The influence of warning signals on the level of alertness is thought to be due to modulation of neural activity by the neurotransmitter norepinepherine (Marrocco & Davidson, 1998).

Orienting involves aligning attention with a source of sensory signals. This may be overt, as in eye movements, or may occur covertly, without any movement. The orienting system for visual events has been associated with posterior brain areas, including the superior parietal lobe, the temporal parietal junction, and, in addition, the frontal eye fields (Corbetta & Shulman, 2002). Orienting can be manipulated by presentation of a cue indicating where in space a person should attend, thereby directing attention to the cued location (Posner, 1980). Event-related fMRI studies have suggested that the superior parietal lobe is associated with orienting after the presentation of a cue (Corbetta & Shulman, 2002). The superior parietal lobe in humans is closely related to the lateral intraparietal area (LIP) in monkeys, which is known to produce eye movements (Anderson, 1989). When a target occurs at an uncued location and attention has to be disengaged and moved to a new location, there is activity in the temporal parietal junction (Corbetta & Shulman, 2002). Lesions of the parietal and superior temporal lobes have been consistently related to difficulties in orienting (Karnath, Ferber, & Himmelbach, 2001).

TABLE 14.1. Brain Areas and Neuromodulators Involved in Attention Networks

Function	Structures	Modulator
Orient	Superior parietal cortex Temporal parietal junction Frontal eye fields Superior colliculus	Acetylcholine
Alert	Locus coeruleus Right frontal and parietal cortex	Norepinephrine
Executive attention	Anterior cingulate Lateral ventral prefrontal Basal ganglia	Dopamine

Executive control of attention is often studied by tasks that involve conflict, such as various versions of the Stroop task (Bush et al., 2000), in which subjects must respond to the color of ink (e.g., red) while ignoring the color word name (e.g., blue). Resolving conflict in the Stroop task activates midline frontal areas (anterior cingulate) and lateral prefrontal cortex (Botvinick et al., 2001; Fan et al., 2003). There is also evidence for the activation of this network in tasks involving conflict between a central target and surrounding flankers that may be congruent or incongruent with the target (Botvinick et al., 2001; Fan et al., 2003). Experimental tasks may provide a means of fractionating the functional contributions of different areas within the executive attention network (MacDonald, Cohen, Stenger, & Carter, 2000).

Regulatory Functions of Attention

The anterior cingulate gyrus, one of the main nodes of the executive attention network, has been linked to a variety of specific functions in attention (Posner & Fan, in press), working memory (Duncan et al., 2000), emotion (Bush et al., 2000), pain (Rainville, Duncan, Price, Carrier, & Bushnell, 1997), and monitoring for conflict (Botvinick et al., 2001) and error (Holroyd & Coles, 2002). These functions have been well documented, but no single rubric seems to explain all of them. In studies of emotion, the cingulate is often seen as part of a network involving orbitofrontal and limbic (amygdala) structures. The frontal areas seem to have an ability to interact with the limbic system (Davidson, Putnam, & Larson, 2000) that might fit well with self-regulation.

A specific test of this idea involved subjects' exposure to erotic films, with the requirement to regulate any resulting arousal. The cingulate activity shown by fMRI was found to be related to the regulatory instruction (Beauregard, Levesque, & Bourgouin, 2001). In a different study, cognitive reappraisal of photographs producing negative affect showed a correlation between extent of cingulate activity and the reduction in negative affect (Ochsner, Bunge, Gross, & Gabrieli, 2002). Similarly, in a study in which hypnotism was used to control the perception of pain, the cingulate activity reflected the perception, not the strength, of the physical stimulus (Rainville et al., 1997). These results indicate a role for this anatomical structure in regulating limbic activity related to emotion, and provide evidence for a role of the cingulate as part of the network controlling affect (Bush et al., 2000).

In tasks such as the Stroop and flanker, conflict is introduced by the need to respond to one aspect of the stimulus, while ignoring another (Bush et al., 2000; Fan et al., 2003). Cognitive activity that involves this kind of conflict activates the dorsal anterior cingulate and lateral prefrontal cortex. Large lesions of the anterior cingulate in either adults (Damasio, 1994) or children (Anderson, Damasio, Tranel, & Damasio, 2000) result in great difficulty in regulating behavior, particularly in social situations. Smaller lesions may produce only a temporary inability to deal with conflict in cognitive tasks (Ochsner et al., 2001; Turken & Swick, 1999).

DEVELOPMENT OF ATTENTIONAL SELF-REGULATION

A major advantage of viewing attention in relation to self-regulation is that it allows one to relate the development of a specific neural network to the ability of children and adults to regulate their thoughts and feelings. Over the first few years of life, the regulation of emotion is a major issue of development. Panksepp (1998) laid out anatomical reasons why the regulation of emotion may pose a difficult problem for the child:

One can ask whether the downward cognitive controls or the upward emotional controls are stronger. If one looks at the question anatomically and neurochemically the evidence seems overwhelming. The upward controls are more abundant and electrophysiologically more insistent: hence one might expect they would prevail if push came to shove. Of course, with the increasing influence of cortical functions as humans develop, along with the pressures for social conformity, the influences of the cognitive forces increase steadily during maturation. We can eventually experience emotions without sharing them with others. We can easily put on false faces, which can make the facial analysis of emotions in real-life situations a remarkably troublesome business. (p. 319)

The ability of attention to control distress can be traced to early infancy (Harman, Rothbart, & Posner, 1997). In infants as young as 3 months, we have found that orienting to a visual stimulus provided by the experimenter produces powerful, if only temporary, soothing of distress. One of the major accomplishments of the first few years is for infants to develop the means to achieve this regulation on their own. At the same time, there emerges in infancy clear evidence of anticipation of predictable locations by eye movements (see Colombo, 2001, for a review).

A sign of the control of cognitive conflict is found in the first year of life. For example, in A, not B tasks, children are trained to reach for a hidden object at location A, and then tested on their ability to search for the hidden object at a new location B. Children younger than 12 months of age tend to look in the previous location A, even though they see the object disappear behind location B. After the first year, children develop the ability to inhibit the prepotent response toward the trained location A and successfully reach for the new location B (Diamond, 1991). During this period, infants develop the ability to resolve conflict between line of sight and line of reach when retrieving an object. At 9 months of age, line of sight dominates completely. If the open side of a box is not in line with the side in view, an infant will withdraw its hand and reach directly along the line of sight, striking the closed side (Diamond, 1991). In contrast, 12-month-old infants can simultaneously look at a closed side and reach through the open end to retrieve a toy.

The ability to use context to reduce conflict can be traced developmentally using the learning of sequences of locations. Infants as young as 4 months can learn to anticipate the location of a stimulus, provided the associations in the sequences are unambiguous (Haith, Hazan, & Goodman, 1988). In unambiguous sequences, each location is invariably associated with another location (e.g., 123; Clohessy, Posner, & Rothbart, 2001). Because the location of the current target is fully determined by the preceding item, only one type of information needs to be attended; therefore, there is no conflict (e.g., location 3 always follows location 2). Adults can learn unambiguous sequences of spatial locations implicitly even when attention is distracted by a secondary task (Curran & Keele, 1993).

Ambiguous sequences (e.g., 1213) require attention to the current association, in addition to the context in which the association occurs (e.g., location 1 may be followed by location 2, or by location 3). Ambiguous sequences pose conflict, because, for any association, there exist two strong candidates that can only be disambiguated by context. When distracted, adults are unable to learn ambiguous sequences of length six (e.g., 123213; Curran & Keele, 1993), a finding that demonstrates the need for higher level attentional resources to resolve this conflict. Even simple ambiguous associations (e.g., 1213) were not performed by children at above-chance level until about 2 years of age (Clohessy et al., 2001).

Gerardi-Caulton (2000) found developmental changes in executive attention during the third year of life, using a conflict key-pressing task. Because children of this age do not read, location and identity, rather than word meaning and ink color, served as the dimensions of conflict (spatial conflict task). Children sat in front of two response keys, one located to their left and one to their right. Each key displayed a picture, and on every trial, a picture identical to one of the pair appeared on either the left or right side of the screen. Children were rewarded for responding to the identity of the stimulus, regardless of its spatial compatibility with the matching response key (Gerardi-Caulton, 2000). Reduced accuracy and slowed reaction times for spatially incompatible relative to spatially compatible trials reflect the effort required to resist the prepotent response and resolve conflict between these two competing dimensions. Performance on this task produced a clear interference effect in adults and activated the anterior cingulate (Fan et al., 2003). Children age 24 months tended to perseverate on a single response, whereas 36-month-old children performed at high accuracy levels, but like adults, responded more slowly and with reduced accuracy to incompatible trials.

At 30 months, when toddlers were first able to perform the spatial conflict task successfully, we found that performance on this task was significantly correlated with their ability to learn the ambiguous associations in the sequence-learning task described earlier (Rothbart, Ellis, Rueda, & Posner, in press). This finding, together with the failure of 4-month-olds to learn ambiguous sequences, holds out the promise of being able to trace the emergence of executive attention during the first years of life.

The importance of being able to study the emergence of executive attention is enhanced, because cognitive measures of conflict resolution in these laboratory tasks have been linked to aspects of children's temperament. Signs of the development of executive attention by cognitive tasks relate to a temperamental individual-differences measure obtained from caregiver reports, called effortful control (see Rothbart et al., Chapter 18, this volume, for a review). Children relatively less affected by spatial conflict received higher parental ratings of temperamental effortful control and higher scores on laboratory measures of inhibitory control (Gerardi-Caulton, 2000). We regard effortful control as reflecting the efficiency with which the executive attention network operates in naturalistic settings.

Empathy is strongly related to effortful control, with children high in effortful control showing greater empathy (Rothbart, Ahadi, & Hershey, 1994). To display empathy toward others requires that we interpret their signals of distress or pleasure. Imaging work in normals indicates that sad faces activate the amygdala. As sadness increases, this activation is accompanied by activity in the anterior cingulate as part of the attention network (Blair, Morris, Frith, Perrett, & Dolan, 1999). It seems likely that the cingulate activity represents the basis for our attention to the distress of others.

Developmental studies have identified different routes to the successful development of conscience. The internalization of moral principles appears to be facilitated in fearful preschool-age children, especially when their mothers use gentle discipline (Kochanska, 1995). A strongly reactive amygdala would provide signals of distress that would easily allow empathic feelings toward others and improve socialization abilities. In the absence of this form of control, development of the cingulate would allow appropriate attention to the signals provided by amygdala activity. Consistent with its influence on empathy, effortful control also appears to play a role in the development of conscience. In addition, internalized control is facilitated in children high in effortful control (Kochanska et al., 1996). Thus, two separable control systems, one reactive (fear) and the other self-regulative (effortful control), appear to regulate the development of conscience.

Individual differences in effortful control are also related to some aspects of metacognitive knowledge, such as theory of mind (i.e., knowing that people's behavior is guided by their beliefs, desires, and other mental states; Carlson & Moses, 2001). Moreover, tasks that require the inhibition of a prepotent response correlate with theory of mind tasks even when other factors, such as age, intelligence, and working memory, are factored out (Carlson & Moses, 2001). Inhibitory control and theory of mind share a similar developmental time course in children, with advances in both areas between the ages of 2 and 5.

One function that has been traced to the anterior cingulate is monitoring of error. In the spatial conflict task, reaction times following an error were 200 msec longer than those following a correct trial at age 30 months, and over 500 msec longer at 36 months, indicating that children were noticing their errors and correcting them (Rothbart et al., in press). In this study, no evidence of slowing after an error was found in children at 24 months. A somewhat more difficult conflict is introduced when subjects must utilize information from one verbal command, while ignoring information from another. In one version of this Simple Simon game, children were asked to execute a response command given by one puppet, while inhibiting commands from a second puppet (Jones, Rothbart, & Posner, in press). Children of 36–38 months showed no ability to inhibit their response, and no slowing after an error, but at 39–41 months, children showed both an ability to inhibit and slowed reaction time after an error. These results suggest that between 30 and 39 months, performance changes based on detecting an error response. Because error detection has been studied with the use of scalp electrical recording (Gehring, Gross, Coles, Meyer, & Donchin, 1993; Luu, Collins, & Tucker, 2000) and has been shown to originate in the anterior cingulate (Bush et al., 2000), we now have the means to examine the emergence of this cingulate function in children at 2.5–3.5 years of age.

The attention network task (ANT; Fan, McCandliss, Sommer, Raz, & Posner, 2002) was developed to assay the efficiency of the three attentional networks. The task was built around the flanker task (Eriksen & Eriksen, 1974) but used cues to vary alertness and orienting. The output of this test are three scores related to the efficiency of each of the networks. In a study of 40 adults, we found fairly high immediate test–retest reliability for the scores of each attentional network provided by the ANT. Furthermore, these scores were not correlated across individuals and showed only small interactions between networks.

We have also developed an ANT specifically for children (Child ANT; see Figure 14.1). Independence between the network scores for the Child ANT is shown both by the lack of correlation between the three scores and the finding of no interactions between cue conditions and target flanker condition. Using the Child ANT, we found clear differences in the development of the attentional networks between 6- and 10-year-old children, and from this period to adulthood.

In a cross-sectional study, we did not find changes in orienting effects in subjects from 6 years of age to adulthood in this task. In conformity with this result, authors of previous orienting studies (Trick & Enns, 1998) have suggested that only voluntary movement speed and the accuracy of termination continue to improve in late childhood. Because we used a peripheral cue that tends to pull attention to the central portion of the target, our task appears to be one whose requirements would suggest an early developmental course.

For alerting, we found a significant decline from 10-year-olds to adults, and some improvement in late childhood, because the 10-year-olds tend to have lower alerting scores than the younger children. In general, large alerting scores appear to arise because children do poorly when there is no cue. We have documented an automatic effect of

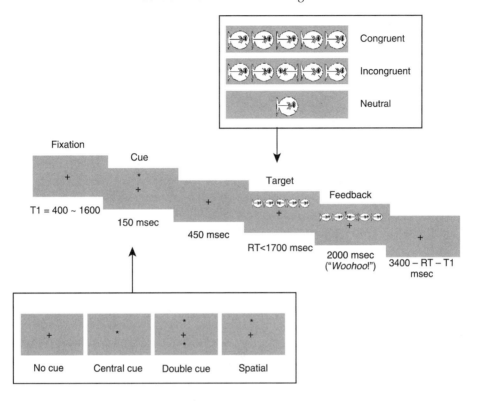

FIGURE 14.1. Schematic presentation of the time course of the Child ANT.

warning signals on performance at age 5 (Berger, Jones, Rothbart, & Posner, 2000), but 5-year-olds have trouble managing the more strategic aspect of alertness that is involved when warning intervals are varied between trials. The presentation of a target without a warning signal in the ANT is relatively rare, and this may reveal the problem children have in maintaining a level of alertness in the face of varying target arrival times. Further work on this aspect of the test may clarify why there is a late development of this system.

More relevant for the purposes of this chapter are results on the executive network. The conflict scores of subjects from age 6 to adulthood are shown in Table 14.2. The conflict score, computed by taking the median reaction time for trials with congruent flankers from the median reaction time for incongruent flanker trials (see Figure 14.1), is considered an index of conflict resolution abilities. Conflict scores showed a marked decrease between ages 6 and 7, but above age 7, there is remarkably little difference in conflict scores (as measured by both reaction time and errors), up to and including adults (Rueda et al., in press). This result is surprising given the general expectation that the executive network would improve until adulthood, as children are able to solve more difficult problems. A previous developmental study of the flanker task (Ridderinkhof, van der Molen, Band, & Bashore, 1997) showed improvement in conflict from ages 5 to 10 then little difference between age 10 and adulthood. Ridderinkhof and colleagues (1997) conclude that the major problem for children in flanker tasks is the translation of the input code into an appropriate response code, particularly when the response is incompatible. It seems likely that such a transformation would involve cingulate activity in monitoring the possible conflict.

TABLE 14.2. Development of Conflict Resolution Ability as Measured by the Child ANT as a Function of Age

Age	Overall performance		Conflict scores	
	Overall RT (msec)	Overall accuracy (% errors)	RT (msec)	Accuracy (% errors)
		Section 1		
6	931	15.8	115	15.6
7	833	5.7	63	0.7
8	806	4.9	71	−0.3
9	734	2.7	67	1.6
10	640	2.2	69	2.1
Adults	483	1.2	61	1.6
		Section 2		
4.5	1,599	12.79	207	5.8
Adults	443	1.4	31	2.3

Note. Section 1 shows overall performance and conflict scores of six groups (*n* = 12) from ages 6 to adulthood. Section 2 shows the same data in a different experiment, also using the Child ANT. In this second experiment, the stimuli were larger than in the experiment in Section 1, which result in slightly smaller conflict scores. RT, reaction time.

Diamond and Taylor (1996) carried out a study in which they evaluated performance of children between 3.5 and 7 years old in the tapping test, in which children are ask to tap once when the experimenter taps twice, and to tap twice when the experimenter taps once. Correct performance on this test is thought to require certain aspects of executive control, such as the ability to hold two rules in mind and to inhibit the tendency to imitate the experimenter. Diamond and Taylor found a steady improvement in both accuracy and speed on the tapping test in subjects ages 3.5 to 7; however, consistent with our result, most of the improvement occurred by 6 years of age, with the 7-year-old group demonstrating an accuracy rate close to 100%.

Our findings of little or no development in the executive network for the resolution of conflict after age 7 may not extend to more difficult executive tasks (e.g., those involving strategic decisions, such as the Tower of Hanoi). A recent imaging study found a common network of brain areas involved in the arrow version of the flanker task (similar to the adult version of the ANT), in the color Stroop task, and in a task involving a conflict between location and identity (Fan, Flombaum, McCandliss, Thomas, & Posner, 2002). Of these tasks, the flanker had the largest conflict effect, as measured by reaction time difference, and the strongest activation within the anterior cingulate area. Moreover, the fish and arrow ANTs differ a great deal in level of difficulty, yet show about the same developmental trend. These findings suggest an earlier than might have been expected development of neural areas related to the resolution of conflict, but this will need to be tested more directly in future work.

Using the Child ANT, while recording brain activity with a high-density scalp electrode array, we have recently compared 4-year-olds and adults. Despite dramatically different reaction times and conflict resolution scores (see Table 14.2), event-related potential (ERP) differences between incongruent and congruent trials were strikingly similar. Consistent with other studies (Kopp, Rist, & Mattler, 1996; van Veen & Carter, 2002), the adults showed differences in the brain waves for congruent and incongruent conditions around 300 msec after the presentation of the target in both child and adult versions of the task. In adults, this effect has been shown to be related to action monitoring processes (Botvinick et al., 2001) and associated with differences in activation localized in the anterior cingulate (van Veen & Carter, 2002). The child data also show a larger negative deflection for the incongruent condition compared to the congruent one, but this difference starts around 600 msec posttarget and extends for a period of 500 msec. Compared to that of adults, this effect covers a larger extent, has greater amplitude, and extends over a longer period of time. Differences between children and adults in ERP amplitude have been related to brain size and skull thickening; however, differences in the latency of components may be more related to the observed differences in conflict resolution between children and adults, as measured by the ANT. Electrophysiological measures can be used relatively easily with young children and will be useful in understanding developmental changes in the brain mechanisms of executive functions.

Above the age of 6, children are more amenable to studies using fMRI. Children ages 5–16 years show a significant correlation between the volume of the area of the right anterior cingulate and the ability to perform tasks requiring focal attention (Casey, Trainor, Giedd, et al., 1997). In a fMRI study, performance of children ages 7–12 and adults was studied in a go/no-go task. In comparison with a control condition in which children responded to all stimuli, the condition requiring inhibitory control activated prefrontal cortex in both children and adults. Also, the number of false alarms in this condition correlated significantly with the extent of cingulate activity (Casey, Trainor, Orendi, et al., 1997).

The ability to measure changes in control networks at varying points in the lifespan may be helpful in both considering disorders of attention and assaying the effectiveness of intervention designed to improve their operation. For example, the relatively late development of alerting, and to a lesser extent, the executive network, may make them likely targets of disorders. It is notable that alerting operation depends heavily on norepinepherine, whereas the conflict network involves dopamine (Marrocco & Davidson, 1998). These are the two transmitters most often implicated in attention-deficit/hyperactivity disorder (ADHD). Studies of children with ADHD, using tasks somewhat similar to the ANT, have shown some evidence of abnormalities in alerting (Swanson et al., 1991). Practice in attention skills has shown some effects in brain injury patients (Sohlberg, McLaughlin, Pavese, Heidrich, & Posner, 2000; Sturm, Willmes, Orgass, & Hartje, 1997), and may provide additional benefits in performance at times when attentional networks are developing. Our current data suggest that children below the age of 7 may be good candidates for training the executive attention network.

These studies provide evidence for the development of an executive network during early childhood. The development of executive attention contributes to the socialization process by increasing the likelihood of learning important behaviors related to self-regulation and understanding the cognitions and emotions of others. It seems likely that fostering the understanding of normal development of this system will also illuminate the comprehension of some pathologies.

ROLE OF GENES AND ENVIRONMENT

The specification of development of a specific neural network related to self-regulation is only one step toward a biological understanding. It is also important to know the genetic and environmental influences that together produce the neural network.

Candidate Genes

To determine whether the executive network is likely to be under genetic control, we conducted a small-scale twin study to determine its heritability (Fan, Wu, Fossella, & Posner, 2001). The study showed impressive correlations among twin pairs in overall reaction time, conflict resolution, and alerting, as well as a substantial heritability for the conflict network. These results show that the network scores are valid, in the sense that they are correlated among pairs of subjects with similar genomes, and encourage the search for candidate genes related to the executive network.

The use of genetic analysis with chronometric studies has been applied to the neuropsychology of reading disorders (Olson, Datta, Gayan, & DeFries, 1999), early Alzheimer's dementia (Greenwood, Sunderland, Friz, & Parasuraman, 2000), and attention deficit disorder (Swanson et al., 2000). Parasuraman, Greenwood, Haxby, and Grady (1992), for example, were able to show a deficit in orienting networks in patients with early Alzheimer's disease. Patients had difficulty in using central orienting cues to improve their orienting toward subsequent targets. This chronometric analysis was supported by a finding of a reduction in blood flow specific to the superior parietal lobe, an area known to be important in orchestrating voluntary shifts of attention toward targets. Patients with early Alzheimer's disease frequently have a characteristic genetic allele related to the tendency to produce deposits of amyloid. In a study of asymptomatic subjects that carried this genetic variant, Parasuraman and colleagues found a small deficit in orienting to central cues that closely resembled what they had reported for early Alzheimer's disease (Greenwood et al., 2000). This remarkable finding suggests that the study of mental chronometry may be useful in dealing with subtle differences in normal function that would not be called pathology but might be useful in directing treatment.

Similarly, we have been using the links between specific neural networks of attention and chemical modulators to investigate the genetic basis of normal attention (Fossella et al., 2002) and psychopathologies (Swanson et al., 2000). In general, we have examined genes related to dopamine, because there is clear evidence that the cingulate gyrus expresses all of the dopamine receptors and is modulated by input from the ventral tegmental dopamine system. We first tested 200 normal persons using the ANT. Because each of our subjects used a kit we provided to collect a DNA sample from cheek cells, we were able to collect genotypic information. We then attempted to relate differences in executive attention performance on the ANT with alleles of various common polymorphisms by testing whether significant differences in the efficiency of the conflict network were found for different alleles. We found that the conflict network operated differently depending on the alleles related to four different dopamine genes, including the dopamine 4-receptor gene (Fossella et al., 2002).

After identifying alleles associated with poor executive attention (Fossella et al., 2002), we can ask whether they are abnormal within any disorder related to that network. As one example of this strategy, we found the patients with borderline personality disorder (BPD) showed a deficit in the executive attention networks (Posner et al., in press). We then examined whether these alleles were overrepresented in patients with BPD, that is, whether these alleles were present at frequencies significantly higher than in a population of control subjects. This simple method provides a rapid means to evaluate the role that candidate genes play in normal cognitive function and, subsequently, whether a genetic risk toward BPD arises from deficits in cognitive performance. In our relatively small sample of patients with BPD, we did not find any abnormal allele frequencies (Posner et al., in press).

DEVELOPMENTAL PATHOLOGIES

By relating the ANT phenotype to genetic variation, it may be possible to obtain insight into developmental pathologies through either genetic links or links to attentional networks. Work currently going on at various centers has already provided some evidence of this. These relationships are still rather tentative, but they do illustrate the possible utility of these approaches discussed in understanding abnormalities of attention and self-regulation.

Studies of autism have provided important links between the disorder and the orienting network (Akshoomoff, Pierce, & Courchesne, 2002; Rodier, 2002). Using a task closely related to that used for orienting in the ANT, it has been found the persons with autism have difficulty in disengaging from a visual event to orient to a new event. This happens even with completely nonsocial stimuli. Rodier has speculated that this may involve an early developing HOX gene. Both parietal and cerebellar areas have been implicated in producing this effect.

In the case of ADHD, the most compelling connection has involved alleles of dopamine 4-receptor gene. In normal subjects the 4 repeat allele has been associated with more difficulty in resolving conflict than shorter or longer repeats of the gene. Substantial evidence has related ADHD symptoms to the 7 repeat allele (Swanson et al., 2000). This same allele has been shown to be related to the personality trait of sensation seeking (Auerbach, Benjamin, Faroy, Geller, & Ebstein, 2001). However, efforts to determine whether the 7 repeat produced a cognitive deficit in the Stroop or other attention tasks have suggested that having the 7 repeat allele does not provide a cognitive deficit; indeed, it might be an advantage in cognitive conflict tasks, as was found with the ANT (Fossella et al., 2002). This puzzling result has been clarified somewhat by two, more recent, findings regarding the molecular genetics of the 7 repeat allele. One study found that the 7 repeat appears to have undergone a relatively recent increase in frequency due to positive selection (Ding et al., 2002). This finding suggests that the 7 repeat allele may convey a positive advantage, which might be in addition to any deficit. A second finding suggests that the 7 repeat is only associated with ADHD when it is accompanied by an additional mutation (Grady et al., 2003). These findings may suggest that the 7 repeat is more associated with seeking out a high variety of input and only leads to a disorder because it may also be more susceptible to new mutations. These findings show how revealing a molecular approach can be, and also how complex the route from genes to behavioral outcomes is likely to be.

The executive network shows a high vulnerability to deficit, and is therefore involved in many forms of pathology. For example, there is evidence that subjects with schizophrenia have not only a difficulty of attention that appears related to the executive network (Posner, Early, Reiman, Pardo, & Dhawan, 1988) but also cellular abnormalities in the anterior cingulate (Benes, 1999). The 22q11 deletion syndrome involves a 1.5-megabase region of chromosome 22. This region includes the COMT gene that has been related to conflict resolution in the ANT experiment with normal adults and also to schizophrenia. BPD, which is frequently found in adults who have undergone abuse as children, also shows an abnormality in executive attention, as measured by the ANT (Posner et al., 2002). These findings suggest that a variety of pathologies may be related to deficits in the cognitive network underlying executive control.

FOSTERING SELF-REGULATION

The strong emphasis on neural networks, and genetic influence on them, may lead the reader to think that these networks are not amenable to interventions involving training or other behavioral therapies. It is not our intention to leave this impression. Indeed, we think that normal socialization is important for the development of these networks, and that specific training may well be an effective way to foster them at particular stages of development.

The executive attention network appears to show substantial development between ages 2 and 7. Recently, several training-oriented programs have resulted in improved executive control within special populations and domains. For example, training of patients with specific brain injury, with the attention process training method, has led to specific improvements in executive attention in tasks quite remote from those for which patients have undergone training (Sohlberg et al., 2000). These effects of practice may depend on first successfully establishing a minimum level of alerting and orienting (Sturm et al., 1997).

Various forms of attention training for children with ADHD have also proven to be successful, for example, the use of attention process training (Kerns, Esso, & Thompson, 1999; Semrud-Clikeman, Nielsen, & Clinton, 1999) or practice related to working memory (Klingberg, Forssberg, & Westerberg, 2002).

In studies of monkeys trained for space flight, a series of training programs has been found to be very appealing to the primates and to result in general improvements in aggression, social relations, and hyperactivity (Rumbaugh & Washburn, 1995). We have now adapted these programs for use with toddlers and young children, and trials are under way to determine the range of improvement possible, and which children and which brain networks are likely to reflect those improvements.

Psychologists have often argued that learning must involve domain specificity (Simon, 1969; Thorndike, 1903). However, viewing attention as an organ system closely related to self-regulation, as we have done in this chapter, suggests a somewhat different view. Attention is domain-general in the sense that any content area can be the subject of modification through attention. If the appropriate methods for training attention in young children can be identified, it is possible that systematic training of attention might be an important addition to preschool education.

ACKNOWLEDGMENTS

The research reported in this chapter was supported by the James S. McDonnell Foundation through a grant to the University of Oregon, in support of research on training of attention. M. Rosario Rueda was supported in part by a grant from La Caixa Foundation—USA Program.

REFERENCES

Akshoomoff, N., Pierce, K., & Courchesne, E. (2002). The neurobiological basis of autism from a developmental perspective. *Development and Psychopathology, 14*, 613–634.

Anderson, R. A. (1989). Visual eye movement functions of the posterior parietal cortex. *Annual Review of Neuroscience, 27*, 377–403.

Anderson, S.W., Damasio, H., Tranel, D., & Damasio, A.R. (2000). Long-term sequelae of prefrontal cortex damage acquired in early childhood. *Developmental Neuropsychology, 18*(3), 281–296.

Auerbach, J. G., Benjamin, J., Faroy, M., Geller, V., & Ebstein, R. (2001). DRD4 related to infant attention and information processing: A developmental link to ADHD? *Psychiatric Genetics*, *11*(1), 31–35.

Baddeley, A. D. (1986). *Working memory*. Oxford, UK: Claredon Press.

Beauregard, M., Levesque, J., & Bourgouin, P. (2001). Neural correlates of conscious self-regulation of emotion. *Journal of Neuroscience*, *21*, RC165.

Benes, F. (1999). Model generation and testing to probe neural circuitry in the cingulate cortex of postmortem schizophrenic brains. *Schizophrenia Bulletin*, *24*, 219–229.

Berger, A., Jones, L., Rothbart, M. K., & Posner, M. I. (2000). Computerized games to study the development of attention in childhood. *Behavioral Research Methods and Instrumentation*, *32*, 299–303.

Blair, R. J., Morris, J. S., Frith, C. D., Perrett, D. I., & Dolan, R. J. (1999). Dissociable neural responses to facial expression of sadness and anger. *Brain*, *122*, 883–893.

Botvinick, M. M., Braver, T. S., Barch, D. M., Carter, C. S., & Cohen, J. D. (2001). Conflict monitoring and cognitive control. *Psychological Review*, *108*, 624–652.

Broadbent, D. E. (1958). *Perception and communication*. London: Pergamon.

Bronson, M. B. (2000). *Self-regulation in early childhood: Nature and nurture*. New York: Guilford Press.

Bush, G., Luu, P., & Posner, M. I. (2000). Cognitive and emotional influences in the anterior cingulate cortex. *Trends in Cognitive Science*, *4*, 215–222.

Carlson, S. M., & Moses, L. J. (2001). Individual differences in inhibitory control in children's theory of mind. *Child Development*, *72*, 1032–1053.

Casey, B. J., Trainor, R., Giedd, J., Vauss, Y., Vaituzis, C. K., Hamburger, S., Kozuch, P., & Rapoport, J. L. (1997). The role of the anterior cingulate in automatic and controlled processes: A developmental neuroanatomical study. *Developmental Psychobiology*, *3*, 61–69.

Casey, B. J., Trainor, R. J., Orendi, J. L., Schubert, A. B., Nystrom, L. E., Giedd, J. N., Castellanos, F. X., Haxby, J. V., Noll, D. C., Cohen, J. D., Forman, S. D., Dahl, R. E., & Rapoport, J. L. (1997). A developmental functional MRI study of prefrontal activation during performance of a go–no-go task. *Journal of Cognitive Neuroscience*, *9*, 835–847.

Clohessy, A. B., Posner, M. I., & Rothbart, M. K. (2001). Development of the functional visual field. *Acta Psychologica*, *106*, 51–68.

Colombo, J. (2001). The development of visual attention in infancy. *Annual Review of Psychology*, *52*, 337–367.

Corbetta, M., & Shulman, G. L. (2002). Control of goal-directed and stimulus-driven attention in the brain. *Nature Neuroscience Reviews*, *3*, 201–215.

Curran, T., & Keele, S. W. (1993). Attentional and non-attentional forms of sequence learning. *Journal of Experimental Psychology: Learning, Memory and Cognition*, *19*, 189–202.

Dale, A. M. Liu, A. K., Fischi, B. R., Ruckner, R., Beliveau, J. W., Lewine, J. D., & Halgren, E. (2000). Dynamic statistical parameter mapping: Combining fMRI and MEG for high resolution cortical activity. *Neuron*, *26*, 55–67.

Damasio, A. (1994). *Descartes error: Emotion, reason and the brain*. New York: Putnam.

Davidson, R. J., Putnam, K. M., & Larson, C. L. (2000). Dysfunction in the neural circuitry of emotion regulation: A possible prelude to violence. *Science*, *289*(5479), 591–594.

Desimone, R., & Duncan, J. (1995). Neural mechanisms of selective visual attention. *Annual Review of Neuroscience*, *18*, 193–222.

Diamond, A. (1991). Neuropsychological insights into the meaning of object concept development. In S. Carey & R. Gelman (Eds.), *The epigenesis of mind: Essays on biology and cognition* (pp. 67–110). Hillsdale, NJ: Erlbaum.

Diamond, A., & Taylor, C. (1996). Development of an aspect of executive control: Development of the abilities to remember what I said and "do as I say, not as I do." *Developmental Psychobiology*, *29*(4), 315–334.

Ding, Y. C., Chi, H. C., Grady, D. L., Morishima, A., Kidd, J. R., Kidd, K. K., Flodman, P., Spence, M. A., Schuck, S., Swanson, J. M., Zhang, Y. P., & Moyzis, R. K. (2002). Evidence of positive selection acting at the human dopamine receptor D4 gene locus. *Proceedings of the National Academy of Sciences, USA, 99*(1), 309–314.

Drevets, W. C., & Raichle, M. E. (1998). Reciprocal suppression of regional blood flow during emotional versus higher cognitive processes: Implications for interactions between emotion and cognition. *Cognition and Emotion, 12,* 353–385.

Driver, J., Eimer, M., & Macaluso, E. (in press). Neurobiology of human spatial attention: Modulation, generation, and integration. In N. Kanwisher & J. Duncan (Eds.), *Attention and performance: Vol. 20. Functional brain imaging of visual cognition.* Amsterdam: North-Holland.

Duncan, J., Seltz, R. J., Kolodny, J., Bor, D., Herzog, H., Ahmed, A., Newell, F. N., & Emslie, H. (2000). A neural basis for general intelligence. *Science, 289,* 457–460.

Eriksen, B. A., & Eriksen, C. W. (1974). Effects of noise letters upon the identification of a target letter in a nonsearch task. *Perception and Psychophysics, 16,* 143–149.

Fan, J., Flombaum, J. I., McCandliss, B. D., Thomas, K. M., & Posner, M. I. (2003). Cognitive and brain mechanisms of conflict. *Neuroimage, 18,* 42–57.

Fan, J., McCandliss, B. D., Sommer, T., Raz, A., & Posner, M. I. (2002). Testing the efficiency and independence of attentional networks. *Journal of Cognitive Neuroscience, 14*(3), 340–347.

Fan, J., Wu, Y., Fossella, J., & Posner, M. I. (2001). Assessing the heritability of attentional networks. *BioMed Central Neuroscience, 2,* 14.

Fonagy, P., & Target, M. (2002). Early intervention and the development of self-regulation. *Psychoanalytic Quarterly, 22,* 307–335.

Fossella, J., Posner, M. I., Fan, J., Swanson, J. M., & Pfaff, D. M. (2002). Attentional phenotypes for the analysis of higher mental function. *Scientific World Journal, 2,* 217–223.

Gehring, W. J., Gross, B., Coles, M. G. H., Meyer, D. E., & Donchin, E. (1993). A neural system for error detection and compensation. *Psychological Science, 4,* 385–390.

Gerardi-Caulton, G. (2000). Sensitivity to spatial conflict and the development of self-regulation in children 24–36 months of age. *Developmental Science, 3,* 397–404.

Grady, D. L., Chi, H.-C., Ding, Y. C., Smith, M., Wang, E., Schuck, S., Flodman, P., Spence, M. A., Swanson, J. M., & Moyzis, R. K. (2003). High prevalence of rare dopamine receptor D4 alleles in children diagnosed with attention-deficit hyperactivity disorder (ADHD). *Molecular Psychiatry, 8,* 536–545.

Greenwood, P. M., Sunderland, T., Friz, J. L., & Parasuraman, R. (2000). Genetics and visual attention: Selective deficits in healthy adult carriers of the epsilon 4 allele of the apolipoprotein E gene. *Proceedings of National Academy of Sciences, USA, 97,* 11661–11666.

Haith, M. M., Hazan, C., & Goodman, G. S. (1988). Expectation and anticipation of dynamic visual events by 3.5 month-old babies. *Child Development, 59,* 467–479.

Harman, C., Rothbart, M. K., & Posner, M. I. (1997). Distress and attention interactions in early infancy. *Motivation and Emotion, 21,* 27–43.

Holroyd, C. B., & Coles, M. G. H. (2002). The neural basis of human error processing: Reinforcement learning, dopamine and the error related negativity. *Psychological Review, 109,* 679–709.

Jones, L., Rothbart, M. K., & Posner, M. I. (in press). Development of inhibitory control in preschool children. *Developmental Science.*

Karnath, H. O., Ferber, S., & Himmelbach, M. (2001). Spatial awareness is a function of the temporal not the posterior parietal lobe. *Nature, 411,* 950–953.

Kerns, K. A., Esso, K., & Thompson, J. (1999). Investigation of a direct intervention for improving attention in young children with ADHD. *Developmental Neuropsychology, 16,* 273–295.

Klingberg, T., Forssberg, H., & Westerberg, H. (2002). Training of working memory in children with ADHD. *Journal of Clinical and Experimental Neuropsychology, 24,* 781–791

Kochanska, G. (1995). Children's temperament, mothers' discipline, and security of attachment: Multiple pathways to emerging internalization. *Child Development, 66,* 597–615.

Kochanska, G., Murray, K., Jacques, T. Y., Koenig, A. L., & Vandegeest, K. A. (1996). Inhibitory control in young children and its role in emerging internationalization. *Child Development, 67,* 490–507.

Kopp, B., Rist, F., & Mattler, U. (1996). N200 in the flanker task as a neurobehavioral tool for investigating executive control. *Psychophysiology*, *33*, 282–294.

Luu, P., Collins, P., & Tucker, D. M. (2000). Mood, personality and self-monitoring: Negative affect and emotionality in relation to frontal lobe mechanisms of error-detection. *Journal of Experimental Psychology—General*, *129*, 43–60.

MacDonald, A. W., Cohen, J. D., Stenger, V. A., & Carter, C. S. (2000). Dissociating the role of the dorsolateral prefrontal and anterior cingulate cortex in cognitive control. *Science*, *288*, 1835–1838.

Marrocco, R. T., & Davidson, M. C. (1998). Neurochemistry of attention. In R. Parasuraman (Ed.), *The attention brain* (pp. 35–50). Cambridge, MA: MIT Press.

Ochsner, K. N., Bunge, S. A., Gross, J. J., & Gabrieli, J. D. E. (2002). Rethinking feelings: An fMRI study of the cognitive regulation of emotion. *Journal of Cognitive Neuroscience*, *14*, 1215–1229.

Ochsner, K. N., Kossyln, S. M., Cosgrove, G. R., Cassem, E. H., Price, B. H., Nierenberg, A. A., & Rauch, S. L. (2001). Deficits in visual cognition and attention following bilateral anterior cingulotomy. *Neuropsychologia*, *39*, 219–230.

Olson, R. K., Datta, H., Gayan, J., & DeFries, J. C. (1999). A behavioral-genetic analysis of reading disabilities and component processes. In R. Klein & P. McMullen (Eds.), *Converging methods for understanding reading and dyslexia* (pp. 133–151). Cambridge, MA: MIT Press.

Panksepp, J. (1998). *Affective neuroscience*. New York: Oxford University Press.

Parasuraman, R., Greenwood, P. M., Haxby, J. V., & Grady, C. L. (1992). Visuospatial attention in dementia of the Alzheimer type. *Brain*, *115*, 711–733.

Posner, M. I. (1980). Orienting of attention: The 7th Sir F. C. Bartlett lecture. *Quarterly Journal of Experimental Psychology*, *32*, 3–25.

Posner, M. I., Early, T. S., Reiman, E., Pardo, P. J., & Dhawan, M. (1988). Asymmetries in hemispheric control of attention in schizophrenia. *Archives of General Psychiatry*, *45*, 814–821.

Posner, M. I., & Fan, J. (in press). Attention as an organ system. In J. Pomerantz (Ed.), *Neurobiology of perception and communication: From synapse to society:. The 4th De Lange Conference*. Cambridge, UK: Cambridge University Press.

Posner, M. I., & Raichle, M. E. (1994). *Images of mind*. Scientific American Books.

Posner, M. I., & Raichle, M. E. (Eds.). (1998). Overview: The neuroimaging of human brain function. *Proceedings of the National Academy of Sciences, USA*, *95*, 763–764.

Posner, M. I., & Rothbart, M. K. (1998). Attention, self-regulation and consciousness. *Philosophical Transactions of the Royal Society of London, B*, *353*, 1915–1927.

Posner, M. I., & Rothbart, M. K. (2000). Developing mechanisms of self-regulation. *Development and Psychopathology*, *12*, 427–441.

Posner, M. I., Rothbart, M. K., Vizueta, N., Levy,K., Thomas, K. M., & Clarkin, J. F. (2002). Attentional mechanisms of borderline personality disorder. *Proceedings of the National Academy of Sciences, USA*, *99*, 16366–16370.

Posner, M. I., Rothbart, M. K., Vizueta, N., Thomas, K. M., Levy, K., Fossella, J., Silbersweig, D. A., Stern, E., Clarkin, J., & Kernberg, O. (2003). An approach to the psychobiology of personality disorders. *Development and Psychopathology*.

Rainville, P., Duncan, G. H., Price, D. D., Carrier, B., & Bushnell, M. C. (1997). Pain affect encoded in human anterior cingulated but not somatosensory cortex. *Science*, *277*, 968–970.

Rensink, R. A., O'Regan, J. K., & Clark, J. J. (1997). To see or not to see: The need for attention to perceive changes in scenes. *Psychological Science*, *8*(5), 368–373.

Ridderinkhof, K. R., van der Molen, M. W., Band, P. H., & Bashore, T. R. (1997). Sources of interference from irrelevant information: A developmental study. *Journal of Experimental Child Psychology*, *65*, 315–341.

Rodier, P. M. (2002). Converging evidence for brain stem injury during autism. *Development and Psychopathology*, *14*, 537–559.

Rothbart, M. K., Ahadi, S. A., & Hershey, K. (1994). Temperament and social behavior in children. *Merrill–Palmer Quarterly*, *40*, 21–39.

Rothbart, M. K., & Bates, J. E. (1998). Temperament. In W. Damon (Series Ed.) & N. Eisenberg (Vol. Ed.), *Handbook of child psychology: Vol. 3. Social, emotional and personality development* (5th ed., pp. 105–176). New York: Wiley.

Rothbart, M. K., Ellis, L. K., Rueda, M. R., & Posner, M. I. (in press). Developing mechanisms of conflict resolution. *Journal of Personality.*

Rueda, M. R., Fan, J., McCandliss, B., Halparin, J. D., Gruber, D. B., Pappert, L., & Posner, M. I. (in press). Development of attentional networks in childhood. *Neuropsychologia.*

Ruff, H. A., & Rothbart, M. K. (1996). *Attention in early development: Themes and variations.* New York: Oxford University Press.

Rumbaugh, D. M., & Washburn, D. A. (1995). Attention and memory in relation to learning: A comparative adaptation perspective. In G. R. Lyon & N. A. Krasengor (Eds.), *Attention, memory and executive function* (pp. 199–219). Baltimore: Brookes.

Semrud-Clikeman, M., Nielsen, K. H., & Clinton, A. (1999). Anintervention approach for children with teacher and parent-identified attentional difficulties. *Journal of Learning Disabilities, 32,* 581–589.

Simon, H. A. (1969). *The sciences of the artificial.* Cambridge, MA: MIT Press.

Sohlberg, M. M., McLaughlin, K. A., Pavese, A., Heidrich, A., & Posner, M. I. (2000). Evaluation of attention process therapy training in persons with acquired brain injury. *Journal of Clinical and Experimental Neuropsychology, 22,* 656–676.

Sturm, W., Willmes, K., Orgass, B., & Hartje, W. (1997). Do specific attention deficits need specific training? *Neuropsychological Rehabilitation, 7,* 81–103.

Swanson, J., Oosterlaan, J., Murias, M., Moyzis, R., Schuck, S., Mann, M., Feldman, P., Spence, M. A., Sergeant, J., Smith, M., Kennedy J., & Posner, M. I. (2000). ADHD children with 7-repeat allele of the DRD4 gene have extreme behavior but normal performance on critical neuropsychological tests of attention. *Proceedings of the National Academy of Sciences, USA, 97,* 4754–4759.

Swanson, J. M., Posner, M. I., Potkin, S., Bonforte, S., Youpa, D., Cantwell, D., & Crinella, F. (1991). Activating tasks for the study of visual–spatial attention in ADHD children: A cognitive anatomical approach. *Journal of Child Neurology, 6,* S119–S127.

Thorndike, E. L. (1903). *Educational psychology.* New York: Teachers College Press.

Titchener, E. B. (1909). *Experimental psychology of the thought processes.* New York: Macmillan.

Trick, L. M., & Enns, J. T. (1998). Lifespan changes in attention: The visual search task. *Cognitive Development, 13*(3), 369–386.

Turken, A. U., & Swick, D. (1999). Response selection in the human anterior cingulate cortex. *Nature Neurosceince, 2*(10), 920–924.

van Veen, V., & Carter, C. S. (2002). The timing of actino-monitoring processes in the anterior cingulate cortex. *Journal of Cognitive Neuroscience, 14*(4), 593–602.

Ventner, J. C., Adams, M. D., Myers, E. W., Li, P. W., Mural, R. J., Sutton, et al. (2001). The sequence of the human genome. *Science, 291,* 1304–1335.

Welch, M. C. (2001). The prefrontal cortex and the development of executive function in childhood. In A. F. Kalverboer & A. Gramsbergen (Eds.), *Handbook of brain and behavior in human development* (pp. 767–790). Dordrecht, The Netherlands: Kluwer Academic.

15

Attention-Deficity/Hyperactivity Disorder and Self-Regulation

Taking an Evolutionary Perspective on Executive Functioning

RUSSELL A. BARKLEY

Current psychiatric taxonomy describes attention-deficit/hyperactivity disorder, or ADHD, as involving developmentally inappropriate degrees of inattention and hyperactive–impulsive behavior. These symptoms frequently arise in early childhood, are relatively pervasive or cross-situational in nature, may persist into adolescence and even adulthood in the majority of clinically diagnosed cases, and result in impairment in major life activities, such as family functioning, developing self-sufficiency, peer relations, and educational and occupational functioning, among others (American Psychiatric Association, 1994; Barkley, 1998). This perspective emphasizes problems in the realms of attention, impulsiveness, and activity level as being central to the disorder. But children with ADHD often demonstrate deficiencies in many other motor and cognitive abilities.

Among these are difficulties with (1) physical fitness, gross and fine motor coordination, and motor sequencing (Breen, 1989; Kadesjo & Gillberg, 2001; Mariani & Barkley, 1997); (2) speed of color naming (Tannock, Martinussen, & Frijters, 2000); (3) verbal and nonverbal working memory and mental computation (Mariani & Barkley, 1997; Murphy, Barkley, & Bush, 2001; Zentall & Smith, 1993); (4) story recall (Lorch et al., 2000); (5) planning and anticipation (Grodzinsky & Diamond, 1992; Klorman et al., 1999); (6) verbal fluency and confrontational communication (Grodzinsky & Diamond, 1992; Zentall, 1988); (5) effort allocation (Douglas, 1983); (6) developing, applying, and self-monitoring organizational strategies (Hamlett, Pellegrini, & Conners, 1987; Purvis & Tannock, 1997); (7) internalization of self-directed speech (Berk & Potts, 1991; Winsler, Diaz, Atencio, McCarthy, & Chabay, 2000); (8) adhering to restrictive instructions (Danforth, Barkley, & Stokes, 1991; Roberts, 1990); and (9) self-regulation of emotion (Braaten & Rosen, 2000; Hinshaw, Buhrmeister, & Heller, 1989; Maedgen &

Carlson, 2000). Several studies have also demonstrated that ADHD may be associated with less mature or diminished moral development (Hinshaw, Herbsman, Melnick, Nigg, & Simmel, 1993; Simmel & Hinshaw, 1993). Many of these cognitive difficulties appear to be specific to ADHD and are not a function of its commonly comorbid disorders, such as learning disabilities, depression, anxiety, or oppositional defiant/conduct disorder (Barkley, Edwards, Lanieri, & Metevia, 2001; Klorman et al., 1999; Murphy et al., 2001; Nigg, 1999; Nigg, Blaskey, Huang-Pollock, & Rappley, 2002).

The commonality among most or all of these seemingly disparate abilities is that all have been considered to fall within the domain of "executive functions" in the field of neuropsychology (Barkley, 1997b; Denckla, 1996) or "metacognition" in developmental psychology (Flavell, 1970; Torgesen, 1994; Welsh & Pennington, 1988), or to be affected by these functions. All seem to be mediated, at least in part, by the frontal cortex, and particularly the prefrontal lobes (Fuster, 1997; Stuss & Benson, 1986). Theorists and clinical scientists have long speculated that problems with executive functioning specifically and self-regulation more generally are at the heart of this disorder and give rise to the more superficial and surface symptoms represented in clinical diagnostic criteria (Barkley, 1997a; Cantwell, 1975; Douglas, 1983; Still, 1902).

As appealing as these speculations have been about ADHD and self-control in seeming to square better with the behavior of children with ADHD, they necessitate that one have a reasonable account of how normal self-regulation develops in children and of how ADHD acts to disrupt that normal developmental process. These necessities have led me to spend the better part of the past decade conceptualizing and investigating the nature of self-control in children and adults with and without ADHD (Barkley, 1997a) and, more recently, conjecturing about the possible adaptive advantages that psychological modules for self-regulation and executive functioning may have served in the course of human evolution (Barkley, 2001b). As I discuss later, such conjecture can serve to suggest testable hypotheses for future research concerning the nature and purposes of self-regulation, and broaden the scope of social domains that developmental disorders such as ADHD, or acquired disorders such as frontal lobe injuries, may disrupt. Space constraints limit this chapter to providing merely an overview of the self-control problems experienced by children and adults with ADHD, and the course I have taken in developing a theory of self-control to try to explain that disorder. Greater coverage of these issues can be found in other sources (Barkley, 1997a, 1997b, 1998, 2001b). Good science and scholarship demand that we define our terms in as operational a way as possible, if we are to avoid conceptual or semantic confusion. Of relevance here, the terms "behavioral inhibition," "self-control," and "executive functioning," which have been employed frequently in the fields of developmental psychology, neuropsychology, and child psychopathology, need some pinning down if we are to get some idea of what they represent and how their functions may be disturbed in individuals with ADHD.

DEFINING INHIBITION, SELF-CONTROL, AND EXECUTIVE FUNCTION

From the perspective taken here, the terms "behavioral" or "response inhibition," "self-control" or "self-regulation," and "executive functioning" define overlapping and interacting human abilities. Defining them carefully shows their interconnectedness. The definitions used here are behavioral rather than cognitive terms, which at least permits them to be more operationally defined, more easily observed and understood, and potentially more easily examined in research. Behavioral terms also make more evident the possible evolutionary continuity or transition from the rudimentary appearance of some aspects of inhibition, self-control, and executive functions (EFs) observed in a few other primates (e.g., nonverbal working memory in rhesus monkeys and chimpanzees) to the complex executive system ascribed to humans. To describe these terms operationally relative to their manifest behavioral equivalents also may clarify their possible path of gradual evolution and their adaptive purpose(s). In this chapter, I take the stance that the initial and overarching purpose of self-control and executive functioning is inherently social. That purpose arose out of the group-living niche that humans occupy, particularly out of social groups comprised of genetically unrelated, or distantly related, individuals who came to depend on forms of reciprocal exchange or altruism and the formation of cooperative coalitions for orchestrating non-zero-sum activities on which their survival likely depended. The essence of such non-zero-sum coalitions is that they attain economic and other survival benefits that cannot be achieved by individuals acting alone (Wright, 2000). From this perspective, nonsocial organisms that live relatively independently of other members of their species (other than for mating/reproductive activities) do not need self-control or the executive system that permits it.

The term "response inhibition," as I use it here, refers to three overlapping yet somewhat distinct processes:

1. Inhibiting the initial prepotent response to an event, so as to create a delay in responding.
2. Interrupting an ongoing response that proves ineffective, thereby permitting a delay in and reevaluation of the decision to continue responding (a sensitivity to error).
3. Protecting not only the self-directed (executive) responses that occur within the delay but also the goal-directed behavior they generate from disruption by competing events and responses (interference control or resistance to distraction) (Barkley, 1997a, 1997b; Fuster, 1997).

I view the first process as the most important, for without a delay in the prepotent response (stopping), any thinking and related goal-directed actions pertinent to that situation are pointless, if they can occur at all (Barkley, 1997a; Bronowski, 1967/1977). It is not only the response that is delayed but also the decision about a response (Bronowski, 1967/1977, 1976). The prepotent response is that response for which immediate reinforcement (positive or negative) is available within a particular context, or which has been previously associated with that context (Barkley, 1997b). Both forms of reinforcement—positive and negative—must be considered in defining a response as being prepotent. Whereas some forms of impulsive behavior function to achieve an immediate reward, others serve to escape or avoid immediate aversive, punitive, or otherwise undesirable events (negative reinforcement). Such escape/avoidance responses are just as much a part of immediate gratification as are responses that result in immediate reward. Both forms of prepotent response will require inhibition if executive functioning, or thinking, and self-regulation are to occur and to be effective.

I employ the definition of "self-control" used in behavior analysis: *Self-control is a response (or series of responses) by the individual that functions to alter the probability of a subsequent response to an event, thereby changing the likelihood of a later consequence related to that event* (Barkley, 1997a, 1997b; Kanfer & Karoly, 1972; Mischel, Shoda, & Rodriguez, 1989; Skinner, 1953). In other words, self-control is any action by individuals directed toward themselves, so as to change their behavior and therein alter future rather than merely immediate consequences. Some have considered self-control to be the choice of a delayed, larger reward over a more immediate, smaller one (Ainslie, 1974; Burns & Powers, 1975; Logue, 1988; Mischel, 1983; Navarick, 1986). But this ignores the self-directed actions in which the individual must engage, so as to value the delayed over the immediate reward and to pursue that delayed consequence.

What then is executive functioning? Neuropsychology seems to view it as being largely comprised of unobservable "cognitive" or mentalistic events mediated chiefly by the prefrontal cortex. That literature is typified by descriptions of various activities thought to be involved in executive functioning, whereas the construct itself goes undefined. For instance, the term "executive function" has been used to encompass the actions of planning, inhibiting responses, developing and using strategy, flexible sequencing of actions, maintaining a behavioral set, resisting interference, and so on (Denckla, 1996; Morris, 1996; Spreen, Risser, & Edgell, 1995). Others simply concluded that the EFs are what the frontal lobes do (Stuss & Benson, 1986). Denckla (1994) defined executive functioning by its components: interference control, effortful and flexible organization, and strategic planning or anticipatory, goal-directed preparedness to act. Dennis (1991) did likewise, recognizing the components of regulatory (mental attention), executive (planning), and social discourse (productive verbal interaction with others). And so did Spreen and colleagues (1995) in their description of EFs as inhibition, planning, organized searching, self-monitoring, and flexibility of thought and action. The underlying theme of EFs seems to be this future orientation as conjectured by Denckla, and which the philosopher Daniel Dennett (1995) has called "the intentional stance." Goal-directed behaviors require a capacity for understanding the temporal ordering of events and of requisite responses to them (Shimamura, Janowsky, & Squire, 1990), including the hierarchical staging of behavior into arrangements of goal–subgoal components (Goel & Grafman, 1995). Those arrangements may form part of a larger capacity for the formation of social scripts (Sirigu et al., 1995) that involve the generation of the sequential steps needed to complete a social goal, such as shopping for groceries, planning a wedding, and so on. As Sirigu and colleagues (1995) found, these scripts are impaired in patients with frontal lobe injuries. Yet all such efforts to describe the EFs seem to fall short of the mark. They merely invite the question of what underlying theme binds these descriptions together.

Neuropsychology has opted for a "cognitive" or mentalistic view of executive functioning, founded on the computer as a metaphor for brain–behavior functioning. This view is incorrect, I believe, for two reasons. First, as I assert later, the EFs are not mental in some impossibly undetectable, otherworldly sense that they take place in something called a mind on some higher than physical plane. *The EFs comprise the principal classes of behavior that we use toward ourselves for purposes of self-regulation (changing our future)*. An "executive act" is any act toward oneself that functions to modify one's own behavior, so as to change one's future outcomes. Such actions may be covert but need not be so to be classified as "executive" actions here. The term "covert" merely means that the outward, publicly observable (musculoskeletal) manifestations of such behavior have been made very difficult to detect by others over the course of human evolution. But those actions still occur, and they can still be thought of as forms of behavior. Second, developments in the technology of neuroimaging and the fine-grained recording of shifts in muscle potential now suggest that this covert behavior-to-the-self is capable of being measured (D'Esposito et al., 1997; Livesay, Liebke, Samaras, & Stanley, 1996; Livesay & Samaras, 1998; Ryding, Bradvik, & Ingvar, 1996). As these studies suggest, when we engage in verbal thought (covert self-speech) and imagined actions, the peripheral muscles and brain substrates ordinarily associated with the public display of these same actions continue to be activated. But the movements of the peripheral muscles are largely imperceptible to others, being reflected chiefly through small changes in muscle electrical potentials at those sites. Thinking is behaving to the self, with the peripheral muscle apparatus being largely suppressed.

The conceptual linkage of inhibition with self-regulation, and of both constructs with executive functioning is now obvious. Response inhibition is a prerequisite to self-regulation, because one cannot direct actions or behavior toward oneself if one has already responded impulsively to an immediate event. The EFs are the general forms or classes of self-directed actions that humans use in self-regulation. I have identified at least four such classes below. The EFs and the self-regulation they create produce a net overall maximization of social consequences when considering both the immediate and delayed outcomes of certain response alternatives. Self-regulation and the EFs that comprise it, in short, function to maximize future consequences over immediate ones, and so are instrumental to purposive, intentional behavior. As I argued earlier, that future is a social one. This resembles the view of Lezak (1995), who described the EFs as "those capacities that enable a person to engage successfully in independent, purposive, self-serving behavior," (p. 42) or that of Denckla (1994), noted earlier, who described them as attention and intention toward the future. Regrettably, neither author specified the nature of those EFs with any precision.

Often unstated is the fact that self-control is nearly impossible if there is not some means by which the individual is capable of perceiving and valuing future over immediate outcomes: No sense of the future—no self-control. A longer term outcome may have greater reward value than a short-term reward, if the two are compared to each other without regard to time. But arranged temporally, as they are, the reward value of the longer term outcome will be discounted by all organisms as a function of the length of the temporal delay involved to get it (Mazur, 1993). Humans demonstrate a remarkable shift over the first three decades of life toward a greater preference for larger, delayed versus smaller, more immediate rewards (Green, Meyerson, Lichtman, Rosen, & Fry, 1996). They discount future outcomes less steeply with age than do younger individuals or other species. This requires some neuropsychological capacity to sense the future, that is, to construct hypothetical futures, particularly for social consequences. It also simultaneously involves the weighing of alternative responses and their temporally proximal and distal outcomes—a calculation of risk–benefit ratios over time. Some neuropsychological mechanism must have evolved that permitted this relatively rapid construction of hypothetical social futures, while engaging in an economic analysis of immediate versus delayed outcomes. Without such an evolved mental mechanism, self-control would not occur. As I discuss below, the first EF to develop in children provides the capacity for just such a cross-temporal economic spreadsheet—visual imagery.

CONSTRUCTING A THEORY
OF THE EXECUTIVE FUNCTIONS AND SELF-CONTROL

I have suggested that humans have at least four means of self-control—four classes of action that they direct toward themselves to change themselves to improve their future. The details of this model of EFs can be found in previous publications (Barkley, 1997a, 1997b), along with the evidence that seems to support their existence. That evidence comes from developmental psychology, neuropsychological studies into the underlying factors or dimensions of executive functioning, and neuroimaging research on the apparent localization of these EFs within the prefrontal lobes. It also comes from a substantial amount of research on executive functioning in children and adults with ADHD, a disorder of inhibition believed to originate in the prefrontal–striatal–cerebellar network (Castellanos et al., 1996; Filipek et al., 1997).

The initial structure of this model is taken from Bronowski (1967/1977), who first proposed it in his discussion of the unique properties of human language that he attributed to the prefrontal cortex. I further elaborated this framework by drawing heavily from Fuster's insights into the functioning of the prefrontal cortex (Fuster, 1995, 1997). To this, I added the findings of Goldman-Rakic (1995) and others on working memory, and also those of Damasio (1994, 1995) on the somatic marker system and the rapid economic (motivational) analysis of hypothetical outcomes it affords. The model of EFs offered here is thereby a hybrid one.

The EFs model is graphically depicted in Figure 15.1. Space here permits only a very brief summary of it; far greater detail is provided elsewhere (Barkley, 1997a, 1998). In this model, inhibition sets the occasion for the occurrence of the EFs and provides the protection from interference that those EFs will require to construct hypothetical futures and direct behavior toward them. Despite being relatively distinct, the three inhibitory functions and the four EFs are interactive in their natural state and share a common pur-

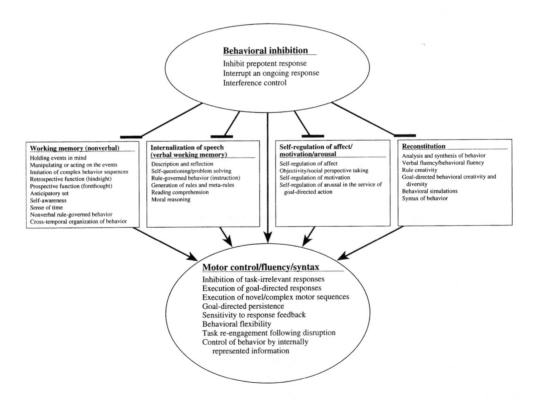

FIGURE 15.1. A schematic model of the relationship of inhibition to four executive functions and the motor control they govern. From Barkley (1997b). Copyright 1997 by The Guilford Press. Reprinted by permission.

pose. That purpose is to "internalize," or make private, certain self-directed behavior, so as to anticipate and prepare for the future, especially the social future. Why such self-directed behaviors had to become covert in form is be noted later. For now, the ultimate utility of the EFs is to maximize net long-term versus short-term social outcomes.

I view the four EFs as developing by a common process. I have borrowed Vygotsky's process for the internalization of speech (Diaz & Berk, 1992; Vygotsky, 1978; Vygotsky & Luria, 1994), which I ascribe to the second EF, and extended it to three other forms of behavior that become self-directed and eventually covert or internalized. All four EFs represent private, covert forms of behavior that at one time in early child development (and in human evolution) were entirely publicly observable and directed toward others and the external world at large. With maturation, this outer-directed behavior becomes turned on the self as a means to control one's own behavior. Such self-behaving then becomes increasingly less observable to others as the suppression of the public musculoskeletal aspects of the behavior progresses. This progressively greater capacity to suppress the publicly observable aspects of behavior is what is meant here by the terms "covert, privatized, or internalized."

Sensing to the Self (Nonverbal Working Memory)

The first executive function has been called nonverbal working memory by others. It is akin to Baddeley's visuospatial sketchpad in his information-processing rendition of working memory (Baddeley, 1986). It originates in the privatization of sensorimotor actions—it is sensing to the self (literally, re-sensing to the self). The most important of the senses to humans are vision and audition, so this executive function may be chiefly comprised of visual imagery and covert audition—seeing and hearing to the self.

This EF has both retrospective (sensory or resensing) and prospective (preparatory motor) elements (Fuster, 1997; Goldman-Rakic, 1995), and requires interference control for its effective performance. Here, then, arises the mental module for sensing the hypothetical future from the experienced past. This serves to generate the private or mental representations (images, auditions, etc.) that bridge the cross-temporal elements within a contingency arrangement (event–response–outcome) that is so crucial for self-control toward the future. Pierce (1897/1955), and later Deacon (1997) and Donald (1993), noted that such private sensorimotor representations are prerequisites for symbolization. They constitute mental icons that can be linked with others to form indexical relations (e.g., smell smoke → iconic smoke → iconic fire → escape) (Deacon, 1997). Symbols can then arise as means of linking such indexical relations to each other (Deacon, 1997). Both private sensory representations (nonverbal working memory) and symbolization (language and verbal working memory) are among the prerequisites for culture (Deacon, 1997; Donald, 1993; Durham, 1991; Lumsden & Wilson, 1982).

Speech to the Self (Verbal Working Memory)

The second EF, verbal working memory, is similar to Baddeley's (Baddeley & Hitch, 1994) construct of the same name. It originates in the developmental internalization of speech. The individual is capable of activating the central or cortical aspects of speech without engaging the actual motor execution of that speech. Such self-speech permits self-description and reflection, self-instruction, self-questioning and problem solving, as well as the invention of rules and metarules to be applied to oneself (Diaz & Berk, 1992). Therefore, it contributes not only to a major form of self-control via language but also likely provides the basis for moral conduct. It also makes possible reading comprehension through silent reading (self-speech) that must be held in mind for the extraction of its semantic (nonverbal) content.

Emotion to the Self
(Self-Regulation of Affect–Motivation–Arousal Emotion)

This EF may occur initially as a mere consequence of the first two (private sensing and speech). Those EFs involve covertly re-presenting forms of visual and verbal information to oneself. These mentally represented events have associated affective and motivational properties or valences, which Damasio (1994, 1995) called "somatic markers." Initially, those affective and motivational valences may have publicly visible counterparts, emotional displays, such as when we laugh out loud in response to a mentally visualized incident. Eventually, though, these affective displays are kept private or covert in form. Hence, originates the third EF of privatizing affect and its motivational properties. In brief, it is feeling (emoting–motivating) to the self. This model argues that this EF forms the wellspring of intrinsic motivation (willpower) so necessary to support future-directed behavior.

Self-Play (Reconstitution)

The fourth EF is self-directed, private (covert) play, or reconstitution. "Fluency," "flexibililty," and "generativity" are some other terms by which this EF is known in neuropsychology. It serves to generate a diversity of new combinations of behavioral units out of old ones through a two-step process: analysis and synthesis. In analysis, old behavior sequences are broken down into smaller units. These units are then recombined (synthesized) into new sequences that can be tested against the requirements of the problem to be solved (Corballis, 1989; Fuster, 1997). It is hypothesized here to arise from the internalization of play (both sensorimotor and symbolic) and serves to create novel future-directed actions. Such novel actions will be needed when obstacles to a goal are encountered (problems), in order to overcome them and successfully attain the goal. The generation of such novel responses has been shown to be especially problematic for patients with frontal lobe injuries (Godefroy & Rosseaux, 1997). It has been blamed on their inability to form and sustain mental referents from instructions, so as to manipulate them to discover a means to achieve a goal. And that, as I have argued, is simply covert play to one's self.

This EF may be subdivided further into verbal and nonverbal components comparable to the working memory system (verbal or nonverbal) on which it acts. Fluency tasks are one means of assessing this function. Recent neuroimaging studies suggest that verbal and nonverbal (design) fluency are mediated by separate (left vs. right) regions of the dorsolateral frontal cortex (Lee et al., 1997; Stuss et al., 1998). That would imply that a bivariate subdivision of this executive function might be useful. However, prior factor-analytic studies of EF measures have found only a single dimension representing both verbal and nonverbal fluency (Levin et al., 1996).

Further Implications of the Theory

Each executive function is also hypothesized to contribute to the following developmental shifts in the sources of control over human behavior:

- From external events to mental representations related to those events.
- From control by others to control by the self.
- From immediate reinforcement to delayed gratification.
- From the temporal now to the conjectured social future.

With maturation, the individual progressively comes to be guided more by covert representations that permit self-control, deferred gratification, and goal-directed actions toward conjectured social futures.

Briefly put, the internalization of sensorimotor action, self-speech, and emotion–motivation, along with the internalization of play (reconstitution), provides an exceptionally powerful set of mind tools that greatly facilitate adaptive functioning. In a sense, these EFs permit the private simulation of actions within specific settings that can be tested out mentally for their probable consequences (somatic markers) before a response is selected for eventual public execution. This, as Karl Popper noted, allows our ideas to die in our place (see Dennett, 1995). It constitutes a form of mental trial-and-error learning that is devoid of real world consequences for one's mistakes.

This use of the EFs for private simulation has led me to consider what might be the ultimate adaptive advantage or evolutionary function for which self-control and the executive system arose in humans (Barkley, 2001b). Why give consideration to an evolutionary perspective on self-control? Because it can be a rich source of testable hypotheses about a set of mental functions and the disorders associated with them, if properly done (Buss, Haselton, Shackelford, Bleske, & Wakefield, 1998).

EVOLUTIONARY CONSIDERATIONS

The importance of taking an evolutionary stance toward child psychopathologies rests in three interrelated ideas. The first derives from the criteria that may be used to define a mental disorder. Wakefield (1999) has championed a simple yet elegant set of useful requirements that must be met for a condition to be considered a valid disorder. These requirements are based, in part, on the definition of a "biological adaptation." For a disorder to be considered as such from this perspective, it must be a "harmful dysfunction." In the first part of these criteria, existent scientific evidence must demonstrate that those experiencing the disorder have a failure or extreme deficiency in a biological adaptation. Adaptations are universal functional mechanisms found in all members of that species under their typical species range or environmental circumstances. Like hearts, lungs, and eyes, brains are an adaptation. But such adaptations are not only physical but also psychological (Barkow, Cosmides, & Tooby, 1992). In a sense, the human brain comes with a large number of inborn psychological adaptations, or mental modules (Pinker, 1997). Mental disorders are therefore defined, in part, as failures or extreme deficiencies in psychological adaptations. The second part of these criteria is the requirement that harm result from the failing adaptation. Harm can consist of increased mortality, morbidity, or substantial impairment in major life activities. This view of disorders requires that a relatively clear understanding of the psychological mechanism exists, along with evidence that it is disrupted in those possessing the disorder. Only evolution provides a means by which to understand the basis for the psychological adaptation, or its adaptive purpose(s). There is no question that ADHD is associated with a significant deficit in a psychological adaptation (response inhibition) and significant impairment in daily life activities (Barkley, 1998). It also contributes to increased morbidity through accidental injury

(Barkley, 2001a) and may result in decreased life expectancy, though the latter is rather speculative at this time (Barkley, 1998).

This raises the second rationale for an evolutionary approach to psychopathology. If disorders are failures of adaptations, then the more one understands the evolutionary history of that adaptation, and especially what functions it serves, the deeper the appreciation for what the disorder has disrupted in the psychological functioning of those so afflicted. Adaptations arise from evolution as a consequence of their solving adaptive problems for the species (Ridley, 1996). To fully understand the adaptation, then, one needs to consider the nature of these problems and how the adaptive mechanism contributes to their reduction or resolution. For instance, I have speculated that behavioral inhibition, and especially the associated executive functions, may have arisen for purposes of reciprocal exchange (delayed altruism), the formation of cooperative coalitions that engage in non-zero-sum activities, and, eventually, imitation and vicarious learning (Barkley, 2001b). By approaching the disorder from the standpoint of evolution, a person is better able to appreciate the purposes of the adaptation and how its failure via the disorder may disrupt normal functioning. Returning to ADHD, an evolutionary analysis would raise the hypothesis that those with ADHD will have substantial difficulty in social realms that involve reciprocal exchange or altruism, development of cooperative coalitions to achieve greater benefits than can be attained by acting alone, and use of vicarious learning for self-management and improvement. None of these directions for future research would have arisen from the purely descriptive and taxonomic view of ADHD as an attention disorder (American Psychiatric Association, 1994).

The third basis for considering an evolutionary stance to disorders comes from the fact that much of a species' development is governed by heritable patterns of structural and functional change. Both the physical and psychological molding of a species to its relatively recognizable and uniform body plan and set of behavioral predispositions have been, to varying degrees, determined by natural selection acting on heritable, recurring patterns of structural and functional development (Barkow, Cosmides, & Tooby, 1992). In short, not only do adaptations arise through the process of natural selection, but so also do their pattern and sequence of development. This being so, one must consider the pattern and sequence for the normal development of an adaptation, including psychological ones, if one is to understand better how they are disrupted by or within a particular form of psychopathology or developmental disability. Just as an evolutionary perspective raises interesting hypotheses about the end purpose of an adaptation, so too can it raise equally interesting hypotheses about the development of that functional mechanism. For ADHD, an evolutionary developmental perspective would provide a fuller account of ADHD through its implications for the pattern and sequence in which normal inhibition and self-regulation emerge in children, and what ADHD may be doing to them.

As noted earlier, I believe that there is little question that self-regulation arose for a social function; thus, self-control is directly related to social relations (see Vohs & Ciarocco, Chapter 20, this volume). I discuss two among several possible adaptive social advantages for which self-control and an executive system might be useful (see Barkley, 2001b, for others).

Reciprocal Altruism (Social Exchange) and Coalition Formation

Among human universal social attributes, reciprocal altruism with nonkin (others with whom one does not share genetic self-interest) stands out as among our most unique behavioral features relative to other species. Humans exchange goods or services now for other ones later, despite having no common genetic self-interests with those with whom they engage in such exchanges. They do it nearly all the time, forming the backbone of human economic systems (Ridley, 1997). Although Williams (1966/1996) prefers the less emotive term "social donors" for those engaged in this practice to Haldane's term "altruism," the point is the same. Genetically unrelated humans live within a social group and frequently exchange benefits and costs now for benefits and costs later. The exchanges are reciprocated, and those reciprocations are delayed in time. Such a delayed exchange of costs and benefits between nonkin constitutes a promise or a social contract. Darwin (see Williams, 1966/1996, p. 94) was apparently well aware of the fact that a group-living species might well come to evolve a form of social exchange (what he termed as "the lowly motive"). He also appreciated that such exchange was an important factor to consider in understanding the evolution of not only human mental functions but also friendship and culture.

Reciprocal exchange, particularly when it is delayed, constitutes a prime candidate for the initial adaptive function of the prefrontal cortex. It requires both inhibition and a representational memory system for sensing past and future occasions—the foundation of self-control, as discussed earlier. Just as with any other form of adaptation, the mental mechanisms affording self-control exact a biological cost to the individual. That cost must be outweighed by some benefit, and such benefit need not be for the good of the species, or even the group, in order to evolve. It must be for the good of the individual and, specifically, the individual's genes. Yet humans voluntarily subject themselves to periods of self-deprivation (as in sharing or even dieting), deferred gratification (such as saving, investing, and education), and even aversiveness (as in getting inoculations against diseases). From the standpoint of selfish gene theory and its related kin, selection theory (Ridley, 1997), these actions make little sense in the context of the moment. According to those theories, individuals should seek as much benefit and advantage now for themselves and their genetic relatives, if only because others will do so if they do not, leaving the former at a disadvantage. Such personal greed is certainly evident in humans and can result in a sort of Tragedy of the Commons, whereby publicly held resources are depleted by self-interested individuals, even if the long-term depletion of the asset is not in those individuals' best interests (Ridley, 1997). In such instances, acts of self-control are losing strategies. The costs of reciprocal altruism and self-control can be substantial, and the individual employing it can be easily cheated out of or outcompeted for the immediate resources. The existence of reciprocal altruism requires that there be some advantage to the self-interested motives of individuals involved in those exchanges.

Delayed reciprocal exchange requires a capacity to perceive long-term sequences of events and their outcomes for one's self and for others, with whom one is trading. Even rudimentary, little-delayed forms of reciprocal exchange would begin to create selection pressures for the evolution of an increasingly longer sense of past and future (nonverbal working memory), so as to evaluate those longer term consequences of the trade. It has been suggested that in the environment of prehistoric humans, such as the grasslands of central Africa, food sources and other resources showed cyclical patterns of availability, as they do even today (Ridley, 1997). Periods of plenty were punctuated by periods of famine. Under such conditions of large swings in resource availability, sharing and its associated reciprocal exchange would have brought great advantage to individuals living in groups as a means of mediating or modulating the personal risks and costs associated with these cycles of feast and famine. Under such circumstances, it would pay those who had been lucky in hunting or scavenging to give up some of their excess bounty to others, in exchange for the same sort of reciprocation later, when those others were more fortunate and the previously successful hunters were not. Like a group-insurance pool today, individuals would chip in resources they did not require at the moment to those who needed them, in exchange for the same treatment later, in their own time of need—a sort of Golden Rule would result. A group of selfish cooperators would evolve, provided that the consequences for cheating on the contracts were made sufficiently harsh by the group to make reneging on those exchanges costly (Ridley, 1997). Indeed, in some modern hunter–gatherer groups, such as Eskimos, it seems that on some occasions, successful hunters' failure to share when their turn came could cost them their lives (Dugatkin, 1999; Ridley, 1997). Under periods of extreme resource variability, reciprocal exchange is a good adaptive strategy to solve the problem, a strategy converged on by other species such as vampire bats (reciprocal blood sharing) and some birds and mammals (reciprocal grooming) in more rudimentary forms (Ridley, 1997; Williams, 1966/1996). Perhaps this is what led to the further development of the EFs.

In essence, social exchange requires a sort of mental spreadsheet that calculates temporal sequences of exchange for which the executive system seems ideally designed. Social exchanges that occur frequently between two selfish cooperators can become the foundation for building not only friendships but also social coalitions for cooperating with or acting against other individuals and coalitions. The executive functions would seem to be well-designed mental modules for mediating this adaptive strategy of social exchange and cooperative coalition formation for greater adaptive advantage. If so, it implies that one of the major detrimental effects of ADHD (and of other frontal lobe injuries) for daily adaptive functioning is the diminution of the capacity for effective social exchange and its attendant cooperative coalition formation in daily social life.

Imitation (Vicarious) Learning

Though rarely mentioned in discussions of EFs, particularly those of nonverbal working memory, the capacity to engage in imitation, particularly delayed imitation, is probably one of the most important capacities for group-living social species such as humans. Many species, as Darwin (1871/1992) noted, are capable of mimicry or even immediate imitation of particular acts. For many reasons, immediate mimicry or imitation is a good adaptive strategy, and other species have converged on it. Delayed imitation, however, especially in generalized form, is a notably human achievement (Donald, 1991, 1993). Our species has an early developing instinct, nay, nearly a compulsion, to do it (Meltzoff, 1988).

Imitation, especially delayed imitation, clearly depends on three cognitive capacities: (1) the inhibition of prepotent responses, (2) an evolved mental mechanism for carrying past sensory perceptions of others' behavior forward in time across a delay interval, and (3) a capacity to construct motor responses on the basis of those mentally reperceived actions of others. The latter two requirements are obviously the retrospective and prospective aspects of the nonverbal working memory system. Initially, it seems likely that the initial delay between the act and its imitation was undoubtedly brief, perhaps owing to the initially fleeting afterimages that occurred from primary sensory impressions. Regardless of how it originated, the capacity to inhibit prepotent responses and to carry forward in time past perceptions (retrospection) that create the template for the later imitative motor act (prospection) form the foundation of self-regulation, as noted earlier. The more highly developed the nonverbal working memory capacity, the lengthier and more hierarchically complex the sequence of actions that can be held in mind for later imitation, and the longer the delay over which it can be carried into the future. And the greater would be the demand for response inhibition during the period when such imitative responses are being programmed and eventually executed. The more complex the sequence, the more its syntax and timing must also be held in mind. The holding of a sequence of events in mind may also form the beginnings of a subjective, or psychological, sense of time (Davies, 1995).

Imitation involves the reproduction of another person's behavior after it is observed. Vicarious learning is a more advanced form of imitation. It involves not just imitation (doing what gained reinforcement for others) but inverse imitation, not doing what another person does (avoiding actions that led to aversive, painful, or even mortal outcomes for others). Note the requirement for oppositional action involved in vicarious learning. The amount of social learning that occurs in humans through imitation and vicarious learning is substantial, to say the least. It is undoubtedly far more than the learning that could occur by operant conditioning or by trial and error alone. Imitation develops very early in childhood; in fact, rudiments of it are present in infants at 9 months of age (Meltzoff, 1988). Its development seems to parallel the development of representational memory, especially visual imagery (Kopp, 1982; Meltzoff, 1988).

No other species comes close to the human capacity for this form of learning. Evolutionary theory demands that explanations for such adaptations initially be considered from a self-interested perspective (the good of the individuals or of their genes), before giving credence to explanations at the group level (for the good of others) (Dawkins, 1976, 1997; Williams, 1966/1996). From that self-interested perspective, vicarious learning constitutes a form of *experiential theft* that is clearly in the imitator's self-interests. More precisely, it is behavioral plagiarism. Through imitation and vicarious learning, the individual profits from the experiences that others may have with real-world contingencies, without the costs, penalties, pitfalls, morbidity, and mortality associated with those contingencies. Vicarious learners gain a considerable adaptive advantage in a group-living species, because they appropriate the experience of another person for their own, with minimal costs. From that vantage point, imitation and vicarious learning are incredibly useful self-interested adaptations.

Imitation also provides for the development of tool manufacture, as well as social communication via gesture (Blackmore, 1999; Donald, 1993). The origin of imitation and later vicarious learning would have set up selection pressure for humans to evolve a covert form of behavioral rehearsal to keep others from copying (plagiarizing) their behavior while it was being rehearsed and further perfected. Though speculative, this may have initiated the need for the internalization or privatization of one's behavior-to-the-self that became the basis for the EFs. Interestingly, this resensing of one's past experiences may also be the origin of "autonoetic awareness," or the awareness of self across time (Barkley, 1997a; Kopp, 1982; Wheeler, Stuss, & Tulving, 1997).

FALSIFYING THE THEORY OF EXECUTIVE FUNCTIONING

One obvious result of redefining the EFs as being relatively covert behavior-to-the-self is that it is testable. When individuals are engaged in each of these forms of private behavior, it may be possible to detect subtle yet measurable aspects of the originally public form of that behavior. This could be done by using very sensitive instruments that can detect fine changes in muscle tension or even movement associated with the covert form of the behavior involved. Livesay and colleagues have done this to show that some changes in muscle tension and even micromovements of the oral-musculature occur during covert verbal thought. And changes in muscle tension in the limbs have been found to occur during acts of visual imagery of imagined manipulative activity (Livesay & Samaras, 1998; Livesay et al., 1996). This prediction also could be tested by neuroimaging studies. Those studies might show that the same or similar zones of cortical activation are involved in both the public and private forms of behavior, except that in the private form, the primary sensory cortex would not be activated, and the primary motor zone associated with the public behavior would need to be suppressed to preclude the actual public execution of the response. Ryding and colleagues (1996) appear to have demonstrated this very finding in their neuroimaging studies of covert self-speech or verbal thought, and D'Esposito and colleagues (1997) have done so for visual imagery. Perhaps this explains the relatively recent discovery that the cerebellum is related in some ways to "cognition," and the planning and execution of motor actions once attributed to just the prefrontal cortex (Diamond, 2000; Houk & Wise, 1995). Not only is the cerebellum important in the execution of overt behavior but it also may be just as important in this form of covert behavior to the self that comprises nonverbal working memory.

This rendering of executive function as covert behavior-to-the-self leads to a further prediction: We should expect that the private forms of the behavior suffer from many of the same constraints, flaws, and qualities as do their public counterparts. For instance, the fact that I am largely color blind to pastel reds and greens would have little or no meaning for a cognitive psychological view of nonverbal working memory, such as that proposed by Baddeley (1986). Yet it would have substantial meaning here as a prediction that my capacity for visual imagery (nonverbal working memory) would be equally deficient in these color hues. Such a prediction has some support in research on visual imagery (Kosslyn, 1994). The same would be true of mentally simulated motor actions that would be afflicted with the same deficits, flaws, and limitations as are the publicly observable movements on which they are based. This seems to be the case for children with developmental motor coordination disorder (Maruff, Wilson, Trebilcock, & Currie, 1999). Such deficits are imminently understandable from the perspective of the present EF theory, but make little or no sense from the viewpoint of the information-processing/ computer metaphor of the EFs. And so, too, would comparable deficits and constraints be predicted to occur in private speech, private emotion–motivation, and private play (reconstitution), if deficits existed in their public counterparts.

Moreover, this perspective on the executive system further argues that an individual could not engage in the public and private action simultaneously, given that many of the same brain regions are employed in both. A moment's reflection will show this to be true for speech. One cannot speak covertly to oneself and publicly to others at the same time. This should be so for the other EFs as well. By adulthood, then, humans have two means of behaving—a public one and a covert one. Behaviors proposed for execution are initially tested out in their covert form, and then one is selected for public execution (Bronowski, 1967/1977). It is the covert form that is impaired by injuries to the frontal lobes, often to the detriment of the effective use of the public form as well.

A third prediction from this model is that of a stagewise hierarchy in the development of these EFs, each requiring that the previous one emerge before it can begin to do so during maturation. So crucial may be nonverbal working memory (sensing to the self) to human development and survival that it seems to arise within the first few months of life. By ages 12–24 months, it far exceeds that of our closest living primate relative (Diamond, Cruttenden, & Niederman, 1994; Hofstader & Reznick, 1996; Kopp, 1982; Zelazo, Kearsley, & Stack, 1995). Thereafter develops the internalization of self-speech, then that of emotion–motivation, eventually leading to that of reconstitution. This sequence is admittedly speculative. Some type of staging in the development of EFs, how-ever, has been suggested in cross-sectional studies of age-related differences in batteries of EF tasks (Hale, Bronik, & Fry, 1997; Levin et al., 1996; Passler, Isaac, & Hynd, 1985; Welsh, Pennington, & Grossier, 1991). None of these were longitudinal designs, however, so these studies cannot speak directly to the slope, rate, and specific staging of the devel-opmental trajectories the EFs may take.

Noteworthy here is the additional implication that the very nature of self-control demonstrates qualitative, not just quantitative, changes throughout child development. From this model comes the prediction that young children may use just one form of self-regulation (sensing to the self, largely imagery), whereas somewhat older children have two forms (now adding self-speech), and even older children manifest three forms (with the addition of self-directed emotion). Eventually, by late childhood to early adolescence, the fourth form of self-control emerges, granting individuals four means by which to reg-ulate their own behavior toward a more effective and successful social future.

THE IMPACT OF ADHD ON SELF-CONTROL

A central problem for persons with ADHD is the lack of capacity for behavioral inhibi-tion (Barkley, 1999; Nigg, 2001; Quay, 1997). Given the importance of such inhibition to executive functioning as described earlier, a deficit in inhibition will result in a cascade of secondary deficits into the four EFs. As extrapolated to those with ADHD, the model pre-dicts that deficits in behavioral inhibition lead to deficiencies in nonverbal working mem-ory, thus resulting in (1) particular forms of forgetfulness (forgetting to do things at cer-tain critical points in time), (2) impaired ability to organize and execute actions relative to time (e.g., time management), and (3) reduced hindsight and forethought, (4) leading to a reduction in the creation of anticipatory action toward future events. Consequently, the capacity for the cross-temporal organization of behavior in persons with ADHD is dimin-ished, disrupting the ability to string together complex chains of actions directed, over time, to a future goal. The greater the degree to which time separates the components of the behavioral contingency (event, response, consequence), the more difficult the task will prove to be for those with ADHD who cannot bind the contingency together across time to use it to govern their behavior as well as others.

Research is beginning to demonstrate some of these deficits in persons with ADHD, such as nonverbal working memory, timing, and forethought (Barkley, 1997a; Barkley, Edwards, Laneri, Fletcher, & Metevia, 2001; Barkley, Murphy, & Bush, 2001; Murphy et al., 2001). Still unstudied is the prediction from this theory that children with ADHD will be delayed in making references to time, to the past, and to the future in their verbal in-teractions with others relative to when normal children begin making such references in their development of sense of time, hindsight, and foresight.

For those with ADHD, the privatization of speech should be delayed, resulting in greater public speech (excessive talking), less verbal reflection before acting, less orga-nized and rule-oriented self-speech, diminished influence of self-directed speech in con-trolling one's own behavior, and difficulties following the rules and instructions given by others (Barkley, 1997a). Substantial accumulated evidence supports this prediction of de-layed internalization of speech (Berk & Potts, 1991; Landau, Berk, & Mangione, 1996; Winsler, 1998; Winsler et al., 2000). Given that such private self-speech is a major basis for verbal working memory (Baddeley, 1986), this domain of cognitive activity should be impaired in ADHD as well. Evidence suggests that this is so; children with ADHD have

difficulties with tasks such as digit span backwards, mental arithmetic, paced auditory serial addition, paired associated learning, and other tasks believed to reflect verbal working memory (Barkley, 1997a; Chang et al., 1999; Grodzinsky & Diamond, 1994; Kuntsi,
Oosterlaan, & Stevenson, 2001).

The impairment in the internalization and self-direction of emotion arising from
ADHD leads to the following predictions: Those with ADHD should display (1) greater
emotional expression in their reactions to events; (2) less objectivity in the selection of a
response to an event; (3) diminished social perspective taking, because the child does not
delay his or her initial emotional reaction long enough to take the view of others and
their needs into account; and (4) diminished ability to induce drive and motivational
states in themselves in the service of goal-directed behavior. Those with ADHD remain
more dependent than do others on the environmental contingencies within a situation or
task to determine their motivation (Barkley, 1997a). Preliminary work has begun to demonstrate that those with ADHD do have significant problems with emotion regulation
(Braaten & Rosen, 2000; Maedgen & Carlson, 2000) and that this may be particularly so
in that subset having comorbid oppositional defiant disorder (Melnick & Hinshaw,
2000).

The model further predicts that ADHD will be associated with impaired reconstitution, or self-directed play, evident in a diminished use of analysis and synthesis in the formation of both verbal and nonverbal responses to events. The capacity to visualize mentally, manipulate, then generate multiple plans of action (options) in the service of goal-
directed behavior and to select from among them those plans with the greatest likelihood
of succeeding should, therefore, be reduced. This impairment in reconstitution will be evident in everyday verbal fluency, when the person with ADHD is required by a task or situation to assemble rapidly, accurately, and efficiently the parts of speech into messages
(sentences) to accomplish the goal or requirements of the task. It will also be evident in
tasks in which visual information must be held in mind and manipulated to generate diverse scenarios to help solve problems (Barkley, 1997a). Evidence for deficiency in verbal
and nonverbal fluency, planning, problem solving, and strategy development more generally in children with ADHD is limited, but what does exist is consistent with the theory
(Barkley, 1997a; Clark, Prior, & Kinsella, 2000; Klorman et al., 1999; Nigg et al., 2002;
Oosterlaan, Scheres, & Sergeant, 2002).

In general, ADHD is predicted to disrupt the aforementioned four transitions in the
source of control over behavior. The child with ADHD will be more under the control of
external events than of mental representations about time and the future, under the influence of others rather than acting to control the self, pursuing immediate gratification over
deferred gratification, and under the influence of the temporal now more than of the
probable social futures that lie ahead. From this vantage point, ADHD is not a disorder
of attention, at least not to the moment or to the external environment, but is more of a
disorder of intention—that is, attention to the future and what one needs to do to prepare
for its arrival. It is also a disorder of time, specifically, time management, in that individuals manifest an inability to regulate their behavior relative to time, as well as do others of
their own developmental level. This creates a sort of temporal myopia in which the individual responds to or prepares only for relatively imminent events rather than ones that
lie further ahead in time, for which others their age are preparing, so as to be ready for
their eventual arrival (Barkley, 1997a).

By implication, this view of ADHD, combined with an evolutionary perspective on
the disorder, suggests that the disorder will interfere with two of the larger social purposes for which executive functioning and self-control may have evolved—reciprocal al-

truism (social exchange) and vicarious learning. These predictions have yet to be tested directly through research on children with ADHD. But there is currently sufficient evidence available to demonstrate significant impairments in the peer relationships of children with ADHD, perhaps for these very reasons. And it is apparent that those with ADHD have a propensity for risk taking, despite having been reasonably informed of the consequences for others who do so.

CONCLUSIONS

In closing, there is obviously much promise in viewing ADHD as a disorder of self-regulation. It encourages child and developmental psychopathologists to develop more fully models of how normal self-control arises across childhood and even into adulthood, and to examine where in these models disorders such as ADHD disrupt the normal structure and processes of self-regulation to produce what is known about the disorder. Moreover, such model building also suggests new hypotheses that can not only be pursued in testing the models but also provide a greater understanding of what is disrupted by the disorder. I have also argued here that taking an evolutionary or adaptive perspective toward self-control and its associated EFs can further enlighten us on the nature of these relatively unique human abilities, and what larger domains and problems of social functioning they evolved to solve. This may also help to demonstrate what social functions may be deficient in persons with ADHD. That perspective implies that self-control may have arisen for a set of largely social functions, such as reciprocal exchange, cooperative coalitions, and vicarious learning. It provides further grounds for the development of testable hypotheses not only about self-control but also about the social deficiencies that arise in disorders of self-regulation such as ADHD.

REFERENCES

Ainslie, G. (1974). Impulse control in pigeons. *Journal of the Experimental Analysis of Behavior, 21*, 485–489.

American Psychiatric Association. (1994). *Diagnostic and statistical manual of mental disorders* (4th ed.). Washington, DC: Author.

Baddeley, A. D. (1986). *Working memory*. London: Clarendon Press.

Baddeley, A. D., & Hitch, G. J. (1994). Developments in the concept of working memory. *Neuropsychology, 8*, 1485–493.

Barkley, R. A. (1997a). *ADHD and the nature of self-control*. New York: Guilford Press.

Barkley, R. A. (1997b). Behavioral inhibition, sustained attention, and executive functions: Constructing a unifying theory of ADHD. *Psychological Bulletin, 121*, 65–94.

Barkley, R. A. (1998). *Attention-deficit hyperactivity disorder: A handbook for diagnosis and treatment* (2nd ed.). New York: Guilford Press.

Barkley, R. A. (1999). Response inhibition in attention deficit hyperactivity disorder. *Mental Retardation and Developmental Disabilities Research Reviews, 5*, 177–184.

Barkley, R. A. (2001a). Accidents and ADHD. *Economics of Neuroscience, 3*, 64–68.

Barkley, R. A. (2001b). The executive functions and self-regulation: An evolutionary neuropsychological perspective. *Neuropsychology Review, 11*, 1–29.

Barkley, R. A., Edwards, G., Laneri, M., Fletcher, K., & Metevia, L. (2001). Executive functioning, temporal discounting, and sense of time in adolescents with attention deficit hyperactivity disorder and oppositional defiant disorder. *Journal of Abnormal Child Psychology, 29*, 541–556.

Barkley, R. A., Murphy, K. R., & Bush, T. (2001). Time perception and reproduction in young adults with attention deficit hyperactivity disorder (ADHD). *Neuropsychology, 15*, 351–360.

Barkow, J. H., Cosmides, L., & Tooby, J. (1992). *The adapted mind: Evolutionary psychology and the generation of culture.* New York: Oxford University Press.

Berk, L. E., & Potts, M. K. (1991). Development and functional significance of private speech among attention-deficit hyperactivity disorder and normal boys. *Journal of Abnormal Child Psychology, 19,* 357–377.

Blackmore, S. (1999). *The mem machine.* New York: Oxford University Press.

Braaten, E. B., & Rosen, L. A. (2000). Self-regulation of affect in attention deficit hyperactivity disorder (ADHD) and non-ADHD boys: Differences in empathic responding. *Journal of Consulting and Clinical Psychology, 68,* 313–321.

Breen, M. J. (1989). Cognitive and behavioral differences in ADHD boys and girls. *Journal of Child Psychology and Psychiatry, 30,* 711–716.

Bronowski, J. (1976). *The ascent of man.* New York: Little, Brown.

Bronowski, J. (1977). Human and animal languages. In P. E. Ariotti (Ed.), *A sense of the future: Essays in natural philosophy* (pp. 104–131). Cambridge, MA: MIT Press. (Original work published 1967)

Burns, D. J., & Powers, R. B. (1975). Choice and self-control in children: A test of Rachlin's model. *Bulletin of the Psychonomic Society, 5,* 156–158.

Buss, D. M., Haselton, M. G., Shackelford, T. K., Bleske, A. L., & Wakefield, J. C. (1998). Adaptations, exaptations, and spandrels. *American Psychologist, 53,* 533–548.

Cantwell, D. (1975). *The hyperactive child.* New York: Spectrum.

Castellanos, F. X., Giedd, J. N., Marsh, W. L., Hamburger, S. D., Vaituzis, A. C., Dickstein, D. P., Sarfatti, S. E., Vauss, Y. C., Snell, J. W., Lange, N., Kaysen, D., Krain, A. L., Ritchhie, G. F., Rajapakse, J. C., & Rapoport, J. L. (1996). Quantitative brain magnetic resonance imaging in attention-deficit hyperactivity disorder. *Archives of General Psychiatry, 53,* 607–616.

Chang, H. T., Klorman, R., Shaywitz, S. E., Fletcher, J. M., Marchione, K. E., Holahan, J. M., Stuebing, K. K., Brumaghim, J. T., & Shaywitz, B. A. (1999). Paired-associate learning in attention-deficit/hyperactivity disorder as a function of hyperactivity–impulsivity and oppositional defiant disorder. *Journal of Abnormal Child Psychology, 27,* 237–245.

Clark, C., Prior, M., & Kinsella, G. J. (2000). Do executive function deficits differentiate between adolescents with ADHD and oppositional defiant/conduct disorder?: A neuropsychological study using the Six Elements Test and Hayling Sentence Completion Test. *Journal of Abnormal Child Psychology, 28,* 405–414.

Corballis, M. C. (1989). Laterality and human evolution. *Psychological Review, 96,* 492–505.

Damasio, A. R. (1994). *Descartes' error: Emotion, reason, and the human brain.* New York: Putnam.

Damasio, A. R. (1995). On some functions of the human prefrontal cortex. In J. Grafma, K. J. Holyoak, & F. Boller (Eds.), *Structure and functions of the human prefrontal cortex: Vol. 769. Annals of the New York Academy of Sciences* (pp. 241–251). New York: New York Academy of Sciences.

Danforth, J. S., Barkley, R. A., & Stokes, T. F. (1991). Observations of parent–child interactions with hyperactive children: Research and clinical implications. *Clinical Psychology Review, 11,* 703–727.

Darwin, C. (1992). *The descent of man and selection in relation to sex.* Chicago: Enclyclopedia Britannica. (Original work published 1871)

Davies, P. (1995). *About time: Einstein's unfinished revolution.* New York: Simon & Schuster.

Dawkins, R. (1976). *The selfish gene.* New York: Oxford University Press.

Dawkins, R. (1997). *Climbing mount improbable.* New York: Oxford University Press.

Deacon, T. W. (1997). *The symbolic species: The co-evolution of language and the brain.* New York: Norton.

Denckla, M. B. (1994). Measurement of executive function. In G. R. Lyon (Ed.), *Frames of reference for the assessment of learning disabilities: New views on measurement issues* (pp. 117–142). Baltimore: Brookes.

Denckla, M. B. (1996). A theory and model of executive function: A neuropsychological perspective. In G. R. Lyon & N. A. Krasnegor (Eds.), *Attention, memory, and executive function* (pp. 263–277). Baltimore: Brookes.

Dennett, D. (1995). *Darwin's dangerous idea: Evolution and the meanings of life*. New York: Simon & Schuster.

Dennis, M. (1991). Frontal lobe function in childhood and adolescence: A heuristic for assessing attention regulation, executive control, and the intentional states important for social discourse. *Developmental Neuropsychology, 7,* 327–358.

D'Esposito, M., Detre, J. A., Aguirre, G. K., Stallcup, M., Alsop, D. C., Tippet, L. J., & Farah, M. J. (1997). A functional MRI study of mental image generation. *Neuropsychologia, 35,* 725–730.

Diamond, A. (2000). Close interrelation of motor development and cognitive development and of the cerebellum and prefrontal cortex. *Developmental Psychology, 71,* 44–56.

Diamond, A., Cruttenden, L., & Neiderman, D. (1994). AB with multiple wells: 1. Why are multiple wells sometimes easier than two wells? 2. Memory or memory + inhibition? *Developmental Psychology, 30,* 192–205.

Diaz, R. M., & Berk, L. E. (1992). *Private speech: From social interaction to self-regulation.* Mahwah, NJ: Erlbaum.

Donald, M. (1991). *Origins of the modern mind: Three stages in the evolution of culture and cognition.* Cambridge, MA: Harvard University Press.

Donald, M. (1993). Precis of origins of the modern mind: Three stages in the evolution of culture and cognition. *Behavioral and Brain Sciences, 16,* 737–791.

Douglas, V. I. (1983). Attention and cognitive problems. In M. Rutter (Ed.), *Developmental neuropsychiatry* (pp. 280–329). New York: Guilford Press.

Dugatkin, L. (1999). *Cheating monkeys and citizen bees: The nature of cooperation in animals and humans.* New York: Free Press.

Durham, W. H. (1991). *Co-evolution: Genes, culture, and human diversity.* Stanford, CA: Stanford University Press.

Filipek, P. A., Semrud-Clikeman, M., Steingard, R. J., Renshaw, P. F., Kennedy, D. N., & Biederman, J. (1997). Volumetric MRI analysis comparing subjects having attention-deficit hyperactivity disorder with normal controls. *Neurology, 48,* 589–601.

Flavell, J. H. (1970). Developmental studies of mediated memory. In H. W. Reese & L. P. Lipsett (Eds.), *Advances in child development and behavior* (pp. 181–211). New York: Academic Press.

Fuster, J. M. (1995). Memory and planning: Two temporal perspectives of frontal lobe function. In H. H. Jasper, S. Riggio, & P. S. Goldman-Rakic (Eds.), *Epilepsy and the functional anatomy of the frontal lobe* (pp. 9–18). New York: Raven.

Fuster, J. M. (1997). *The prefrontal cortex: Anatomy, physiology, and neuropsychology of the frontal lobe* (3rd ed.). Philadelphia: Lippincott-Raven.

Godefroy, O., & Rosseaux, M. (1997). Novel decision making in patients with prefrontal or posterior brain damage. *Neurology, 49,* 695–701.

Goel, V., & Grafman, J. (1995). Are the frontal lobes implicated in "planning" functions?: Interpreting data from the Tower of Hanoi. *Neuropsychologia, 33,* 623–642.

Goldman-Rakic, P. S. (1995). Architecture of the prefrontal cortex and the central executive. In J. Grafman, K. J. Holyoak, & F. Boller (Eds.), *Structure and functions of the human prefrontal cortex: Vol. 769. Annals of the New York Academy of Sciences* (pp. 71–83). New York: New York Acdemy of Sciences.

Green, L., Myerson, J., Lichtman, D., Rosen, S., & Fry, A. (1996). Temporal discounting in choice between delayed rewards: The role of age and income. *Psychology and Aging, 11,* 79–84.

Grodzinsky, G. M., & Diamond, R. (1992). Frontal lobe functioning in boys with attention-deficit hyperactivity disorder. *Developmental Neuropsychology, 8,* 427–445.

Hale, S., Bronik, M. D., & Fry, A. F. (1997). Verbal and spatial working memory in school-age children: Developmental differences in susceptibility to interference. *Developmental Psychology, 33,* 364–371.

Hamlett, K. W., Pellegrini, D. S., & Conners, C. K. (1987). An investigation of executive processes in the problem-solving of attention deficit disorder-hyperactive children. *Journal of Pediatric Psychology, 12,* 227–240.

Hinshaw, S. P., Buhrmeister, D., & Heller, T. (1989). Anger control in response to verbal provocation: Effects of stimulant medication for boys with ADHD. *Journal of Abnormal Child Psychology, 17,* 393–408.

Hinshaw, S. P., Herbsman, C., Melnick, S., Nigg, J., & Simmel, C. (1993, February). *Psychological and familial processes in ADHD: Continuous or discontinuous with those in normal comparison children?* Paper presented at the Society for Research in Child and Adolescent Psychopathology, Santa Fe, NM.

Hofstadter, M., & Reznick, J. S. (1996). Response modality affects human infant delayed-response performance. *Child Development, 67,* 646–658.

Houk, J. C., & Wise, S. P. (1995). Distributed modular architectures linking basal ganglia, cerebellum, and cerebral cortex: Their role in planning and controlling action. *Cerebral Cortex, 2,* 95–110.

Kadesjo, B., & Gillberg, C. (2001). The comorbidity of ADHD in the general population of Swedish school-age children. *Journal of Child Psychology and Psychiatry, 42,* 487–492.

Kanfer, F. H., & Karoly, P. (1972). Self-control: A behavioristic excursion into the lion's den. *Behavior Therapy, 3,* 398–416.

Klorman, R., Hazel-Fernandez, H., Shaywitz, S. E., Fletcher, J. M., Marchione, K. E., Holahan, J. M., Stuebing, K. K., & Shaywitz, B. A. (1999). Executive functioning deficits in attention-deficit/hyperactivity disorder are independent of oppositional defiant or reading disorder. *Journal of the American Academy of Child and Adolescent Psychiatry, 38,* 1148–1155.

Kopp, C. B. (1982). Antecedents of self-regulation: A developmental perspective. *Developmental Psychology, 18,* 199–214.

Kosslyn, S. (1994). *Image and the brain.* Cambridge, MA: MIT Press.

Kuntsi, J., Oosterlaan, J., & Stevenson, J. (2001). Psychological mechanisms in hyperactivity: I. Response inhibition deficit, working memory impairment, delay aversion, or something else? *Journal of Child Psychology and Psychiatry, 42,* 199–210.

Landau, S., Berk, L. E., & Mangione, C. (1996, March). *Private speech as a problem-solving strategy in the face of academic challenge: The failure of impulsive children to get their act together.* Paper presented at the meeting of the National Association of School Psychologists, Atlanta, GA.

Lee, G. P., Strauss, E., Loring, D. W., McCloskey, L., Haworth, J. M., & Lehman, R. A. W. (1997). Sensitivity of figural fluency on the Five-Point Test to focal neurological dysfunction. *Clinical Neuropsychologist, 11,* 59–68.

Levin, H. S., Fletcher, J. M., Kufera, J. A., Harward, H., Lilly, M. A., Mendelsohn, D., Bruce, D., & Eisenberg, H. M. (1996). Dimensions of cognition measured by the Tower of London and other cognitive tasks in head-injured children and adolescents. *Developmental Neuropsychology, 12,* 17–34.

Lezak, M. D. (1995). *Neuropsychological assessment* (3rd ed.). New York: Oxford University Press.

Livesay, J. R., Liebke, A. W., Samaras, M. R., & Stanley, S. A. (1996). Covert speech behavior during a silent language recitation task. *Perceptual and Motor Skills, 83,* 1355–1362.

Livesay, J. R., & Samaras, M. R. (1998). Covert neuromuscular activity of the dominant forearm during visualization of a motor task. *Perceptual and Motor Skills, 86,* 371–374.

Logue, A. W. (1988). Research on self-control: An integrating framework. *Behavioral and Brain Sciences, 11,* 665–709.

Lorch, E. P., Milich, M., Sanchez, R. P., van den Broek, P., Baer, S., Hooks, K., Hartung, C., & Welsh, R. (2000). Comprehension of televised stories in boys with attention deficit/hyperactivity disorder and nonreferred boys. *Journal of Abnormal Psychology, 109,* 321–330.

Lumsden, C. J., & Wilson, E. O. (1982). Precis of *Genes, Mind, and Culture. Behavioral and Brain Sciences, 5,* 1–37.

Maedgen, J. W., & Carlson, C. L. (2000). Social functioning and emotion regulation in the attention deficit hyperactivity disorder subtypes. *Journal of Clinical Child Psychology, 29,* 30–42.

Mariani, M., & Barkley, R. A. (1997). Neuropsychological and academic functioning in preschool children with attention deficit hyperactivity disorder. *Developmental Neuropsychology, 13,* 111–129.

Maruff, P., Wilson, P., Trebilcock, M., & Currie J. (1999). Abnormalities of imagined motor sequences in children with developmental coordination disorder. *Neuropsychologia, 37,* 1317–1324.

Mazur, J. E. (1993). Predicting the strength of a conditioned reinforcer: Effects of delay and uncertainty. *Current Directions in Psychological Science, 2,* 70–74.

Melnick, S. M., & Hinshaw, S. P. (2000). Emotion regulation and parenting in AD/HD and comparison boys: Linkages with social behaviors and peer preference. *Journal of Abnormal Child Psychology, 28,* 73–86.

Meltzoff, A. N. (1988). Infant imitation and memory: Nine-month-olds in immediate and deferred tests. *Child Development, 59,* 217–225.

Mischel, W. (1983). Delay of gratification as process and as person variable in development. In D. Magnusson & V. L. Allen (Eds.), *Human development: An interactional perspective* (pp. 149–166). New York: Academic Press.

Mischel, W., Shoda, Y., & Rodriguez, M. I. (1989). Delay of gratification in children. *Science, 244,* 933–938.

Morris, R. D. (1996). Relationships and distinctions among the concepts of attention, memory, and executive function: A developmental perspective. In G. R. Lyon & N. A. Krasnegor (Eds.), *Attention, memory, and executive function* (pp. 11–16). Baltimore: Brookes.

Murphy, K. R., Barkley, R. A., & Bush, T. (2001). Executive functioning and olfactory identification in young adults with attention deficit hyperactivity disorder. *Neuropsychology, 15,* 211–220.

Navarick, D. J. (1986). Human impulsivity and choice: A challenge to traditional operant methodology. *Psychological Record, 36,* 343–356.

Nigg, J. T. (1999). The ADHD response-inhibition deficit as measured by the stop task: Replication with DSM-IV combined type, extension, and qualification. *Journal of Abnormal Child Psychology, 27,* 393–402.

Nigg, J. T. (2001). Is ADHD an inhibitory disorder? *Psychological Bulletin, 125,* 571–596.

Nigg, J. T., Blaskey, L. G., Huang-Pollock, C. L., & Rappley, M. D. (2002). Neuropsychological executive functions in DSM-IV ADHD subtypes. *Journal of the American Academy of Child and Adolescent Psychiatry, 41,* 59–66.

Oosterlaan, J., Scheres, A., & Sergeant, J. A. (2002). Verbal fluency, working memory, and planning in children with ADHD, ODD/CD, and comorbid ADHD+ODD/CD: Specificity of executive functioning deficits. *Journal of Abnormal Psychology.*

Passler, M. A., Isaac, W., & Hynd, G. W. (1985). Neuropsychological development of behavior attributed to frontal lobe functioning in children. *Developmental Neuropsychology, 1,* 349–370.

Pierce, C. S. (1955). Logic as semiotic: The theory of signs. In J. Buchler (Ed.), *The philosophical writings of Peirce* (pp. 98–119). New York: Dover. (Original work published in 1897)

Pinker, S. (1997). *How the mind works.* New York: Norton.

Purvis, K. L., & Tannock, R. (1997). Language abilities in children with attention deficit hyperactivity disorder, reading disabilities, and normal controls. *Journal of Abnormal Child Psychology, 25,* 133–144.

Quay, H. C. (1997). Inhibition and attention deficit hyperactivity disorder. *Journal of Abnormal Child Psychology, 25,* 7–13.

Ridley, Mark. (1996). *Evolution* (2nd ed.). Cambridge, MA: Blackwell Science.

Ridley, Matt. (1997). *The origins of virtue.* New York: Viking.

Roberts, M. A. (1990). A behavioral observation method for differentiating hyperactive and aggressive boys. *Journal of Abnormal Child Psychology, 18,* 131–142.

Ryding, E., Bradvik, B., & Ingvar, D. H. (1996). Silent speech activates prefrontal cortical regions asymmetrically, as well as speech-related areas in the dominant hemisphere. *Brain and Language, 52*, 435–451.

Shimamura, A. P., Janowsky, J. S., & Squire, L. R. (1990). Memory for the temporal order of events in patients with frontal lobe lesions and amnesic patients. *Neuropsychologia, 28*, 803–813.

Simmell, C., & Hinshaw, S. P. (1993, March). *Moral reasoning and antisocial behavior in boys with ADHD*. Poster presented at the biennial meeting of the Society for Research in Child Development, New Orleans, LA.

Sirigu, A. Zalla, T., Pillon, B., Grafman, J., DuBois, B., & Agid, Y. (1995). Planning and script analysis following prefrontal lobe lesions. In J. Grafman, K. J. Holyoke, & F. Boller (Eds.), *Structure and functions of the human prefrontal cortex: Volume 769. Annals of the New York Academy of Sciences* (pp. 277–288). New York: New York Academy of Sciences.

Skinner, B. F. (1953). *Science and human behavior*. New York: Macmillan.

Spreen, O., Risser, A. H., & Edgell, D. (1995). *Developmental neuropsychology*. New York: Oxford University Press.

Still, G. F. (1902). Some abnormal psychical conditions in children. *Lancet, 1*, 1008–1012, 1077–1082, 1163–1168.

Stuss, D. T., Alexander, M. A., Hamer, L., Palumbo, C., Dempster, R., Binns, M., Levine, B., & Izukawa, D. (1998). The effects of focal anterior and posterior brain lesions on verbal fluency. *Journal of the International Neuropsychological Society, 4*, 265–278.

Stuss, D. T., & Benson, D. F. (1986). *The frontal lobes*. New York: Raven.

Tannock, R., Martinussen, R., & Frijters, J. (2000). Naming speed performance and stimulant effects indicate effortful, semantic processing deficits in attention-deficit/hyperactivity disorder. *Journal of Abnormal Child Psychology, 28*, 237–252.

Tooby, J., & Cosmides, L. (1992). The psychological foundations of culture. In J. Barkow, L. Cosmides, & J. Tooby (Eds.), *The adapted mind: Evolutionary psychology and the generation of culture* (pp. 19–136). New York: Oxford University Press.

Torgesen, J. K. (1994). Issues in the assessment of executive function: An information-processing perspective. In G. R. Lyon (Ed.), *Frames of reference for the assessment of learning disabilities: New views on measurement issues* (pp. 143–162). Baltimore: Brookes.

Vygotsky, L. S. (1978). *Mind in society*. Cambridge, MA: Harvard University Press.

Vygotsky, L. S. (1987). Thinking and speech. In *The collected works of L. S. Vygotsky: Vol. 1. Problems in general psychology* (N. Minick, Trans.). New York: Plenum Press.

Vygotsky, L. S., & Luria, A. (1994). Tool and symbol in child development. In R. van der Veer & J. Valsiner (Eds.), *The Vygotsky reader* (pp. 99–174). Cambridge, MA: Blackwell Science.

Wakefield, J. C. (1999). Evolutionary versus prototype analyses of the concept of disorder. *Journal of Abnormal Psychology, 108*, 374–399.

Welsh, M. C., & Pennington, B. F. (1988). Assessing frontal lobe functioning in children: Views from developmental psychology. *Developmental Neuropsychology, 4*, 199–230.

Welsh, M. C., Pennington, B. F., & Grossier, D. B. (1991). A normative-developmental study of executive function: A window on prefrontal function in children. *Developmental Neuropsychology, 7*, 131–149.

Wheeler, M. A., Stuss, D. T., & Tulving, E. (1997). Toward a theory of episodic memory: The frontal lobes and autonoetic consciousness. *Psychological Bulletin, 121*, 331–354.

Williams, G. C. (1996). *Adaptation and natural selection: A critique of some current evolutionary thought*. Princeton, NJ: Princeton University Press. (Original work published 1966)

Winsler, A. (1998). Parent–child interaction and private speech in boys with ADHD. *Applied Developmental Science, 2*, 17–39.

Winsler, A., Diaz, R. M., Atencio, D. J., McCarthy, E. M., & Chabay, L. A. (2000). Verbal self-regulation over time in preschool children at risk for attention and behavior problems. *Journal of Child Psychology and Psychiatry, 41*, 875–886.

Wright, R. (2000). *Nonzero: The logic of human destiny*. New York: Vintage Books.

Zelazo, P. R., Kearsley, R. B., & Stack, D. M. (1995). Mental representations for visual sequences: Increased speed of central processing from 22 to 32 months. *Intelligence, 20,* 41–63.

Zentall, S. S. (1988). Production deficiencies in elicited language but not in the spontaneous verbalizations of hyperactive children. *Journal of Abnormal Child Psychology, 16,* 657–673.

Zentall, S. S., & Smith, Y. S. (1993). Mathematical performance and behavior of children with hyperactivity with and without coexisting aggression. *Behaviour Research and Therapy, 31,* 701–710.

16

Early Attachment Processes and the Development of Emotional Self-Regulation

SUSAN D. CALKINS

In the developmental psychology literature, the construct of emotional self-regulation and its role in successful adaptation has been examined quite extensively, particularly for the early childhood period. Emotional self-regulation refers to processes that serve to manage emotional arousal and support adaptive social and nonsocial responses (Calkins, 1994; Kopp, 1992; Thompson, 1994). The capacity to exercise self-control over the expression of emotions, particularly negative emotions, develops over the first years of life and has particular importance for the unfolding of appropriate and adaptive social behavior during the preschool and school years (Eisenberg, Murphy, Maszk, Smith, & Karbon, 1995; Eisenberg et al., 1996; Thompson, 1994). Furthermore, the lack of adequate development of control over emotion (as well as, in some instances, overcontrol of emotion) may be a precursor to the development of psychopathology (Calkins & Dedmon, 2000; Calkins & Fox, 2002; Keenan, 2000).

The broad construct of emotional self-regulation has been studied in many ways, including the examination of specific strategies and their effects on affective experience and expression. For example, research reveals that specific emotion regulation strategies, such as self-comforting, help seeking, and distraction, may assist the young child in managing early temperament-driven frustration and fear responses in situations in which the control of negative emotions may be necessary (Stifter & Braungart, 1995). Moreover, emotion regulation skills may be useful in situations that elicit positive affective arousal in that they allow the child to keep such arousal within a manageable and pleasurable range (Grolnick, Cosgrove, & Bridges, 1996; Stifter & Moyer, 1991). Because the lack of emotion regulation skills contributes to adjustment difficulties (Calkins, 1994; Calkins & Dedmon, 2000; Cicchetti, Ackerman, & Izard, 1995; Keenan, 2000; Rubin, Coplan, Fox, & Calkins, 1995), failure to acquire these skills may lead to difficulties in areas such as social competence and school adjustment. Thus, the acquisition of emotion regulation skills and strategies is considered a critical achievement of early childhood (Bronson, 2000; Sroufe, 1996).

One important assumption in much of the research on the acquisition of emotional self-regulation is that parental caregiving practices may support or undermine such development and contribute to observed individual differences among young children's emotional skills (Thompson, 1994). Infants almost exclusively rely on parents for the regulation of emotion. Over time, interactions with parents in emotion-laden contexts teach children that the use of some particular strategies rather than others may be more useful for the reduction of emotional arousal (Sroufe, 1996). Although caregiving practices are often attributed a role in the development of emotion regulation, the specific processes by which these practices affect children's development are often left unspecified (Fox & Calkins, 2003).

One hypothesis about the way in which caregiving practices affect developing emotion regulation is through the emerging attachment relationship and the experience, over the course of infancy, of attachment-related processes. Attachment processes are often activated in emotionally evocative contexts and serve specific emotion regulatory functions. Thus, it is likely that they contribute to the acquisition of the repertoire of self-regulated emotional skills that develop in the child over the course of infancy and toddlerhood.

In this chapter, I examine the early development of emotional self-regulation processes across the first 2 years of life. First, I briefly review the emergence of these processes as a function of normative development in the affective, motor, and cognitive domains. Next, I address the role of specific types of attachment experiences within the family context, and examine both short- and long-term emotional consequences of attachment processes. Despite much advancement in our knowledge of these processes, specific questions remain about the ways in which attachment processes affect self-regulatory processes on multiple levels. Recommendations for future research include an examination of the integration of different levels of self-regulation and a focus on the mechanisms that explain the effects of attachment processes on these multiple levels.

EMOTION REGULATION IN EARLY CHILDHOOD: NORMATIVE DEVELOPMENT

Dramatic developments are observed during the infancy and toddlerhood periods of development in terms of emotional self-regulation skills and abilities. The process may be broadly described as one in which the relatively passive and reactive neonate becomes a child capable of self-initiated behaviors that serve a regulatory function (Calkins, 1994; Kopp, 1982; Sroufe, 1996). In addition, this process has also been described as one in which the infant progresses from near-complete reliance on caregivers for regulation to independent self-regulation. As the infant makes this transition, the use of specific strategies and behaviors become organized into the infant's repertoire of emotional self-regulation that may be used in a variety of contexts.

Kopp (1982) provides an excellent overview of the early developments in emotional self-regulation. This description has been verified by studies of both normative development (Buss & Goldsmith, 1998; Rothbart, Ziaie, & O'Boyle, 1992) and individual differences (Stifter & Braungart, 1995). These descriptions provide an explanation of how infants develop and utilize a rich behavioral repertoire of strategies in the service of reducing, inhibiting, amplifying, and balancing different affective responses. Moreover, it is also clear from these descriptions that functioning in a variety of nonemotional domains, including motor, language and cognition, and social development, is implicated in these changes (Kopp, 1989, 1992).

Early efforts at emotional self-regulation—those occurring prior to about 3 months of age—are thought to be controlled largely by innate physiological mechanisms (Kopp, 1982). By 3 months, primitive mechanisms of self-soothing, such as sucking, simple motor movements, such as turning away, and reflexive signaling in response to discomfort, often in the form of crying, are the primary processes that operate independently of caregiver intervention (Kopp, 1982; Rothbart et al., 1992).

The period between 3 and 6 months of age marks a major transition in infant development. First, sleep–wake cycles and eating and elimination processes have become more predictable, signaling an important biological transition. Second, the ability of the infant to voluntarily control arousal levels begins to emerge. This control depends largely on attentional control mechanisms and simple motor skills (Rothbart et al., 1992; Ruff & Rothbart, 1996), and leads to coordinated use of attention engagement and disengagement, particularly in contexts that evoke negative affect. Infants are now capable of engaging in self-initiated distraction, moving attention away from the source of negative arousal to more neutral, nonsocial stimuli. For example, the ability to shift attention away from a negative event (such as something frightening) to a positive distracter may lead to decreases in the experience of negative affect. Importantly, though, there are clear individual differences in the ability to utilize attention to control emotion and behavior successfully. Rothbart (1981, 1986) found increases in positive affect and decreases in distress from 3 to 6 months during episodes of focused attention, which suggest that attentional control is tied to affective experience. Moreover, the experience of negative affect is believed to interfere with the child's ability to explore and learn about the environment (Ruff & Rothbart, 1996). Consequently, there are clear implications of early emotional self-regulation for development in a range of domains.

By the end of first year of life, infants become much more active and purposeful in their attempts to control affective arousal (Kopp, 1982). First, they begin to employ organized sequences of motor behavior that enable them to reach, retreat, redirect, and self-soothe in a flexible manner that suggests they are responsive to environmental cues. Second, infants' signaling and redirection become explicitly social as they recognize that caregivers and others may behave in a way that will assist them in the regulation of affective states (Rothbart et al., 1992).

During the second year of life, the transition from passive to active methods of emotional self-regulation is complete (Rothbart et al., 1992). Although infants are not entirely capable of controlling their own affective states by this age, they are capable of using specific strategies to attempt to manage different affective states, albeit sometimes unsuccessfully (Calkins & Dedmon, 2000; Calkins, Gill, Johnson, & Smith, 1999). Moreover, during this period, infants begin to respond to caregiver directives and, as a consequence of this responsivity, compliance and behavioral self-control begin to emerge (Kopp, 1989). This shift is supported by developments in the motor domain, as well as changes in representational ability and the development of language skills. Brain maturation contributes as well, and by the end of toddlerhood, children have executive control abilities that allow control of arousal, regulation of affective expression, and inhibition and activation of behavior (Bronson, 2000).

The description of the developmental process of emerging self-regulation, including emotional self-regulation, has been subject to inquiry regarding the role of the factors that contribute to these developments. Like investigations of other areas of self-control

(Sethi, Mischel, Aber, Shoda, & Rodriguez, 2000), understanding the development of control of emotions necessitates examination of both intrinsic and extrinsic factors (Calkins, 1994). Intrinsic factors include the temperamental disposition of the child, certain cognitive skills, and the underlying neural and physiological systems that support and are engaged in the processes of control (Calkins, 1994; Fox, 1994; Fox, Henderson, & Marshall, 2001). Extrinsic factors include the manner in which caregivers shape and socialize emotional responses of the child (Thompson, 1994). Caregivers may utilize specific strategies to enhance the development of self-control by providing environments that are supportive and responsive to the child's needs, and by socializing culturally appropriate behavior (Thompson, 1990, 1994). In addition, other socializing agents, including siblings and peers, influence the extent to which children utilize self-control strategies and the success of these strategies (Fox & Calkins, 2003).

Empirical evidence supports the theoretical notion that both biological and innate dispositions and environmental experiences contribute to emerging emotional self-regulation (Calkins, Dedmon, Gill, Lomax, & Johnson, 2002; Calkins & Johnson, 1998; Stifter & Braungart, 1995). Clearly, though, emotional self-regulatory processes begin to develop in the context of dyadic interactions (Sroufe, 1996). Such interactions contribute to normative developments in emotional self-regulation and create opportunities for individual variability in such skills and abilities to emerge (Cassidy, 1994). Although multiple dimensions of caregiving may contribute to the development of self-regulation (Kopp, 1982; Thompson, 1994), one important dimension of the dyadic relationship is the attachment relationship that develops between caregivers and infants over the first year of life. This relationship is viewed as the primary context for infants to internalize expectations regarding their own emotional functioning, and environmental support of such functioning. In the next section, I briefly review attachment theory, with a specific emphasis on the way attachment processes affect developing emotional self-regulation.

ATTACHMENT PROCESSES IN EARLY EMOTIONAL DEVELOPMENT

Current theorizing about childhood attachment and its role in emotional functioning and behavioral adjustment has its roots in the work of John Bowlby (1969/1982), whose evolutionary theory of attachment emphasized the biological adaptedness of specific attachment behaviors displayed during the infancy period. Such behaviors permit the infant to initiate and maintain contact with the primary caregiver, which serves a survival purpose (Bowlby, 1988). In typical development, infants exhibit a repertoire of behaviors, including looking, crying, and clinging, that allows them to signal and elicit support from the primary caregiver in times of external threat. Bowlby argued that, by the end of the first year of life, the interactive history between the infant and caregiver, including during times of stress or external threat, produces an attachment relationship that provides a sense of security for the infant and significantly influences the child's subsequent adaptation to a variety of developmental challenges.

Bowlby (1988) hypothesized that the mechanism through which early parent–child attachment affects later functioning involves a psychological construct having to do with expectations of self and other. Bowlby's notion of an "internal working model" referred to cognitive representations of the self and the caregiver that were constructed out of repeated early interactions. Such representations provide the infant and young child with a guide to expectations about his or her own emotional responding, and the likelihood and success of caregiver intervention in managing this affective responding. Thus, the experience of sensitive caregiving was hypothesized to lead to a secure attachment and expectations that emotional needs would either be met by the caregiver or managed with skills developed through interactions with the caregiver.

Numerous developmental scientists have tested Bowlby's theory, though Mary Ainsworth is likely the most noted of these. Ainsworth's pioneering naturalistic and observational studies of attachment processes in a longitudinal study of infants and mothers in Baltimore focused on individual differences in mother–infant attachment relationships (Ainsworth, Blehar, Waters, & Wall, 1978). She theorized that although all infants become attached to primary caregivers, the quality of this attachment varies as a function of the relationship history. She developed an empirical paradigm that examined infant responses as a function of this relationship history. In her "Strange Situation" laboratory procedure, she constructed a series of brief, but increasingly stressful, episodes designed to activate the infant's attachment system. These episodes consisted of interactions with a stranger, and separations and reunions from the caregiver, that elicit individual variation in exploratory and security-seeking behaviors.

On the basis of infants' behaviors in the Strange Situation, particularly those that reflected the dyad's ability to manage stress, she characterized infants as securely attached or insecurely attached, with either resistant or avoidant profiles. Ainsworth characterized secure infants as those comfortable with exploration and sharing positive affect during the low-stress context, and proximity seeking and the ability to be comforted in the high-stress context of separation. In contrast, insecurity was indexed by either heightened distress and difficulty calming (referred to as resistance or ambivalence) or active avoidance of the caregiver during the high-stress context of separation. Importantly, Ainsworth reported that the quality of different types of attachment relationships could be predicted by the quality of maternal caregiving observed in the home across the first year of life. She argued that the experience of consistent sensitive and responsive caregiving teaches the infant about appropriate expectations regarding others, and allows the infant to experience a reduction in arousal level as a consequence of the caregiver's behaviors (Ainsworth et al., 1978). In this way, her findings provided empirical support for Bowlby's internal working model construct and supported the hypothesized link between attachment and emotional processes.

This early theoretical and empirical work makes clear, then, why the recent interpretations of Bowlby's attachment theory attribute significance to the role of attachment processes in the development of emotional self-regulation. Sroufe (1996), for example, argued that emotional development is inextricably linked with social development, with the course of emotional development described as the transition from dyadic regulation of affect to self-regulation of affect. He argued that the ability to self-regulate arousal levels is embedded in affective interactions between the infant and caregiver. These interactions provide infants with the experience of arousal escalation and reduction as a function of caregiver interventions, distress reactions that are relieved through caregiver actions, and positive interactions with the caregiver (Sroufe, 1996). Such experiences contribute to the working model of affect-related expectations that transfer from the immediate caregiving environment to the larger social world of peers and others.

Cassidy (1994) has also addressed the role of attachment processes in the development of emotional self-regulation. She focuses on the adaptive function of different patterns of emotional responding in the context of the attachment relationship, and argues that these patterns of affective responding are actually strategies that infants use to allow their attachment needs to be met. The open and flexible emotional communication that is characteristic of a secure attachment allows the infant to comfortably and safely express both positive and negative affect, ensuring proximity and comfort from the responsive caregiver. Moreover, the different strategies of insecure infants also provide these infants with a means of meeting their own needs within the context of a less-than-optimal care-giving environment. The heightened distress that characterizes some insecure infants also serves as a clear signal to gain the attention of the inconsistent or unresponsive caregiver. In a similar manner, avoidant behavior serves the adaptive purpose of minimizing the at-tachment relationship and has the effect of allowing the infant to maintain the needed proximity, without threatening the relationship with the caregiver through displays of overt sadness or anger. Importantly, though, these short-term adaptations of the different patterns displayed by insecure infants may lead to long-term difficulties in other contexts. For example, heightened emotional expression, in the context of peer relationships, may lead to problematic peer interactions and has implications for the development of social competence (Cassidy, 1994).

Other theoretical perspectives focus on the biological processes involved in the regu-lation of attachment and emotional processes (Field, 1994; Fox & Card, 1999; Hofer, 1994; Schore, 2000). For example, Hofer (1994; Polan & Hofer, 1999) addressed the multiple psychobiological roles that the caregiver plays in regulating infant behavior and physiology early in life. Based on his research with infant rat pups, he described these "hidden regulators" as operating at multiple sensory levels (e.g., olfactory, tactile, and oral) and influencing multiple levels of behavioral and physiological functioning in the in-fant. So, for example, maternal tactile stimulation may have the effect of lowering the in-fant's heart rate during a stressful situation, which in turn may support a more adaptive behavioral response. Moreover, removal of these regulators, during separation, for exam-ple, disrupts the infant's functioning at multiple levels as well. Clearly, then, opportunities for individual differences in the development of emotional self-regulation may emerge from differential rearing conditions providing more or less psychobiological regulation.

The psychobiological interpretation of attachment theory also offers insight into the mechanism by which interactive experiences across the first year of life become integrated into the internal working model that Bowlby articulated. For example, Hofer (1994) de-scribed how the biological experience of infant–caregiver interactions becomes a repre-sentational structure that guides affective functioning. He argued that these early interac-tions are, in fact, regulatory experiences that contribute to an inner affective experience composed of sensory, physiological, and behavioral responses. Over time, these affective experiences lead to organized representations, the integration of which is the internal working model. These organized mental representations rather than the individual sen-sory and physiological components to which the infant responded earlier in infancy are ultimately what guide the child's behavior (Hofer, 1994).

Schore (2000) extends these psychobiological ideas even further in arguing that the interactive experiences between caregiver and child that are the essential elements of the emerging attachment relationship also affect the development of the prefrontal cor-tex. The right hemisphere, in particular, he notes, is especially influenced by experi-ences in the social world, and in turn determines the regulation and coping skills that young children develop. Support for the role of the right frontal cortex in human behavioral and emotion regulation has emerged over the last several years (Fox, 1994; Fox & Card, 1999), but evidence of the role of social experience in its development is still lacking. Nevertheless, there appears to be a compelling conceptual rationale for in-vestigating whether and how caregivers affect infants' emerging self-regulatory system at multiple levels.

From this brief review of current theorizing in the area of attachment and emotional self-regulation, it is clear that multiple possible pathways to the development of emotional self-regulation in infancy and early childhood likely involve attachment processes. Moreover, these theoretical perspectives suggest that empirical evidence for the role of attachment processes in the development of emotional self-regulation may come from a number of different directions. First, attachment processes may be predictive of specific emotional responses in the context of the relationship dyad itself, and may be observed empirically in behavioral and emotional responses to the Strange Situation or in other interactions between the caregiver and the infant. Second, attachment processes may affect the development and function of physiological processes that support emotional self-regulation. Third, attachment processes may be implicated in the development and use of specific strategies outside the context of the attachment relationship, such as during tasks requiring more independent self-regulation of emotion. Fourth, attachment processes may be implicated in the patterns of behavioral and social adaptation children display as they move from the social world of the family to that of school and peers. These patterns are often considered to be proxies for self-regulatory skills. In the next section, I examine evidence for each of these propositions.

ATTACHMENT PROCESSES
AND THE DEVELOPMENT OF EMOTIONAL SELF-REGULATION

In examining the multiple indices of regulation that may be a consequence of attachment processes, then, one may focus on indicators that are more rather than less proximal to these processes. So, for example, research has addressed the more proximal relation of attachment processes and emotion regulation under conditions with relationship-relevant challenges, such as the Strange Situation, maternal separation contexts, and stranger exposure paradigms (Braungart & Stifter, 1991; Fox, Bell, & Jones, 1992). Moreover, these studies have examined both physiological and affective indices of regulation. In addition, a number of studies have examined the emergence of autonomous emotional and behavioral regulation, as well as the even less proximal regulation that occurs in the context of the peer and academic world. Illustrative examples of this work are now described.

Attachment and Emotion Regulation in Dyadic Contexts

The research examining attachment and emotion regulation processes in contexts that activate the attachment system is consistent in its findings. In multiple studies conducted in different laboratories, researchers have demonstrated that infants with secure attachment relationships utilize strategies that include social referencing and express a need for social intervention (Braungart & Stifter, 1991; Nachmias, Gunnar, Manglesdorf, Parritz, & Buss, 1996). These same researchers report that insecure–avoidant children are more likely to use self-soothing and solitary exploration with toys (Nachmias et al., 1996; Stifter & Braungart, 1991). The strategies of both secure and insecure infants seem to reflect a history of experiences and expectations regarding the availability of the caregiver as an external source of emotional self-regulation. These expectations are clearly important when the attachment system becomes activated during the stressful context of the Strange Situation. Such work provides direct support for the notion that patterns of emotional self-regulation are evident quite early in development and are an integral component of the dyadic interactions that produce secure attachment.

Attachment and Physiological Self-Regulation

Researchers have examined whether attachment processes also affect physiological indices of emotional self-regulation when the attachment system is activated. Much of this work is reviewed by Fox (Fox & Card, 1999), who noted that multiple physiological indices have been examined, including measures of heart rate, cortisol, and brain electrical activity. One difficulty with this work, in general, is that the extent to which the measures reflect emotional tone or reactivity versus emotional self-regulation is often unclear. For example, most studies report elevated heart rate in response to both the Strange Situation and maternal separation (Donovan & Leavitt, 1985; Sroufe & Waters, 1977), but because separation distress alone is not indicative of attachment, it is difficult to know whether these measures can reveal much about individual differences in the nature of the attachment relationship and developing emotion regulation. Clearly, though, they support the notion that specific components of the normative attachment process are physiological in nature.

Studies of endocrine system responding reveal similar relations as the heart rate work. Cortisol findings indicate that infants who are stressed during the Strange Situation also experience elevated cortisol. In one study, elevated cortisol was found among infants who were both highly fearful, as measured using a different empirical paradigm, and insecurely attached, suggesting that perhaps their experience of a lack of external arousal regulation has produced heightened arousal during the Strange Situation (Nachmias et al., 1996).

Evidence for the role of the activation of the frontal cortex in contexts in which the attachment system is activated comes from the work on brain electrical activity (EEG) and maternal separation. This work suggests that the frontal brain regions involved in affective expression and regulation (Fox, 1994) are differentially activated during maternal separation, with the right frontal region being more activated in infants who were more distressed during separation (Fox et al., 1992). Again, though, the specificity of these findings to emotional self-regulation versus emotional reactivity is unclear, as are implications for individual differences in security of attachment.

Attachment and Emerging Autonomous Emotional Self-Regulation

The research examining direct links between attachment and emotional self-regulation in situations that activate the attachment system reveals clear behavioral differences between secure and insecure infants. This work also indicates that specific physiological response systems come into play when the attachment system is activated. An additional question addressed in this literature is whether these attachment processes have less proximal effects. Attachment theory would predict that the child's internal working model of self and others would affect his or her emotion regulatory skills outside the context of the caregiver–child relationship interactions. Researchers have examined this proposition both directly, by focusing on specific emotion regulatory strategies, and indirectly, by studying adaptive functioning that is presumed to have regulatory underpinnings (Lewis & Miller, 1990).

Interestingly, studies assessing direct relations between attachment and emotion regulatory skills and strategies are relatively rare. Three recent studies, though, support the notion that relations between the two domains are observable outside the immediate dyadic context. First, Diener, Manglesdorf, McHale, and Frosch (2002) observed that attachment classification, as observed in the Strange Situation, did predict regulatory strategies in a situation in which the infant is required to regulate negative affect, but that did not explicitly activate the attachment system. Their findings were quite consistent with work examining emotional self-regulation within the context of the Strange Situation. Infants in secure attachment relationships with both parents used strategies emphasizing social orientation. Thus, security of attachment leads to infants' expectations of caregivers that extend beyond the immediate parent–child interactional context. In turn, these expectations lead to the use of specific kinds of emotion regulation strategies in situations that place demands on the child.

Gilliom, Shaw, Beck, Schonberg, and Lukon (2002) conducted a study that examined specific emotion regulation strategy use beyond the infancy period. The focus of this investigation was on preschoolers' use of specific anger control strategies during a waiting paradigm. Specific strategies involving the control of attention were found to predict the anger reactions of the children in this situation. In addition, though, secure attachment in infancy was predictive of the use of specific strategies, including the use of attentional distraction, that lead to successful waiting. By preschool, young children are capable of controlling their attention in a manner that leads to successful emotional and behavioral control. This study demonstrated that the effects of attachment beyond the infancy period are observable in the development and use of such strategies.

In another recent examination of the relation between attachment and emotional functioning beyond the dyadic context, Kochanska (2001) conducted an extensive longitudinal study of the development of fear, anger, and joy across the first 3 years of life. Her rationale for this investigation was that attachment processes should be implicated in the development of different emotion systems, and that children with different attachment histories should display different patterns of functioning in these systems. Moreover, she argued that evidence for such a developmental process would provide an explanation of how early attachment processes might be linked to the range of outcomes and indices of adjustment that have been studied.

Differences in the emotional functioning of secure and insecure infants in Kochanska's study were apparent at the end of the first year of life. Consistent with other research (Calkins & Fox, 1992), Kochanska found that insecure–resistant infants were more fearful than other infants. In addition, across the second and third year of life, insecure infants displayed a different pattern with respect to the display of both positive and negative affect. Secure infants showed a predictable decline in the display of negative affect, whereas insecure infants displayed an increase, as well as a decrease, in positive affect. A notable finding of this study that pertains to the development of emotional self-regulation concerns the pattern of insecure–avoidant children. Recall that these children are likely to minimize their emotional reactions in the context of the Strange Situation. However, Kochanska observed that, over time, these infants display an increase in fear reactions, a finding that supports Cassidy's notion that such a strategy, while effective in the short term, may lead to difficulties later in development. Clearly, the strategy of minimization is either ineffective over time or leads to repeated experiences of internal arousal that eventually become difficult to contain.

These data provide support for the notion that early attachment processes are implicated in the development of affective functioning, an important component of which is self-regulation. Presumably, by the age of 3, decreases in the expression of negative affect observed among securely attached children are, at least in part, a function of emerging control of such expression. Similarly, appropriate positive engagement and affective expression, which are critical elements of successful dyadic interaction in the peer domain, are also a reflection of emerging affective control (Calkins, 1994).

Although data on the relation between attachment and emotional self-regulation strategies are limited, a few studies have examined the relations between aspects of parenting thought to be linked to attachment and emotional self-regulation. These studies are worth noting because they are conducted with toddlers, children for whom there are clear expectations of emerging autonomous emotional control. In one study of mothers and toddlers, for example, we examined the relations between maternal behavior across a variety of different situations and child emotional self-control in frustrating situations (Calkins, Smith, Gill, & Johnson, 1998). Our analyses indicated that maternal negative and controlling behavior (thought to be reflective of intrusive behavior characteristic of insecure attachment relationships) was positively related to the use of orienting to or manipulating the object of frustration (a barrier box containing an attractive toy) and negatively related to the use of distraction techniques. These data are important in light of findings that the ability to control attention and engage in distraction (such that ruminating over the object of denial is minimized) has been related to the experience of less emotional arousal and reactivity (Calkins, 1997; Grolnick et al., 1996), and to the display of early externalization of behavior problems (Calkins & Dedmon, 2000).

Attachment and Behavioral Self-Regulation

In examining the relation between attachment processes and emotion regulation that is less proximal to the dyadic caregiver–child relation, it is important to examine the behavior problem literature. Within this literature, problems of both an internalizing and externalizing nature are often defined by self-regulatory difficulties (Barkley, 1997; Calkins & Howse, in press; Keenan, 2000). For example, in characterizing the behavior of children with early externalizing behavior problems, there is often reference to a lack of control, undercontrol, or poor regulation (Campbell, 1995). In characterizing the behavior of children with internalizing disorders, there is often a discussion of overcontrol (Calkins & Fox, 2002). Rarely do these investigations examine specific emotion regulation strategies or processes (but see Calkins & Dedmon, 2000, and Gilliom et al., 2002, for exceptions). Rather, it is often assumed that the behavioral symptoms themselves (e.g., aggression, in the case of externalizing, or withdrawal, in the case of internalizing) are either strategies for regulation (Calkins, 1994) or behaviors that reflect a lack of adaptive strategies (Keenan, 2000). The child behavior problem literature, then, is an appropriate place to examine the relation between attachment processes and emerging emotional self-regulation.

A large empirical literature has examined the relations between parenting behavior and child behavior problems, particularly the more salient and disruptive externalizing behavior problems. Many of these studies have focused on early attachment and its relation to aggression or oppositional defiant disorder (ODD). Several studies have shown that insecure infant attachment is predictive of later externalizing behavior problems in children (Booth, Rose-Krasnor, & Rubin, 1991; Shaw, Owens, Giovanelli, & Winslow, 2001; Shaw, Owens, Vondra, Keenan, & Winslow, 1996). In contrast, though, Bates and colleagues (Bates & Bayles, 1988; Bates, Maslin, & Frankel, 1985) failed to show that 13-month-old infants' attachment security predicted later behavior problems at 3, 5, or 6 years of age. These researchers concluded that the link between externalizing behavior and attachment could not be supported. However, it is important to note that attachment classifications may not consistently predict later behavior problems, because attachment status can change as children move beyond infancy (Cicchetti, Cummings, Greenberg, & Marvin, 1990). An examination of concurrent relations between attachment status and child behavior problems, as opposed to early attachment security as a predictor of later behavior problems, may be more useful in understanding the processes underlying the display and maintenance of problematic behavior. For example, in an extensive study of the concurrent correlates of preschool boys, with and without a clinical diagnosis of ODD, Greenberg and colleagues (DeKlyen, Speltz, & Greenberg, 1998; Greenberg, Speltz, DeKlyen, & Endriga, 1991; Speltz, Greenberg, & DeKlyen, 1990) found that the preschool boys with a clinical diagnosis of ODD were more likely than the boys in the control group to be insecurely attached.

In examining attachment processes as predictors of internalizing spectrum problems, results have been even less consistent. Three studies have found relations, but the types of insecurity that predict outcomes differ, as does the developmental lag between attachment predictors and outcomes. For example, Shaw and colleagues found that toddler insecurity predicted both internalizing and externalizing problems at preschool age (Vondra, Shaw, Swearingen, Cohen, & Owens, 2001), but that disorganized attachment in infancy predicted toddler internalizing (Shaw, Keenan, Vondra, Delliquadri, & Giovanelli, 1997). In addition, Lyons-Ruth, Easterbrooks, and Cibelli (1997) observed that avoidant attachment in infancy predicted internalizing problems at age 7 years.

Thus, across studies examining the relations between attachment processes and behavioral self-regulation disorders of an internalizing and externalizing nature, the more proximal measures of attachment seem, in general, to be better predictors of difficulties. This is probably due to changes in the nature of the attachment relationship and the differential effects of other environmental factors that may serve either to exacerbate or to ameliorate the effects of the child's attachment history.

Summary

This review of research examining the effects of early relationships on the development of emotional self-regulation seems to demonstrate that the proximal effects of this relationship are quite evident. Infants in secure attachment relationships utilize effective and appropriate caregiver-directed behaviors to elicit supportive caregiving in times of stress. In addition, the psychophysiological literature indicates that predictable biological responses can be expected from infants in contexts that activate the attachment system, as well as more limited evidence for the effects of attachment security on this responding. Beyond this immediate dyadic context, though, are also effects of the attachment relationship on emotional self-regulation. Secure infants and children use effective strategies when engaged in tasks that require more autonomous emotional control, rather than the anticipated external control provided in dyadic regulation. More distal effects of attachment on behavioral and emotional self-regulation that underlie adaptive functioning in preschool and early childhood have also been observed. However, clear interpretation of these data may require a more systematic evaluation of both the timing of the effects of attachment, the influence of other environmental factors, and the role of mediational and moderational variables.

FUTURE DIRECTIONS IN THE STUDY OF ATTACHMENT PROCESSES AND EMOTIONAL SELF-REGULATION

The theoretical and empirical work reviewed to this point suggest clear implications of attachment processes for the development of emotional self-regulation. Based on the work conducted to date, associations are strongest concurrently and in contexts that activate the attachment system. Longer term relations and relations to emotional functioning in other contexts are more modestly supported. Nevertheless, there is reason to think that future studies of these phenomena might clarify the nature and extent of these relations.

First, empirical work that is more focused on process, rather than on simple associations, might be more informative for elucidating the complex ways that attachment and emotion regulation influence development. For example, it might be useful to examine the role of emotion regulation as a mediator of the relations between early attachment and other, more complex kinds of self-regulation. In one of the few studies that examined such a hypothesis, Contreras, Kerns, Weimer, Gentzler, and Tomich (2000) observed that specific dimensions of emotion regulation, including arousal and attention deployment, mediated the relation between attachment and peer social behavior. emotion regulation processes may mediate a variety of outcomes that have self-regulatory components. Thus, a movement away from use of the broad definition of "self-regulation" as adaptive functioning that includes an array of outcomes, and toward a focus on specific styles or strategies of emotional control might provide greater specificity with respect to the role of attachment in behavioral adjustment.

A second step that might help to illuminate these processes would be to address the issues of moderators of the relation between attachment and regulation. It is clear from some of the behavior problem literature (Shaw et al., 1997) that the direct relations are likely to be observed under some conditions but perhaps not others. For example, environmental factors that place even greater stress on the attachment relationship are also likely to undermine the child's own efforts to develop a self-regulatory repertoire. A focus on moderated effects will provide greater specificity in prediction, while preserving the important role of attachment processes in emotional functioning.

Third, it is clear that the direction of effects in development is not always from parent to child. Transactional influences from the environment to the child, and back again, are clearly responsible for some pathways in development. Moreover, it must be acknowledged that the child plays an important role in the dyadic interactions with caregivers that lead to the development of attachment relationships (Calkins, 1994). Consequently, these transactional influences may obscure the identification of longer term effects of attachment on emotional processes but are clearly important to understanding developmental pathways (Cicchetti, 1984, 1993).

Finally, it may be more useful to adopt an approach that considers multiple levels of analysis of self-regulation (Calkins & Fox, 2002). Bowlby's original theory of attachment and subsequent elaboration of the theory placed emotional development at the center of attachment processes. For this reason, the theory has clear implications for the emergence of early emotional self-regulation. It has been noted, however, that self-regulation occurs on a number of different, and likely interrelated, levels (Calkins & Fox, 2002; Eisenberg et al., 2001; Posner & Rothbart, 2000). Clearly, a rationale is provided by the empirical literature reviewed here for examining emotion-related processes across a number of interrelated levels of analysis.

For example, one way to conceptualize the self-regulatory system is to describe it as adaptive control that may be observed at the level of physiological, attentional, emotional, behavioral, cognitive, and interpersonal or social processes (Calkins & Fox, 2002). Control at these various levels emerges, at least in primitive form, across the prenatal, infancy, toddler, and early childhood periods of development. Importantly, though, the mastery of earlier regulatory tasks becomes an important component of later competencies, and, by extension, the level of mastery of these early skills may constrain the development of later skills. Thus, understanding the development of specific regulatory processes, such as emotion regulation, becomes integral to understanding how regulatory deficits across multiple levels affect the emergence of childhood behavior and behavior problems (Calkins & Fox, 2002). Embedding emotional self-regulation in a larger self-regulatory framework has the advantage of allowing researchers to understand the multiple levels of infants and child functioning that may be influenced by the emerging attachment relationship.

ACKNOWLEDGMENTS

The writing of this chapter was supported by National Institute of Health Grant Nos. MH 55584 and MH 58144 to Susan D. Calkins. Thanks to Martha J. Cox for helpful comments on an earlier draft of this chapter.

REFERENCES

Ainsworth, M., Blehar, M., Waters, E., & Wall, S. (1978). *Patterns of attachment*. Hillsdale, NJ: Erlbaum.

Barkley, R. A. (1997). *ADHD and the nature of self-control*. New York: Guilford Press.

Bates, J. E., & Bayles, K. (1988). Attachment and the development of behavior problems. In J. Belsky & T. Nezworski (Eds.), *Clinical implications of attachment* (pp. 253–299). Hillsdale, NJ: Erlbaum.

Bates, J. E., Maslin, C. A., & Frankel, K. A. (1985). Attachment security, mother–child interaction and temperament as predictors of behavior-problem ratings at age three years. In I. Bretherton & E. Waters (Eds.), *Growing points of attachment theory and research: Monographs of the Society for Research in Child Development*, 50(1–2, Serial No. 209), 167–193.

Booth, C. L., Rose-Krasnor, L., & Rubin, K. H. (1991). Relating preschoolers' social competence and their mothers' parenting behaviors to early attachment security and high-risk status. *Journal of Social and Personal Relationships*, 8, 363–382.

Bowlby, J. (1982). *Attachment and loss: Vol. 1. Attachment*. New York: Basic Books. (Original work published 1969)

Bowlby, J. (1988). *A secure base*. New York: Basic Books.

Braungart, J. M., & Stifter, C. A. (1991). Regulation of negative reactivity during the Strange Situation: Temperament and attachment in 12-month-old infants. *Infant Behavior and Development*, 14, 349–367.

Bronson, M. B. (2000). *Self-regulation in early childhood: Nature and nurture*. New York: Guilford Press.

Buss, K. A., & Goldsmith, H. H. (1998). Fear and anger regulation in infancy: Effects on the temporal dynamics of affective expression. *Child Development*, 69, 359–374.

Calkins, S. D. (1994). Origins and outcomes of individual differences in emotion regulation. In N. A. Fox (Ed.), *Emotion regulation: Behavioral and biological considerations: Monographs of the Society for Research in Child Development*, 59(240), 53–72.

Calkins, S. D. (1997). Cardiac vagal tone indices of temperamental reactivity and behavioral regulation in young children. *Developmental Psychobiology*, 31, 125–135.

Calkins, S. D., & Dedmon, S. A. (2000). Physiological and behavioral regulation in two-year-old children with aggressive/destructive behavior problems. *Journal of Abnormal Child Psychology*, 2, 103–118.

Calkins, S. D., Dedmon, S., Gill, K., Lomax, L., & Johnson, L. (2002). Frustration in infancy: Implications for emotion regulation, physiological processes, and temperament. *Infancy*, 3, 175–198.

Calkins, S. D., & Fox, N. A. (1992). The relations among infant temperament, security of attachment and behavioral inhibition at 24 months. *Child Development*, 63, 1456–1472.

Calkins, S. D., & Fox, N. A. (2002). Self-regulatory processes in early personality development: A multilevel approach to the study of childhood social withdrawal and aggression. *Development and Psychopathology, 14*, 477–498.

Calkins, S. D., Gill, K. A., Johnson, M. C., & Smith, C. (1999). Emotional reactivity and emotion regulation strategies and predictors of social behavior with peers during toddlerhood. *Social Development, 8*, 310–341.

Calkins, S. D., & Howse, R. (in press). Individual differences in self-regulation: Implications for childhood adjustment. In P. Philipot & R. Feldman (Eds.), *The regulation of emotion*. Mahwah, NJ: Erlbaum.

Calkins, S. D., & Johnson, M. C. (1998). Toddler regulation of distress to frustrating events: Temperamental and maternal correlates. *Infant Behavior and Development, 21*, 379–395.

Calkins, S. D., Smith, C. L., Gill, K. L., & Johnson, M. C. (1998). Maternal interactive style across contexts: Relations to emotional, behavioral and physiological regulation during toddlerhood. *Social Development, 7*(3), 350–369.

Campbell, S. B. (1995). Behavior problems in preschool children: A review of recent research. *Journal of Child Psychology and Psychiatry, 36*, 113–149.

Cassidy, J. (1994). Emotion regulation: Influences of attachment relationships. In N. A. Fox (Ed.), *Emotion regulation: Behavioral and biological considerations: Monographs of the Society for Research in Child Development, 59*(240), 228–249.

Cicchetti, D. (1984). The emergence of developmental psychopathology. *Child Development, 55*, 1–7.

Cicchetti, D. (1993). Developmental psychopathology: Reactions, reflections, projections. *Developmental Review, 13*, 471–502.

Cicchetti, D., Ackerman, B., & Izard, C. (1995). Emotions and emotion regulation in developmental psychopathology. *Development and Psychopathology, 7*, 1–10.

Cicchetti, D., Cummings, E. M., Greenberg, M. T., & Marvin, R. S. (1990). An organizational perspective on attachment beyond infancy: Implications for theory, measurement, and research. In M. T. Greenberg, D. Cicchetti, & E. M. Cummings (Eds.), *Attachment in the preschool years* (pp. 3–50). Chicago: University of Chicago Press.

Cicchetti, D. & Rogosch, , F. A. (1996). Equifinality and multifinality in developmental psychopathology. *Development and Psychopathology, 8*, 597–600.

Cole, P., Michel, M. K., & Teti, L. (1994). The development of emotion regulation and dysregulation. In N. A. Fox (Ed.), *Emotion regulation: Behavioral and biological considerations: Monographs of the Society for Research in Child Development, 59* (Nos. 2–3, Serial No. 240), 73–100.

Contreras, J., Kerns, K. A., Weimer, B., Gentzler, A., & Tomich, P. (2000). Emotion regulation as a mediator of associations between mother–child attachment and peer relationships in middle childhood. *Journal of Family Psychology, 14*, 111–124.

DeKlyen, M., Speltz, M. L., & Greenberg, M. T. (1998). Fathering and early onset conduct problems: Positive and negative parenting, father–son attachment, and the marital context. *Clinical Child and Family Psychology Review, 1*, 3–21.

Diener, M., Mangelsdorf, S., McHale, J., & Frosch, C. (2002). Infants' behavioral strategies for emotion regulation with fathers and mothers: Associations with emotional expressions and attachment quality. *Infancy, 3*, 153–174.

Donovan, W. L., & Leavitt, L. A. (1985). Physiologic assessment of mother–infant attachment. *Journal of the American Academy of Child Psychiatry, 24*, 65–70.

Eisenberg, N., Fabes, R., Guthrie, I., Murphy, B., Maszk, P., Holmgren, R., & Suh, K. (1996). The relations of regulation and emotionality to problem behavior in elementary school. *Development and Psychopathology, 8*, 141–162.

Eisenberg, N., Fabes, R. A., Shepard, S. A., Murphy, B. C., Guthrie, I. K., Jones, S., Freidman, J., Poulin, R., & Maszk, P. (1997). Contemporaneous and longitudinal prediction of children's social functioning from regulation and emotionality. *Child Development, 68*, 642–664.

Eisenberg, N., Guthrie, I. K., Fabes, R. A., Shepard, S., Losoya, S., Murphy, B. C., Jones, S., Poulin,

R., & Reiser, M. (2000). Prediction of elementary school children's externalizing problem behaviors from attention and behavioral regulation and negative emotionality. *Child Development, 71*(5), 1367–1382.

Eisenberg, N., Murphy, B. C., Maszk, P., Smith, M., & Karbon, M. (1995). The role of emotionality and regulation in children's social functioning: A longitudinal study. *Child Development, 66*, 1360–1384.

Field, T. (1994). The effects of mother's physical and emotional unavailability on emotion regulation. In N. A. Fox (Ed.), *Emotion regulation: Behavioral and biological considerations: Monographs of the Society for Research in Child Development, 59*(240), 208–227.

Fox, N. A. (1994). Dynamic cerebral process underlying emotion regulation. In N. A. Fox (Ed.), *Emotion regulation: Behavioral and biological considerations: Monographs of the Society for Research in Child Development, 59*(240), 152–166.

Fox, N. A., Bell, M. A., & Jones, N. A. (1992). Individual differences in response to stress and cerebral asymmetry. *Developmental Neuropsychology, 8*, 165–184.

Fox, N., & Calkins, S. D. (2003). The development of self-control of emotion: Intrinsic and extrinsic influences. *Motivation and Emotion, 27*, 7–26.

Fox, N. A., & Card, J. A. (1999). Psychophysiological measures in the study of attachment. In J. Cassidy & P. R. Shaver (Eds.), *The handbook of attachment: Theory, research, and clinical applications* (pp. 226–245). New York: Guilford Press.

Fox, N. A., Henderson, H. A., & Marshall, P. J. (2001). The biology of temperament: An integrative approach. In C. A. Nelson & M. Luciana (Eds.), *The handbook of developmental cognitive neuroscience* (pp. 631–646). Cambridge, MA: MIT Press.

Gilliom, M., Shaw, D. S., Beck, J. E., Schonberg, M. A., & Lukon, J. L. (2002). Anger regulation in disadvantaged preschool boys: Strategies, antecedents, and the development of self-control. *Developmental Psychology, 38*, 222–235.

Greenberg, M. T., Speltz, M. L., DeKlyen, M., & Endriga, M. C. (1991). Attachment security in preschoolers with and without externalizing behavior problems: A replication. *Development and Psychopathology, 3*, 413–430.

Grolnick, W., Cosgrove, T., & Bridges, L. (1996). Age-graded change in the initiation of positive affect. *Infant Behavior and Development, 19*, 153–157.

Hofer, M. (1994). Hidden regulators in attachment, separation, and loss. In N. A. Fox (Ed.), *Emotion regulation: Behavioral and biological considerations: Monographs of the Society for Research in Child Development, 59*(240), 192–207.

Keenan, K. (2000). Emotion dysregulation as a risk factor for child psychopathology. *Clinical Psychology: Science and Practice, 7*, 418–434.

Kochanska, G. (2001). Emotional development in children with different attachment histories: The first three years. *Child Development, 72*, 474–490

Kopp, C. (1982). Antecedents of self-regulation: A developmental perspective. *Developmental Psychology, 18*, 199–214.

Kopp, C. (1989). Regulation of distress and negative emotions: A developmental view. *Developmental Psychology, 25*, 243–254.

Kopp, C. (1992). Emotional distress and control in young children. In N. Eisenberg & R. Fabes (Eds.), *Emotion and its regulation in early development* (pp. 7–23). San Francisco: Jossey-Bass/Pfeiffer.

Lewis, M., & Miller, S. M. (1990). *Handbook of developmental psychopathology*. New York: Plenum Press.

Lyons-Ruth, K., Easterbrooks, M., & Cibelli, C. (1997). Infant attachment strategies, infant mental lag, and maternal depressive symptoms: Predictors of internalizing and externalizing problems at age 7. *Developmental Psychology, 33*, 681–692.

Nachmias, M., Gunnar, M., Mangelsdorf, S., Parritz, R., H., & Buss, K. (1996). Behavioral inhibition and stress reactivity: The moderating role of attachment security. *Child Development, 67*, 508–522.

Polan, H. J., & Hofer, M. A. (1999). Psychobiological origins of infant attachment and separation responses. In J. Cassidy & P. R. Shaver (Eds.), *Handbook of attachment: Theory, research, and clinical applications* (pp. 162–180). New York: Guilford Press.

Posner, M. I., & Rothbart, M. K. (2000). Developing mechanisms of self-regulation. *Development and Psychopathology*, 12, 427–441.

Rothbart, M. K. (1981). Measurement of temperament in infancy. *Child Development*, 52, 569–578.

Rothbart, M. K. (1986). Longitudinal observation of infant temperament. *Developmental Psychology*, 22, 356–365.

Rothbart, M., Ziaie, H., & O'Boyle, C. (1992). Self-regulation and emotion in infancy. In N. Eisenberg & R. Fabes (Eds.), *Emotion and its regulation in early development* (pp. 7–23). San Francisco: Jossey-Bass/Pfeiffer.

Rubin, K. H., Coplan, R. J., Fox, N. A., & Calkins, S. D. (1995). Emotionality, emotion regulation and preschooler's social adaptation. *Development and Psychopathology*, 7, 49–62.

Ruff, H., & Rothbart, M. K. (1996). *Attention in early development*. New York: Oxford University Press.

Schore, A. N. (2000). Attachment and the regulation of the right brain. *Attachment and Human Development*, 2, 23–47.

Sethi, A., Mischel, W., Aber, J. L., Shoda, Y., & Rodriguez, M. L. (2000). The role of strategic attention deployment in development of self-regulation: Predicting preschoolers' delay of gratification from mother–toddler interactions. *Developmental Psychology*, 36(6), 767–777.

Shaw, D., Owens, E., Giovannelli, J., & Winslow, E. (2001). Infant and toddler pathways leading to early externalizing disorders. *Journal of the American Academy of Child and Adolescent Psychiatry*, 40, 36–43.

Shaw, D. S., Keenan, K., Vondra, J., Delliquadri, E., & Giovanelli, J. (1997). Antecedents of preschool children's internalizing problems: A longitudinal study of low-income families. *Journal of the American Academy of Child and Adolescent Psychiatry*, 36, 1760–1767.

Shaw, D. S., Owens, E. B., Vondra, J. I., Keenan, K., & Winslow, E. B. (1996). Early risk factors and pathways in the development of early disruptive behavior problems. *Development and Psychopathology*, 8, 679–699.

Speltz, M. L., Greenberg, M. T., & DeKlyen, M. (1990). Attachment in preschoolers with disruptive behavior: A comparison of clinic-referred and nonproblem children. *Development and Psychopathology*, 2, 31–46.

Sroufe, A. L. (1996). Emotional development: The organization of emotional life in the early years. New York: Cambridge University Press.

Sroufe, A. L., & Waters, E. (1977). Heart rate as a convergent measures in clinical and developmental research. *Merrill–Palmer Quarterly*, 23, 3–27.

Stifter, C. A., & Braungart, J. M. (1995). The regulation of negative reactivity in infancy: Function and development. *Developmental Psychology*, 31(3), 448–455.

Stifter, C. A., & Moyer, D. (1991). The regulation of positive affect: Gaze aversion activity during mothernfant interaction. *Infant Behavior and Development*, 14(1), 111–123.

Thompson, R. A. (1994). Emotion regulation: A theme in search of definition. In N. A. Fox (Ed.), *The development of emotion regulation: Biological and behavioral considerations: Monographs of the Society for Research in Child Development*, 59(240), 25–52.

Thompson, R. A. (1998). Emotion and self-regulation. In R. A. Thompson (Ed.). *Socioemotional development: Nebraska Symposium on Motivation*, 36, 367–468. Lincoln: University of Nebraska Press.

Vondra, J. I., Shaw, D. S., Swearingen, L., Cohen, M., & Owens, E. B. (2001). Attachment stability and emotional and behavioral regulation from infancy to preschool age. *Development and Psychopathology*, 13, 13–33.

17

The Development of Self-Regulation in Young Children

Individual Characteristics and Environmental Contexts

LISA A. MCCABE
MARISOL CUNNINGTON
JEANNE BROOKS-GUNN

Four-year-old Jacob sits cross-legged on the floor of the large, indoor space of his child care center. He and a developmental psychologist, Maria, are the only ones present. They have been playing together for about 20 minutes. Maria gives Jacob the following instructions: "I have a present for you. But I need to wrap it first so it will be a surprise. You need to help me. Try not to look so that I can wrap your surprise for you. I'll let you know when I'm ready to give you the present. OK? Try not to look!" Maria then walks behind Jacob. Standing about 5 feet from him, she crinkles the wrapping paper noisily so as to attract Jacob's attention. Almost immediately Jacob turns around to look at Maria. "Are you done yet?" he asks. Maria reminds him that the rule of the game is not to look. Jacob turns back. Five seconds later, as Maria continues to make wrapping noises, Jacob turns around again. He grins slyly at Maria. "Remember, no looking," says Maria. Jacob ignores this reminder and continues to watch Maria until, after 60 seconds, she hands him a wrapped gift. He reaches for it with a big smile on his face.

Janelle, also 4 years old, now has her turn with Maria. She has just been given the same instructions about a surprise gift and not to look while it is being wrapped. While Maria busies herself making wrapping noises, Janelle sits quietly, fiddling with the laces on her sneakers. She does not say anything, nor does she turn to see what Maria is doing. After 60 seconds, Maria announces, "I'm done." Janelle turns around, smiling, and accepts the wrapped gift Maria hands her.

A few weeks later, Jacob and Janelle sit with two of their peers in the child care center. The four children sit in a line facing the wall. Maria, the developmental psychologist, gives them the following instructions: "Do you like presents? I have a present for each of you in this

340

bag. I need to wrap them first so they will be a surprise. You need to help me. Don't look so that I can wrap your presents for you. I'll let you know when I'm ready to give you the presents. OK? Remember, no looking!" She then walks behind the four children and begins to loudly crinkle wrapping paper. As soon as she does, Jacob turns his head to look at her. "Ready?" he asks. Maria reminds him that the rule of the game is no peeking. Janelle reaches out to place her open palm on Jacob's cheek. She gently pushes his face away from Maria. "No looking!" she reprimands her friend. A few seconds later Jacob quickly glances over his shoulder at Maria again. Janelle takes a quick peek of her own. Then she says, "I'm looking at the bicycle," while pointing to a bike pushed against the wall. "I'm looking at the door," responds one of the other children. "I'm looking at the garbage can," says Jacob. The children continue to search the room, identifying things to look at. After 45 seconds of waiting, two of the children turn to look at Maria. Janelle reminds them in a stern voice, "She said no looking!" Both children quickly turn to face the wall again. After 60 seconds, Maria announces that she's ready and hands a wrapped gift to each child.

What can be learned from situational assessments such as these? The Gift Wrap task, described here, has been adapted for use with individual and groups of children in nonlaboratory settings (McCabe, Rebello-Britto, Hernandez, & Brooks-Gunn, in press). It provides a window into children's ability to regulate their own impulses in the face of temptation. For Jacob, waiting to receive a gift is a difficult challenge. When assessed both in an individual and a group context, he fails to follow directions to not look while Maria wraps a gift for him. Repeated peeks, as well as verbal communications, reveal his inability to self-regulate his own impulsive behaviors. Janelle, on the other hand, when faced with the same challenging situation, appears very capable of waiting for a present and resisting, for the most part, the urge to peek at it before it is wrapped. In the group context, she even helps her peers by reminding them to not look during the assessment. Note, however, that in the more challenging group context, even Janelle gives in to the impulse to peek at Maria before the time is up.

Self-regulation assessments such as the Gift Wrap task have long been used to assess young children's self-regulatory capacities. Previous work has reviewed the diverse assessments used to explore particular aspects of self-regulation. These include laboratory and clinical assessments, and more recently, assessments appropriate for home and classroom use, in areas such as delay of gratification, cognitive control, motor control, and sustained attention (McCabe et al., in press). Based on this extensive work with varied methodological techniques, links between the ability to regulate one's own emotions and behaviors and later developmental outcomes have repeatedly been demonstrated. In particular, the ability to self-regulate has been associated with secure attachments (Vondra, Shaw, Swearingen, Cohen, & Owens, 2001), and is also predictive of emotional knowledge (Schultz, Izard, Ackerman, & Youngstrom, 2001), social competence (Denham et al., 2003; Eisenberg et al., 2003; Fabes et al., 1999), conscience (Kochanska, Murray, & Coy, 1997), and resiliency (Eisenberg, Guthrie, et al., 1997) in early to middle childhood. Similarly, early regulatory difficulties predict later problematic social behavior (Campbell, Pierce, March, Ewing, & Szumowski, 1994; Newman, Caspi, Moffitt, & Silva, 1997). Longitudinal research has also shown a relation between self-regulation in the preschool years and later cognitive achievement (Shoda, Mischel, & Peake, 1990).

Given the importance of self-regulation to both social and cognitive development, it is essential to understand how these capacities develop in young children. In this chapter, we begin with a brief review of what it means to self-regulate from infancy through age 5, prior to formal schooling. Next, such development is explored from a bioecological perspective (Bronfenbrenner & Ceci, 1994). In the bioecological model, development is viewed as a function of both the person and the environment in which he or she lives. "Proximal processes," or interactions between the individual and his or her environment, are key to understanding developmental outcomes. Thus, we first review what is known about individual or "person" characteristics as they relate to the development of a broad rubric of self-regulation skills. Then the development of self-regulation in ecological contexts is considered, with specific attention paid to how home, nonparental child care, peer, neighborhood, and cultural environments can influence and shape the development of self-regulation in young children.

WHAT IS SELF-REGULATION?

Though the study of self-regulation has captured the interest of child development researchers for more than three decades, only recently has the field begun to acknowledge definitional issues and overlap among similar constructs (for reviews, see Cole, Martin, & Dennis, in press; Kochanska, Murray, & Harlan, 2000; Welsh, 2002). For the purpose of this chapter, the term "self-regulation" is used to refer to a wide variety of capacities involved in regulating emotion and behavior of the self. For example, drawing from Mischel's classic work in the field (Mischel & Rodriguez, 1993), we consider delay of gratification, or the ability to control impulses to wait for a future reward, to represent one aspect of self-regulation. Also included in this broad rubric is the ability to inhibit automated responses in favor of a less dominant behavior. Because this capacity reflects the ability to think before acting, we have used the term "cognitive control." Others in the field refer to similar abilities as "effortful attention" (Kochanska et al., 2000). Suppressing/initiating activity to a signal also reflects cognitive and motor self-regulatory capacities (Kochanska et al., 2000; Livesey & Morgan, 1991) in that the child must learn under what conditions an action is appropriate. Motor control, or the ability to slow down motor activity, should also be included when considering self-regulation research (Kochanska et al., 2000; Lee, Brooks-Gunn, & Schnur, 1988). In addition, sustained attention (National Institute of Child Health and Human Development Early Child Care Research Network, 2003a), that is, the ability to filter out extraneous information and focus on a task at hand, is also encompassed within our conceptualization of self-regulation. These individual self-regulation capacities do not represent an exhaustive list. Rather, they are meant to convey the diversity in skills and terminology used in the developmental literature on self-regulation. They also highlight the capacities that have been the focus of recent work to review existing self-regulation measures. Specifically, tables summarizing measures in the areas of delay of gratification, cognitive control, motor control, and sustained attention are available to researchers and practitioners interested in further study of self-regulation in young children (McCabe et al., in press).

In examining these specific kinds of capacities for this chapter, we have drawn from a diverse literature base of more global concepts related to self-regulation. These include executive functions (Barkley, 1997; Espy & Kaufmann, 2002), ego control (Block & Block, 1980; Eisenberg et al., 2003), inhibitory or effortful control (Eisenberg et al., 2003; see also Eisenberg et al., Chapter 13, this volume; Kochanska et al., 1997; Kochanska, Murray, Jacques, Koenig, & Vandegeest, 1996; Rothbart, Ahadi, & Hershey, 1994), emotion regulation (Kopp, 1989), and externalizing behavioral problems (Bates, Pettit, Dodge, & Ridge, 1998; Rubin, Coplan, Fox, & Calkins, 1995), among others. As such, an attempt was made to integrate across somewhat disparate fields, while still acknowledging the diversity of capacities encompassed within the general term "self-regulation."

CHANGE IN SELF-REGULATION IN THE FIRST FIVE YEARS

Much development occurs in the area of self-regulation over the first 5 years of life. In this section, early regulatory capabilities and strategies are reviewed from infancy through the preschool years.

Infancy

Rudimentary self-regulation skills are evident as early as the first year of life. Using A-not-B tasks, in which an object is hidden first in one location (A) and then another (B), researchers have documented young infants' difficulty in searching location B after having previously retrieved the object from location A. This impulsive A-not-B error occurs even when the infant observes the object being hidden in location B. Baillargeon and her colleagues, however, have demonstrated that as early as 5½ months of age, children look longer (i.e., visually search) at the correct hiding place (Baillargeon & Graber, 1988; Baillargeon, Graber, DeVos, & Black, 1990). Furthermore, by about 7–8 months of age, the majority of infants overcome the impulse to continue erroneously searching in location A and manually search in the correct location, if the delay between hiding and retrieval is minimal (Bell & Fox, 1992; Diamond, 1985). Similar improvement in controlling impulsive reaching has been demonstrated in infants between 6 and 12 months of age through the use of a Plexiglas-top box with a toy inside. For this assessment, the infant must inhibit reaching through the glass top and instead reach through an opening in the side of the box to retrieve the object (Diamond, 1990).

In the first year of life, gaze aversion and fussiness are two of the few self-regulatory strategies available to the infant. In fact, 6-month-old infants are more likely than 12- and 18-month-olds to use these strategies and less likely to demonstrate self-soothing and self-distraction (Mangelsdorf, Shapiro, & Marzolf, 1995).

Toddlerhood

Early demonstrations of self-regulation continue to develop through the toddler years. For example, young children continue to improve their performance on AB error tasks, with longer delay times (10 sec) through the toddler and preschool years (Espy, Kaufmann, McDiarmid, & Glisky, 1999). Rudimentary abilities to delay gratification are also evident by 18 months, with significant improvement between 2 and 3 years (Vaughn, Kopp, & Krakow, 1984; Vaughn, Krakow, Kopp, Johnson, & Schwartz, 1986). Grolnick, Bridges, and Connell (1996) also documented toddlers' abilities to delay gratification, especially when using active engagement with a substitute object as a waiting strategy. Improvement on broader executive function tasks, such as spatial conflict (in which children are instructed to press a button corresponding to a spatially compatible or incompatible picture on a computer screen), is also evident between ages 2 and 3. On this type of task, toddlers between 24 and 36 months of age showed improvements in accuracy and reaction time (Gerardi-Caulton, 2000).

Preschool Years

The preschool years represent a key period in the continued development of self-regulation. Using a variety of assessments, researchers have documented improvements in self-regulatory behaviors among children during these years. For example, young preschoolers (age 3) typically have difficulty in child versions of the classic Stroop task. Specifically, they demonstrate longer response latencies and fewer correct responses when asked to say "day" to a card with a moon and stars, and "night" to a picture of a sun (Gerstadt, Hong, & Diamond, 1994). By age 5, children's inhibitory control improves on this task. Three-year-olds also perform more poorly than older preschoolers on the tapping task (in which children are instructed to tap once if the experimenter taps twice, and vice versa; Diamond & Taylor, 1996). Similarly, older preschoolers (5- and 6-year-olds) perform better than younger preschoolers on go/no-go tasks, such as being asked to locate a toy in a box, based on cues placed on the box lid (e.g., colors or shapes; Bell & Livesey, 1985; Livesey & Morgan, 1991). Three-year-olds also commit more perseverative errors on the Dimensional Change Card Sort task than do 4- and 5-year-old children; that is, when asked to first sort cards by one criterion (e.g., color), then by a second criterion (e.g., shape), younger preschoolers tend to continue to sort using the first set of rules (Frye, Zelazo, & Palfai, 1995; Zelazo, Frye, & Rapus, 1996). Finally, results from the Attention Network Test, used to measure alerting, orienting, and executive attention, tell us that children show greater responsiveness to alerting cues and are less hindered by competing demands during cognitive tasks as they get older (Mezzacappa, 2003).

What is it that makes young preschoolers struggle with the ability to perform well on these varied self-regulation assessments while older preschoolers perform them with relative ease? Preschoolers' increasing capacity for selecting appropriate self-regulation strategies may help to explain some of the improvement. For example, self-distraction, a strategy seen during toddlerhood, continues to be an important strategy for facilitating self-regulation in the preschool years (Raver, Blackburn, Bancroft, & Torp, 1999). By age 5, children also begin to realize that removing a reward from view (e.g., by placing a cover over it) will help them to wait longer before receiving the reward (Mischel & Mischel, 1983).

Using experimental techniques in laboratory settings, researchers have also identified additional strategies that facilitate improved performance on self-regulation tasks. Specifically, Diamond, Kirkham, and Amso (2002) found that imposing a delay between presenting a Stroop-like stimulus and requiring a response helped younger children perform well, even when a distraction task was present during the delay. Reducing the inhibitory demand of the task (e.g., by asking the child to say "dog" and "pig" instead of "night" and "day" on the child version of the Stroop task) also helped, whereas reducing memory load by "chunking rules" (e.g., instructing the child to "say the opposite" instead of say "night" or "day") did not. Mischel's work on delay of gratification suggests that strategies that encourage "psychological distance" from the desired object facilitate longer delay times. For example, when children were told to think about "cool" or abstract features of the reward (e.g., how pretzel sticks look like thin, brown logs), they were able to wait for longer periods of time. Thinking about "hot" or salient aspects of the reward (e.g., the crunchy, salty taste of pretzels) had the opposite effect (Mischel & Rodriguez, 1993).

Beyond strategy use, researchers have also looked at the more specific abilities needed to successfully complete preschool self-regulation assessments. It is not simply that younger preschoolers have difficulty remembering two rules (as is required in the Day–Night Stroop task), because they perform adequately on control assessments (in which they are asked to say "day" and "night" to pictures of squiggles or checks; Gerstadt et al., 1994). Instead, it may be that inhibition in the face of cognitive interference is a difficult skill for the youngest preschoolers. This may be due in part to an immature frontal lobe, which develops slowly over the course of childhood and adolescence (Nelson & Luciana, 2001; Shonkoff & Phillips, 2000). Neurobiological research has demonstrated that the development and integration of the frontal lobe, especially the prefrontal regions, facilitates executive functions through increased self-monitoring and behavioral inhibition (Aman, Roberts, & Pennington, 1998; Shonkoff & Phillips, 2000). In particular, the anterior attention system (the neural system encompassing the anterior cingulated gyrus) has been linked to the capacity to self-regulate (Davis, Bruce, & Gunnar, 2002).

Evidence is mixed, however, regarding whether regulatory problems may also reflect performance rather than cognitive difficulties. In Livesey and Morgan's work (1991) 4-year-old children performed better in conditions requiring a verbal response as opposed to a task requiring children to actually search for a toy in boxes with cues on the lids. In contrast, children's errors on the Dimensional Change Card Sort task persisted even under conditions in which a motor response was not required (e.g., in which children judged the correctness of a puppet's response), thus indicating that the difficulty may lie in the ability to select rules flexibly, not in motor response control (Jacques, Zelazo, Kirkham, & Semcesen, 1999). Such seemingly contradictory findings may reflect the varied nature of the specific assessments, or the inherent complexity in self-regulatory capacities. Future research should further illuminate the specific self-regulatory abilities under development during the preschool years.

INDIVIDUAL CHARACTERISTICS

Thus far, we have reviewed general developmental trends in self-regulation. But what about characteristics that may differ across individuals? In the bioecological model (Bronfenbrenner & Ceci, 1994), the person remains central to development over time. Identifying and exploring innate or biological characteristics are critical to understanding developmental outcomes, such as the ability to self-regulate behaviors and emotions. What follows is a brief review of the literature base examining individual characteristics as they relate to the development of self-regulation.

Gender

Gender has often been identified as a factor in the ability to self-regulate. Beginning in infancy, girls are better able to regulate affect during the still face paradigm (in which mothers maintain a still face and do not smile, touch, or talk while looking at the infant) than are boys (Weinberg, Tronick, Cohn, & Olson, 1999). Girls also perform better on AB error tasks than do boys (Diamond, 1985). Some evidence suggests gender differences in the use of self-regulation strategies in the toddler years, with boys more likely to use distraction, and girls more likely to seek comfort from their mothers (Raver, 1996). Girls also show more self-regulated compliance to adults (Feldman & Klein, 2003; Kochanska, Tjebkes, & Forman, 1998) and better effortful control (Kochanska et al., 1997, 2000) than do boys. In the preschool years and beyond, differences in self-regulatory abilities are evident in the higher prevalence of externalizing behaviors in boys and decreased impulsivity in girls (Zahn-Waxler, Schmitz, Fulker, Robinson, & Emde, 1996), in the continuity in physical aggression in boys over time (Broidy et al., 2003), and in more socially competent responding by girls (Fabes et al., 1999). Thus, there seems to be a general trend for girls to demonstrate better self-regulation than boys in early childhood.

Temperament

Numerous researchers posit that self-regulation capacities reflect genetic or temperamental characteristics (Eisenberg et al., 2003; Kochanska et al., 1997; Rothbart, Derryberry, & Posner, 1994; Zahn-Waxler et al., 1996). In particular, stability in "effortful control," defined as the ability to inhibit a prepotent response in favor of a less dominant behavior, has been documented from toddlerhood to early school age (Kochanska et al., 1997). Researchers have also examined negative emotionality as a temperamental construct. Here, the focus is on the regulation of negative emotions. Children who are better able to regulate negative emotions (e.g., to show less distress) are less likely to use aggressive behaviors in frustrating situations as toddlers (Calkins & Johnson, 1998), and more likely to use self-distraction in delay of gratification paradigms (Raver, 1996). Better emotion regulation also predicts self-regulated compliance to parents and caregivers (Feldman & Klein, 2003). Thus, high levels of distress may interfere with children's ability to use optimal strategies for dealing with challenging tasks and situations that require self-regulation.

Evidence for the temperamental nature of self-regulation also comes from studies examining how temperamental characteristics early in life relate to later developmental outcomes reflecting self-regulatory capacities. A difficult temperament at age 2 has been found to predict behavior problems at age 4 (Pettit & Bates, 1989). Similarly, teacher reports of regulatory behavior in early elementary school predict social functioning at ages 8–10 (Eisenberg, Fabes, et al., 1997). Taken together, these varied studies indicate that self-regulatory capacities do in fact reflect, as least in part, temperamental or inborn characteristics.

Clinical Conditions

Individual self-regulatory capacities may also be influenced by the presence of diverse clinical conditions. For example, children with the genetic disorder phenylketonuria (PKU) show difficulty with tasks requiring inhibition and flexibility in action (Diamond, Prevor, Callender, & Druin, 1997). Autistic children also demonstrate inhibition and flexibility problems (Pennington, 1998), whereas children with attention-deficit/hyperactivity disorder (ADHD) struggle with impulsivity and sustained attention problems (Barkley, 1997; see also Barkley, Chapter 15, this volume), perhaps in part due to motivation and decisions about when to inhibit (Taylor, 1999). Finally, cognitive and language delays in children have been linked to regulatory problems, such as externalizing behaviors (Dionne, Tremblay, Boivin, Laplante, & Perusse, 2003; Kaiser, Hancock, Cai, Foster, & Hester, 2000) and the use of less effective regulation strategies in challenging social situations (Wilson, 1999).

ENVIRONMENTAL CONTEXTS

Literature reviewed thus far reveals how a variety of individual characteristics relate to the development of self-regulation in young children. An individual, however, does not develop in the absence of context. The bioecological model, in fact, stresses the importance of interactions between biological and environmental factors in explaining development (Bronfenbrenner & Ceci, 1994). In his ecological systems theory, Bronfenbrenner (1989) identifies four environmental systems in which development occurs: micro-, meso-, exo-, and macrosystems. In this section, we examine two of these levels,[1] the micro- and macrolevel contexts, as they relate to the development of self-regulation in young children.

Microenvironment

According to Bronfenbrenner, the microsystem is made up of the "pattern of activities, roles, and interpersonal relations experienced by the developing person in a given face-to-face setting with particular physical and material features and containing other persons with distinctive characteristics of temperament, personality, and systems of belief" (1989, p. 227). As such, the microlevel environment represents a key setting for the proximal processes thought to drive individual development. What follows is a description of some of the more common microlevel settings or environmental conditions in which young children live, and how they relate to the development of self-regulation.

Home

A wealth of research has examined how aspects of the home environment relate to the development of self-regulation in young children. More specifically, higher family socioeconomic status has been linked to better performance on the aforementioned Attention Network Test in 6-year-old children assessed in their homes (Mezzacappa, 2003). The quality of the family environment (in this case, a composite measure including physical and social resources, maternal sensitivity, and maternal cognitive stimulation) has also been shown to predict sustained attention and impulsivity on the Continuous Performance Task in preschool children (National Institute of Child Health and Human Development Early Child Care Research Network, 2003a).

In looking at the development of self-regulation, much evidence suggests that parenting behaviors represent a key facet of the home environment. For example, early in a child's life the use of kangaroo care (i.e., mother–child skin-to-skin contact) for premature infants has been associated with increased sustained attention in a play session at 6 months of age (Feldman, Weller, Sirota, & Eidelman, 2002). Throughout early childhood, positive and/or sensitive parenting also seems to promote the development of self-regulation in young children. In particular, Raver's (1996) work demonstrates an association between social contingency in mother–child interactions (i.e., joint attention) and 2-year-olds' use of distraction as a strategy for self-regulation while waiting for a gift. Similarly, positive maternal affect is related to committed compliance (i.e., internalized self-control) at age 2 (Kochanska & Aksan, 1995) and fewer behavior problems at age 4 (Pettit & Bates, 1989). Additionally, when parents utilize positive guidance (e.g., praise, physical affection, and encouragement), children tend to use more constructive coping strategies in challenging or frustrating tasks (Calkins & Johnson, 1998).

On the other hand, parental behaviors can also have a negative impact on a young child's developing self-regulation skills. Research suggests that when parents provide too much guidance (e.g., doing tasks for a child), children may have difficulty learning to regulate on their own (Calkins & Johnson, 1998; see also Calkins, Chapter 16, this volume; Grolnick, Kurowski, McMenamy, Rivkin, & Bridges, 1998). Furthermore, the absence of guidance, as may occur in depressed parents, may contribute to self-regulatory difficulties, as expressed in externalizing behaviors (Dawson et al., 2003; Shaw, Gilliom, Ingoldsby, & Nagin, 2003). Finally, rejecting, intrusive, or hostile–controlling parenting has also been linked to externalizing behaviors in young children (Marchand, Hock, & Widaman, 2002; Shaw et al., 2003), especially for young children who displayed high levels of negativity as infants (Belsky, Hsieh, & Crnic, 1998). Thus, it seems that responsive parenting that assists children when needed, but also gives room to grow, facilitates children's self-regulation better than absent or overcontrolling discipline techniques.

The links between parenting and child self-regulation, however, also need to be examined in terms of child characteristics. In some cases, parenting behavior may moderate the association between child temperamental characteristics and behavioral outcomes. For example, Kochanska (1995, 1997) found that highly fearful children were more likely to demonstrate conscience (i.e., internalized self-control) when mothers used gentle as opposed to harsh discipline. Similarly, parental restrictive control (e.g., prohibitions, scoldings, and warnings) can moderate the relation between child resistance to control (i.e., noncompliance) and externalizing behavior. Specifically, child resistance to control predicts externalizing behavior better in children with parents who have low rather than high restrictive control behaviors (Bates et al., 1998). Evidence also suggests that in cases of high maternal control, children's ability to deploy attention strategically (i.e., independent exploration) in toddlerhood is related to longer delay times and "cool ideation" strategies in a delay of gratification situation at age 5. When mothers are not controlling, focusing attention on the caregiver is associated with better self-regulatory capacities at age 5 (Sethi, Mischel, Aber, Shoda, & Rodriguez, 2000).

Nonparental Care Settings

Literature examining non-parental-care settings as a microcontext for the development of self-regulation presents a complex picture. Studies of Head Start suggest that participation in this program for low-income children may be associated with better motor control and fewer behavior problems, especially for African American children (Lee, Brooks-Gunn, & Schnur, 1988) and temperamentally undercontrolled children with multiple risk factors (Hart, Atkins, & Fegley, 2003). Research on child care settings in general (as opposed to Head Start programs in particular), however, suggests that participation in such programs may lead to more externalizing behaviors in the preschool and kindergarten years (National Institute of Child Health and Human Development, 2003b, 2003c). The generalizability of such findings, however, have been called into question by researchers who have examined more diverse samples and a broader range of experiences (including families from countries other than the United States, samples with wider variations in the quality of child care programs, and families with more diverse characteristics). Specifically, Love and colleagues (2003) contend that quality and stability of child care (as opposed to quantity of child care) may moderate the relation between child care experience and the development of externalizing behavior problems in young children.

Peer Group

Research on older children suggests that children who interact with peers who engage in antisocial behavior (e.g., substance abuse) are more likely to engage in this behavior themselves (Farrell & White, 1998). Yet very few studies have examined how the peer group influences self-regulatory behaviors in early childhood. In our own work, the Games as Measurement for Early Self-Control (GAMES) project, we provide one of the few examinations of early childhood self-regulation in the peer context. In particular, we explored how children's self-regulatory capacities differ when assessed one-on-one with an adult tester versus with a group of four familiar peers (McCabe & Brooks-Gunn, 2002; McCabe et al., in press). Findings reveal that across four different situational assessments (tapping four components of self-regulation: delay of gratification, impulse control, motor control, and cognitive control), children seem less well regulated in a group context than they do when assessed individually. Specifically, children tended to peek less while waiting for a gift, to wait for longer periods of time for a desired reward, to slow down their gross motor behaviors while walking on a line, and to demonstrate more cognitive control (e.g., to touch their heads when the experimenter said "feet" and touch their feet when the experimenter said "head") when they were assessed individually than in a group. Thus, it appears that self-regulatory behaviors, skills that are underdevelopment during the preschool years, are much more difficult to maintain in the presence of peers. It may be that peers serve as distracters during these varied tasks, thus making it more difficult for young children to employ the concentration needed to demonstrate self-regulation. Another possibility is that peers decrease the motivation for displaying optimal self-regulation skills. For example, in some cases, we observed children making up games that involved dysregulatory behaviors (e.g., touching the M&M during the snack-delay task) while waiting for the desired reward. Finally, peers may "teach" dysregulation by modeling less than optimal behaviors during self-regulation assessments. Further research is needed to understand fully the exact mechanisms through which the presence of peers makes self-regulation more difficult in young children.

Additional research on self-regulation in the context of the peer group suggests that the tendency to approach or to interact with peers moderates the association between emotion regulation and social competence with peers (Rubin et al., 1995). Specifically, children who are high in social interaction but are poor regulators of their own emotions tend to show more externalizing behaviors than do children who are high in social interaction but better with emotion regulation. In contrast, children who are less prone to social interaction and are also poor emotional regulators demonstrate more internalizing problems than do low-social-interaction children with good or average emotion regulation skills.

Play among children not only allows researchers to learn about self-regulation through observation but also facilitates its development. In fact, Vygotsky's (1930–1935/1978) sociocultural theory describes self-regulation as a fundamental outcome of sociodramatic play, or pretend play, because the social interactions involved lead children to internalize social norms and behaviors. This theory was tested in a longitudinal study that used naturalistic observations to assess sociodramatic play and the development of self-regulation in two preschool classroom contexts (cleanup and group circle time; Elias & Berk, 2002). Findings supported Vygotsky's hypothesis and suggested a particularly strong link between complex sociodramatic play and self-regulation in impulsive children. Joint make-believe play requires children to react continually against their own impulses in order to follow social rules and coordinate their behavior with that of others. Thus, it facilitates the development of important self-regulatory capacities.

Macroenvironment

Bronfenbrenner defines the macrosystem as "a societal blueprint for a particular culture, subculture, or other broader social context" (1989, p. 228). Thus, the focus here is on the belief systems, opportunities, resources, and social patterns of a particular group. Very few studies have in fact looked at the relationship between macrolevel environmental characteristics and the development of self-regulation. This section, therefore, reviews the scant research that does exist, as well as highlights a study under way, with the potential to contribute to our knowledge of self-regulation development in the context of the macroenvironment.

Neighborhoods

In recent years, researchers have begun to examine associations between neighborhood-level characteristics and child outcomes (Leventhal & Brooks-Gunn, 2000). Very few, however, have looked at neighborhood context and the development of self-regulation. In one of the rare examples of such research, Kupersmidt, Griesler, DeRosier, Patterson, and Davis (1995) found that living in a middle-socioeconomic-status neighborhood served as a protective factor for at-risk, black, grade school children (from low income, single-parent homes), in that children were less likely to demonstrate aggressive behaviors.

Other research also demonstrates a link between the presence of poor families in a neighborhood and externalizing problems in early childhood (Duncan, Brooks-Gunn, & Klebanov, 1994). The quality of the neighborhood (e.g., safety, social involvement, satisfaction with public services) has also been shown to predict externalizing behavior problems in first grade (Greenberg, Lengua, Coie, Pinderhughes, & the Conduct Problems Prevention Research Group, 1999).

Though these studies demonstrate the importance of considering neighborhood context when investigating the development of self-regulation, they tend to focus on older children and self-regulation that is broadly conceived (i.e., they examine general externalizing difficulties). Future research should address how features of the neighborhood environment relate to the development of more specific self-regulatory capacities in young children. The Project on Human Development in Chicago Neighborhoods (Brooks-Gunn, Berlin, Leventhal, & Fuligni, 2000; Leventhal & Brooks-Gunn, 2003) aims to meet both these goals. Data on motor control, sustained attention, and delay of gratification have been gathered from approximately 850 four-year-old children, who have been followed from birth. Analyses are currently under way to explore how neighborhood characteristics such as socioeconomic status and racial composition relate to the development of self-regulation in young children.

Culture

Very few researchers have investigated the development of self-regulation in young children cross-culturally. A small number of studies, however, provide some evidence that, in fact, culture does play a role in children's ability to self-regulate. For example, parent reports of hyperactivity are lower in Hong Kong than in London, perhaps in part because cultural values in Hong Kong stress lower levels of tolerance for uncontrolled behavior (Leung et al., 1996).

Difficulties in self-regulation development have also been documented in studies in China and the United States. Specifically, effortful control was negatively related to extraversion in China (with no such relation found in the United States), but negatively related to negative affectivity in the United States. No relation was found between effortful control and negativity in China (Ahadi, Rothbart, & Ye, 1993).

CONCLUSIONS AND FUTURE DIRECTIONS

Decades of research, including a recent proliferation in self-regulation studies, have revealed much about the development of self-regulation in young children. This large body of literature indicates that beginning in the first year of life, children demonstrate rudimentary self-regulatory abilities, with continued development of these capacities in toddlerhood. The preschool years are critical to self-regulation development, because they seem to represent a time of rapid self-regulatory growth, especially in areas such as inhibitory control, motor control, and delay of gratification. These increasing abilities likely reflect brain maturation, as well as more sophisticated use of strategies to facilitate self-regulation of behaviors and emotions. Some evidence also suggests that gender may play a role in the development of self-regulation, with girls generally being better regulators than boys.

Although strong evidence indicates the temperamental nature of the ability to self-regulate, studies also clearly show the malleability of such capacities. Characteristics of both the micro- and macrolevel environment can shape how innate characteristics are expressed and developed in real-world settings. On the positive side, sensitive parenting seems to facilitate self regulation, as does participation in high-quality early care and education settings, such as Head Start. Opportunities for sociodramatic play with peers can also foster the development of self-regulation, especially for impulsive children. On the negative side, overcontrolling or absent parenting, extensive non-maternal-care experience (especially of low quality), and a less than ideal neighborhood environment (e.g., poverty or safety concerns) may hinder young children's efforts to regulate their own behavior and emotions.

This review suggests that the exploration of both inborn characteristics and environmental contexts is essential to understanding the development of self-regulation in young children. Much work, however, remains to be done to fully understand how children develop the capacity to regulate behaviors and emotions. At the individual level, future research might, for example, further explore how improvements in general self-regulation performance during the preschool years relate to the development of specific regulatory capacities, such as motor control and cognitive control. In addition, at the microenvironmental level, research could examine the particular features of child care settings (e.g., opportunities for sociodramatic play, curricula that promote social development) that may promote or hinder development of self-regulation skills. Finally, as is evident from the scant macrolevel research reviewed here, much more work is needed to understand how features of the macroenvironment (e.g., neighborhood and culture) influence the development of self-regulation.

Although a few studies presented here examine interactions between person-and-environment characteristics (e.g., Bates et al., 1998), more work is needed to understand better how innate characteristics *interact* with environmental context to promote the self-regulatory capacities essential to later positive social and cognitive outcomes. Such studies, though more complex to conduct, would provide a more complete picture of how individuals develop such vital self-regulation skills.

ACKNOWLEDGMENTS

Support for the writing of this chapter was provided by the Administration on Children, Youth, and Families and the National Institute of Mental Health (Grant No. 90YM0001). We would like to thank data collectors (Aurelie Athan, Rebecca Fauth, Sandraluz Lara-Cinisomo, Otoniel Lopez, and Eva Medina); data coders (Aurelie Athan, Helen Rozelman, and Stephanie Tom); and the early childhood programs, families, and children who participated in the GAMES project.

NOTE

1. Most research on the development of self-regulation falls within either the micro- and macrolevel environment. Thus, a discussion of the meso- and exosystems is beyond the scope of this chapter. For additional information, see Bronfenbrenner (1989).

REFERENCES

Ahadi, S. A., Rothbart, M. K., & Ye, R. M. (1993). Child temperament in the U.S. and China: Similarities and differences. *European Journal of Personality, 7,* 359–378.

Aman, C. J., Roberts, R. J., & Pennington, B. F. (1998). A neuropsychological examination of the underlying deficit in attention deficit hyperactivity disorder: Frontal lobe versus right parietal lobe theories. *Developmental Psychology, 34*(5), 956–969.

Baillargeon, R., & Graber, M. (1988). Evidence of location memory in 8-month-old infants in a nonsearch AB task. *Developmental Psychology*, *24*(4), 502–511.

Baillargeon, R., Graber, M., DeVos, J., & Black, J. (1990). Why do young infants fail to search for hidden objects? *Cognition*, *36*, 255–284.

Barkley, R. A. (1997). Behavioral inhibition, sustained attention, and executive functions: Constructing a unifying theory of ADHD. *Psychological Bulletin*, *121*, 65–94.

Bates, J. E., Pettit, G. S., Dodge, K. A., & Ridge, B. (1998). Interaction of temperamental resistance to control and restrictive parenting in the development of externalizing behavior. *Developmental Psychology*, *34*(5), 982–995.

Bell, J. A., & Livesey, P. J. (1985). Cue significance and response regulation in 3- to 6-year-old children's learning of multiple choice discrimination tasks. *Developmental Psychobiology*, *18*(3), 229–245.

Bell, M. A., & Fox, N. A. (1992). The relations between frontal brain electrical activity and cognitive development during infancy. *Child Development*, *63*, 1142–1163.

Belsky, J., Hsieh, K., & Crnic, K. (1998). Mothering, fathering, and infant negativity as antecedents of boys' externalizing problems and inhibition at age 3 years: Differential susceptibility to rearing experience? *Development and Psychopathology*, *10*, 301–319.

Block, J. H., & Block, J. (1980). The role of ego-control and ego-resiliency in the organization of behavior. In W. A. Collins (Ed.), *The Minnesota Symposium on Child Psychology: Development of cognition, affect, and social relations* (Vol. 13, pp. 39–101). Hillsdale, NJ: Erlbaum.

Broidy, L. M., Nagin, D. S., Tremblay, R. E., Bates, J. E., Brame, B., Dodge, K., et al. (2003). Developmental trajectories of childhood disruptive behaviors and adolescent delinquency: A six-site, cross-national study. *Developmental Psychology*, *39*(2), 222–245.

Bronfenbrenner, U. (1989). Ecological systems theory. In R. Vasta (Ed.), *Annals of child development: Vol 6. Six theories of child development: Revised formulations and current issues* (pp. 187–249). Greenwich, CT: JAI Press.

Bronfenbrenner, U., & Ceci, S. (1994). Nature–nurture re-conceptualized in developmental perspective: A bio-ecological model. *Psychological Review*, *101*(4), 568–586.

Brooks-Gunn, J., Berlin, L. J., Leventhal, T., & Fuligni, A. (2000). Depending on the kindness of strangers: Current national data initiatives and developmental research. *Child Development*, *71*(1), 257–267.

Calkins, S. D., & Johnson, M. C. (1998). Toddler regulation of distress to frustrating events: Temperamental and maternal correlates. *Infant Behavior and Development*, *21*(3), 379–395.

Campbell, S. B., Pierce, E. W., March, C. L., Ewing, L. J., & Szumowski, E. K. (1994). Hard-to-manage preschool boys: Symptomatic behavior across contexts and time. *Child Development*, *65*, 836–851.

Cole, P. M., Martin, S. E., & Dennis, T. A. (in press). Emotion regulation as a scientific construct: Methodological challenges and directions for child development research. *Child Development*.

Davis, E. P., Bruce, J., & Gunnar, M. R. (2002). The anterior attention network: Associations with temperament and neuroendocrine activity in 6-year-old children. *Developmental Psychobiology*, *40*(1), 43–56.

Dawson, G., Ashman, S. B., Panagiotides, H., Hessl, D., Self, J., Yamada, E., et al. (2003). Preschool outcomes of children of depressed mothers: Role of maternal behavior, contextual risk, and children's brain activity. *Child Development*, *74*(4), 1158–1175.

Denham, S. A., Blair, K. A., DeMulder, E., Levitas, J., Sawyer, K., Auerbach-Major, S., et al. (2003). Preschool emotional competence: Pathway to social competence? *Child Development*, *74*(1), 238–256.

Diamond, A. (1985). Development of the ability to use recall to guide action, as indicated by infants' performance on AB. *Child Development*, *56*, 868–883.

Diamond, A. (1990). Developmental time course in human infants and infant monkeys, and the neural bases of inhibitory control in reaching. *Annals of the New York Academy of Sciences*, *608*, 673 676.

Diamond, A., Kirkham, N., & Amso, D. (2002). Conditions under which young children can hold two rules in mind and inhibit a prepotent response. *Developmental Psychology, 38*(3), 352–362.

Diamond, A., Prevor, M. V., Callender, G., & Druin, D. P. (1997). Prefrontal cortex cognitive deficits in children treated early and continuously for PKU. *Monographs of the Society for Research in Child Development, 62*(4, Serial No. 252).

Diamond, A., & Taylor, C. (1996). Development of an aspect of executive control: Development of the abilities to remember what I said and to "Do as I say, not as I do." *Developmental Psychobiology, 29,* 315–334.

Dionne, G., Tremblay, R., Boivin, M., Laplante, D., & Perusse, D. (2003). Physical aggression and expressive vocabulary in 19-month-old twins. *Developmental Psychology, 39*(2), 261–273.

Duncan, G. J., Brooks-Gunn, J., & Klebanov, P. K. (1994). Economic deprivation and early-childhood development. *Child Development, 65*(2), 296–318.

Eisenberg, N., Fabes, R. A., Shepard, S. A., Murphy, B. C., Guthrie, I., Jones, S., et al. (1997). Contemporaneous and longitudinal prediction of children's social functioning from regulation and emotionality. *Child Development, 68*(4), 642–664.

Eisenberg, N., Guthrie, I. K., Fabes, R. A., Reiser, M., Murphy, B. C., Holgren, R., et al. (1997). The relations of regulation and emotionality to resiliency and competent social functioning in elementary school children. *Child Development, 68*(2), 295–311.

Eisenberg, N., Zhou, Q., Losoya, S. H., Fabes, R., Shepard, S., Murphy, B. C., et al. (2003). The relations of parenting, effortful control, and ego control to children's emotional expressivity. *Child Development, 74*(3), 875–895.

Elias, C. L., & Berk, L. E. (2002). Self-regulation in young children: Is there a role for sociodramatic play? *Early Childhood Research Quarterly, 17,* 216–238.

Espy, K. A., & Kaufmann, P. M. (2002). Individual differences in the development of executive function in children: Lessons from the delayed response and A-not-B tasks. In D. L. Molfese & V. J. Molfese (Eds.), *Developmental variations in learning: Applications to social, executive function, language, and reading skills* (pp. 113–137). Mahwah, NJ: Erlbaum.

Espy, K. A., Kaufmann, P. M., McDiarmid, M. D., & Glisky, M. L. (1999). Executive functioning in preschool children: A-not-B and other delayed response format task performance. *Brain and Cognition, 41,* 178–199.

Fabes, R. A., Eisenberg, N., Jones, S., Smith, M., Guthrie, I., Poulin, R., et al. (1999). Regulation, emotionality, and preschoolers' socially competent peer interactions. *Child Development, 70*(2), 432–442.

Farrell, A., & White, K. (1998). Peer influences and drug use among urban adolescents: Family structure and parent–adolescent relationship as protective factors. *Journal of Consulting and Clinical Psychology, 66,* 248–258.

Feldman, R., & Klein, P. S. (2003). Toddlers' self-regulated compliance to mothers, caregivers, and fathers: Implications for theories of socialization. *Developmental Psychology, 39*(4), 680–692.

Feldman, R., Weller, A., Sirota, L., & Eidelman, A. I. (2002). Skin-to-skin contact (kangaroo care) promotes self-regulation in premature infants: Sleep–wake cyclicity, arousal modulation, and sustained exploration. *Developmental Psychology, 38*(2), 194–207.

Frye, D., Zelazo, P. D., & Palfai, T. (1995). Theory of mind and rule-based reasoning. *Cognitive Development, 10*(4), 483–527.

Gerardi-Caulton, G. (2000). Sensitivity to spatial conflict and the development of self-regulation in children 24–36 months of age. *Developmental Science, 3*(4), 397–404.

Gerstadt, C. L., Hong, Y. J., & Diamond, A. (1994). The relationship between cognition and action: Performance of children 31/2–7 years old on a Stroop-like day–night test. *Cognition, 53,* 129–153.

Greenberg, M. T., Lengua, L. J., Coie, J. D., Pinderhughes, E. E., & the Conduct Problems Prevention Research Group. (1999). Predicting developmental outcomes at school entry using a multiple-risk model: Four American communities. *Developmental Psychology, 35*(2), 403–417.

Grolnick, W. S., Bridges, L. J., & Connell, J. P. (1996). Emotion regulation in two-year-olds: Strategies and emotional expression in four contexts. *Child Development, 67,* 928–941.

Grolnick, W. S., Kurowski, C. O., McMenamy, J. M., Rivkin, I., & Bridges, L. (1998). Mothers' strategies for regulating their toddlers' distress. *Infant Behavior and Development, 21,* 437–450.

Hart, D., Atkins, R., & Fegley, S. (2003). Personality and development in childhood: A person-centered approach. *Monographs of the Society for Research in Child Development, 68*(1, Serial No. 272).

Jacques, S., Zelazo, P. D., Kirkham, N. Z., & Semcesen, T. K. (1999). Rule selection versus rule execution in preschoolers: An error-detection approach. *Developmental Psychology, 35,* 770–780.

Kaiser, A. P., Hancock, T. B., Cai, X., Foster, E. M., & Hester, P. P. (2000). Parent-reported behavioral problems and language delays in boys and girls enrolled in Head Start classrooms. *Behavioral Disorders, 26*(1), 26–41.

Kochanska, G. (1995). Children's temperament, mothers' discipline, and security of attachment: Multiple pathways to emerging internalization. *Child Development, 66,* 597–615.

Kochanska, G. (1997). Multiple pathways to conscience for children with different temperaments: From toddlerhood to age 5. *Developmental Psychology, 33,* 228–240.

Kochanska, G., & Aksan, N. (1995). Mother–child mutually positive affect, the quality of child compliance to requests and prohibitions, and maternal control as correlates of early internalization. *Child Development, 66*(1), 236–254.

Kochanska, G., Murray, K. T., & Coy, K. C. (1997). Inhibitory control as a contributor to conscience in childhood: From toddler to early school age. *Child Development, 68,* 263–277.

Kochanska, G., Murray, K. T., & Harlan, E. T. (2000). Effortful control in early childhood: Continuity and change, antecedents, and implications for social development. *Developmental Psychology, 36*(2), 220–232.

Kochanska, G., Murray, K. T., Jacques, T. Y., Koenig, A. L., & Vendergeest, K. (1996). Inhibitory control in young children and its role in emerging internalization. *Child Development, 67,* 490–507.

Kochanska, G., Tjebkes, T. L., & Forman, D. R. (1998). Children's emerging regulation of conduct: Restraint, compliance, and internalization from infancy to the second year. *Child Development, 69*(5), 1378–1389.

Kopp, C. B. (1989). Regulation of distress and negative emotions: A developmental view. *Developmental Psychology, 25*(3), 343–354.

Kupersmidt, J. B., Griesler, P. C., DeRosier, M. E., Patterson, C. J., & Davis, P. W. (1995). Childhood aggression and peer relations in the context of family and neighborhood factors. *Child Development, 66,* 360–375.

Lee, V. E., Brooks-Gunn, J., & Schnur, E. (1988). Does Head Start work?: A 1-year follow-up comparison of disadvantaged children attending Head Start, no preschool, and other preschool programs. *Developmental Psychology, 24*(2), 210–222.

Leung, P. W. L., Luk, S. L., Ho, T. P., Taylor, E. Mak, F. L., & Bacon-Shone, J. (1996). The diagnosis and prevalence of hyperactivity in Chinese schoolboys. *British Journal of Psychiatry, 168,* 486–496.

Leventhal, T., & Brooks-Gunn, J. (2000). The neighborhoods they live in: The effects of neighborhood residence upon child and adolescent outcomes. *Psychological Bulletin, 126*(2), 309–337.

Leventhal, T., & Brooks-Gunn, J. (2003). Neighborhood-based initiatives. In J. Brooks-Gunn, A. S. Fuligni, & L. Berlin (Eds.), *Early child development in the 21st century: Profiles of current research initiatives* (pp. 279–295). New York: Teachers College Press.

Livesey, D. J., & Morgan, G. A. (1991). The development of response inhibition in 4- and 5-year-old children. *Australian Journal of Psychology, 43*(3), 133–137.

Love, J. M., Harrison, L., Sagi-Schwartz, A., van IJzendoorn, M. H., Ross, C., Ungerer, J. A., et al.

(2003). Child care quality matters: How conclusions may vary with context. *Child Development, 74*(4), 1021–1033.

Manglesdorf, S. C., Shapiro, J. R., & Marzolf, D. (1995). Developmental and temperamental differences in emotion regulation in infancy. *Child Development, 66,* 1817–1828.

Marchand, J., Hock, E., & Widaman, K. (2002). Mutual relations between mothers' depressive symptoms and hostile-controlling behavior and young children's externalizing and internalizing behavior problems. *Parenting: Science and Practice, 2*(4), 335–353.

McCabe, L. A., & Brooks-Gunn, J. (2002, June). Self-regulation tasks for preschool children: Addressing issues to valid assessment in less "regulated" environments. In L. A. McCabe (Chair), *Innovations in the study of self-regulation: New methods, ecologically valid contexts, and diverse populations.* Symposium conducted at Head Start's Sixth National Research Conference, Washington, DC.

McCabe, L. A., Rebello-Britto, P., Hernandez, M., & Brooks-Gunn, J. (in press). Games children play: Observing young children's self-regulation across laboratory, home, and school settings. In R. DelCarmen-Wiggins & A. Carter (Eds.), *Handbook of infant, toddler, and preschool mental health assessment.* New York: Oxford University Press.

Mezzacappa, E. (2003). *Alerting, orienting, and executive attention: Developmental and sociodemographic properties in an epidemiological sample of young, urban children.* Manuscript submitted for publication.

Mischel, H. N., & Mischel, W. (1983). The development of children's knowledge of self-control strategies. *Child Development, 54,* 603–619.

Mischel, W., & Rodriguez, M. L. (1993). Psychological distance in self-imposed delay of gratification. In R. R. Cocking & K. A. Renniger (Eds.), *The development and meaning of psychological distance* (pp. 109–121). Hillsdale, NJ: Erlbaum.

National Institute of Child Health and Human Development Early Child Care Research Network. (2003a). Do children's attention processes mediate the link between family predictors and school readiness? *Developmental Psychology, 39*(3), 581–593.

National Institute of Child Health and Human Development Early Child Care Research Network. (2003b). Does amount of time spent in child care predict socioemotional adjustment during the transition to kindergarten? *Child Development, 74*(4), 976–1005.

National Institute of Child Health and Human Development Early Child Care Research Network. (2003c). Does quality of child care affect child outcomes at age 4½? *Developmental Psychology, 39,* 451–469.

Nelson, C. A., & Luciana, M. (2001). *Handbook of developmental cognitive neuroscience.* Cambridge, MA: MIT Press.

Newman, D. L., Caspi, A., Moffitt, T. E., & Silva, P. A. (1997). Antecedents of adult interpersonal functioning: Effects of individual differences in age 3 temperament. *Developmental Psychology, 33*(2), 206–217.

Pennington, B. F. (1998). Dimensions of executive functions in normal and abnormal development. In N. A. Krasnegor, G. R. Lyon, & P. S. Goldman-Rakic (Eds.), *Development of the prefrontal cortex: Evolution, neurobiology, and behavior* (pp. 265–281). Baltimore: Brookes.

Pettit, G. S., & Bates, J. E. (1989). Family interaction patterns and children's behavior problems from infancy to 4 years. *Developmental Psychology, 25*(3), 413–420.

Raver, C. C. (1996). Relations between social contingency in mother–child interaction and 2-year-olds' social competence. *Developmental Psychology, 32*(5), 850–859.

Raver, C. C., Blackburn, E. K., Bancroft, M., & Torp, N. (1999). Relations between effective emotional self-regulation, attentional control, and low-income preschoolers' social competence with peers. *Early Education and Development, 10*(3), 333–350.

Rothbart, M. K., Ahadi, S. A., & Hershey, K. L. (1994). Temperament and social behavior in childhood. *Merrill–Palmer Quarterly, 40*(1), 21–39.

Rothbart, M. K., Derryberry, D., & Posner, M. I. (1994). A psychobiological approach to the development of temperament. In J. E. Bates & T. D. Wachs (Eds.), *Temperament: Individual differ-*

ences in biology and behavior (pp. 83–116). Washington, DC: American Psychological Association.

Rubin, K. H., Coplan, R. J., Fox, N. A., & Calkins, S. D. (1995). Emotionality, emotion regulation, and preschoolers' social adaptation. *Development and Psychopathology, 7,* 49–62.

Schultz, D., Izard, C. E., Ackerman, B. P., & Youngstrom, E. A. (2001). Emotion knowledge in economically disadvantaged children: Self-regulatory antecedents and relations to social difficulties and withdrawal. *Development and Psychopathology, 13,* 53–67.

Sethi, A., Mischel, W., Aber, J. L., Shoda, Y., & Rodriguez, M. L. (2000). The role of strategic attention deployment in development of self-regulation: Predicting preschoolers' delay of gratification from mother–toddler interactions. *Developmental Psychology, 36*(6), 767–777.

Shaw, D. S., Gilliom, M., Ingoldsby, E. M., & Nagin, D. S. (2003). Trajectories leading to school-age conduct problems. *Developmental Psychology, 39*(2), 189–200.

Shoda, Y., Mischel, W., & Peake, P. K. (1990). Predicting adolescent cognitive and self regulatory competencies from preschool delay of gratification: Identifying diagnostic conditions. *Developmental Psychology, 26,* 978–986.

Shonkoff, J. P., & Phillips, D. A. (Eds.). (2000). *From neurons to neighborhoods: The science of early childhood development.* Washington, DC: National Academy Press.

Taylor, E. (1999). Developmental neuropsychopathology of attention deficit and impulsiveness. *Development and Psychopathology, 11,* 607–628.

Vaughn, B. E., Kopp, C. B., & Krakow, J. B. (1984). The emergence and consolidation of self-control from 18 to 30 months of age: Normative trends and individual differences. *Child Development, 55,* 990–1004.

Vaughn, B. E., Krakow, J. B., Kopp, C. B., Johnson, K., & Schwartz, S. S. (1986). Process analysis of the behavior of very young children in delay tasks. *Developmental Psychology, 22,* 752–759.

Vondra, J. I., Shaw, D. S., Swearingen, L., Cohen, M., & Owens, E. B. (2001). Attachment stability and emotional and behavioral regulation from infancy to preschool age. *Development and Psychopathology, 13,* 13–33.

Vygotsky, L. S. (1978). The role of play in development. In M. Cole, V. John-Steiner, S. Scribner, & E. Souberman (Eds. & Trans.), *Mind in society: The development of higher mental processes* (pp. 92–104). Cambridge, MA: Harvard University Press. (Original work published 1930–1935)

Weinberg, M. K., Tronick, E. Z., Cohn, J. F., & Olson, K. (1999). Gender differences in emotional expressivity and self-regulation during early infancy. *Developmental Psychology, 35*(1), 175–188.

Welsh, M. C. (2002). Developmental and clinical vairiations in executive functions. In D. L. Molfese & V. J. Molfese (Eds.), *Developmental variations in learning: Applications to social, executive function, language, and reading skills* (pp. 139–185). Mahwah, NJ: Erlbaum.

Wilson, B. J. (1999). Entry behavior and emotion regulation abilities of developmentally delayed boys. *Developmental Psychology, 35*(1), 214–222.

Zahn-Waxler, C., Schmitz, S., Fulker, D., Robinson, J., & Emde, R. (1996). Behavior problems in 5-year-old monozygotic and dizygotic twins: Genetic and environmental influences, patterns of regulation, and internalization of control. *Development and Psychopathology, 8,* 103–122.

Zelazo, P. D., Frye, D., & Rapus, T. (1996). An age-related dissociation between knowing rules and using them. *Cognitive Development, 11,* 37–63.

18

Temperament and Self-Regulation

MARY K. ROTHBART
LESA K. ELLIS
MICHAEL I. POSNER

Concepts of temperament have ancient roots, linking observations of individual differences to an underlying physiology. Many of us are familiar with the Greco-Roman typology of temperament based on the body humors, in which the melancholic person is described as anxious and moody, with a predominance of black bile; the sanguine person, as cheerful and good natured, with a predominance of blood; the choleric, as prone to anger and irritability, with a predominance of yellow bile; and the phlegmatic, as slow to arousal, with a predominance of phlegm. The ancient typology demonstrated concepts of temperament that persist to the present day. First, the typology reflected observed consistencies in individual feelings and behavior; second, these individual differences could be observed early in life. Third, temperament types were linked to individual physiology, as it was understood at the time, in terms of the humors. In modern times, attempts to relate temperament to an underlying physiology have continued, with recent links to physiology in brain imaging studies (Canli, Sivers, Whitfield, Gotlib, & Gabrieli, 2002) and molecular genetics (Swanson et al., 2000). Fourth, the typology was associated with the development of psychopathology, especially in the melancholic and choleric types.

The ancient typology also focused on the primary emotions and self-regulatory action tendencies related to them: positive affect and sociability for the sanguine; fear and sadness for the melancholic; anger, irritability, and aggression for the choleric; and a general slowness to emotion and action for the phlegmatic. Although some current definitions of temperament limit the temperament domain to the emotions, we also include activity level, orienting and executive attention, thus establishing even stronger connections with self-regulation. We have defined temperament as constitutionally based individual differences in reactivity and self-regulation, as seen in the emotional, motor, and attentional domains (Rothbart & Bates, 1998; Rothbart & Derryberry, 1981). By "constitutional," we refer to the biological bases of temperament, influenced over time by genes, environment, and experience. By "reactivity," we mean the onset, intensity, and duration of emotional, motor, and attentional reactions. Reactivity may apply to quite general behavioral dimensions, as in negative emotional reactivity, or more specific physiological reactions, such as heart rate reactivity.

Self-regulation is also a major part of our view of the organization of temperament. "Self-regulation" is defined as processes that serve to modulate reactivity, including fearful inhibition, surgent or extraverted approach, and the effortful control of behavior based on the executive attention system. Whereas some aspects of attention are almost entirely self-regulatory, as in effortful control, the reactive emotions themselves include behavioral tendencies with self-regulatory aspects. Fear, for example, involves regulation of motor and autonomic circuits in the support of avoidance, inhibition of action, and modulation of perceptual pathways to enhance information about locations of safety and threat (Derryberry & Rothbart, 1997). Thus, not only is fear a reactive system, but it also involves motivational systems of self-regulation. As we describe some of the recent history of theory of temperament, we hope that the special contributions of attention to self-regulation become apparent.

TEMPERAMENT AND PERSONALITY

Temperament involves evolutionarily conserved systems seen in both humans and other animals (Strelau, 1983). These systems are commonly shared by all humans, but individuals differ in the strength and sensitivity of the dispositions and the efficiency of their attentional capacities. Temperament can be seen as part of the broader domain of personality. "Personality" may be defined as patterns of thought and behavior that show consistency across situations and stability over time, affecting the individual's adaptation to the internal and social environment. In addition to temperamental dispositions, personality includes many additional characteristics, including self-concept, perceptions of others, personal values, morals, expectations, defenses, coping strategies, attitudes, and beliefs. Many of these characteristics are strongly self-regulatory, for example, the influences of self-related thought on emotion (Beck, 1976). Temperament can be seen as forming the evolutionarily conserved core from which personality develops. Temperament also refers to the individual differences in personality that characterize the infant and young child, before many of the more cognitive and highly socialized aspects of personality listed earlier have yet developed.

THEORETICAL APPROACHES
TO TEMPERAMENT AND SELF-REGULATION

Theoretical approaches to temperament have often included strong self-regulative components. Temperamental self-regulation, however, almost always has been seen as being driven by individual differences in arousal or affective-motivational reactivity. Two examples of this approach are the theories of Eysenck and Gray. Eysenck's (1967) theory of temperament identified three major dimensions. The first, Extraversion (vs. Introversion), was tied to self-regulation through a theory of arousal and its relation to pleasure and distress. Eysenck postulated that the introvert is more sensitive and arousable to stimulation than the extravert. As stimulation increases in quantity, intensity, or duration, the introvert more rapidly reaches a level of pleasant stimulation. Introverts are seen to enjoy low-intensity pleasures to a greater extent than do extraverts, who are likely to be bored with low levels of stimulation. The introvert, however, will reach and then exceed an optimal level of stimulation at lower levels than the extravert, experiencing distress to overstimulation. The extravert, therefore, is a stimulation seeker, whereas the introvert seeks to avoid overstimulation. Eysenck's model is very similar to that of Strelau (1975, 1983) and his colleagues, whose self-regulatory model is also based on individual arousability or reactivity. Eysenck's dimension of Neuroticism (vs. Emotional Stability), seen as orthogonal to Extraversion–Introversion, is tied less closely to aspects of self-regulation. By crossing the axes of Extraversion and Neuroticism, Eysenck generated the ancient fourfold typology. Eysenck's third dimension, Psychoticism, includes aspects of psychopathy or disinhibition; it is therefore related to the ability to inhibit action (Watson & Clark, 1993).

Jeffrey Gray (1970) followed in Eysenck's general tradition, but his model modified Eysenck's structure: He rotated the axes of Eysenck's Extraversion–Neuroticism structure and postulated an approach system labeled Impulsivity, ranging from low Extraversion-low Neuroticism to high Extraversion–high Neuroticism, and a behavioral inhibition system labeled Anxiety, ranging from high Extraversion–low Neuroticism to low Extraversion–high Neuroticism. More impulsive individuals were seen as having a more reactive approach system, with underlying brain circuits involving the median forebrain bundle and the lateral hypothalamus, and a greater sensitivity to reward or nonpunishment. Individuals high on behavioral inhibition or anxiety were hypothesized to have more reactive orbitofrontal cortex, medial septal area, and hippocampus, and to be more sensitive to punishment or nonreward. Behavioral approach (BAS) and inhibition (BIS) systems were both seen as having a positive input into the arousal system, increasing the behavioral intensity of the selected response and related at high levels to negative affect. Gray (1981) postulated that when a mismatch between expectation and outcome is detected, the control mode of the BIS comes into play, interrupting the current execution of behavioral programs, and identifying stimuli mentally to resolve the mismatch. Gray further postulated a fight-versus-flight system. Gray's dimensions, like Eysenck's, are reactive, although they include aspects of attention. Similar models, which are all based on reactive systems and identify underlying physiology of temperament, have been developed by Zuckerman (1991), Depue and his associates (Depue & Collins, 1999; Depue & Iacono, 1989), and Panksepp (1998).

TEMPERAMENT IN INFANCY AND CHILDHOOD

Thomas and Chess's (1977) pioneering work described individual differences in temperament during infancy. Content analyses of parents' interviews describing their infants' reactions to a number of situations yielded nine temperament dimensions: Activity Level, Approach–Withdrawal, Mood, Attention Span–Persistence, Intensity, Distractibility, Adaptability, Threshold, and Rhythmicity (Thomas, Chess, Birch, Herzig, & Korn, 1963). Although Thomas and Chess's nine dimensions have not held up well in factor analyses (Rothbart & Bates, 1998), item-level factor analyses of New York Longitudinal Study (NYLS)-based questionnaires, along with other approaches to rational scale development, have yielded a smaller number of dimensions in infancy (Rothbart & Mauro, 1990), including Activity Level, Positive Affect and Approach, Fear, Frustration or Irritability, and Attentional Persistence. These dimensions are intriguing, because they involve emotional and attentional systems that, even in early infancy, demonstrate self-regulative qualities.

At the University of Oregon, we have developed a comprehensive and highly differentiated parent-report instrument called the Children's Behavior Questionnaire (CBQ) for children ages 3–7 years (Ahadi, Rothbart, & Ye, 1993; Rothbart, Ahadi, Hershey, & Fisher, 2001). Over a number of studies in several laboratories using the CBQ, three broad factors of children's temperament have emerged. The first factor, called Surgency, or Extraversion, is defined by scales assessing positive emotionality and approach, including positive anticipation, high-intensity pleasure (sensation seeking), impulsivity, activity level, and a negative loading for shyness. The second broad factor, called Negative Affectivity, is defined by discomfort, fear, anger/frustration, and sadness, with a secondary loading for shyness, and a negative loading for soothability–falling reactivity. The third broad factor, Effortful Control, is defined by inhibitory control, attentional focusing, low–intensity pleasure, and perceptual sensitivity. Discovery of the Effortful Control factor was very interesting, because it identified a latent variable involved in the control of behavior that was either orthogonal to, or negatively related to, fearfulness, another system of temperamental control of action.

In the United States in both child and adult samples, Effortful Control was also inversely related to Negative Affectivity, and independent of Surgency/Extraversion. In a Chinese sample of children, however, these relations were not found (Ahadi et al., 1993). Effortful Control in the Chinese sample was negatively related to measures of Surgency/Extraversion and independent of Negative Affectivity, suggesting that effortful control might serve to enhance or suppress reactive behavior in keeping with the values of the culture.

Gartstein and Rothbart (2003) have further investigated the factor structure of parent-reported infant temperament, assessing several dimensions derived from research on temperament in childhood. These broad dimensions were revealed in factor analysis: Surgency/Extraversion, with loadings for approach, vocal reactivity, high-intensity pleasure, smiling and laughter, activity level, and perceptual sensitivity; Negative Affectivity, with positive loadings for sadness, frustration, fear, and, loading negatively, falling reactivity. Finally, a third factor, Orienting/Regulation, included loadings for low-intensity pleasure, cuddliness, duration of orienting, and soothability, with a secondary loading for smiling and laughter.

Thus, as early as infancy, there is evidence for a broad dimension of positive reactivity and approach, negative affectivity, and a regulative factor that appears to include contributions of both caregiver and individual self-regulation. Infant orienting to distractors presented by the caregiver affords an early example of this kind of regulation of emotion. Harman, Rothbart, and Posner (1997) showed that infants were soothed while orienting their attention to a visual and/or auditory stimulus, but when orienting was broken, they returned to the prior level of distress even though the distressing event was no longer present. This illustrates how orienting of attention blocks the expression of the brain's computations of emotion, which appear to remain stored, probably in limbic areas. Not until early childhood do we see clear signs of another attentional regulation dimension that we call effortful control, discussed later in this chapter.

In our infant laboratory research, we used parent-report and laboratory measures in a longitudinal study of infants seen at 3, 6.5, 10, and 13.5 months (Rothbart, Derryberry, & Hershey, 2000). Infants' reactions were videotaped during presentation of nonsocial- and social-eliciting stimuli. For example, smiling and laughter in response to visual and auditory stimuli was coded for its latency, intensity, and duration, then aggregated into positive affect measures. Approach was assessed in infants' latency to grasp low-intensity toys such as small squeeze toys, blocks, and a cup, and activity level was assessed in children's movement among toys distributed across a grid-lined floor. At 7-year follow-up, parents of a subset of these infants filled out the CBQ (Rothbart et al., 2001), describing their children's temperamental tendencies in childhood. Smiling and Laughter in infancy predicted concurrent infant and 7-year-olds' Approach tendencies. Infant approach at 6, 10, and 13 months also predicted later maternal reports of high approach, impulsivity, anger and aggression, and low sadness at age 7. These findings suggest that approach tendencies may contribute both to externalizing negative emotionality and positive emotionality (Derryberry & Reed, 1994; Rothbart, Ahadi, & Hershey, 1994). These findings are consonant with the idea that more active children can become more frequently frustrated, and indeed, positive relations between anger and activity levels are found throughout infancy (Rothbart, 1981, 1986; Rothbart et al., 2001).

Questionnaire measures of approach have also shown stability from toddlerhood to early childhood years (Pedlow, Sanson, Prior, & Oberklaid, 1993), and both approach and activity level have demonstrated stability from 2 to 12 years (Guerin & Gottfried, 1994). Caspi and Silva (1995) found that children high on confidence or approach at age 3–4 years were high on social potency and impulsiveness at age 18.

FEAR AND SELF-REGULATION

Late in their first year, some infants begin to demonstrate fear in their inhibited approach to unfamiliar and intense stimuli (Rothbart, 1988; Schaffer, 1974), and this inhibition can be predicted by a measure of crying and motor reactivity to stimulation at 4 months (Calkins, Fox, & Marshall, 1996; Kagan, 1994). Fear-related inhibition also shows considerable stability across childhood and into adolescence (Kagan, 1998). Fearful inhibition developing within the first year of life allows inhibitory control of behavior.

Stability of fearful inhibition has been found from 2 to 4 years (Lemery, Goldsmith, Klinnert, & Mrazek, 1999), 2 to 8 years (Kagan, Reznick, & Snidman, 1988), 3–4 years to age 18 (Caspi & Silva, 1995), and 8–12 years to early adulthood (17–24 years) (Gest, 1997). In our longitudinal work, infant fear in the laboratory predicted fear, sadness, and shyness, as well as low-intensity pleasure at 7 years (Rothbart et al., 2001). Fear did not predict later frustration/anger, and was negatively related to later approach, impulsivity, and aggression, suggesting that fear may be involved in the regulation of those tendencies (Gray & McNaughton, 1996). More fearful infants also showed greater empathy, guilt, and shame in childhood (Rothbart, Ahadi, et al., 1994). These findings suggest that fear is involved in the early development of conscience, and Kochanska (1995, 1997) has found that temperamental fearfulness predicts emerging conscience development. Fearful children whose mothers made use of gentle socialization techniques developed particularly highly internalized conscience, demonstrating an interaction between temperament and socialization in the development of internal control. Later in development, attentionally based effortful control becomes more influential in the operation of children's conscience (Kochanska, Murray, & Harlan, 2000).

Other studies indicate the further regulative influence of fearfulness. Children with concurrent attention-deficit/hyperactivity disorder (ADHD) and anxiety show reduced impulsivity compared to children with ADHD alone (Pliszka, 1989), and young children with internalizing patterns of behavior demonstrate declines in aggressiveness between kindergarten and first grade (Bates, Pettit, & Dodge, 1995). Kerr, Tremblay, Pagani, and Vitaro (1997) have found that inhibition has a protective effect against the development of delinquent behavior. Finally, Raine, Reynolds, Venables, Mednick, and Farrington (1998) found that lack of fear at age 3 predicted higher aggression at age 11. High autonomic arousal and electrodermal orienting at age 15, typically associated with fearfulness, were also protective factors for the development of criminal behavior at age 29 (Raine, Venables, & Williams, 1995).

When high approach is linked with low fear, approach may not be inhibited under circumstances that might lead to punishment. Children with strong approach tendencies who are also fearful, on the other hand, can inhibit approach tendencies when they might lead to negative outcomes. Because anxiety is linked to enhanced attention to threats (Derryberry & Reed, 1994, 1996; Vasey, Daleiden, Williams, & Brown, 1995), fear may enhance sensitivity to potential negative events and allow the child to avoid problems. On the other hand, extreme fear may lead to problems with rigid overcontrol of behavior, as reflected in the Blocks' description of overcontrolled patterns that can limit positive experiences (Block & Block, 1980; Kremen & Block, 1998). Thus, the dimension of fearfulness within the first year of life allows the first major control system of behavior, a reactive one.

EFFORTFUL CONTROL AND SELF-REGULATION

A behavioral system also develops, beginning late in infancy and continuing through the early years, that allows voluntary control of behavior and emotion, and which we have labeled effortful control, defined as the ability to inhibit a dominant response in order to perform a subdominant response. A broad dimension of "effortful control" was identified in parent-report measures of temperament in childhood (Rothbart & Bates, 1998) and in a review of the literature on temperament and development (Rothbart, 1989). Kochanska and colleagues (2000) characterized this construct of effortful control as being "situated at the intersection of the temperament and behavioral regulation literatures" (p. 220).

In further study of the link between self-regulatory temperament and the ability to focus attention consciously, we hypothesized that executive attention might underlie effortful control (Posner & Rothbart, 1998; Rothbart, Derryberry, & Posner, 1994). This hypothesis was also influenced by the correlations we had found among attentional focusing, attentional shifting, and inhibitory control in self-reports of adults (Derryberry & Rothbart, 1988). The resulting hypothesis led to studies in Oregon on the early development of attentional control under conflict conditions (Gerardi-Caulton, 2000; Posner & Rothbart, 1998, 2000; Rothbart, Ellis, Rueda, & Posner, in press). In a basic measure of executive attention, the Stroop task, subjects are asked to report the color of ink in which a word is written when the color word (e.g., red) might conflict with the ink color (e.g., blue). Adult brain imaging studies have found a variety of Stroop-like tasks to activate a midline brain structure in the anterior cingulate gyrus that has been associated with other executive attention activities (Bush, Luu, & Posner, 2000). We developed a marker task to assess executive attention in young children by creating a conflict between the identity of an object and its location. Children's performance on this task demonstrated considerable improvement between 27 and 36 months of age (Gerardi-Caulton, 2000). Children who performed well on the task were described by their parents as more skilled at attentional control, less impulsive, and less prone to frustration reactions.

As described in our other chapter (Rueda, Posner, & Rothbart, Chapter 14, this volume), we also developed and tested a Child Attention Network Test. Employing this measure, we found that the executive attention network developed strongly between 4 and 7 years of age. In addition, Diamond and Taylor (1996) evaluated performance of children between ages 3.5 and 7 in the tapping test developed by Luria. They found steady improvement in both accuracy and speed on the tapping test over the ages 3.5 to 7. Most of the improvement occurred by 6 years, with the 7-year-old group showing an accuracy rate close to 100%.

We recently assessed toddlers 24, 30, and 36 months old using the spatial conflict task we had used to mark development of effortful control (Gerardi-Caulton, 2000; Rothbart et al., in press). We replicated a significant improvement on the task with increasing age. Children performing relatively better on the task were also rated by their parents as having relatively higher levels of effortful control and lower levels of negative affectivity. The children in this study also completed a conflict task involving anticipatory eye movements to ambiguous locations (Clohessy, Posner, & Rothbart, 2001). This task, which is thought to involve the executive attention system, provides a measure suitable for use with very young children. Performance on the task was related to performance on the spatial conflict task and also to parent-reported effortful control.

Finally, the children completed a block tower–building task and a nested cup-stacking task, both of which involve volitional skills, such as task orientation, error detection and correction, and goal completion. Scores for the two tasks were combined to form a composite measure of volitional skills, and compared to parent-reported temperament scores within each age group. At age 24 months, scores on the volitional skills composite were positively related to parent-reported effortful control, and negatively related to both surgency and negative affect. At 30 months, composite scores were negatively related to impulsivity and, at a trend level, negatively related to surgency. At 36 months, composite scores were positively related, at trend level, to attention focusing. These results suggest that emerging self-regulation at 24 months may play an important role in the development of volitional skills, allowing a child greater control as he or she waits or searches for appropriate opportunities to act, resists distractions, detects and corrects errors, overcomes obstacles, and completes a goal. As these skills become practiced with age, self-regulation may play a lesser role.

TEMPERAMENT AND KOPP'S MODEL
OF THE DEVELOPMENT OF SELF-REGULATION

In Claire Kopp's (1982, 1989) analysis of the development of self-regulation, she notes that during the first 3 months, innate physiological mechanisms and preadapted action systems help to regulate the physiological state of the infant. During the next developmental phase of about 3–9 months, infants engage in sensorimotor activities that are shaped by the environment and voluntarily make contact with others; from 9 to 12 months, infants become better able to engage in goal-directed action and come to respond to commands from others.

During the second year, language and increasing impulse control become available to the child, along with increased understanding that the self is an independent being in potential control of events. Children now attempt to influence both objects and others. However, children of this age have few self-regulatory skills and little patience, and when their expectations are not met, they frequently respond with anger. They may cry or show temper tantrums (Kopp, 1992). Bronson (2000) notes the importance of the toddler's increasing awareness of the possibility of control; the actual skills of inhibition and activation of behavior under conscious control will develop during the preschool years.

In Kopp's model, self-control does not emerge until age 3–4 years, when children are able to comply with the requests of caregivers and show control in the absence of caregiver monitoring. We have suggested that the changes occurring over this period are related to development of the executive attention system and shown in the child's effortful control (Rothbart & Posner, 2001). Individual differences in effortful control allow the child to go beyond fearfully reactive self-regulation in order to inhibit dominant responses and to perform subdominant responses.

In general, the stages described in Kopp's model fit well with our new findings. However, it is unlikely to be true that preadapted genetic effects are confined to the first stage of development of self-regulation. Rather, genetic and environment together probably exert influence throughout all of the stages. In our companion chapter (Rueda et al., Chapter 14, this volume), we describe some preliminary efforts to study gene–environment interactions in development.

To examine the possibility that effortful control, as assessed by temperament questionnaires, and conflict, as measured by performance in reaction time tasks, remain correlated during adolescence, Ellis (2002), using two Stroop-like computerized tasks, measured executive attention in 100 adolescents. Effortful control and other temperament variables were measured with the use of parent- and self-report versions of the Early Adolescent Temperament Questionnaire—Revised (Ellis & Rothbart, 2002). Performance on the computerized measures of executive attention was related to mother-reported adolescent effortful control and (negatively) to negative affectivity. In addition, teacher assessment of risk for deviant behaviors was negatively related to scores on the tasks. Derryberry and Reed (1998), who used a similar spatial conflict task with adults, found that participants with poor performance tended to have low self-reported attentional control and high anxiety.

Kochanska and colleagues (2000) have developed a battery of effortful control tasks for use in the laboratory with children between 22 months and 5 years. Beginning at age 2.5 years, children's performance showed considerable consistency across tasks, indicating that the tasks measured a common underlying capacity. Children showed improvements in their performance on the battery but were also remarkably stable in their individual performance over time, with correlations ranging from .44 for the youngest children (22 to 33 months) to .59 (from 32 to 46 months), to .65 (from 46 to 66 months).

Additional evidence for stability of effortful control constructs has been found in research by Mischel and his colleagues (Mischel, Shoda, & Peake, 1988; Shoda, Mischel, & Peake, 1990; for a review, see Mischel & Ayduk, Chapter 6, this volume). Preschoolers' ability to continue to wait for a delayed treat that was preferable to a readily accessible, but less preferred treat, was measured. Delay of gratification in seconds predicted parent-reported attentiveness, concentration, competence, planfullness, and intelligence during adolescence. In addition, preschoolers better able to delay gratification were seen in adolescence as having better self-control and an increased ability to deal with stress, frustration, and temptation. Preschoolers' seconds of delay also predicted Scholastic Aptitude Test (SAT) scores, even when controlling for intelligence. In additional follow-up studies, preschoolers' delay behavior predicted goal-setting and self-regulatory abilities when participants reached their early 30s (Ayduk et al., 2000), suggesting extensive continuity in self-regulatory tendencies.

Sethi, Mischel, Aber, Shoda, and Rodriguez (2000) found that toddlers who, at 18 months, used attentional distraction techniques during a brief separation from their mothers were, at age 5, better able to delay immediate gratification. This use of attentional distraction was viewed as an attempt at self-regulating the distress brought about by maternal separation, as evidenced by lower levels of negative affect in children deploying such strategies.

Effortful control plays an important role in the development of conscience, with internalized conscience being greater in children high in effortful control (Kochanska, Murray, & Coy, 1997; Kochanska, Murray, Jacques, Koenig, & Vandegeest, 1996; Kochanska et al., 2000). Thus, both the reactive temperamental control system of fear and the attentionally based system of effortful control appear to regulate the development of conscientious thought and behavior, with the influence of fear being found earlier in development. At the University of Oregon, we found that children age 6–7 years who were high in effortful control were also high in empathy and guilt–shame, and low in aggressiveness (Rothbart, Ahadi, et al., 1994). Effortful control may support empathy by allowing a child to attend to another child's condition, instead of focusing only on his or her own sympathetic distress. Eisenberg et al. (1994; see also Eisenberg, Smith, Sadovsky, & Spinrad, Chapter 13, this volume) found that 4- to 6-year-old boys with good attentional control dealt with anger using nonhostile verbal methods rather than overt aggression.

Although effortful control is a fairly recent addition to the domain of temperament, it is proving to be an important one. Eisenberg and Fabes (1992) for example, proposed a model in which emotionality and regulation combine or interact to affect social behavior. The model distinguishes between emotion regulation, in which regulation of attention and cognition acts to regulate internal states and processes, and behavioral regulation, involving inhibition or activation of emotion-linked behavior. The model further suggests that children high in negative affectivity and low in regulation will be most likely to exhibit externalizing behavior problems.

Eisenberg and colleagues (1996) examined kindergarten through third grade children, measuring both negative emotionality and a composite measure of attentional regulation. As predicted, children high in negative emotionality and low in regulation were most likely to concurrently exhibit externalizing behavior problems. Furthermore, regulation appeared to be a stronger predictor of behavior problems in children with higher levels of negative affectivity. In a 2-year longitudinal follow-up study (Eisenberg, Fabes, Guthrie, & Reiser, 2000), children were also assessed for behavioral regulation in completing a puzzle box task. Results suggesting that attentional control was an effective predictor of behavioral problems in children with higher levels of negative emotionality replicated the results of the previous study. Children low in negative emotionality were generally low in externalizing behaviors, and individual differences in attention regulation did not appear to have an effect. In children high in negative emotionality, however, greater variability existed in levels of problem behavior, and this variability appeared to be associated with levels of attention regulation. In addition, behavioral dysregulation, as measured by the puzzle box task, was associated with problem behaviors in children both high and low in negative emotionality.

Eisenberg and colleagues (1997) also examined socially appropriate and prosocial behaviors in the same sample. At all levels of emotional intensity, regardless of valence, children high in regulation exhibited higher levels of social competence. However, this relationship was strongest for children higher in general emotional intensity. In addition, attentional control was related to resiliency, but it was particularly important for children prone to negative affect.

Eisenberg, Shepard, Fabes, Murphy, and Guthrie (1998) studied the role of internalizing negative emotionality and regulation in shyness. Children high in parent-reported fear, sadness, anxiety, and autonomic reactivity, combined with poor regulation, were seen as high in shyness by both parents and teachers. However, children with internalizing behaviors were seen to differ in some types of regulation from children with externalizing behavior (Eisenberg et al., 2001). Children high in internalizing behaviors were lower in impulsivity and higher in inhibitory control than were children high in externalizing behaviors. However, there was little difference in attentional regulation.

We (Ellis & Rothbart, 2002) also found evidence of poor effortful control in both externalizing (aggression) and internalizing (depressive mood) in a group of young adolescents. Low effortful control and high approach tendencies best predicted aggression, whereas low effortful control and high levels of affiliative needs, combined with gender (being female), best predicted depressive mood. In an additional study involving both early and late adolescent samples (Ellis, 2002), low effortful control and high frustration predicted aggression, with low effortful control and high affiliative need predicting depressive mood in both samples.

Effortful control adds a very important self-regulation dimension to the domain of temperament. Going beyond the models described here that find us moved chiefly by affect or arousal, effortful control allows us to resist the immediate influence of affect and either approach situations we fear or resist actions we desire in a flexible way. We expect, however, that the efficiency of effortful control will depend on the strength of the dominant response. Our only predictor of effortful control from infancy, given that we were not directly measuring this system during the early months, was the speed with which children grasped high-intensity toys in the laboratory (Rothbart et al., 2000). Those who grasped the toys quickly showed higher impulsivity, anger/frustration, and aggression at 7 years, and tended to be lower in attentional and inhibitory control. We have suggested that strong approach tendencies may constrain the application of effortful control (Rothbart et al., 2000). If we use an analogy of approach tendencies as the "accelerator" and inhibition tendencies, both fear and effortful control, as the "brakes" on behavior and emotional expression, stronger acceleration would be expected to weaken the braking influence of fear and effortful control.

Effortful control provides a voluntary basis for self-regulation that goes beyond the earlier inhibitory influences of fear. Differences among individuals in the degree to which they can exercise effortful control have a dramatic influence on behavior, particularly in later childhood, adolescence, and adulthood. The ability to measure and study the correlates and outcomes of these individual differences by questionnaire, observation, and laboratory tasks provides a strong basis for future understanding of the developing mechanisms of self-regulation.

REFERENCES

Ahadi, S. A., Rothbart, M. K., & Ye, R. (1993). Children's temperament in the U.S. and China: Similarities and differences. *European Journal of Personality*, 7, 359–378.

Ayduk, O., Mendoza-Denton, R., Mischel, W., Downey, G., Peake, P., & Rodriguez, M. (2000). Regulating the interpersonal self: Strategic self-regulation for coping with rejection sensitivity. *Journal of Personality and Social Psychology*, 79, 776–792.

Bates, J. E., Pettit, G. S., & Dodge, K. A. (1995). Family and child factors in stability and change in children's aggressiveness in elementary school. In J. McCord (Ed.), *Coercion and punishment in long-term perspectives* (pp. 124–138). New York: Cambridge University Press.

Beck, A. T. (1976). *Cognitive therapy and the emotional disorders*. New York: International Universities Press.

Block, J. H., & Block, J. (1980). The role of ego control and ego-resiliency in the organization of behavior. In W. A. Collins (Ed.), *Minnesota Symposium on Child Psychology* (Vol. 13, pp. 39–101). Hillsdale, NJ: Erlbaum.

Bronson, M. B. (2000). *Self-regulation in early childhood: Nature and nurture.* New York: Guilford Press.

Bush, G., Luu, P., & Posner, M. I. (2000). Cognitive and emotional influences in anterior cingulate cortex. *Trends in Cognitive Sciences, 4*(6), 215–222.

Calkins, S. D., Fox, N. A., & Marshall, T. R. (1996). Behavioral and psychological antecedents of inhibition in infancy. *Child Development, 67,* 523–540.

Canli, T., Sivers, H., Whitfield, S. L., Gotlib, I. H., & Gabrieli, J. D. E. (2002). Amygdala response to happy faces as a function of extraversion. *Science, 296*(5576), 2191.

Caspi, A., & Silva, P. A. (1995). Temperamental qualities at age three predict personality traits in young adulthood: Longitudinal evidence from a birth cohort. *Child Development, 66,* 486–498.

Clohessy, A. B., Posner, M. I., & Rothbart, M. K. (2001). Development of the functional visual field. *Acta Psychologica, 106*(1–2), 51–68.

Depue, R. A., & Collins, P. F. (1999). Neurobiology of the structure of personality: Dopamine, facilitation of incentive motivation, and extraversion. *Behavioral and Brain Sciences, 22,* 491–569.

Depue, R. A., & Iacono, W. G. (1989). Neurobehavioral aspects of affective disorders. In M. R. Rosenzweig & L. Y. Porter (Eds.), *Annual review of psychology* (Vol. 40, pp. 457–492). Palo Alto, CA: Annual Reviews.

Derryberry, D., & Reed, M. A. (1994). Temperament and the self-organization of personality. *Development and Psychopathology, 6,* 653–676.

Derryberry, D., & Reed, M. A. (1996). Regulatory processes and the development of cognitive representations. *Development and Psychopathology, 8,* 215–234.

Derryberry, D., & Reed, M. A. (1998). Anxiety and attentional focusing: Trait, state and hemispheric influences. *Personality and Individual Difference, 25,* 745–761.

Derryberry, D., & Rothbart, M. K. (1988). Arousal, affect, and attention as components of temperament. *Journal of Personality and Social Psychology, 55,* 958–966.

Derryberry, D., & Rothbart, M. K. (1997). Reactive and effortful processes in the organization of temperament. *Development and Psychopathology, 9,* 633–652.

Diamond, A., & Taylor, C. (1996). Development of an aspect of executive control: Development of the abilities to remember what I said and to "Do as I say, not as I do." *Developmental Psychobiology, 29,* 315–334.

Eisenberg, N., Cumberland, A., Spinrad, T. L., Fabes, R. A., Shepard, S. A., Reiser, M., Murphy, B. C., Losoya, S. H., & Guthrie, I. K. (2001). The relations of regulation and emotionality to children's externalizing and internalizing problem behavior. *Child Development, 72*(4), 1112–1134.

Eisenberg, N., & Fabes, R. A. (Eds.). (1992). *Emotion and its regulation in early development.* San Francisco: Jossey-Bass.

Eisenberg, N., Fabes, R. A., Guthrie, I. K., Murphy, B. C., Poulin, R., & Shepard, S. (1996). The relations of regulation and emotionality to problem behavior in elementary school children. *Development and Psychopathology, 8*(1), 141–162.

Eisenberg, N., Fabes, R. A., Guthrie, I. K., & Reiser, M. (2000). Dispositional emotionality and regulation: Their role in predicting quality of social functioning. *Journal of Personality and Social Psychology, 78*(1), 136–157.

Eisenberg, N., Fabes, R. A., Murphy, B., Karbon, M., Maszk, P., Smith, M., O'Boyle, C., & Suh, K. (1994). The role of emotionality and regulation in children's social functioning: A longitudinal study. *Child Development, 66,* 1360–1384.

Eisenberg, N., Fabes, R. A., Shepard, S. A., Murphy, B. C., Guthrie, I. K., Jones, S., Friedman, J., Poulin, R., & Maszk, P. (1997). Contemporaneous and longitudinal prediction of children's social functioning from regulation and emotionality. *Child Development, 68,* 642–664.

Eisenberg, N., Shepard, S. A., Fabes, R. A., Murphy, B. C., & Guthrie, I. K. (1998). Shyness and children's emotionality, regulation, and coping: Contemporaneous, longitudinal, and across-context relations. *Child Development, 69,* 767–790.

Ellis, L. K. (2002). Individual differences and adolescent psychosocial development. *Dissertation Abstracts International, 63*(08B), 3956. (UMI No. 3061943)

Ellis, L. K., & Rothbart, M. K. (2002). *Revision of the Early Adolescent Temperament Questionnaire.* Manuscript in preparation.

Eysenck, H. J. (1967). *The biological basis of personality.* Springfield, IL: Thomas.

Gartstein, M., & Rothbart, M. K. (2003). Studying infant temperament via a revision of the Infant Behavior Questionnaire. *Infant Behavior and Development, 26,* 64–86.

Gerardi-Caulton, G. (2000). Sensitivity to spatial conflict and the development of self-regulation in children 24–36 months of age. *Developmental Science, 3*(4), 397–404.

Gest, S. D. (1997). Behavioral inhibition: Stability and associations with adaptation from childhood to early adulthood. *Journal of Personality and Social Psychology, 72*(2), 467–475.

Gray, J. A. (1970). The psychophysiological basis of introversion–extraversion. *Behaviour Research and Therapy, 8,* 249–266.

Gray, J. A. (1981). A critique of Eysenck's theory of personality. In H. J. Eysenck (Ed.), *A model for personality* (pp. 246–276). Berlin: Springer-Verlag.

Gray, J. A., & McNaughton, N. (1996). The neuropsychology of anxiety: Reprise. In D. A. Hope (Ed.), *Nebraska Symposium on Motivation: Perspectives on anxiety, panic, and fear* (Vol. 43, pp. 61–134). Lincoln: University of Nebraska Press.

Guerin, D. W., & Gottfried, A. W. (1994). Temperamental consequences of infant difficultness. *Infant Behavior and Development, 17*(4), 413–421.

Harman, C., Rothbart, M. K., & Posner, M. I. (1997). Distress and attention interactions in early infancy. *Motivation and Emotion, 21,* 27–43.

Kagan, J. (1994). *Galen's prophecy: Temperament in human nature.* New York: Basic Books.

Kagan, J. (1998). Biology and the child. In W. S. E. Damon & N. V. E. Eisenberg (Eds.), *Handbook of child psychology: Vol. 3. Social, emotional and personality development* (5th ed., pp. 177–235). New York: Wiley.

Kagan, J., Reznick, J. S., & Snidman, N. (1988). Biological bases of childhood shyness. *Science, 240,* 167–171.

Kerr, M., Tremblay, R. E., Pagani, L., & Vitaro, F. (1997). Boys' behavioral inhibition and the risk of later delinquency. *Archives of General Psychiatry, 54,* 809–816.

Kochanska, G. (1995). Children's temperament, mothers' discipline, and security of attachment: Multiple pathways to emerging internalization. *Child Development, 66,* 597–615.

Kochanska, G. (1997). Multiple pathways to conscience for children with different temperaments: From toddlerhood to age five. *Developmental Psychology, 33,* 228–240.

Kochanska, G., Murray, K., & Coy, K. C. (1997). Inhibitory control as a contributor to conscience in childhood: From toddler to early school age. *Child Development, 68,* 263–277.

Kochanska, G., Murray, K. T., & Harlan, E. (2000). Effortful control in early childhood: Continuity and change, antecedents, and implications for social development. *Developmental Psychology, 36,* 220–232.

Kochanska, G., Murray, K., Jacques, T. Y., Koenig, A. L., & Vandegeest, K. A. (1996). Inhibitory control in young children and its role in emerging internalization. *Child Development, 67,* 490–507.

Kopp, C. B. (1982). Antecedents of self-regulation: A developmental perspective. *Developmental Psychology, 18,* 199–214.

Kopp, C. B. (1989). Regulation of distress and negative emotions: A developmental view. *Developmental Psychology, 25,* 343–354.

Kopp, C. (1992). Emotional distress and control in young children. In N. Eisenberg & R. A. Fabes (Eds.), *Emotion and its regulation in early development* (pp. 41–56). San Francisco: Jossey-Bass.

Kremen, A. M., & Block, J. (1998). The roots of ego-control in young adulthood: Links with parenting in early childhood. *Journal of Personality and Social Psychology, 75,* 1062–1075.

Lemery, K. S., Goldsmith, H. H., Klinnert, M. D., & Mrazek, D. A. (1999). Developmental models of infant and childhood temperament. *Developmental Psychology, 35,* 189–204.

Mischel, W., Shoda, Y., & Peake, P. (1988). The nature of adolescent competencies predicted by preschool delay of gratification. *Journal of Personality and Social Psychology, 54,* 687–696.

Panksepp, J. (1998). *Affective neuroscience: The foundations of human and animal emotions.* New York: Oxford University Press.

Pedlow, R., Sanson, A., Prior, M., & Oberklaid, F. (1993). Stability of maternally reported temperament from infancy to 8 years. *Developmental Psychology, 29,* 998–1007.

Pliszka, S. R. (1989). Effect of anxiety on cognition, behavior, and stimulant response in ADHD. *Journal of the American Academy of Child and Adolescent Psychiatry, 28,* 882–887.

Posner, M. I., & Rothbart, M. K. (1998). Developing attentional skills. In J. Richards (Ed.), *Cognitive neuroscience of attention: A developmental perspective* (pp. 317–323). Mahwah, NJ: Erlbaum.

Posner, M. I., & Rothbart, M. K. (2000). Developing mechanisms of self-regulation. *Development and Psychopathology, 12,* 427–441.

Raine, A., Reynolds, C., Venables, P. H., Mednick, S. A., & Farrington, D. P. (1998). Fearlessness, stimulation-seeking, and large body size at age 3 years as early predispositions to childhood aggression at age 11 years. *Archives of General Psychiatry, 55,* 745–751.

Raine, A., Venables, P. H., & Williams, M. (1995). High autonomic arousal and electrodermal orienting at age 15 years as protective factors against criminal behavior at age 29 years. *American Journal of Psychiatry, 152,* 1595–1600.

Rothbart, M. K. (1981). Measurement of temperament in infancy. *Child Development, 52,* 569–578.

Rothbart, M. K. (1986). Longitudinal observation of infant temperament. *Developmental Psychology, 22,* 356–365.

Rothbart, M. K. (1988). Temperament and the development of inhibited approach. *Child Development, 59,* 1241–1250.

Rothbart, M. K. (1989). Temperament in childhood: A framework. In G. Kohnstamm, J. Bates, & M. K. Rothbart (Eds.), *Temperament in childhood* (pp. 59–73). Chichester, UK: Wiley.

Rothbart, M. K., Ahadi, S. A., & Hershey, K. L. (1994). Temperament and social behavior in childhood. *Merrill–Palmer Quarterly, 40,* 21–39.

Rothbart, M. K., Ahadi, S. A., Hershey, K. L., & Fisher, P. (2001). Investigations of temperament at three to seven years: The Children's Behavior Questionnaire. *Child Development, 72,* 1394–1408.

Rothbart, M. K., & Bates, J. E. (1998). Temperament. In W. Damon (Series Ed.) & N. Eisenberg (Vol. Ed.), *Handbook of child psychology: Vol. 3. Social, emotional, and personality development* (5th ed., pp. 105–176). New York: Wiley.

Rothbart, M. K., & Derryberry, D. (1981). Development of individual differences in temperament. In M. E. Lamb & A. L. Brown (Eds.), *Advances in developmental psychology* (Vol. 1, pp. 37–86). Hillsdale, NJ: Erlbaum.

Rothbart, M. K., Derryberry, D., & Hershey, K. (2000). Stability of temperament in childhood: Laboratory infant assessment to parent report at seven years. In V. J. Molfese & D. L. Molfese (Eds.), *Temperament and personality development across the life span* (pp. 85–119). Hillsdale, NJ: Erlbaum.

Rothbart, M. K., & Derryberry, D., & Posner, M. I. (1994). A psychobiological approach to the development of temperament. In J. E. Bates & T. D. Wachs (Eds.), *Temperament: Individual differences at the interface of biology and behavior* (pp. 83–116). Washington, DC: American Psychological Association.

Rothbart, M. K., Ellis, L. K., Rueda, M. R., & Posner, M. I. (in press). Developing mechanisms of temperamental effortful control. *Journal of Personality.*

Rothbart, M. K., & Mauro, J. A. (1990). Questionnaire approaches to the study of infant temperament. In J. W. Fagen & J. Colombo (Eds.), *Individual differences in infancy: Reliability, stability and prediction* (pp. 411–429). Hillsdale, NJ: Erlbaum.

Schaffer, H. R. (1974). Cognitive components of the infant's response to strangeness. In M. Lewis & L. A. Rosenblum (Eds.), *The origins of fear* (pp. 11–24). New York: Wiley.

Sethi, A., Mischel, W., Aber, J. L., Shoda, Y., & Rodriguez, M. L. (2000). The role of strategic attention deployment in development of self-regulation: Predicting preschoolers' delay of gratification from mother–toddler interactions. *Developmental Psychology, 36*(6), 767–777.

Shoda, Y., Mischel, W., & Peake, P. (1990). Predicting adolescent cognitive and self-regulatory competencies from preschool delay of gratification: Identifying diagnostic conditions. *Developmental Psychology, 26*, 978–986.

Strelau, J. (1975). Reactivity and activity style in selected occupations. *Polish Psychological Bulletin, 6*(4), 199–206.

Strelau, J. (1983). *Temperament personality activity.* New York: Academic Press.

Swanson, J., Oosterlaan, J., Murias, M., Moyzis, R., Schuck, S., Mann, M., Feldman, P., Spence, M. A., Sergeant, J., Smith, M., Kennedy, J., & Posner, M. I. (2000). ADHD children with 7-repeat allele of the DRD4 gene have extreme behavior but normal performance on critical neuropsychological tests of attention. *Proceedings of the National Academy of Sciences, USA, 97*, 4754–4759.

Thomas, A., Chess, S., Birch, H. G., Herzig, M. E., & Korn, S. (1963). *Behavioral individuality in early childhood.* New York: New York University Press.

Thomas, A., & Chess, S. (1977). *Temperament and development.* New York: Brunner/Mazel.

Vasey, M. W., Daleiden, E. L., Williams, L. L., & Brown, L. M. (1995). Biased attention in childhood anxiety disorders: A preliminary study. *Journal of Abnormal Child Psychology, 23*, 267–279.

Watson, D., & Clark, L. A. (1993). Behavioral disinhibition versus constraint: A dispositional perspective. In D. M. Wegner & J. W. Pennebaker (Eds.), *Handbook of mental control* (pp. 506–527). Englewood Cliffs, NJ: Prentice-Hall.

Zuckerman, M. (1991). *Psychobiology of personality.* New York: Cambridge University Press.

IV

The Interpersonal Dimension of Self-Regulation

19

The Sociometer, Self-Esteem, and the Regulation of Interpersonal Behavior

MARK R. LEARY

Most theoretical and empirical analyses of self-regulation have focused on the generic psychological processes that allow people to control their thoughts, emotions, and behaviors (Baumeister, Heatherton, & Tice, 1994; Carver & Scheier, 1981; Mischel, 1996; Wegner & Pennebaker, 1993). I refer to these processes as "generic" because they seem to be nonspecific with regard to the action being regulated. For example, TOTE (test–operate–test–exit) and other cybernetic models of self-control (Carver & Scheier, 1981) can be applied to many behavioral domains, and the same basic processes are presumably involved regardless of the nature of the self-control task at hand. Indeed, Baumeister and his colleagues have shown that exerting self-control in one behavioral arena can undermine self-regulation in unrelated domains, suggesting that all efforts at self-regulation may involve the same underlying mechanism (Baumeister & Vohs, 2003). Whether one is trying to persevere on a difficult task, resist the temptation to overeat, restrain one's anger, or ignore disturbing thoughts, self-control often involves similar psychological processes.

In addition to these general-purpose self-regulatory systems, people also possess mechanisms that are dedicated to particular functions. Such mechanisms operate in a circumscribed range of situations and handle only one kind of regulatory problem. This chapter examines one such self-regulatory mechanism—the *sociometer*—that appears to be involved in the control of interpersonal behavior. Most previous writing and research regarding the sociometer have emphasized its connection to self-esteem (e.g., Leary & Downs, 1995) but, as we will see, its functions go far beyond simply leading people to feel good or bad about themselves.

According to evolutionary psychologists, the human mind is composed of a number of distinct, domain-specific modules that evolved because they solved recurrent problems involving survival and reproduction in the prehistoric past (Buss, 1995; Cosmides &

Tooby, 1994; Samuels, 2000). Recurrent challenges in the ancestral environment would have led to the evolution of systems designed to meet those challenges. So, for example, theorists have posited the existence of regulatory modules that help people to avoid toxic substances, identify the "best" potential mates, detect group members who cheat, and ostracize those who may be infected with parasites (Cosmides & Tooby, 1992; Kurzban & Leary, 2001; Rozin & Fallon, 1987).

Many of these systems—such as mechanisms involving fear and disgust—undoubtedly serve to protect people from physical threats directly. Other systems, however, evolved to serve interpersonal functions by helping people behave toward others in ways that facilitated their own survival and reproduction. Perhaps the best known module of this kind involves the attachment system by which infants and parents bond with one another (Bowlby, 1969). Such systems have clear adaptive effects, but their effects on the individual's well-being are indirect, being mediated by the responses of other people.

THE SOCIOMETER

Perhaps the fundamental prerequisite of interpersonal life is that a person be minimally accepted by other people while avoiding wholesale rejection. Virtually all social affordances—such as friendship, social support, coalition membership, social influence, and pair bonds—require the individual to be minimally accepted by other people. Furthermore, only those who have established mutually supportive relationships with other people can count on others' assistance in terms of food sharing, physical protection, and care when ill, injured, or old. An individual who does not maintain a minimal level of social acceptance is at a decided disadvantage compared to one who is warmly accepted. Because of the numerous adaptive advantages of being accepted by other people, human beings are not only highly social animals but also possess a strong and pervasive need for acceptance and belongingness (Baumeister & Leary, 1995). Thus, given the vital importance of social acceptance and the disastrous consequences of rejection throughout human evolution, human beings developed a psychological system for regulating their relationships with other people—a psychological module that monitors and responds to events that are relevant to interpersonal acceptance and rejection.

Regulatory systems generally possess three features. They monitor the internal or external environment for certain stimuli or cues that signal advantageous or disadvantageous circumstances, evoke positive or negative feelings when these cues are detected, and motivate behaviors that help the individual to capitalize on the opportunity or avert the threat that presents itself. To offer a biological example (Rozin & Fallon, 1987), the regulatory mechanisms that underlie disgust respond to visual and olfactory cues that tend to be associated with toxic substances (e.g., the sight or smell of decaying matter), evoke an emotional reaction to the stimulus (i.e., subjective feelings of disgust), and produce an action tendency to avoid the threat (e.g., to steer clear of disgusting things). In the same way, a module that evolved to facilitate acceptance and avoid rejection would be expected to respond to cues indicating real or potential rejection, evoke feelings that alert the individual to the threat of rejection, and motivate the person to behave in ways that minimize the probability of rejection and promote acceptance.

Elsewhere, I have described evidence to support the view that the self-esteem system is essentially a sociometer that serves precisely these functions (Leary, 1999; Leary & Baumeister, 2000; Leary & Downs, 1995; Leary, Tambor, Terdal, & Downs, 1995). In this chapter, however, I focus specifically on the role of the sociometer in regulating inter-personal behavior.

Detecting Threats to Relational Value

As noted, regulatory systems monitor the internal and/or external environment for cues that connote a particular class of threat or opportunity. The function of the sociometer is to monitor the interpersonal environment for cues that are relevant to a person's *relational value* in the eyes of other people. Although I initially described the sociometer as a mechanism that reacts to indications of social acceptance and rejection (Leary & Downs, 1995), the sociometer's function can be more precisely described as one of monitoring and responding to cues that reflect the individual's relational value—the degree to which other people regard their relationships with the individual as valuable or important (Leary, 2002; Leary, Cottrell, & Phillips, 2001).

In describing the function of the sociometer, the term "relational value" is preferred over "acceptance" and "rejection" for two reasons. First, "acceptance," "rejection," and their synonyms reflect an artificial dichotomy that makes it difficult to talk about degrees of accepting and rejecting reactions (e.g., it is awkward to talk about being "half-accepted" or "partly ostracized"). What we colloquially call "rejection" and "acceptance" are actually end points along a continuum of relational value (Leary, 2001).

Second, the term "relational value" makes it easier to conceptualize instances in which people *feel* rejected even though they are being objectively accepted, such as when a woman who knows her husband loves and accepts her nonetheless feels rejected when he chooses to watch sports on television rather than go to dinner with her. Such cases arise not because people are actually rejected, but because they perceive that their relational value is not as high as they desire (i.e., the woman may believe that if her husband valued his relationship with her enough, he would not choose to watch television instead of going to dinner).

People are exceptionally sensitive to events that have implications for their relational value and seem to monitor the environment for cues relevant to relational value on a preattentive level. For example, the classic "cocktail party phenomenon," in which a person orients toward his or her name in the otherwise babbling hubbub of a loud party (Cherry, 1953), demonstrates a preattentive vigilance for indications of one's relational value. When people experience the cocktail party phenomenon, they invariably wonder (and may even ask) what is being said about them and whether it is evaluatively positive or negative. In addition, people spend a good deal of time thinking about other people's perceptions and evaluations of them, and trying to anticipate how others will react to them in future situations. Some of these imaginings are idle ruminations, but others evoke deep concern, if they suggest that one's past, present, or future relational value is lower than desired. People regularly, easily, and often automatically monitor their relational value to others (see Leary & Baumeister, 2000, for a review of relevant evidence).

The Warning System

At least since Darwin, theorists have agreed that the affective overlay on our lives serves to alert us to dangers, challenges, opportunities, and other events with implications for our well-being. Among other things, emotions shift our attention to critical features of our environment; it is difficult not to think about threats and opportunities that evoke strong emotion. In addition, emotions motivate behaviors that respond to these events and serve to reinforce, either positively or negatively, actions that deal effectively with them. So, for example, threatening stimuli evoke fear that is accompanied by an action tendency to avoid or escape the feared stimulus, and such actions are reinforced by a decline in the aversive fearful feelings. Of course, a functional analysis of emotion does not imply that all emotions are adaptive. Clearly, people may react dysfunctionally when they misappraise a situation or misjudge the most effective response to it. Even so, emotions evolved because they were adaptive in helping people to regulate their behavior. To say it differently, feelings are fundamentally involved in effective self-regulation (Carver & Scheier, 1981).

The affective output of the sociometer serves precisely this warning function. Indications that the individual is approved of or accepted—that his or her relational value is high—lead to positive affect. Indications that the individual is disapproved of or rejected—that his or her relational value is low (or declining)—lead to negative affect. Dozens of studies have shown that perceived rejection (i.e., low relational value) is associated with negative emotions such as anxiety, sadness, hurt feelings, and jealousy, and with focused attention to the problematic interpersonal situation (Leary, Koch, & Hechenbleikner, 2001).

Typically, whenever people experience pleasant or unpleasant emotions as the result of interpersonal acceptance and rejection, they also feel good or bad *about themselves*. The sociometer model suggests that these self-relevant feelings—what we typically call state self-esteem—are part of this regulatory system. When the sociometer detects cues that connote actual or potential rejection (i.e., unacceptably low relational value), it not only triggers negative affect but also instigates a process to assess whether one's low relational value is due to some personal action, shortcoming, or deficiency. In most cases, people at least entertain the possibility that others' low appraisal of their relational value is partly their own fault, which leads them to feel bad about themselves, that is, to experience low state self-esteem. However, when people are certain that their exclusion by other people does not reflect on them personally, their state self-esteem is unaffected (Leary, Tambor, et al., 1995).

The (So-Called) Self-Esteem Motive

Most conceptualizations of self-esteem have made no effort to explain what self-esteem does or why it is important (Leary, 1999). The assumption has been that people's positive and negative feelings about themselves are related to a variety of important outcomes (such as achievement, positive interpersonal relations, and psychological well-being; Mecca, Smelser, & Vasconcellos, 1989), but few efforts have been made to explain why people have feelings about themselves or what function they might serve. To complicate matters, most psychologists have assumed that people possess a *need* for self-esteem, without ever asking why people would need to feel good about themselves.

Sociometer theory answers this question by proposing that, contrary to how it may appear, people do not need to feel good about themselves at all. Stated baldly, people do not have a need for self-esteem (Leary & Downs, 1995). Rather, people only appear to seek self-esteem, because they typically try to behave in ways that maintain or increase their relational value to other people. The various behaviors that have been attributed to people's efforts to maintain self-esteem reflect their efforts to maintain relational value in other people's eyes. They appear to be seeking self-esteem, because self-esteem is the internal, subjective gauge that monitors their success in promoting relational value (see Leary & Baumeister, 2000). This is not to say that people do not occasionally try to override the sociometer to avoid negative feelings about themselves, but these intrapsychic, self-serving reactions reflect a hedonistic effort to avoid negative affect rather than a need for self-esteem per se. I return to this point later in the chapter.

Two Key Questions Regarding Sociometer Theory

Before proceeding, I wish to address two common questions about the sociometer that are relevant to understanding its regulatory function.

Why Is the "Self" Needed in This System?

Some critics of sociometer theory have correctly observed that a regulatory system with the properties of a sociometer need not involve any connection to the self. After all, other species of social animals possess systems that help them to regulate interactions with conspecifics, both with respect to dominance–submission and inclusion–exclusion (Gilbert & Trower, 1990). For example, other species of monkeys and apes are quite attuned to others' reactions to them vis-à-vis dominance and acceptance. Yet despite the fact that some of these species show a rudimentary capacity for self-awareness (Mitchell, 2003), we would probably not wish to invoke the concept of *self-esteem* in accounting for their reactions.

This objection is partially correct. An animal does not need self-esteem, or even a self, to regulate its social behavior effectively. In fact, prior to the appearance of the self during human evolution, our self-less hominid ancestors presumably interacted effectively and generally avoided interpersonal problems involving social rejection, even though they lacked the capacity for conscious self-reflection. In the absence of self-reflection, however, this system could respond only to cues in the immediate social environment. Responses to some of these cues, such as certain facial expressions (e.g., stares, frowns) or gestures (Ohman, 1986), may have been innate, whereas others were conditioned reactions to otherwise neutral stimuli that became associated with negative interpersonal consequences (e.g., learning that a particular group member performed a particular action whenever he or she was displeased). In either case, the detection of certain "rejection" cues would likely have elicited negative affect and motivated behavioral efforts to appease, ingratiate, or withdraw. All of this could have happened without a self.

With the appearance of full-blown self-awareness and the modern conceptual self, however, people's reactions to rejection-relevant cues became more complex. Although early human beings would still have responded to natural and learned cues relevant to acceptance and rejection, changes in three features of the self would have built a new layer of cognitive processing on top of the older self-less sociometer. First, improvements in the extended self, which processes information about the individual over time, would have allowed people to ponder past rejections and anticipate possible rejections in the future (Leary & Buttermore, 2003). As a result, they could have evoked rejection-related thoughts and feelings in themselves in the absence of immediate feedback and, thus, have felt "good" or "bad" about past and future events. This would have been an important development in self-regulation, because it would have allowed people to anticipate others' future reactions to them. The negative feelings that such imaginings evoked would then have served to deter actions that might result in rejection.

Second, although other great apes may possess a weak theory of mind that allows them to infer others' reactions (Mitchell, 2003), modern human beings are far more capable of getting into the heads of other people than any ape (and, presumably, than our prehuman ancestors). Many theorists have suggested that the ability to infer other people's thoughts, feelings, and intentions is linked to the ability to reflect on one's own internal states. We can draw inferences about the private states of others only by extrapolating from our own. As Humphrey (1986) observed, we can "imagine what it's like to be them, because we know what it's like to be ourselves" (p. 71). With enhancements in reflexive self-awareness, human beings were able to imagine how they were being perceived and evaluated by other people and to think consciously about how others might react if they acted in certain ways. Among other things, this ability would have allowed them to imagine whether particular actions would ultimately lead to acceptance or rejection.

Third, modern human beings are able to think about themselves in abstract, conceptual, and symbolic ways that are not characteristic of any other animal or, I presume, our prehuman ancestors. With a modern conceptual (or symbolic) self, they could consciously think about and evaluate themselves. They could also use other people's (often symbolic) reactions to them to assess their abilities and worth, and judge themselves according to other people's abstract standards. As a result, thinking about other people's reactions to them could evoke positive and negative feelings about symbolic aspects of the self.

Prior to the time that human beings became fully capable of modern forms of self-related thought, people would have had a sociometer of sorts, but it would have responded only to concrete social cues in the immediate situation and would have functioned based exclusively on affect. Only after people could think about themselves over time, adopt others' perspectives of them, and conceptualize themselves symbolically would they have had a modern sociometer that led them to feel good and bad *about themselves* as a result of the real or imagined evaluations of other people, including evaluations that had implications for acceptance and rejection.

Do All Changes in Self-Esteem Involve Only Acceptance and Rejection?

A second common question is whether state self-esteem is ever affected by events that do not involve social acceptance or rejection. The traditional conceptualization views self-esteem as an individual's personal self-evaluation—an assessment of whether one has achieved one's personal goals or lived up to one's personal standards. Such a view can be traced to the James (1890) formula that portrayed self-esteem as the ratio of one's successes to one's pretensions.

Conceptualizing self-esteem as a person's private self-evaluation has had important (and, in my view, unfortunate) consequences for the study of self-esteem. If we start with the assumption that self-esteem is a person's private self-evaluation based on a comparison of him- or herself with personal standards, it is but a short step to conclude that healthy self-esteem *ought not* to be affected by other people's opinions and evaluations of the person. Several theorists have taken this step, suggesting that self-esteem that is affected by other people is not "true" or "healthy" self-esteem (Deci & Ryan, 1995). Furthermore, many people protest that how they feel about themselves is not affected by other people's reactions to them.

The data tell a different story, however, suggesting that events with implications for acceptance and rejection affect self-esteem in most normal individuals. In two studies (Leary et al., 2003), we preselected extreme groups of participants who either believed that their self-esteem was affected by acceptance and approval or strongly denied that acceptance and approval had any effect whatsoever on how they felt about themselves. Then, in a laboratory experiment, we gave both groups feedback indicating a low or high degree of approval/acceptance from other participants and measured their state self-esteem. The results of both studies unequivocally showed that the two groups did not respond differently to the acceptance–rejection manipulation. The fact that the sociometer detects and responds to rejection even among people who adamantly deny it (and who may be unaware of it) not only suggests that contingent self-esteem is an inherent and normal feature of human nature but also that it often works outside people's conscious awareness.

The traditional conceptualization of self-esteem as a private, inner judgment can neither account easily for why self-esteem is so sensitive to interpersonal appraisals nor explain the function of self-esteem. (What is the adaptive value of judging oneself by one's idiosyncratic personal standards?) Sociometer theory provides the straightforward, though perhaps tautological, answer that other people's appraisals affect self-esteem because that is what the sociometer/self-esteem system evolved to do.

However, even if we accept the claim that self-esteem naturally responds to perceived relational value from others, we may ask whether self-esteem is ever affected by events that have no real or potential implications for social acceptance–rejection. Certainly, people's self-efficacy and self-concepts can be affected by outcomes that have no interpersonal implications, but self-efficacy and self-concepts involve beliefs or expectations about oneself rather than the self-relevant feelings that lie at the heart of self-esteem (Brown, 1993; James, 1890; Leary & Baumeister, 2000). Is self-esteem ever affected by events that have no implications for the individual's relational value?

One possible candidate is situations in which people feel good about themselves when they achieve or do good deeds even though no one else is privy to their behavior, or, conversely, feel bad about themselves when they do (or even contemplate) some dark and reprehensible thing that no one else will ever know. Where are the implications for acceptance and rejection of private behaviors such as these? The answer is that, as a regulatory mechanism, the sociometer cannot afford to wait until one is already rejected to respond. Just as the mechanism that elicits fear and avoidance cannot always wait until a threat is immediately present, the sociometer must warn people *in advance* whenever the possibility of low relational value arises (Haupt & Leary, 1997). Thus, the sociometer should warn us that our relational value is potentially in jeopardy even when we have only contemplated performing some dark and reprehensible act. Only then can it deter us from engaging in behaviors that might ultimately jeopardize our relational value to other people.

In brief, people appear to possess a psychological mechanism (a sociometer) that monitors their interpersonal worlds for information relevant to relational value, alerts them through unpleasant emotions and lowered state self-esteem when their relational value is lower than desired or declining, and motivates behavior that helps to enhance relational value (and, hence, self-esteem). This system is essential for helping people to regulate their interpersonal behavior in ways that minimize the potential for rejection.

THE CALIBRATION OF THE SOCIOMETER AND INTERPERSONAL SELF-REGULATION

Self-regulatory systems function optimally only to the degree to which they accurately monitor relevant aspects of the organism's world and, thus, "know" the true state of the environment in which the organism is operating. Unfortunately, like all other meters and gauges, the sociometer may be calibrated in such a manner that it does not accurately reflect the person's relational value to other people. It may, for example, be calibrated to be biased toward false positives (detecting threats to relational value that are not there) or false negatives (failing to detect real threats to relational value). It may also be unstable and overly responsive to cues that connote relational value, or be "stuck" and unresponsive to such cues. In each case, miscalibration undermines the sociometer's ability to regulate people's interpersonal behaviors in ways that help them to maintain an acceptable level of interpersonal acceptance. As we will see, many interpersonal and psychological difficulties can be conceptualized as miscalibrations of the sociometer.

To discuss ways in which a person's sociometer may be miscalibrated, we must first consider what a well-calibrated sociometer looks like. One might expect that a properly calibrated sociometer would respond to relational evaluation in a linear fashion, with equal increments or decrements in relational value resulting in equal changes in state self-esteem. However, Leary, Haupt, Strausser, and Chokel (1998) showed that this is not the case. In four experiments, participants imagined or actually received one of several levels of evaluative feedback, ranging from extreme rejection to neutrality to extreme acceptance. Although state self-esteem increased with relational value, the function was curvilinear (ogival, to be precise).

Figure 19.1 shows the general form of the relationship between relational value (i.e., acceptance–rejection) and state self-esteem. As can be seen, the sociometer is not equally sensitive throughout the entire possible range of interpersonal feedback. In general, it is more sensitive to small changes in relational value in the neutral to moderately positive range of relational value than in the rejecting and highly accepting ranges. So, for example, with declining relational value, state self-esteem hits its lowest point long before feedback is maximally rejecting. Or, to say it differently, people respond as strongly to feedback that reflects slightly negative relational value as to feedback reflecting maximally negative value. One possible explanation for this pattern is that once relational value drops to a point just below neutral, further decrements in relational value have few, if any, tangible consequences. Generally, people simply ignore or ostracize individuals whose relationships they do not value, no matter how strongly they devalue those individuals. As a result, being greatly devalued is not much more troubling than being moderately devalued.

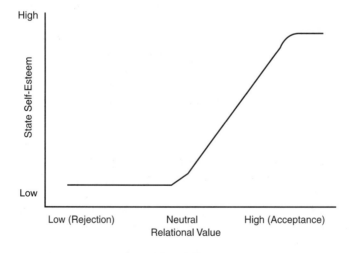

FIGURE 19.1. The relationship between relational value and state self-esteem.

By the same token, once relational value reaches a moderately high level, further increases in relational value do not affect state self-esteem, probably for the same reason. Once people value and accept us moderately, increases in our relational value rarely have additional benefits. Thus, beyond a certain point, there is little reason for the system to respond to increasing acceptance.

Between neutral and moderately high relational value, however, small changes in relational value have notable practical consequences. Being relationally valued just a little is certainly more advantageous than being viewed neutrally, and being valued moderately is better than being valued just a little. As a result, people are sensitive to gradations in relational value in this range.

Trait Self-Esteem

As we have seen, the sociometer is responsible for fluctuations in affect and state self-esteem as a function of events that have implications for one's relational value. In addition, what is commonly called trait self-esteem—a person's typical or chronic level of self-esteem—is also relevant to the workings of the sociometer and interpersonal self-regulation. If we think of the sociometer as a meter or gauge that assesses relational value, trait self-esteem may be conceptualized as the resting position of the sociometer in the absence of incoming interpersonal feedback. Metaphorically speaking, it is where the indicator on the gauge rests when explicit cues relevant to one's relational value are not present.

The sociometer of a person with high trait self-esteem rests at a relatively high position, indicating a high degree of relational value when it is in "standby mode"(Figure 19.2A). Because of past experiences, such individuals implicitly assume that they are generally acceptable individuals with whom others value having relationships. As a result, they move through life feeling generally valued and having relatively high self-esteem even when direct evidence regarding their relational value is not available. Research shows that trait self-esteem correlates highly with the degree to which people believe that they are acceptable individuals who possess attributes that other people value (see Leary & MacDonald, 2003; Leary, Tambor, et al., 1995; MacDonald, Saltzman, & Leary, 2003).

In contrast, the sociometer of a person with low trait self-esteem rests at a point indicating a low to moderate degree of relational value (Figure 19.2B). Several theorists have noted that people who score "low" on measures of trait self-esteem rarely possess truly

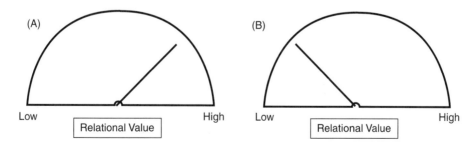

FIGURE 19.2. (A) The sociometer of a person with high trait self-esteem rests in a position that indicates relatively high relational value in the absence of incoming interpersonal feedback. (B) The sociometer of a person with low trait self-esteem rests in a relatively low position in the absence of incoming interpersonal feedback.

low self-esteem. Rather, their feelings about themselves are neutral or mixed, often with some combination of positive and negative reactions (Baumeister, Tice, & Hutton, 1989). This fact suggests that very few people have sociometers that chronically register no relational value, probably because most people have a least a few people who value having relationships with them.

Viewed from the sociometer perspective, what are typically regarded as effects of trait self-esteem are more accurately conceptualized as the effects of a sociometer that tends to operate in a particular range of relational value. Because of the set point of their sociometers, people with low versus high self-esteem react to acceptance and rejection differently (Nezlek, Kowalski, Leary, Blevins, & Holgate, 1997). For example, people with low trait self-esteem are not anxious, depressed, jealous, lonely, or rejection-sensitive *because* they have low self-esteem. Rather they are anxious, depressed, jealous, lonely, or rejection-sensitive because they go through life detecting a relatively low degree of relational value. Similarly, people with low self-esteem do not conform, abuse alcohol or drugs, or join gangs because they have low self-esteem (e.g., Heaven, 1986; Kaplan, 1980; Rosenberg, Schooler, & Schoenbach, 1981; Vega, Zimmerman, Warheit, & Apospori, 1993), but rather because they regularly detect an inadequate amount of acceptance in their interpersonal environments and, thus, resort to extreme measures to boost their relational value (Leary, 1999; Leary, Schreindorfer, & Haupt, 1995).

It may be tempting to conclude that people who score low on measures of trait self-esteem suffer from a poorly calibrated sociometer, but that is not necessarily the case. Many people with low trait self-esteem have well-calibrated sociometers that accurately detect that they have a relatively low degree of relational value. However, some people with low self-esteem probably detect lower relational evaluation from others than actually exists, and their sociometers can be viewed as miscalibrated. In the following sections, I examine ways in which a miscalibrated sociometer may lead to emotional distress and problems with self-regulation.

When the Sociometer Is Set Low

One type of miscalibration occurs when the sociometer is set "too low"—that is, when it detects a lower amount of relational value in the interpersonal environment than actually exists. This situation, which is shown in Figure 19.3, is comparable to a thermostat that reports a lower temperature than is the case (and, thus, turns on the heat prematurely), or

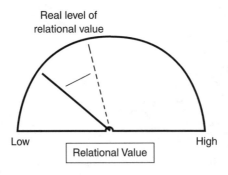

FIGURE 19.3. A person with a sociometer that is calibrated low chronically experiences less relational value (and, thus, lower self-esteem) than is warranted by the situation.

a fuel gauge that indicates less gas in the tank than there really is (causing the driver to be more anxious about running out of gas than is warranted).

The primary consequence of this kind of miscalibration is an oversensitivity to cues that connote potential relational devaluation. In the language of signal detection theory, the system will have a high proportion of false positives, registering benign (or even somewhat favorable) interpersonal events as potential threats to acceptance. As a result of the sociometer responding as if relational value is unacceptably low, the individual will experience frequent episodes of low self-esteem, along with rejection-related emotions such as social anxiety, jealousy, guilt, and embarrassment (Leary, Koch, et al., 2001; Leary & MacDonald, 2003). Furthermore, the individual will often overreact to situations that pose a risk to relational value, either in terms of shy withdrawal or angry defensiveness.

For example, people who are high in rejection sensitivity seem to possess a sociometer that is calibrated in this fashion. Walking through life detecting a lower level of relational value that actually exists makes them hypersensitive to any indication of potential rejection and leads them to experience a large number of interpersonal encounters as rejecting. As a result, they often see rejection where none exists, and overreact to real and imagined relational devaluation (see Downey & Feldman, 1996; Levy, Ayduk, & Downey, 2001). Viewed in this fashion, it is not surprising that rejection sensitivity correlates negatively with self-esteem. Given that self-esteem is a reflection of perceived acceptance, a sociometer that is calibrated low will result in both heightened sensitivity to rejection and lower self-esteem.

Evidence also suggests that some people with low trait self-esteem have a sociometer that is calibrated too low. Although some people with low self-esteem may be accurately perceiving a low level of relational value, others may be biased to perceive less acceptance than actually exists. Koch (2002), for example, found that people who scored low in trait self-esteem tended to respond to evaluatively ambiguous primes as though they were negative (see also Baldwin & Sinclair, 1996). In light of their low relational value set point, it is not surprising that people with low trait self-esteem tend to be more jealous (Buunk, 1982) and lonely (Vaux, 1988; White, 1981) than people with high self-esteem.

Having such an improperly calibrated sociometer compromises the person's ability to self-regulate optimally. By responding to interpersonal events as though they connote lower relational value than is the case, people overreact, both emotionally and behaviorally, to such situations. And, as research has shown, such reactions can become a self-fulfilling prophecy, because the person who often feels devalued either pulls back from or attacks relational partners, leading those individuals to withdraw (Downey, Freitas, Michealis, & Khouri, 1998; Murray, Holmes, MacDonald, & Ellsworth, 1998).

When the Sociometer Is Set High

The sociometer may also be set "too high"—like a fuel gauge that indicates more gas than is actually in the tank (see Figure 19.4). In this case, people chronically detect that others value them more as social interactants and relational partners than they actually do.

Subjectively, such a situation may seem beneficial, because the person has high self-esteem and rarely experiences the aversive emotions associated with feeling devalued or rejected. In fact, the prevailing view for many years has been that holding positive illusions regarding one's acceptability and worth is psychologically beneficial (Murray, Holmes, & Griffin, 1996; Taylor & Brown, 1988).

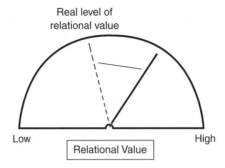

FIGURE 19.4. A person with a sociometer that is calibrated high chronically experiences greater relational value (and, thus, higher self-esteem) than is warranted by the situation.

However, if we think of self-esteem and affect as features of a sociometer designed for interpersonal self-regulation, the fallacy of this view becomes apparent. A sociometer that is calibrated too high (as in Figure 19.4) will lead people to overestimate their relational value to others and, thus, show inadequate concern for how others perceive and evaluate them. Such a miscalibrated sociometer will fail to warn them when their acceptance by other people is in jeopardy. Although a driver on a lonely stretch of desolate highway may take great comfort in seeing that the fuel gauge is well above "Empty," this consolation is badly misplaced if the gas tank is actually running dry, particularly if the malfunctioning gas gauge leads the driver to drive past a gas station without stopping, under the false belief that there is plenty of gas in the tank.

Social life requires that people be attentive to how they are perceived, evaluated, and accepted by others. Although it is sometimes wise to disregard others' evaluations, effective interpersonal behavior cannot be predicated on erroneous perceptions of other people's reactions. Believing that one's relational value is higher than is the case results in a number of negative consequences, both for the individual and for those with whom he or she interacts.

At minimum, the person whose sociometer is calibrated too high will be disparaged, if not rejected, for being haughty, conceited, or snobbish (Leary, Bednarski, Hammon, & Duncan, 1997). People dislike those who think that they are more relationally valuable than they are. Worse, people who overestimate their relational value (and, thus, have undeservedly high self-esteem) tend to influence, dominate, and exploit other people (Emmons, 1984). They also tend to respond defensively and aggressively to suggestions that they are not as wonderful as their sociometers suggest (Baumeister, Smart, & Boden, 1996; Emmons, 1984). People whose sociometers typically indicate that they are valuable and acceptable are understandably miffed when people do not give them the respect or affection they think they deserve. Furthermore, people who believe they have generally high relational value may be insufficiently restrained in mistreating or hurting other people, because they assume they are so highly valued. In part, a well-placed concern for potential rejection helps to keep our behavior within socially acceptable bounds.

The extreme case of this kind of miscalibration is narcissism, in which people feel more special, important, and self-satisfied than the objective feedback warrants (Raskin, Novacek, & Hogan, 1991; Rhodewalt & Eddings, 2002). Conceptualizing narcissism as arising from a sociometer that is calibrated too high helps to explain the long-standing paradox of why narcissists have high, if not grandiose, levels of self-esteem yet react so strongly to criticism (see Rhodewalt & Sorrow, 2003, for an excellent discussion of this paradox). The answer may be that, with a sociometer that is set too high, narcissists chronically feel better about themselves than they objectively ought to feel. When they receive clear-cut feedback indicating that other people do not fully value and accept them, there is a clear discrepancy between how they feel about themselves and how they know other people feel about them. Because the powerful, subjective reality of their miscalibrated sociometer convinces them that they are important or valuable, they essentially have no alternative than to conclude that other people's negative evaluations of them are biased and unfair, and this sense of being devalued unfairly produces their extreme defensiveness and anger. On occasion, when narcissists are unable to discount negative interpersonal feedback and rejection, they may suddenly realize that their relational value is not as high as they had assumed, resulting in a devastating crash in self-esteem.

The problems that arise for people whose sociometers are calibrated too high highlight the risks of raising people's self-esteem artificially. Although psychologists, educators, and politicians have advocated raising self-esteem as a way to improve mental health, decrease maladaptive behavior, and eliminate social problems (Mecca et al., 1989), raising self-esteem in a manner that is not commensurate with one's true relational value is a recipe for disaster. Convincing people that they are acceptable, worthy, and lovable individuals despite the fact that they regularly treat others in unacceptable ways is analogous to adjusting one's fuel gauge so that it shows more gas in the tank than there is. The person may feel temporarily good about circumstances but suffer negative consequences in the long run (Robins & Beer, 2001).

When the Sociometer Is Excessively or Insufficiently Sensitive

Some sociometers underreact or overreact to cues that are relevant to relational value. Having a sociometer that is excessively or insufficiently sensitive to interpersonal appraisals creates yet other problems with interpersonal self-regulation.

Hypersensitivity

An overactive sociometer leads people to experience extreme swings in affect and state self-esteem on the basis of relatively minor changes in the interpersonal environment. Mild signs of acceptance may evoke high self-esteem and euphoria, and mild signs of disinterest or disapproval may crush self-esteem and elicit despair. Such a sociometer responds disproportionately to changes in the interpersonal environment (see Figure 19.5).

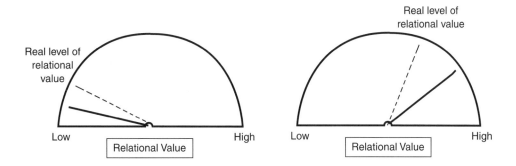

FIGURE 19.5. A person with a hypersensitive sociometer experiences greater swings in perceived relational value (and, thus, self-esteem) than are warranted by the situation.

This seems to be the case for people with highly variable or unstable self-esteem, what Rosenberg (1986) referred to as "barometric instability." Kernis and his colleagues suggest that unstable self-esteem reflects "fragile, vulnerable feelings of immediate self-worth that are influenced by potentially self-relevant events" (Kernis & Goldman, 2003, p. 114). This view is undoubtedly correct, and sociometer theory helps to explain the source of highly variable self-esteem. When the sociometer overresponds to events that are relevant to relational value, people display swings in self-esteem that are out of proportion to the evaluative implications of those events. Indeed, the personality factors associated with unstable self-esteem are those that characterize a person with an unstable sociometer. For example, high degree of dependence on other people makes others' reactions vis-à-vis acceptance and rejection particularly important; an impoverished self-concept fails to provide an anchor from which one can assess one's relational value independently of immediate social feedback, and an overreliance on social approval renders one's relational value in other people's eyes more important than it needs to be (see Butler, Hokanson, & Flynn, 1994; Kernis, Paradise, Whitaker, Wheatman, & Goldman, 2000). The extensive literature on self-esteem instability (see Kernis & Goldman, 2003, for a review) can be integrated, if we assume that people with unstable self-esteem have hyperactive sociometers.

Hyposensitivity

A hypoactive sociometer is relatively insensitive to changes in relational value (see Figure 19.6). Large changes in one's relational value to other people result in only slight movement in the sociometer and negligible changes in state self-esteem. A sociometer that does not react to interpersonal feedback cannot adequately assess the person's relational value to others. Although there are obviously instances in which people ought to disregard other people's reactions, chronically failing to do so will lead people to be ostracized by everyone, because they regularly fail to react intelligently to situations that ought to convey that their relational value is low or declining. Such individuals may be able to recognize devaluing feedback when they think consciously about it, but they do not automatically pick up on such cues easily.

In extreme cases, some people's sociometers are essentially out of service. If being valued and adored has largely the same subjective effect as being devalued and detested, then the person is incapable of interpersonal self-regulation. People who rarely experience anxiety, hurt feelings, or guilt in situations in which others dislike, detest, or ostracize them may have a broken sociometer. Although no direct evidence has a bearing on

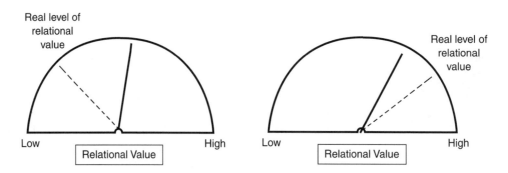

FIGURE 19.6. A person with a hyposensitive sociometer experiences smaller changes in perceived relational value (and, thus, self-esteem) than are warranted by the situation.

this point, one exemplar of an insensitive (if not "stuck" sociometer) would seem to be the antisocial (or sociopathic) personality, which is characterized by impaired empathy and a weak conscience. The selfish, manipulative, and hurtful behaviors of a person with antisocial personality disorder often seem to stem from an indifference to how their actions are perceived and evaluated by other people, and to the ostracism that often results. For example, people with an antisocial personality are repeatedly deceitful, egocentric, irresponsible, and manipulative (Lykken, 1995; Seto, Khattar, Lalumiere, & Quinsey, 1997)—characteristics that most people try to avoid, because they likely lead to rejection. This is not to say that an out-of-order sociometer lies at the heart of sociopathy (although it might), but it does suggest that sociopaths have broken sociometers.

SECONDARY SATISFACTION OF SELF-ESTEEM

As noted, sociometer theory suggests that rather than possessing an inherent need for self-esteem, people's apparent efforts to protect their self-esteem stem from an interest in maintaining their relational value to other people. Although it is easy to see how publicly self-serving behaviors—such as self-handicapping, excuse making, and self-serving attributions—may enhance one's image and apparent value to other people, one can reasonably ask whether people sometimes try to maintain self-esteem in their own heads. Do people not also try to protect their self-esteem intrapsychically, in ways that have no direct implications for relational value or interpersonal acceptance?

The answer is clearly "yes." The human ability to self-reflect allows people to override their natural and immediate reactions by cognitively reconstruing the personal meaning of events. As a result, people sometimes interpret interpersonal events in ways that allow them to maintain self-esteem even in the face of events that objectively "ought" to make them feel bad about themselves. In essence, people can cognitively override the sociometer.

There has been considerable debate regarding whether these private self-serving biases or positive illusions are beneficial or detrimental to people's well-being (Colvin & Block, 1994; Robins & Beer, 2001; Taylor & Brown, 1988). Viewing self-esteem as a sociometer that is involved in self-regulation suggests that these biases and illusions are probably detrimental. The sociometer effectively regulates interpersonal relations only to the extent that it provides a reasonably accurate picture of other people's reactions to the individual vis-à-vis acceptance and rejection. In overriding and fooling the system, positive illusions increase the likelihood of serious misregulation.

Positive illusions about the self undoubtedly make people feel better and, occasionally, allow them to maintain a positive attitude and motivation in the face of adversity. But over the long haul, positive illusions circumvent the sociometer's function. Convincing oneself that one is more acceptable than one actually is makes no more sense than convincing oneself that the car's gas tank contains more gasoline than it really does. It may make one feel better temporarily but, to the extent that it deters appropriate or remediative action, the ultimate outcome will often be negative.

CONCLUSIONS

The concept of the sociometer as a psychological mechanism that monitors people's social environments and helps them minimize the likelihood of rejection is helpful in thinking about the self-regulation of interpersonal behavior (see also Vohs & Ciarocco, Chapter 20, this volume). Research supports the idea that, in fact, people do possess a regulatory mechanism that responds to changes in relational value, and the concept of a sociometer provides an overarching framework for conceptualizing a variety of phenomena, such as self-esteem, interpersonal emotions (e.g., social anxiety, jealousy, hurt feelings, anger), reactions to rejection, individual differences in rejection sensitivity, and personality disorders (particularly the narcissistic and antisocial disorders). Importantly, the metaphor of the sociometer as a psychological gauge of relational value may also provide insights into what goes wrong when people self-regulate in dysfunctional ways that damage their relationships with other people.

REFERENCES

Baldwin, M. W., & Sinclair, L. (1996). Self-esteem and "if . . . then" contingencies of interpersonal acceptance. *Journal of Personality and Social Psychology, 71,* 1130–1141.

Baumeister, R. F., Heatherton, T. F., & Tice, D. M. (1994). *Losing control: How and why people fail at self-regulation.* San Diego, CA: Academic Press.

Baumeister, R. F., & Leary, M. R. (1995). The need to belong: Desire for interpersonal attachments as a fundamental human motivation. *Psychological Bulletin, 117,* 497–529.

Baumeister, B. F., Smart, L., & Boden, J. M. (1996). Relation of threatened egotism to violence and aggression: The dark side of high self-esteem. *Psychological Review, 103,* 5–33.

Baumeister, R. F., Tice, D. M., & Hutton, D. G. (1989). Self-presentational motivations and personality differences in self-esteem. *Journal of Personality, 57,* 547–579.

Baumeister, R. F., & Vohs, K. D. (2003). Self-regulation and the executive function of the self. In M. R. Leary & J. P. Tangney (Eds.), *Handbook of self and identity* (pp. 197–217). New York: Guilford Press.

Bowlby, J. (1969). *Attachment and loss: Vol. 1. Attachment.* New York: Basic Books.

Brown, J. D. (1993). Self-esteem and self-evaluations: Feeling is believing. In J. Suls (Ed.), *Psychological perspectives on the self* (Vol. 4, pp. 27–58). Hillsdale, NJ: Erlbaum.

Buss, D. M. (1995). Evolutionary psychology: A new paradigm for psychological science. *Psychological Inquiry, 6,* 1–49.

Butler, A. C., Hokanson, J. E., & Flynn, H. A. (1994). A comparison of self-esteem lability and low self-esteem as vulnerability factors for depression. *Journal of Personality and Social Psychology, 66,* 166–177.

Buunk, B. P. (1982). Anticipated sexual jealousy: Its relationship to self-esteem, dependency, and reciprocity. *Personality and Social Psychology Bulletin, 8,* 310–316.

Carver, C. S., & Scheier, M. F. (1981). *Attention and self-regulation: A control theory approach to human behavior.* New York: Springer-Verlag.

Cherry, E. C. (1953). Some experiments on the recognition of speech with one and two ears. *Journal of the Acoustical Society of America, 25,* 975–979.

Colvin, C. R., & Block, J. (1994). Do positive illusions foster mental health?: An examination of the Taylor and Brown formulation. *Psychological Bulletin, 116,* 3–20.

Cosmides, L., & Tooby, J. (1992). Cognitive adaptations for social exchange. In J. Barkow, L. Cosmides, & J. Tooby (Eds.), *The adapted mind* (pp. 163–228). New York: Oxford University Press.

Cosmides, L., & Tooby, J. (1994). Origins of domain specificity: The evolution of functional organization. In L. A. Hirschfeld & S. A. Gelman (Eds.), *Mapping the mind: Domain specificity in cognition and culture* (pp. 85–117). Cambridge, UK: Cambridge University Press.

Deci, E. L., & Ryan, R. M. (1995). Human agency: The basis for true self-esteem. In M. H. Kernis (Ed.), *Efficacy, agency, and self-esteem* (pp. 31–50). New York: Plenum Press.

Downey, G., & Feldman, S. (1996). Implications of rejection sensitivity for intimate relationships. *Journal of Personality and Social Psychology, 70,* 1327–1343.

Downey, G., Freitas, A. L., Michealis, B., & Khouri, H. (1998). The self-fulfilling prophecy in close relationships: Do rejection sensitive women get rejected by romantic partners? *Journal of Personality and Social Psychology, 75,* 545–560.

Emmons, R. A. (1984). Factor analysis and construct validity of the Narcissistic Personality Inventory. *Journal of Personality Assessment, 48,* 291–300.

Gilbert, P., & Trower, P. (1990). The evolution and manifestation of social anxiety. In W. R. Crozier (Ed.), *Shyness and embarrassment* (pp. 144–177). New York: Cambridge University Press.

Haupt, A. L., & Leary, M. R. (1997). The appeal of worthless groups: Moderating effects of trait self-esteem. *Group Dynamics: Theory, Research, and Practice, 1,* 124–132.

Heaven, P. C. (1986). Correlates of conformity in three cultures. *Journal of Personality and Social Psychology, 54,* 883–887.

Humphrey, N. (1986). *The inner eye.* London: Faber & Faber.

James, W. (1890). *The principles of psychology.* New York: Dover.

Kaplan, H. B. (1980). *Deviant behavior in defense of self.* New York: Academic Press.

Kernis, M. H., & Goldman, B. M. (2003). Stability and variability in self-concept and self-esteem. In M. R. Leary & J. P. Tangney (Eds.), *Handbook of self and identity* (pp. 106–127). New York: Guilford Press.

Kernis, M. H., Paradise, A. W., Whitaker, D., Wheatman, S., & Goldman, B. (2000). Master of one's psychological domain?: Not likely if one's self-esteem is unstable. *Personality and Social Psychology Bulletin, 26,* 1297–1305.

Koch, E. J. (2002). Relational schemas, self-esteem, and the processing of social stimuli. *Self and Identity, 1,* 271–279.

Kurzban, R., & Leary, M. R. (2001). Evolutionary origins of stigmatization: The function of social exclusion. *Psychological Bulletin, 127,* 187–208.

Leary, M. R. (1999). The social and psychological importance of self-esteem. In R. M. Kowalski & M. R. Leary (Eds.), *The social psychology of emotional and behavioral problems: Interfaces of social and clinical psychology* (pp. 197–221). Washington, DC: American Psychological Association.

Leary, M. R. (2001). Toward a conceptualization of interpersonal rejection. In M. R. Leary (Ed.), *Interpersonal rejection* (pp. 3–20). New York: Oxford University Press.

Leary, M. R. (2002). The interpersonal basis of self-esteem: Death, devaluation, or deference? In J. Forgas & K. D. Williams (Eds.), *The social self: Cognitive, interpersonal, and intergroup perspectives* (pp. 143–159). New York: Psychology Press.

Leary, M. R., & Baumeister, R. F. (2000). The nature and function of self-esteem: Sociometer theory. In M.P. Zanna (Ed.), *Advances in experimental social psychology* (Vol. 32, pp. 1–62). San Diego: Academic Press.

Leary, M. R., Bednarski, R., Hammon, D., & Duncan, T. (1997). Blowhards, snobs, and narcissists: Interpersonal reactions to excessive egotism. In R. M. Kowalski (Ed.), *Aversive interpersonal behaviors* (pp. 111–131). New York: Plenum Press.

Leary, M. R., & Buttermore, N. (in press). The evolution of the human self: Tracing the natural history of self-reflection. *Journal for the Theory of Social Behaviour.*

Leary, M. R., Cottrell, C. A., & Phillips, M. (2001). Deconfounding the effects of dominance and social acceptance on self-esteem. *Journal of Personality and Social Psychology, 81,* 898–909.

Leary, M. R., & Downs, D.L. (1995). Interpersonal functions of the self-esteem motive: The self-esteem system as a sociometer. In M. Kernis (Ed.), *Efficacy, agency, and self-esteem* (pp. 123–144). New York: Plenum Press.

Leary, M. R., Gallagher, B., Fors, E. H., Buttermore, N., Baldwin, E., Lane, K. K., & Mills. A. (2003). The invalidity of personal claims about self-esteem. *Personality and Social Psychology Bulletin, 29,* 623–636.

Leary, M. R., Haupt, A. L., Strausser, K. S., & Chokel, J. T. (1998). Calibrating the sociometer: The relationship between interpersonal appraisals and state self-esteem. *Journal of Personality and Social Psychology, 74,* 1290–1299.

Leary, M. R., Koch, E., & Hechenbleikner, N. (2001). Emotional responses to interpersonal rejection. In M. R. Leary (Ed.), *Interpersonal rejection* (pp. 145–166). New York: Oxford University Press.

Leary, M. R., & MacDonald, G. (2003). Individual differences in self-esteem: A review and theoretical integration. In M. R. Leary & J. P. Tangney (Eds.), *Handbook of self and identity* (pp. 401–418). New York: Guilford Press.

Leary, M. R., Schreindorfer, L. S. & Haupt, A. L. (1995). The role of low self-esteem in emotional and behavioral problems: Why is low self-esteem dysfunctional? *Journal of Social and Clinical Psychology, 14*, 297–314.

Leary, M. R., Tambor, E., Terdal, S., & Downs, D.L. (1995). Self-esteem as an interpersonal monitor: The sociometer hypothesis. *Journal of Personality and Social Psychology, 68*, 518–530.

Levy, S. R., Ayduk, O., & Downey, G. (2001). The role of rejection sensitivity in people's relationships with significant others and valued social groups. In M. R. Leary (Ed.), *Interpersonal rejection* (pp. 251–289). New York: Oxford University Press.

Lykken, D. T. (1995). *The antisocial personalities.* Hillsdale, NJ: Erlbaum.

MacDonald, G., Saltzman, J. L., & Leary, M. R. (2003). Social approval and trait self-esteem. *Journal of Research in Personality, 37*, 23–40.

Mecca, A. M., Smelser, N. J., & Vasconcellos, J. (1989). *The social importance of self-esteem.* Berkeley: University of California Press.

Mischel, W. (1996). From good intentions to willpower. In P. M. Gollwitzer & J. A. Bargh (Eds.), *The psychology of action: Linking cognition and motivation to behavior* (pp. 197–218). New York: Guilford Press.

Mitchell, R. W. (2003). Subjectivity and self-recognition in animals. In M. R. Leary & J. P. Tangney (Eds.), *Handbook of self and identity* (pp. 567–593). New York: Guilford Press.

Murray, S. L., Holmes, J. G., & Griffin, D. W. (1996). The benefits of positive illusions: Idealization and the construction of satisfaction in close relationships. *Journal of Personality and Social Psychology, 70*, 79–98.

Murray, S. L., Holmes, J. G., MacDonald, G., & Ellsworth, P. C. (1998). Through the looking glass darkly?: When self-doubts turn into relationship insecurities. *Journal of Personality and Social Psychology, 75*, 1459–1480.

Nezlek, J. B., Kowalski, R. M., Leary, M. R., Blevins, T., & Holgate, S. (1997). Personality moderators of reactions to interpersonal rejection: Depression and trait self-esteem. *Personality and Social Psychology Bulletin, 23*, 1235–1244.

Ohman, A. (1986). Face the beast and fear the face: Animal and social fears as prototypes for evolutionary analyses of emotion. *Psychophysiology, 23*, 123–145.

Raskin, R., Novacek, J., & Hogan, R. (1991). Narcissism, self-esteem, and defensive self-enhancement. *Journal of Personality, 59*, 19–38.

Rhodewalt, F., & Eddings, S. (2002). Narcissus reflects: Memory distortion in response to ego relevant feedback in high and low narcissistic men. *Journal of Research in Personality, 36*, 97–116.

Rhodewalt, F., & Sorrow, D. L. (2003). Interpersonal self-regulation: Lessons from the study of narcissism. In M. R. Leary & J. P. Tangney (Eds.), *Handbook of self and identity* (pp. 519–535). New York: Guilford Press.

Robins, R. W., & Beer, J. S. (2001). Positive illusions about the self: Short-term benefits and long-term costs. *Journal of Personality and Social Psychology, 80*, 340–352.

Rosenberg, M. (1986). Self-concept from middle childhood through adolescence. In J. Suls & A. G. Greenwald (Eds.), *Psychological perspectives on the self* (Vol. 2, pp. 107–136). Hillsdale, NJ: Erlbaum.

Rosenberg, M., Schooler, C. & Schoenbach, C. (1989). Self-esteem and adolescent problems: Modeling reciprocal effects. *American Sociological Review, 54*, 1004–1018.

Rozin, R., & Fallon, A. E. (1987). A perspective on disgust. *Psychological Review, 94*, 23–41.

Samuels, R. (2000). Massively modular minds: Evolutionary psychology and cognitive architecture. In P. Carruthers & A. Chamberlain (Eds.), *Evolution and the human mind* (pp. 13–46). Cambridge, UK: Cambridge University Press.

Seto, M., Khattar, N. A., Lalumiere, M. L., & Quinsey, V. L. (1997). Deception and sexual strategy in psychopathy. *Personality and Individual Differences, 22,* 301–307.

Taylor, S. E., & Brown, J. D. (1988). Illusion and well-being: A social psychological perspective on mental health. *Psychological Bulletin, 116,* 193–210.

Vaux, A. (1988). Social and emotional loneliness: The role of social and personal characteristics. *Personality and Social Psychology Bulletin, 14,* 722–735.

Vega, W. A., Zimmerman, R. S., Warheit, G. J., & Apospori, E. (1993). Risk factors for early adolescent drug use in four ethnic and racial groups. *American Journal of Public Health, 83,* 185–189.

Wegner, D. M., & Pennebaker, J. W. (Eds.). (1993). *Handbook of mental control.* Englewood Cliffs, NJ: Prentice-Hall.

White, G. L. (1981). Some correlates of romantic jealousy. *Journal of Personality, 49,* 129–147.

20

Interpersonal Functioning Requires Self-Regulation

KATHLEEN D. VOHS
NATALIE J. CIAROCCO

Forming and maintaining social relationships are two of the most difficult tasks of human life, but they are clearly also among the most rewarding. In this chapter, we provide evidence for the idea that the ability to self-regulate holds the key to both the joys and pains of social relationships. Consider the following scenarios: You are in the final stretches of negotiating the purchase of a new car, when the car dealer approaches you with a list of tempting options for the car. You had decided in advance to say "no" to all but the most basic options, but the salesman pressures you to consider each tempting choice. At first you are able to say "no," but the more you hear, the more you find yourself agreeing with him.

A female friend has been complaining for weeks about the many new demands at work and all the pressures that have been put on her. One Friday night, you are out to dinner with your friend and her husband, and you notice that she seems annoyed at every comment her husband makes and repeatedly snaps at him without provocation.

A woman starts to notice that her long-term boyfriend has been looking lasciviously at every attractive woman he sees. This behavior is a recent occurrence, and it is causing problems in the relationship. The man contends that his longing gazes are the result of his new and highly restrictive diet, which has him constantly calculating calories, keeping track of portions, and monitoring every morsel that goes into his mouth. He feels totally taxed by the new diet and cannot seem to inhibit his staring at other women.

A white man and a black man waiting at a bus stop have a lengthy conversation about everyday topics, such as sports, news, and weather. The white man keeps up the conversation but displays a controlled and inhibited style. After getting off the bus to go home, he decides to stop in first at his favorite bar. He plans on having only a few tonics, but a few hours later, he finds himself intoxicated, much drunker than he intended.

These scenarios illustrate a few of the research areas that link interpersonal relations to self-control. The areas of inquiry covered by this research on interpersonal processes range from individual (e.g., self-presentation) to dyadic interpersonal effects to phenomena that occur at the group level. In addition to the broad range of topics that relate self-regulation to social functioning, several theoretical interpersonal models now include regulatory mechanisms as key components.

Is it plausible that self-regulation aids people in gaining and maintaining interpersonal acceptance? Heatherton and Vohs (1998) argued that self-control may promote dyadic and group relations. They postulated that, from an evolutionary standpoint, people who were able to restrain their responses and modify their behaviors and conform to group criteria to gain acceptance would be less likely to be ousted from social groups and relationships. Furthermore, by virtue of their relationships with others, these self-controlled people would derive numerous benefits from their social connections (e.g., physical protection, shared responsibilities, more reproductive opportunities; see Baumeister & Leary, 1995). We posit that the formation and maintenance of strong social bonds is based in part on the degree to which people can achieve appropriate self-regulation. In our estimation, self-control provides a means for people to increase their belongingness by overriding their own selfish impulses for the good of others and adhering to societal rules for the purpose of inclusion.

WITHIN-PERSON INTERPERSONAL PROCESSES REQUIRE REGULATORY CONTROL

The first area we address examines self-regulation in interpersonal phenomena that occur within the psyche of the individual. In particular, the role of self-regulation in regulatory focus, persuasion, social orientation, self-presentation, social inference, and self-evaluation is discussed. In each of these constructs, researchers have made great strides in demonstrating the interrelatedness of intrapersonal self-regulation and interpersonal processes.

Social Orientation and Self-Regulatory Ability

One view of self-regulation posits that knowing the rules relative to where, when, and in what ways to control oneself is crucial to being an accepted member of society (Heatherton & Vohs, 1998). If this is the case, then people who are responsive to societal self-regulation rules may, as a result, become more practiced at self-regulation. If the capacity for self-regulation can be increased through practice, then those who judiciously exercise their self-control abilities may become better overall self-regulators.

To determine whether some people are better at self-control because they are sensitive to societal regulatory demands, Seeley and Gardner (2003) investigated social orientation and self-regulation during interpersonal interactions. They believed that people high in social orientation would be more practiced at regulating themselves during everyday interactions, and would therefore better withstand situational forces that would otherwise undermine their self-regulatory abilities. They assessed societal orientation at a trait level by examining the cultural values (e.g., individualistic vs. collectivist) and individual differences in interpersonally focused self-monitoring both in participants from collectivist cultures and in highly other-directed, socially oriented participants.

The results of the two studies demonstrated that being attuned to others' or society's demands is related to better self-regulation; participants who were high in social orientation performed better on self-regulation tasks than did participants who were low in social orientation. Specifically, high socially oriented participants showed more regulatory ability than did low socially oriented participants when they were required to squeeze a handgrip after having suppressed thoughts of a white bear. Participants who were low in social orientation replicated prior findings of depletion after self-regulation; suppressing thoughts of a white bear subsequently led to decreased ability to squeeze a handgrip in later attempts.

Thus, securing and maintaining belongingness are motivating forces in self-regulation. It may be that high societal orientation necessitates chronic self-regulation, which in turn boosts people's ability to self-regulate through repeated practice.

Self-Regulation and Self-Presentation

Impression management is another area in which self-regulation follows from sensitivity to social demands. Using a resource model of self-regulation, Vohs, Ciarocco, and Baumeister (2003) conducted a series of studies to demonstrate that some forms of self-presentation require self-regulation. In particular, unfamiliar or atypical self-presentations appear to deplete self-regulatory resources.

The self-regulatory resource model (see Schmeichel & Baumeister, Chapter 5, this volume; Vohs & Schmeichel, 2003) proposes that self-regulatory abilities are overseen by a finite pool of resources expended with each act of self-regulation performed. This pool of resources is conceptualized as managing all varieties of self-regulation, from cognitive to emotional, and from behavioral to impulse-control responses; thus, countless situational and personal demands can potentially drain the pool. According to this model, each act of self-regulation leads subsequently to weaker self-regulatory ability, presumably because there are fewer available regulatory resources to apply to the current task. In the Vohs and colleagues (2003) research, performance of an unfamiliar or atypical self-presentation task was predicted to result in reduced self-regulation, presumably because self-regulatory resources would become depleted after the impression management task. Also, based on a limited-resource conceptualization, they predicted that participants' ability to achieve self-presentational goals would be impaired after a prior act of self-regulation.

One study tested the idea that unfamiliar forms of self-presentation require self-regulation. Participants were given an impression management goal that ran counter to normative impression management goals. Past research has shown that when people interact with their friends, they behave modestly, because their friends' knowledge and memories of past events keep their overly aggrandizing statements in check. Conversely, a positive, self-enhancing style is mainly adopted with strangers, because only a small window of opportunity exists in which to make a positive impression on a new acquaintance (Tice, Butler, Muraven, & Stillwell, 1995). Hence, in one study, participants were induced to act modestly with strangers and very positively with friends. These atypical self-presentation conditions were predicted to result in poorer self-regulation. Participants were then asked to complete a long series of math problems, for as long as they were able, as a measure of self-regulatory ability. This study revealed that people acted modestly with a stranger and positively with a friend were less able to persist on the math task compared to participants who engaged in the typical forms of self-presentation (modestly with friends and positively with strangers). In another study, participants were asked to display a self-image that ran counter to gender-related self-presentation norms. Past research has shown that, typically, women emphasize their social skills, whereas men emphasize their competencies (Leary et al., 1994). Hence, in this study, women who were asked to discuss their outstanding competencies and men who were asked to discuss their outstanding interpersonal qualities were predicted to have poorer subsequent self-regulation relative to participants who engaged in the typical styles of self-presentation. Participants' efforts in squeezing a handgrip exerciser were used as a measure of their self-control capacities. The results showed that women who featured their competencies and men who featured their interpersonal skills were the poorest at overriding the desire to quit squeezing the handgrip. Taken together, the results of these two studies indicate that engaging in new, unusual, or unfamiliar forms of self-presentation requires increased self-regulation, which, consequently, reduces self-regulatory capacity for additional goal pursuits.

An additional set of studies showed that previous depletion of self-regulatory resources leads to impairment in self-presentational abilities. In one such study, some participants were first asked to perform an attention control task to deplete self-regulatory resources, whereas others were not asked to do so. Subsequently, narcissism scores were assessed as a measure of ability to moderate one's public impressions. Narcissism is socially off-putting and is one of the most self-centered and egotistical personality characteristics (Morf & Rhodewalt, 2001). The results showed that after being depleted of regulatory resources, participants described themselves more narcissistically, because they were less able to regulate their self-perceptions to conform to a socially desirable image.

In summary, these results support the idea that self-presentation and self-regulation are crucially linked. Putting forth a positive or desired social impression is perhaps one of the most important tasks involved in initiating social relationship, and it requires the orchestration of impulsive, emotional, and cognitive responses.

Resistance as a Form of Self-Control

It is axiomatic to say that one major function of interpersonal interactions is to achieve social influence. Analyses of influence attempts show that influence tactics can be split into two different types: alpha attempts (which involve boosting approach forces) and omega attempts (which involve reducing opposition). Presumably, it takes self-control to keep up one's resistance while others are trying to wear it down. Thus, the concept of omega strategies suggests that self-regulation may be involved in combating others' attempts to influence. One line of research demonstrates that self-regulation, as guided by a self-regulatory resource model, is a central determinant of people's ability to defend against others' attempts to persuade.

This research tested the idea that the effectiveness of omega strategies depends in part on the strength of the recipient's self-regulatory abilities. According to the resource model, people should be less resistant to later persuasion attempts relative to earlier attempts, because they will have used some of their regulatory resources in refusing the earlier requests. To test this hypothesis, Knowles, Brennan, and Linn (2002) monitored people's reactions to political advertisements. Some participants saw a target political ad first in a series of ads, a situation that should have allowed for a great deal of resistance and thus predicted less favorable (i.e., more skeptical) ratings. Other participants saw the target ad last in a series of ads, a situation predicted to yield higher (i.e., less skeptical) favorable ratings, because participants' ability to resist would have been depleted as a result of skepticism about the prior ads.

In another set of conditions, participants were either given a task to perform before rating the political ad. In both conditions, participants saw the target political ad last. Just prior to seeing the last ad, participants were asked either to state which activities they liked from a video of a vacation in Fiji or to list all the potential pitfalls of the vacation. Allowing participants to list what they liked about the vacation was predicted to re-build resistance, which was hypothesized to bring about more skeptical ratings of the final political ad compared to ratings of participants who continued to be critical by condemning the vacation.

The Knowles and colleagues (2002) study showed that people were skeptical when they saw target ad came first, but their resistance dropped as the series of ads went on, such that when the target ad appeared in the last position, it was rated quite favorably. However, this effect was only found among participants who reported that they typically had relatively little resistance to political ads. When these low-resistance participants got a rest from having to be skeptical, they were able to criticize the final political ad. By comparison, when they were critical for an extra 12 minutes, their resistance wore thin, and they were favorably disposed to the target ad. In short, people who repeatedly re-sisted pressures to change—especially those who were unaccustomed to defending against persuasion attempts—became exhausted and were no longer able to be skeptical. This limited resource pattern suggests that resistance can be depleted, then gradually replen-ished. It appears that resisting others' attempts to change one's attitudes uses the same re-source as do intrapsychic forms of self-regulation.

Social Inference and Self-Regulation

As social creatures, our ability to perceive and process information about others is of ut-most importance. One theory about how humans make social inferences posits that peo-ple first characterize others by making dispositional inferences about them, and must then engage in effortful cognitive correction to account for situational demands (Gilbert, Krull, & Pelham, 1988). Given that correction requires overriding a personal attribution and replacing it with a situational attribution, it seems to require self-regulatory abilities to inhibit and replace a dispositional attribution. Accordingly, if a person is in a state of depleted regulatory capacity, characterization may occur without correction, thereby leading to inaccurate perceptions of others.

In two studies, Gilbert and colleagues (1988) tested the idea that self-regulation is a necessary component of social inferences. In one experiment, an attention control manip-ulation was used to deplete self-control resources. Subsequently, participants watched a video in which a woman being interviewed acted listless and depressed. Participants were led to believe that the interviewee was answering either sadness-inducing or happiness-inducing questions, which tested whether self-regulation enables people to correct for sit-uational constraints.

Participants who were not depleted attributed the interviewee's sad behavior to her disposition only when they thought she was answering happiness-inducing questions; when these participants thought she was responding to sad questions, they were able to attribute her sad behavior to the situation. Participants who were depleted, however, made dispositional inferences about the interviewee's behavior in both conditions, thus failing to correct for situational demands (i.e., sadness-inducing questions). This finding confirms the idea that self-regulatory resources are indispensable to making accurate in-ferences about others' behavior.

In the other experiment, Gilbert and colleagues (1988) asked participants to ingrati-ate themselves to a confederate during an interview. Before the interview, the confederate was instructed to be either very likable or rather aloof and unlikable. The latter condition was meant to induce participants to exert a great deal of regulatory effort to be ingratiat-ing to an unlikable person. As a measure of social inference, participants' goal was to determine the interviewee's true attitudes, while believing that the confederate would be reading experimenter-generated responses to the questions.

As expected, interviewers who were ingratiating to the unlikable confederate made more dispositional inferences about the confederate's attitudes than did those who were ingratiating to a likable confederate. This finding suggests that being nice to someone unlikable undermines the ability to correct for situational effects, presumably because regulatory resources have been depleted. The ability to perceive and incorporate situational features, as well as personality characteristics, into social inferences is governed by self-regulation processes and frees people from mistakenly seeing only dispositional characteristics in others' behaviors.

Regulatory Focus

People approach goal-related activities in all manner of styles and strategies, most of which may be ultimately boiled down to responses aimed at approaching positives or backing away from negatives. The framework of regulatory goals describes goal pursuit via the use of promotion and prevention strategies. Promotion involves achieving ideals, whereas prevention involves avoiding disaster. Research by Higgins (1996, 1997, 2000; see Higgins & Spiegel, Chapter 9, this volume) has shown that there are both stable individual differences in people's dominant regulatory focus and situational influences that change moment-to-moment regulatory focus.

In a recent study, the idea of regulatory focus was applied to people's motivations to achieve a goal inspired by role models who demonstrated either promotion or prevention orientations. Using the logic of regulatory focus theory, Lockwood, Jordan, and Kunda (2002) surmised that promotion-focused people, who prefer a strategy of zealously pursuing their goals, would be best motivated by positive role models who emphasized strategies for reaching success. Conversely, they hypothesized that prevention-focused people, who prefer to avoid undesirable outcomes, would be best inspired by role models who reminded them of strategies for avoiding failure. In two studies, participants were primed with either a positive role model (i.e., a person who had achieved lofty goals) or a negative role model (i.e., a person who had suffered defeat when trying to reach a goal). They then reported on the strength of their motivation in an important life domain (viz., academics). As suspected, promotion-focused participants had more academic motivation after being primed by a positive role model who had reached his or her dreams, whereas prevention-focused participants had more motivation after being primed by a negative role model who reminded them of the possibility of failure.

The idea that people are motivated by outstanding others who have regulatory strategies similar to their own suggests several implications for self-regulation in an interpersonal context. First, these studies suggest that people detect, at some level, variability in how others pursue their goals and also can recognize whether others have adopted a regulatory focus similar to their own. Second, people gravitate to those who will best inspire them and not, coincidentally, people who have a particular regulatory focus. In short, people are affected by the regulatory goals of others, and these effects influence goal motivations and personal inspiration.

Summary

Self-regulation influences a variety of intrapsychic interpersonal behaviors. Social psychologists have begun to elucidate the importance of self-regulation for phenomena such as being inspired by certain types of role models, persuasion attempts, social orientation, impression management, social inference, and self-evaluation. These diverse phenomena illustrate the influence of regulatory control within the domain of intrapsychic, interpersonally oriented responses.

DYADIC INTERPERSONAL FUNCTIONING USES SELF-CONTROL

It is imperative that people form close ties and create intimate bonds with others to secure the reproductive and survival benefits of belongingness (Baumeister & Leary, 1995). In this section, we review evidence that good self-control is a crucial component of maintaining social ties and, conversely, that poor self-control has the potential to damage intimate relationships. A host of interpersonal phenomena depend on emotional regulation, cognitive control, and behavioral management; to best illustrate this point, we concentrate on direct and explicit tests of self-regulatory processes within the context of close relationships.

Regulatory Goals Can Be Primed by Relationships

We begin with a discussion of new research on the entrenchment of regulatory goals within specific dyadic relationships. Most relationships are not maintained through unconditional positive regard of partners for one another, suggesting that goals for securing love and acceptance in a specific relationships likely become embedded in the concept of the relationship itself. If this notion is true, the relationship may serve as a primer for specific regulatory goals that partners have routinely sought during the course of the relationship. This proposition was tested by Fitzsimmons and Bargh (2003), who tracked people's typical goals as a function of the relationship (e.g., having achievement goals with mothers; having caring goals with friends). They found that knowing the goals typically enacted in the context of a particular relationship allows for prediction of specific behaviors when the relationship is primed in memory. Across four experimental studies, Fitzsimmons and Bargh found that activating the idea of a certain relationship (e.g., activation of the concept "mother") led to behavioral outcomes that mapped onto the higher order goal represented by the relationship. The behaviors and the priming of a goal state by the memory of an intimate partner occurred without participants' awareness, and without the actual presence of the relationship partner. These exciting new results speak volumes about how relationships act as goal-priming devices that can instigate a repertoire of goal-pursuit behaviors outside of awareness or intent.

Accommodative Responses

It is perhaps impossible to avoid conflict in a romantic relationship, which means that it is crucial for the health of the relationship that couples find a way to deal with conflict. "Accommodation" refers to a person's response in situations in which his or her partner has behaved in a manner that has the potential to damage the relationship. In these situations (called "accommodative dilemmas"), the responding partner has the choice to behave in kind by engaging in another destructive behavior or to respond in a constructive manner by trying to ameliorate potential interpersonal trouble. The hypothesis that accommodation requires self-regulation arises from the idea that it is natural or habitual to defend the self in times of conflict by responding to an unkind act from one's partner with another unkind response. Finkel and Campbell (2001) and, later, Vohs (2003) postulated that it takes self-control to override these selfish responses and behave in a kind, selfless manner.

In these studies, accommodative tendencies were measured by a standard questionnaire in which participants were asked to describe how they would behave during an accommodative dilemma. Responses were grouped into four categories: voice, exit, loyalty, and neglect. The category voice is active and relationship-oriented, and typically involves a person wanting to talk about issues constructively, whereas exit is active and self-oriented, and describes people's behaviors that emphasize leaving the relationship. Loyalty is passive and relationship-oriented, and characterizes a person who benignly hopes that the conflict will resolve itself, whereas neglect is passive and self-oriented, and characterizes a person who may display laxity and carelessness about the relationship. Voice and loyalty are considered accommodative responses, and exit and neglect are nonaccommodative responses.

Across four studies, Finkel and Campbell (2001) found that participants in committed romantic relationships with higher trait self-control scores also reported more accommodative tendencies. Moreover, using a narrative recall task in which participants remembered a time when they had been accommodating or nonaccommodating, Finkel and Campbell found that accommodation was less likely when self-regulatory abilities were low, a finding they confirmed using an experimental design that manipulated self-regulatory resources. In summary, these studies revealed that accommodation within current romantic relationships requires strong self-regulatory capacity.

The findings regarding depletion and accommodative responses were replicated by Vohs (2003), who used an experimental design that manipulated regulatory resources. In addition to finding significant depletion effects for accommodation to current relationship partners, this study also found fewer accommodative responses among participants who thought of a past or a hypothetical relationship partner when considering the accommodative dilemmas. These initial results hint that self-control's importance in overcoming selfish (i.e., nonaccommodative responses) may span types of relationships (e.g., family, friendships). Hence, regardless of relationship status, participants lower in regulatory resources reported an increased likelihood of reacting to their real, past, and imagined relationship partners' misbehaviors with less constructive and more destructive acts.

Overcoming the Self-Serving Bias in Relationships

The tendency for people to make internal, dispositional attributions for positive outcomes but make situational attributions for negative outcomes (labeled the "self-serving bias," or SSB) is one of the most predictable findings in the attribution literature. In the context of a relationship, this tendency can be problematic when the "situation" that gets blamed for a negative outcome involves the actions of an intimate partner. Initial data suggest that better self-control relates to a diminished SSB in the context of romantic relationships.

In an initial questionnaire study, Vohs (2003) found that trait self-control scores correlated significantly with scores on an SSB scale that measured the tendency to give credit to the self rather than to one's partner (Sicoly & Ross, 1977). The scale items ranged from "taking care of each other when not feeling well" to "doing chores," and were all positively worded, such that making a self-oriented attribution indicated something akin to the SSB. This correlation held even when self-esteem scores (which are highly and positively related to the SSB; see Campbell & Sedikides, 1999) were used as a covariant.

In an additional study, relationship partners were first asked to watch a comedic film, with instructions either to suppress their reactions or to act naturally. These instructions were used to vary self-regulatory resources, with the former group presumably depleting their resources by having to quell their reactions. Afterward, the couple was asked to build a structure from a set of Lego blocks. Participants were given either positive or negative feedback after building their structure, feedback indicating that theirs was among the most or least creative structures. The dependent measure was the credit or blame placed on the self as opposed to the partner after hearing the feedback about the structure. The findings supported the self-control hypothesis in that participants who had earlier contained their reactions to the film were more likely to take credit for the positive feedback or to blame their partner for the negative feedback, depending on condition. Participants who had not previously expended their regulatory resources were able to keep their impulses in check and showed an attenuated SSB.

These data suggest that the ability to overcome the SSB in relationships is a result of good self-control. There is a strong desire to think well of the self and to take responsibility for positive outcomes, while placing blame on others when outcomes are negative. In close relationships, however, it is beneficial to put aside this bias and acknowledge others' roles in producing good outcomes, or to release them from culpability for bad outcomes. Not incidentally, research shows that maladaptive attributions (such as the SSB) are a warning sign of a troubled relationship (Bradbury, Beach, Fincham, & Nelson, 1996). Vohs's (2003) data indicate that low self-control may be a significant factor in determining relationship-relevant attributions.

Controlling Impulses and Attraction to Alternates

People who believe that they have alternatives to their romantic partner are more likely to be dissatisfied with their current partner and to have their current relationship fail. Miller (1997) studied gaze length as a sign of attraction to possible alternate partners, which he considered important, because longer gaze length indicates a deeper processing of a person's attributes and allows for consideration of the person at a more than superficial level. To test the influence of gaze length (as a proxy for consideration of alternate partners) on relationship status, Miller asked participants to view a series of slides of attractive, opposite-sex people for as long as they liked. He then measured the amount of time participants spent gazing at the photos. Miller found that participants' length of time gazing at the slides was a significant predictor of relationship dissolution 2 months later.

Vohs (2003) further hypothesized that turning oneself away from a tempting alternative requires self-control (similar to the mechanism by which dieters turn away from tempting, but off-limits, foods). In her study, participants were asked to read aloud a set of boring historical narratives, with instructions either to act natural or to read with exaggerated emotional and facial expressions. The latter was presumed to require more behavioral control, thus taxing self-regulatory resources. Afterwards, all participants were surreptitiously videotaped while paging through a booklet of photos of scantily clad men and women. Time spent leafing through the booklet (and specifically, looking at the pages of the gender to whom the participant was attracted) was the dependent measure. Consistent with expectations, participants who had earlier drained their resources reading the narratives with exaggerated tone and movements were more likely to leaf slowly through those pages. Moreover, this was especially true for participants involved in a current romantic relationship. Turning away from an attractive alternative partner requires self-regulatory resources, and the lack of these resources may render the relationship vulnerable to eventual dissolution.

Self-Disclosure to a New Acquaintance

We tend to like people who tell us personal information about themselves (Collins & Miller, 1994). To boost being liked by a new acquaintances, it is best to tell a moderate amount about oneself—too little information communicates disinterest in forming a relationship, whereas too much overwhelms the listener. One individual difference that predicts degree of self-disclosure is attachment style: People with a secure attachment style favor moderate disclosures, people with an anxious–ambivalent style favor highly intimate disclosures, and people with a dismissive style favor nonintimate disclosures. Given that people strive to be liked and accepted, Vohs and colleagues (2003) hypothesized that people likely attempt to achieve a moderate level of disclosure. However, insecurely attached people would have to override preexisting tendencies to achieve a moderate level of disclosure, a process hypothesized to require self-regulatory resources. Hence, Vohs and colleagues predicted that attachment-related self-disclosure differences would be attenuated when people had enough regulatory resources, and magnified when they were low in resources.

Participants in these studies were given self-control or non-self-control instructions and were then asked to report preferences in conversational intimacy for an upcoming interaction. Participants watched an emotionally charged film and were asked to exaggerate, suppress, or show their natural emotional reactions. The researchers assumed that the two former groups would exert their regulatory resources performing these tasks (see Vohs & Schmeichel, 2003). Participants were told that they would converse with another participant in a different experiment, that the experimenter would choose some topics as a conversational guide, and that they would be allowed to rate the conversation topics according to their degree of interest in discussing them. The topics ranged from high- to moderate- to low-disclosure topics (on the basis of work by Sedikides, Campbell, Reeder, & Elliot, 1998); thus, participants' ratings of their interest in discussing them served as a measure of the preferred level of intimacy for the conversation.

Participants' preferences for conversational intimacy were significantly predicted by their self-regulatory resource availability and attachment style. Participants of all attachment styles, who were not depleted, tended toward a moderate disclosure style, whereas depleted (both suppressed and exaggerated conditions) participants reverted to their usual tendencies: The dismissives preferred to underdisclose, and the anxious–ambivalents preferred to overdisclose. Securely attached participants remained in the middle, although they tended somewhat to prefer more intimacy when depleted. Giving out information about oneself is thus affected by self-regulatory ability, with disclosure patterns of people with insecure attachment styles being most impaired by low self-control.

Social Rejection

To make a point, to punish someone for a misdeed, or when relationship problems grow too great, people sometimes resort to social rejection. However, given that people have a fundamental need to belong and be close to others (Baumeister & Leary, 1995), rejecting another person may require self-regulation, because it involves overriding the inborn tendency for relatedness. Ciarocco, Sommer, and Baumeister (2001) surmised that to ostracize someone effectively, one must spend some time in close proximity, while refusing to speak or respond to the person. Ciarocco and colleagues predicted, and demonstrated, that ostracizing another person would hinder people's ability to self-regulate during a later task. People who were asked to ostracize a confederate later displayed decrements in their ability to self-regulate on tasks of physical and mental stamina (e.g., persistence in gripping a handgrip exerciser and attempts to solve unsolvable anagrams). Failure to persist was independent of liking the ostracism target, suggesting that the tendency to reject another person goes against basic tendencies for relatedness and is therefore a regulated interpersonal response.

Mixed-Race Interactions

As a segue to the group processes section, we review research on the role of self-control in dyadic, mixed-race interactions. Although white and black people come into frequent contact, this contact may not be benign in its effects on the psychological system; it may, in fact, be perceived as threatening. In a provocative study, Richeson and Shelton (2003) hypothesized that there may be a detrimental effect of mixed-race interactions on the subsequent availability of self-regulatory resources. They predicted, and found, that because these interactions often prompt overcontrolled and inhibited responses, there may be fewer self-regulatory resources available for subsequent self-control tasks, and that this effect would be especially strong among people who held racial biases. Specifically, white participants gave their opinions on one of two topics in response to questions asked by either a white or black experimenter (otherwise, the experimenter did not comment during the interaction). Subsequently, participants' self-control abilities were tested by reaction-time performance on the Stroop task. Participants who held implicitly negative attitudes toward blacks were significantly impaired in performing the Stroop task after their (rather superficial) interaction with the black experimenter. There was some suggestion that those who held implicit biases also exhibited behaviors that were more controlled and inhibited, and that these tendencies can predict poor Stroop performance. Thus, interactions with people of a different race can create stressful regulatory demands, particularly for those whose racial interactions are most infused with (nonconscious) negativity.

Summary

Self-regulation seems to have numerous and diverse effects for dyadic interpersonal relationships. When people are unable to control their behaviors and responses, they present themselves in a less socially acceptable manner (e.g., they become narcissistic), care less about gaining social approval, gaze longer at a potential alternative partner, and are less accommodative and more destructive during a romantic conflict. Likewise, research in this section has demonstrated that people's self-control faculties are impaired after they take part in a mixed-race interaction or are forced to present themselves in an atypical manner (e.g., being modest in front of a stranger).

GOOD SELF-REGULATION AIDS GROUP MEMBERSHIP

Being accepted into groups is an essential component of social and cultural life. In this last section, we turn to an examination of group-related phenomena and self-regulation. Here, we examine self-regulation's influence on conformity, stigma, rejection, and prejudice.

Conforming to the Group

Although thinking of oneself as unique can have its advantages, it can at times be painful and socially damaging to go against group norms. Herman and Polivy (1980) posited that the motivation to conform to societal and personal appearance ideals underlies chronic dieters' self-imposed restriction of caloric consumption. However, despite strong motivation and good intentions, chronic dieters often fail in attempts to control their food intake. One possible explanation for these failed attempts lies in the self-regulatory resource model. In a series of studies, Vohs and Heatherton (2000) found that a depletion of resources as a result of overriding the temptation of chocolate candies or emotion regulation led to more ice-cream eating among dieters but not nondieters. Thus, many everyday self-regulatory tasks—including interpersonally related tasks—may deplete dieters' ego strength and undermine their ability to restrict food intake.

To test an interpersonal account for dieting failure, Kahan, Polivy, and Herman (2003) used an Asch-type conformity task. Dieting and nondieting participants were allowed to respond to a visual task either by themselves or under the influence of others' unanimously incorrect responses (i.e., which compelled them to conform). The conformity task was expected to use up regulatory strength, because it would be difficult for people to go along with a clearly incorrect decision. Being depleted was expected to undermine dieters' ability to restrict their eating in the presence of palatable food. However, among nondieters, no differences in eating were expected after conforming—not because the conformity was any less depletion, but because participants were not trying to regulate their food intake (Vohs & Heatherton, 2000). Only for the dieters was the conformity task expected to affect food consumption.

The results showed that nondieters ate the same amount of cookies whether subjected to the conformity task or allowed to choose on their own, whereas dieters, as expected, ate more in the conformity condition than in the condition in which they were not compelled to conform. These results support the resource model of self-regulation as an explanation for dieting failure. More germane to the current analysis, these finding indicate that feeling the pressure to conform is a depleting activity. Pressure from groups can subsequently undermine our ability to regulate ourselves on any activity requiring self-control.

Rejection from the Group

Ask anyone who has been rejected from a group, and he or she will tell you that it is a painful experience. Yet what sort of impact does it have on subsequent behavior? Recent research has determined that social exclusion leads to both self-defeating and antisocial behavior (Twenge, Baumeister, Tice, & Strucke, 2001; Twenge, Catanese, & Baumeister, 2002). One possible mechanism for these ill effects is that rejection leads to self-regulation failure, which in turn gives rise to self-destructive and antisocial responses.

Using a resource model of self-regulation, Baumeister, Twenge, and Ciarocco (2003) sought to determine whether self-regulation is impaired by social rejection. In one study, each participant was told that no one in a group of newly acquainted peers had elected to work with him or her on an upcoming task. In other studies, researchers manipulated social exclusion by telling people that their scores on a personality questionnaire indicated that they would be alone later in life. Participants' subsequent self-regulation was measured in several ways: They were given the opportunity to eat as many cookies as they desired; they were asked to work on unsolvable puzzle-tracing tasks; or they were asked to consume as many 1-ounce cups of vinegar-infused Kool-Aid as possible. All these tasks required them to override a natural or automatic tendency, such as not wanting to drink sour-tasting beverages, to perform the task.

In all three experiments, rejected participants displayed poorer self-regulation than did participants who were not rejected. When rejected, participants ate more cookies, gave up sooner on unsolvable puzzles, and drank fewer cups of vinegar-infused Kool-Aid. Together, these experiments revealed that self-regulation is impaired by social exclusion, a necessary step in determining whether self-control failure accounts for increased antisocial tendencies among people who feel socially rejected.

Stereotyping Group Members

The mere sight of another person prompts a cascade of categorization and evaluative processes. Using observable, outward characteristics, people make associations between an individual and different social groups. Stereotyping and implicit prejudice are automatically activated when one encounters a member of another group and are often applied without awareness or conscious intent (Devine, 1989). Despite their automatic evocations, people can and do attempt to control stereotypical applicability through devices such as thought suppression, use of individuating information, substitution of a stereotypical response with an egalitarian response, or behaving in a direction opposite to the stereotype.

One element underlying these various methods of overriding stereotyped application tendencies appears to be self-regulation. Monteith (1993) postulated, and found evidence, that people activate a regulatory system when attempting to override a prejudiced response. In two studies, Monteith induced low-prejudiced participants to believe that that they had responded in a prejudiced manner. When these participants believed they had violated their personal standards against prejudice, they appeared to respond by triggering an inhibitory self-regulation system. Specifically, these participants experienced heightened self-awareness regarding their prejudiced responding, reported increased negative affect, showed greater attention to information about this discrepancy, and exhibited slower motor responses.

Despite the ready activation of stereotypes, people learn strategies to interrupt and eventually change their automatic responses. After the initiation of a stereotype occurs, the person must make a conscious decision or effort to override that response. This process surely relies on self-control, because the path of least resistance is to allow the stereotype to proceed, and one must use control processes to subvert the application of a prejudiced response. Arguably, people may be able to change their stereotypical responses if they frequently seek to overcome this tendency.

Summary

People want to belong to groups and to be good group members. The ability to keep one's actions in line with group standards, to substitute group preferences for one's personal desires, and to change the self in response to signs of social rejection requires that people exert control over their responses to secure group membership. Although researchers have not observed many direct connections between group processes and self-control, we predict that the importance of group functioning, combined with the recent influence of ideas on cultural differences, will spark many of the research findings on self-regulation in the upcoming years.

CONCLUSIONS, CLOSING COMMENTS,
AND A CALL FOR MORE RESEARCH

We end this chapter with the overall conclusion that people do indeed use self-regulation skills and resources in interpersonal processes. A wide spectrum of findings from the interpersonal and social inclusion literatures suggests that social functioning is aided by a host of self-control strategies: When people actively control their emotions, guide their mental contents, override incipient impulses, and direct their behaviors, they increase their social belongingness. When people fail in these self-control endeavors, they are more likely to be ousted from groups and relationships. People who fail at self-regulation become narcissistic (Vohs et al., 2003), retaliate in conflicted dyadic interactions (Finkel & Campbell, 2001), gaze longingly at an attractive alternative partner (Vohs, 2003), engage in demeaning and harmful social behaviors (e.g., they are more likely to stereotype others; Monteith, 1993), over- or underdisclose personal information (Vohs et al., 2003), fail to live up to the standards set by positive role models (Lockwood et al., 2002), fall prey to others' influence attempts (Knowles et al., 2002), and spoil a mixed-race interaction (Richeson & Shelton, 2003).

We see a multitude of avenues for future research and would like to see scholars who study interpersonal processes incorporate self-regulatory processes in their models, who take into account the role of domain-specific (e.g., mental control) regulatory strategies as one pathway of achieving (or eroding) interpersonal inclusion.

One area that we would especially like to see investigated is the link between sexuality and self-regulation (see Wiederman, Chapter 27, this volume). Sex is one of the most basic and highly regulated interpersonal behaviors within persons and within societies. As such, one would think that the interface between self-regulation and sex would be a prime area for fruitful research. However, there is a dearth of research on how self-regulatory processes affect sexual tendencies, preferences, and patterns.

At a broader level, we also suggest that interpersonal researchers and social psychologists look for the operation of self-control processes in their own research. Self-regulatory demands are pervasive; consequently, their effects may be underappreciated in interpersonal research. That the effects of self-control processes have been unearthed in the study of person perception, stereotyping, and influence research suggests that some of these connections are already being made. In writing this chapter, we have seen tantalizing signs of the ways in which self-regulation and interpersonal processes are interrelated, and we feel the excitement that this budding new area inspires.

REFERENCES

Baumeister, R. F., & Leary, M. R. (1995). The need to belong: Desire for interpersonal attachments as a fundamental human motivation. *Psychological Bulletin, 117*, 497–529.

Baumeister, R. F., Twenge, J. M., & Ciarocco, N. (2003). *Rejection and ego depletion.* Manuscript in preparation.

Bradbury, T. N., Beach, S. R. H., Fincham, F. D., & Nelson, G. M. (1996). Attributions and behavior in functional and dysfunctional marriages. *Journal of Consulting and Clinical Psychology, 64*, 569–576.

Campbell, W. K., & Sedikides, C. (1999). Self-threat magnifies the self-serving bias: A meta-analytic integration. *Review of General Psychology, 3*, 23–43.

Ciarocco, N. J., Sommer, K. L., & Baumeister, R. F. (2001). Ostracism and ego depletion: The strains of silence. *Personality and Social Psychology Bulletin, 27*, 1156–1163.

Collins, N. L., & Miller, L. C. (1994). Self-disclosure and liking: A meta-analytic review. *Psychological Bulletin, 116,* 457–475.

Devine, P. G. (1989). Stereotypes of prejudice: Their automatic and controlled components. *Journal of Personality and Social Psychology, 56,* 5–18.

Gilbert, D. T., Krull, D. S., & Pelham, B. W. (1988). Of thoughts unspoken: Social inference and the self-regulation of behavior. *Journal of Personality and Social Psychology, 55,* 685–694.

Finkel, E. J., & Campbell, W. K. (2001). Self-control and accommodation in close relationships: An interdependence analysis. *Journal of Personality and Social Psychology, 81,* 263–277.

Fitzsimons, G. M., & Bargh, J. A. (2003). Thinking of you: Nonconscious pursuit of interpersonal goals associated with relationship partners. *Journal of Personality and Social Psychology, 84,* 148–163.

Heatherton, T. F., & Vohs, K. D. (1998). Why is it so difficult to inhibit behavior? *Psychological Inquiry, 9,* 212–215.

Herman, C. P., & Polivy, J. (1980). Restrained eating. In A. J. Stunkard (Ed.), *Obesity* (pp. 208–225). Philadelphia: Saunders.

Higgins, E. T. (1996). The "self digest": Self-knowledge serving self-regulatory functions. *Journal of Personality and Social Psychology, 71,* 1062–1083.

Higgins, E. T. (1997). Beyond pleasure and pain. *American Psychologist, 52,* 1280–1300.

Higgins, E. T. (2000). Making a good decision: Value from fit. *American Psychologist, 55,* 1217–1230.

Kahan, D., Polivy, J., & Herman, C. P. (2003). Conformity and dietary disinhibition: A test of the ego-strength model of self-regulation. *International Journal of Eating Disorders, 32,* 165–171.

Knowles, E. S., Brennan, M., & Linn, J. A. (2002). *Consuming resistance to political ads.* Manuscript in preparation, University of Arkansas, Fayetteville.

Leary, M. R., Nezlek, J. B., Downs, D., Radford-Davenport, J., Martin, J., & McMullen, A. (1994). Self-presentation in everyday interactions: Effects of target familiarity and gender composition. *Journal of Personality and Social Psychology, 67,* 664–673.

Lockwood, P., Jordan, C. H., & Kunda, Z. (2002). Motivation by positive or negative role models: Regulatory focus determines who will inspire us. *Journal of Personality and Social Psychology, 83,* 854–864.

Miller, R. S. (1997). Inattentive and contented: Relationship commitment and attention to alternatives. *Journal of Personality and Social Psychology, 73,* 758–766.

Monteith, M. J. (1993). Self-regulation of prejudiced responses: Implications for progress in prejudice-reduction efforts. *Journal of Personality and Social Psychology, 65,* 469–485.

Morf, C. C., & Rhodewalt, F. (2001). Unraveling the paradoxes of narcissism: A dynamic self-regulatory processing model. *Psychological Inquiry, 12,* 177–196.

Richeson, J. A., & Shelton, N. J. (2003). When prejudice doesn't pay: Effects of interracial contact on executive function. *Psychological Science, 14,* 287–290.

Sedikides, C., Campbell, W. K., Reeder, G. D., & Elliot, A. J. (1998). The self-serving bias in relational context. *Journal of Personality and Social Psychology, 74,* 378–386.

Seeley, E. A., & Gardner, W. L. (2003). The "selfless" and self-regulation: The role of chronic other-orientation in averting self-regulatory depletion. *Journal of Self and Identity, 2,* 103–117.

Sicoly, F., & Ross, M. (1977). The facilitation of ego-biased attributions by means of self-serving, observer feedback. *Journal of Personality and Social Psychology, 35,* 734–741.

Tice, D. M., Butler, J. L., Muraven, M. B., & Stillwell, A. M. (1995). When modesty prevails: Differential favorability of self-presentation to friends and strangers. *Journal of Personality and Social Psychology, 69,* 1120–1138.

Twenge, J. M., Baumeister, R. F., Tice, D. M., & Stucke, T. S. (2001). If you can't join them, beat them: Effects of social exclusion on aggressive behavior. *Journal of Personality and Social Psychology, 81,* 1058–1069.

Twenge, J. M., Catanese, K. R., & Baumeister, R. F. (2002). Social exclusion causes self-defeating behavior. *Journal of Personality and Social Psychology, 83,* 606–615.

Vohs, K. D. (2003). *Self-regulatory resources and romantic relationships.* Unpublished manuscript. University of British Columbia, Vancouver.

Vohs, K. D., Ciarocco, N., & Baumeister, R. F. (2003). *Self-regulation and self-presentation: Regulatory resource depletion impairs management and effortful self-presentation depletes regulatory resource.* Manuscript under review.

Vohs, K. D., & Heatherton, T. F. (2000). Self-regulatory failure: A resource-depletion approach. *Psychological Science, 11,* 249–254.

Vohs, K. D., & Schmeichel, B. J. (2003). Self-regulation and the extended now: Controlling the self alters the subjective experience of time. *Journal of Personality and Social Psychology, 85,* 217–230.

V

Individual Differences
and Self-Regulation

21

Gender and Self-Regulation

SUSAN NOLEN-HOEKSEMA
COLLEEN CORTE

The many specific domains in which we can examine possible gender differences in self-regulation include eating behavior, sexual behavior, and interpersonal functioning (see Vohs & Ciarocco, Chapter 20, for a review of self-regulation and interpersonal functioning, and Wiederman, Chapter 27, this volume, for a review of self-regulation and sex). We focus on two domains in which there is considerable research on gender differences in self-regulation: negative mood and alcohol use. On the one hand, women appear more likely than men to use a passive, self-focused response to negative mood, which we have labeled "rumination." On the other hand, it has been argued that men are more likely than women to use psychoactive substances, particularly alcohol, to regulate negative moods. We review the literature on the uses of rumination and alcohol to regulate mood, and the gender differences in these self-regulatory styles.

RUMINATION

We have conducted extensive research on the role of gender differences in mood regulatory strategies in producing gender differences in depression and, to some extent, anxiety disorders (Nolen-Hoeksema, 2003). This research has focused on a mood regulatory strategy known as "rumination," which is the tendency to focus on one's symptoms of distress, and think about the causes and consequences of these symptoms in a passive and repetitive manner. People who are ruminating engage in thoughts such as "I feel so down and blue. Will I ever snap out of this?"; "I'm overwhelmed and I don't know what to do!"; and "What's wrong with me that I feel this way?" They do not go on to engage in active problem solving, however (Nolen-Hoeksema & Morrow, 1991), and even when they do attempt to generate solutions to their problems, these solutions are lower quality than those they are capable of generating when not ruminating (Lyubomirsky & Nolen-Hoeksema, 1995). Although most people may ruminate at least somewhat when they are sad or depressed, longitudinal, community-based studies have shown that the tendency to engage in rumination when distressed is a stable individual difference characteristic (Nolen-Hoeksema & Davis, 1999). Specifically, whereas many individuals may engage in some rumination when depressed or sad, some people ruminate a great deal; others engage in little or no rumination, and these individual differences tend to be stable over time, even as depressed moods wax and wane.

Gender Differences in Rumination

Several self-report studies have found that women are more likely than men to report ruminating in response to sad mood (Butler & Nolen-Hoeksema, 1994; Nolen-Hoeksema & Larson, 1999; Nolen-Hoeksema, Larson, & Grayson, 1999). Importantly, the gender difference in rumination remains significant when gender differences in levels of depressed mood are statistically controlled (Nolen-Hoeksema et al., 1999), suggesting that gender difference in rumination is not just a product of gender differences in depression.

We have also shown in experimental studies that women are more likely than men to focus on their emotions and self-related thoughts when they are in a sad mood (Butler & Nolen-Hoeksema, 1994). In these studies, a sad mood was first induced in women and men. Then, they were given the opportunity to engage in one of two tasks: One task required participants to focus on their current emotions. The other task had nothing to do with emotions, but instead required that they focus on geographic information. Among participants in the sad mood, women were significantly more likely than men to choose to focus on their emotions. Women were also more likely than men to choose the emotion-focused task when in a neutral mood. Women do not always choose to focus on emotion, however. Rusting and Nolen-Hoeksema (1998) induced angry moods in participants, and found that men were significantly more likely than women to choose to focus on emotion in the context of this mood.

Effects of Rumination on Depression and Anxiety

People who ruminate in response to sad or anxious mood show longer periods of sadness or anxiety and are more likely to develop major depression (Nolen-Hoeksema, 2003). One study demonstrating this was conducted around the time of the major earthquake that hit the San Francisco Bay area in 1989 (Nolen-Hoeksema & Morrow, 1991). Rumination and emotional well-being had been assessed in 137 college students just before the earthquake. We returned to these students at both 10 days and 7 weeks after the earthquake to reassess their levels of distress. Students who were ruminators before the earthquake had more severe levels of depressive symptoms both at 10 days and at 7 weeks after the earthquake, even after we statistically controlled for both their levels of depression before the earthquake and the earthquake-related stress they endured. Ruminators were also more likely than nonruminators to have symptoms of posttraumatic stress disorder after the earthquake, even after we statistically controlled for the presence of these symptoms before the earthquake.

In another study, we followed more than 300 adults who lost a loved one to a terminal illness to assess the impact of a ruminative response style on bereavement-related depression (Nolen-Hoeksema & Larson, 1999; Nolen-Hoeksema, Parker, & Larson, 1994). The participants in this study were interviewed once before their loved one died, and then again at 1, 6, 13, and 18 months postloss. Again, ruminators were consistently more likely than nonruminators to experience elevated depressive symptoms over the course of this study, even after we statistically controlled for previous levels of depression and a number of other variables previously shown to predict bereavement-related depression, such as social support.

In both this bereavement study and in a subsequent study of 1,300 adults chosen randomly from the community, we found that rumination predicts not only depressive symptoms but also episodes of major depression (Nolen-Hoeksema, 2000; Nolen-Hoeksema & Larson, 1999); that is, ruminators were significantly more likely to develop episodes of major depression over time, even after we statistically controlled for previous levels of depression.

Rumination also predicts anxiety and may be particularly strongly associated with a mixed anxiety–depression syndrome, in which people vacillate between anxiety and depressive symptoms. In a 1-year study of community-dwelling adults, we found that ruminators were just as likely to develop severe anxiety symptoms as to develop severe depressive symptoms (Nolen-Hoeksema, 2000). Moreover, rumination was especially strongly related to the development of a mixed anxiety–depression syndrome.

Why would rumination predict mixed anxiety–depression particularly well? Content analyses of people's ruminations suggest that many of these thoughts reflect uncertainty over whether important situations will be manageable or controllable (e.g., "What if I can't pull myself together?" and "What did my spouse's comment mean?"; Lyubomirsky, Tucker, Caldwell, & Berg, 1999). In addition, we found in an experimental study that ruminators expressed more uncertainty than nonruminators, both verbally and nonverbally, in discussing their plans for overcoming a difficult interpersonal situation (Ward, Lyubomirsky, Sousa, & Nolen-Hoeksema, 2003). Several theorists have argued that uncertainty over whether one will be able to control one's environment is key to anxiety (Alloy, Kelly, Mineka, & Clements, 1990; Barlow, 1988; Garber, Miller, & Abramson, 1980). Yet rumination also contributes to hopelessness about the future and negative evaluations about the self, as we describe later, and these cognitions are key to depression (Abramson, Metalsky, & Alloy, 1989; Beck, 1967). Ruminators may vacillate between anxiety and depression as their cognitions vacillate between uncertainty and hopelessness (see Alloy et al., 1990; Garber et al., 1980; Mineka, Watson, & Clark, 1998).

Sources of Gender Difference in Rumination

Social, psychological, and, potentially, biological factors may contribute to the gender difference in rumination (Nolen-Hoeksema, 2002). Regarding social contributors, women report more chronic stressors, such as low income and unsatisfying marriages, than do men, and this gender difference in chronic stressors partially mediates the gender difference in rumination (Nolen-Hoeksema et al., 1999). Women are also more likely than men to suffer certain traumatic events, particularly sexual abuse, and in turn, a history of major stressors, such as childhood sexual abuse, is associated with the tendency to ruminate. Specifically, women who reported they had been abused as children were more likely to be ruminators as adults, again, even after we controlled for their levels of depression (Nolen-Hoeksema, 1998). Experiences of abuse can shatter assumptions about the safety of the world and the trustworthiness of others, which in turn can feed ruminations.

Regarding personality contributors, we found that a trio of personality characteristics tied to women's social roles may also contribute to the gender difference in rumination (Nolen-Hoeksema & Jackson, 2001). First, women were more likely than men to believe that negative emotions, such as sadness, fear, and anger, are difficult to control. In turn, difficulty in controlling negative emotions was related to a greater tendency to ruminate, and helped to account for the gender difference in rumination. Women may believe that they are highly emotional compared to men, and that the sources of their negative emotions (e.g., hormones) are less controllable than the sources of men's negative emotions.

Second, women were more likely than men to report feeling responsible for the emotional tone of their relationships and for maintaining positive relationships with others at all costs; feeling too responsible was also associated with greater rumination. Feeling responsible for the emotional tone of relationships may lead women to attend to every nuance of their relationships, always vigilant for trouble, always wondering what others' comments or behaviors mean, always thinking of how they might make others happier. This, in turn, may make women vigilant to their own emotional states as barometers of how their relationships are going, thus contributing to rumination.

Third, women were more likely than men to report feeling little control over important events in their lives, and people who were lower on mastery reported more rumination. In turn, low perceived mastery helped to mediate the gender difference in rumination. Indeed, low perceived mastery appeared to be the strongest partial mediator of the gender difference in rumination. This suggests that women's sense that they have less control over important events in their lives, compared to men's, is a particularly important contributor to the gender difference in rumination.

None of these three variables fully mediated the gender difference in rumination on its own. This suggests that women both high and low on beliefs about the controllability of emotions and perceived mastery, and who feel responsible for relationships, may be more prone to rumination than men. But the combination of these three characteristics together did mediate the gender difference in rumination. Many women may carry some, but not all three, of these risk factors for rumination. For example, even women who are high in perceived mastery may have a tendency to ruminate, perhaps because they are concerned about the emotional tone and vigilant to problems in their relationships. In addition, even women who believe that the events in their lives are controllable may feel that negative emotions, when they inevitably arise, are not so controllable, and this contributes to their tendency to ruminate.

Biological factors may also play a role in the development of gender differences in rumination. Children who are more physiologically reactive to stress may find their negative emotional states more compelling and more difficult to overcome, leading them to focus on these states and feel helpless to cope with them. Recent evidence suggests that children with a history of sexual or physical abuse, who are more often girls than boys, may develop more dysregulated stress responses, as measured by cortisol levels, adrenocorticotropic hormone levels, and cardiac measures, compared to people who did not suffer child abuse or neglect (Heim et al., 2000; Zahn-Waxler, 2000). In turn, this greater biological reactivity is associated with a greater adult prevalence of major depression. It may also be that greater biological reactivity resulting from childhood abuse or neglect could lead to a ruminative style. Children who have more poorly regulated biological responses to stress find it more difficult to engage in efficacious behavioral responses to new stressors and, thus, may fall into a ruminative pattern.

An anxious temperament may interact with parents' socialization practices around self-regulation to contribute to more rumination in girls. It is unlikely that parents directly reinforce rumination in their daughters. Instead, parents may simply not encourage mastery-oriented problem solving when their daughters are sad or distressed to the same degree they do when their sons are sad or distressed. Parents appear very concerned that their sons not express stereotypically feminine emotions, such as sadness or fear, and that they "be strong" and "act like a little man" when distressed (Maccoby & Jacklin, 1974). Sanctions against males displaying sadness continue in adulthood. Siegel and Alloy (1990) found that depressed men were evaluated much more negatively than depressed women. These social reinforcements and punishments may motivate boys and men to develop active styles of responding to their depressed moods. At times, these active responses may be inappropriate (e.g., engaging in reckless behavior to avoid thinking about one's depressed mood). But much of the time, these active strategies may involve using either positive distractions or constructive problem solving. On the other hand, parents appear more likely to allow and even encourage the expression of sadness and distress in their daughters. Although this may help girls develop a greater appreciation of, and ability to express, negative emotions, it may also prevent girls from developing a repertoire of active strategies to regulate their moods. Indeed, their learning history may be one reason that women are more likely than men to say that negative emotions such as sadness and fear are uncontrollable once a person have them (Nolen-Hoeksema & Jackson, 2001).

ALCOHOL USE

Another domain in which there is evidence of gender differences in self-regulation is alcohol use. Whereas the majority of adults drink alcohol at least periodically (Substance Abuse and Mental Health Service Administration/Office of Applied Studies, 1997), there is a great deal of evidence that men drink alcohol more frequently and in greater quantities than women (Wilsnack & Wilsnack, 1997). In addition, men have a higher prevalence of alcohol use disorders compared to women. Data from the National Household Survey on Drug Abuse show that 12.5% of men and 6.4% of women meet lifetime criteria for alcohol abuse, and a larger percentage (20% of men and 8% of women) meet lifetime criteria for alcohol dependence (Brady & Randall, 1999; Kessler et al., 1997). Alcohol abuse is a less severe alcohol use disorder (AUD) diagnosis based on social and/or legal consequences of maladaptive alcohol use, whereas alcohol dependence is a more severe AUD diagnosis based on a cluster of cognitive, behavioral, and physiological manifestations of the inability to control alcohol use (American Psychiatric Association, 2000).

Although a variety of biological, psychological, and social models have been advanced to explain gender differences in alcohol use and alcohol abuse/dependence (for a review, see Hesselbrock, Hesselbrock, & Epstein, 1999), there has been increasing interest in understanding the nature of gender differences in the use of alcohol for the purposes of regulating negative affect states (Greeley & Oei, 1999; Hussong, Hicks, Levy, & Curran, 2001; Kushner, Sher, Wood, & Wood, 1994). Research has shown that some people use alcohol as a method of affect regulation, whereas others do not (Cooper, Frone, Russell, & Mudar, 1995; see also Hull & Sloane, Chapter 24, this volume, for another approach to alcohol and self-regulation). Clearly, the motivation to cope with negative affect states exerts an important influence on alcohol consumption for some people.

Gender has been identified as an important individual-difference factor that may contribute to the use of alcohol to cope with negative affect (Cooper et al., 1995; Hussong, et al., 2001). Interestingly, when examining alcohol use as an affect regulation strategy, different gender patterns seem to emerge for nonalcoholics (referred to as social drinkers in this chapter) and those with AUD. More specifically, there is some suggestion that among social drinkers, more men than women tend to use alcohol to cope with negative affect, whereas among persons with AUD, it appears that more women than men tend to use alcohol to cope with negative affect states.

Social Drinkers

Among social drinkers, most of the studies to date have used self-report measures of negative mood and alcohol consumption. The alcohol variables generally reflect recent or current alcohol consumption, but some studies focus on measures of heavy drinking, drinking problems, or reasons for drinking. The affect measures generally reflect short-term mood states rather than stable dispositional or trait measures of negative affect. Study samples have included college students, as well as community- and population-based samples of adults.

The most compelling tests of the affect regulation hypothesis—those in which the mood and alcohol measures are in relatively close proximity to each other—have tended to find a stronger relationship between negative mood and alcohol use among male than among female social drinkers. In a longitudinal study based on a large community-based sample of adults, Aneshensel and Huba (1983) found that, particularly for men, depressive symptoms positively predicted alcohol consumption 4 months later, which in turn predicted a decrease in depressive symptoms 4 months later. Cross-sectional studies have also found that male social drinkers exhibit a stronger relationship between alcohol consumption and anxiety (Kushner et al., 1994), stress (Timmer, Veroff, & Colten, 1985), and depressed mood (Berger & Adesso, 1991; Peirce, Frone, Russell, & Cooper, 1994) compared to female social drinkers. Other researchers that focus more specifically on reasons for drinking have found that men more frequently than women report drinking both to relieve depressive symptoms (Olenick & Chalmers, 1991) and to escape (Ratliff & Burkhart, 1984).

Recent studies using experience sampling methodology also converge to suggest that among social drinkers, men tend to use alcohol to regulate negative mood more than do women. Swendsen and colleagues (2000) measured three types of negative mood states at random intervals, three times daily, using handheld computers in a community-based sample of adults. Alcohol consumption was recorded "on-line" as it occurred. A particular strength of this study is the fact that the investigators focused on the relationship between negative mood and alcohol consumption over time intervals not longer than a few hours to more confidently establish the link between these variables. They found that nervousness predicted increases in alcohol consumption, which in turn reduced nervousness. This finding was stronger for male than for female social drinkers. They did not, however, find similar effects for sad mood, bored mood, or for global negative mood.

More recently, Hussong and colleagues (2001) used daily diaries to examine the pattern of relationships between different types of negative mood and alcohol consumption in college students. In this study, participants answered questions about mood in response to a randomly timed pager signal, multiple times daily for 4 weeks, and completed questionnaires about alcohol consumption once a day. Average daily mood scores were constructed for each type of negative mood, and weekday and weekend alcohol consumption scores were computed based on daily data. For men, sadness over the weekend led to high alcohol consumption during the following week, which in turn predicted sadness the following weekend. This pattern was not observed among women, and it was not found for feelings of hostility, fear, or guilt. Although these results differed from those of the previous experience sampling study in terms of the findings for sadness and alcohol consumption, Hussong's operationalization of sadness in terms of a daily average, rather than an average over a period of a few hours, may account for this difference. Because sadness was the only type of negative mood common to both studies, no other comparisons to specific negative moods could be made. Perhaps of more relevance to this chapter, however, is the fact that male social drinkers more often than female social drinkers tended to use alcohol to regulate negative mood in both experience sampling studies.

The studies that did not support the affect regulation hypothesis among male social drinkers either had a very wide temporal gap between the mood and alcohol measures or used trait rather than state measures of affect. For example, a meta-analysis based on eight population-based studies of adults found a stronger relationship between depressive symptoms and alcohol use among women than among men; however, alcohol use was measured 2–10 *years* after depressive symptoms were measured (Hartka et al., 1991). Such a large time interval between measurements is not an ideal test of the affect regulation hypothesis. Studies that measured trait anxiety found that both male and female college students with stably high anxiety reported more frequent use of alcohol to cope with their anxiety (Stewart, Karp, Pihl, & Peterson, 1997) and had higher alcohol consumption (Kalodner, Delucia, & Ursprung, 1989) compared to men and women with lower levels of trait anxiety. This perhaps suggests that whereas chronically high negative affect may motivate alcohol use for both men and women, short-term negative affect may be more of a motivator for men than for women, at least among social drinkers.

The findings across studies are somewhat mixed, yet when considered together, the strongest evidence suggests that among social drinkers, men more often than women tend to use alcohol to cope with negative mood. This is not to say that women do not use alcohol for this purpose; rather, there appears to be a greater tendency, at least among social drinkers, for men to use alcohol as a coping strategy more than do women. This effect was most evident in studies that focused on the association between alcohol and mood state over very short time spans, raising interesting questions about the possible differential influence of chronic versus intermittent negative affect on alcohol use in social drinkers. As can be seen in the next section, a different pattern of findings emerges for persons with AUD.

Persons with Alcohol Abuse and Alcohol Dependence

Although some of the work to date among persons with AUD has focused on negative mood states among alcoholics in treatment, or among those referred for assessment of alcohol problems, much of this work has been in the form of comorbidity studies of psychiatric or alcoholism inpatients or outpatients, or large population-based samples. The findings across studies are similar despite these methodological differences, however.

A key difference in the relationship between negative mood and alcohol consumption in persons with AUD compared to social drinkers is the gender pattern. More specifically, in persons with AUD, a stronger relationship between these variables exists for women compared to men. For example, Windle and Miller (1989) administered a diagnostic interview and self-report measures of current depressive symptoms and alcohol consumption to adult men and women who were sent for court-mandated assessment of alcohol problems. Interestingly, across both men and women, depressive symptoms over the last month were significantly higher in persons with alcohol dependence compared to those with alcohol abuse or no diagnosis, but this effect was substantially stronger for women than for men.

A similar pattern of findings emerged from a study of inpatient alcoholics across the lifespan, which focused on a different alcohol-related outcome variable (Rubonis et al., 1994). In this study, the investigators induced a negative mood state, then measured the urge to drink, after giving participants an alcoholic beverage and instructing them to hold the glass and smell the alcohol for several minutes. Results showed that in the presence of negative mood, women reported stronger urges to drink in response to being exposed to the alcoholic beverage, whereas men actually reported a reduced urge to drink.

Perhaps the most convincing support for the affect regulation hypothesis in women with AUD and, more specifically, for the opposite gender pattern than that noted in social drinkers, comes from a study that compared approximately equal numbers of male and female social drinkers and outpatients with AUD (Olenick & Chalmers, 1991). Variables of interest in this study were the self-reported use of alcohol to decrease negative mood, and drinking in response to marital conflict. A very interesting pattern of findings across gender and diagnostic group, and within gender, emerged. First, a significant gender × diagnostic group interaction revealed that female alcoholics drank more to change their mood and in response to marital conflict than did male alcoholics, but the reverse pattern was found among social drinking men and women. It should also be noted that despite the opposite-gender pattern found for persons with AUD and social drinkers, the means related to alcohol use to decrease negative mood and drinking in response to marital conflict were higher for both of the groups with AUD (men and women) than for the social drinking groups (men and women). This raises an interesting question about whether those who use alcohol to regulate negative affect may in fact be more likely to develop AUD. Second, the pattern of means related to motivations to drink revealed a much larger within-gender difference for women than for men. Women with AUD had the highest means, and women social drinkers had the lowest means, whereas the means for both groups of men were more moderate. Future researchers may wish to address the factors that may contribute to this interesting pattern of gender differences.

Studies designed to examine comorbidity between alcoholism and mood and anxiety disorders also provide some evidence for a stronger relationship between negative affect and alcoholism in women compared to men. These studies generally show that women with AUD experience more mood and anxiety disorders, and men with AUD experience more antisocial personality disorders, as well as dependence on other substances (Hesselbrock, Meyer, & Keener, 1985; Kessler et al., 1997; Sannibale & Hall, 2001) despite the higher base rates of mood and anxiety disorders among women, and antisocial personality disorders and other-substance dependence among men (Brady & Randall, 1999).

Gender differences related to the issue of temporal primacy between AUD and the comorbid disorder(s) have been investigated in an effort to help clarify causal direction. The findings clearly suggest that AUD is generally the primary disorder among men, whereas it is generally the secondary disorder among women (Kessler et al., 1997; Sannibale & Hall, 2001). Whereas this might suggest that women are more likely to develop AUD as a function of maladaptive alcohol use in an effort to cope with symptoms of preexisting mood or anxiety disorders, it might also suggest that women have more biased recall about the onset of mood and alcohol symptoms given that, among women, negative affect is much more acceptable than heavy alcohol use.

Unlike the gender pattern among social drinkers, the findings across studies among persons with AUD quite consistently suggest that the relationship between negative affect and alcohol is stronger for women than for men. This is not to say that no relationship exists between negative affect and alcohol consumption among men with AUD; rather, a stronger relationship appears to exist between these variables in women with AUD compared to men. In fact, there is some suggestion that both men and women with AUD use alcohol for affect regulation purposes more than do male and female social drinkers, and that this is particularly true among those with alcohol dependence rather than alcohol abuse.

CONCLUSIONS

Women appear more likely than men to use rumination to regulate their negative moods. In contrast, among social drinkers, men appear more likely than women to use alcohol to regulate their negative moods. Among people with AUD, however, women may be more likely than men to use alcohol for negative mood regulation. Some explanations for the gender difference in rumination have been explored. The reasons for the pattern of relationships between gender and the use of alcohol to regulate negative mood that we have described here have not been explored. Future research might benefit from a dual focus on rumination and alcohol use as strategies for responding to negative mood, in an effort to understand the social, psychological, and biological forces contributing to gender differences.

REFERENCES

Abramson, L. Y., Metalsky, G. L., & Alloy, L. B. (1989). Hopelessness depression: A theory based subtype of depression. *Psychological Review, 96*, 358–372.

Alloy, L., Kelly, K., Mineka, S., & Clements, C. (1990). Comorbidity in anxiety and depressive disorders: A helplessness/hopelessness perspective. In J.D. Maser & C.R. Cloninger (Eds.), *Comorbidity of mood and anxiety disorders* (pp. 3–12). Washington, DC: American Psychiatric Association Press.

American Psychiatic Association. (2000). *Diagnostic and statistical manual of mental disorders* (4th ed., text rev.). Washington, DC: Author.

Aneshensel C., & Huba, G. (1983). Depression, alcohol use, and smoking over one year: A four-wave longitudinal causal model. *Journal of Abnormal Psychology, 92*, 134–150.

Barlow, D. H. (1988). *Anxiety and its disorders: The nature and treatment of anxiety and panic.* New York: Guilford Press.

Beck, A. T. (1967). *Depression: Clinical, experimental and theoretical aspects.* New York: Harper & Row.

Berger, B., & Adesso, V. (1991). Gender differences in using alcohol to cope with depression. *Addictive Behaviors, 16*, 315–327.

Brady, K., & Randall, C. (1999). Gender differences in substance use disorders. *Psychiatric Clinics of North America: Addictive Disorders* [Special issue], *22*, 241–252.

Butler, L. D., & Nolen-Hoeksema, S. (1994). Gender differences in responses to a depressed mood in a college sample. *Sex Roles, 30*, 331–346.

Cooper, L., Frone, M., Russell, M., & Mudar, P. (1995). Drinking to regulate positive and negative emotions: A motivational model of alcohol use. *Journal of Personality and Social Psychology, 69*, 990–1005.

Garber, J., Miller, S. M., & Abramson, L. Y. (1980). On the distinction between anxiety states and depression: Perceived control, certainty, and probability of goal attainment. In J. Garber & M. E. P. Seligman (Eds.), *Human helplessness: Theory and applications* (pp. 131–169). New York: Academic Press.

Greeley, J., & Oei, T. (1999). Alcohol and tension reduction. In K. E. Leonard & H. T. Blane (Eds.), *Psychological theories of drinking and alcoholism* (2nd ed., pp. 14–53). New York: Guilford Press.

Hartka, E., Johnstone, B., Leino, E., Motoyoshi, M., Temple, M., & Middleton Fillmore, K. (1991). A meta-analysis of depressive symptomatology and alcohol consumption over time. *British Journal of Addiction, 86*, 1283–1298.

Heim, C., Newport, J., Heit, S., Graham, Y., Wilcox, M., Bonsall, R., et al. (2000). Pituitary–adrenal and autonomic responses to stress in women after sexual and physical abuse in childhood. *Journal of the American Medical Association, 284*, 592–596.

Hesselbrock, M., Hesselbrock, V., & Epstein, E. (1999). Theories of the etiology of alcohol and other drug use disorders. In B. S. McCrady & E. E. Epstein (Eds.), *Addictions: A comprehensive guidebook* (pp. 50–72). New York: Oxford University Press.

Hesselbrock, M., Meyer, R., & Keener, J. (1985). Psychopathology in hospitalized alcoholics. *Archives of General Psychiatry, 42,* 1050–1055.

Hussong, A., Hicks, R., Levy, S., & Curran, P. (2001). Specifying the relations between affect and heavy alcohol use among young adults. *Journal of Abnormal Psychology, 110,* 449–461.

Kalodner, C., Delucia, J., & Ursprung, A. (1989). An examination of the tension reduction hypothesis: The relationship between anxiety and alcohol in college students. *Addictive Behaviors, 14,* 649–654.

Kessler, R., Crum, R., Warner, L., Nelson, C., Schulenberg, J., & Anthony, J. (1997). Lifetime co-occurrence of DSM-III-R alcohol abuse and dependence with other psychiatric disorders in the National Comorbidity Survey. *Archives of General Psychiatry, 54,* 313–321.

Kushner, M. G., Sher, K. J., Wood, M. D., & Wood, P. K. (1994). Anxiety and drinking behavior: Moderating effects of tension-reduction alcohol outcome expectancies. *Alcoholism: Clinical and Experimental Research, 18,* 852–860.

Lyubomirsky, S., & Nolen-Hoeksema, S. (1995). Effects of self-focused rumination on negative thinking and interpersonal problem solving. *Journal of Personality and Social Psychology, 69,* 176–190.

Lyubomirsky, S., Tucker, K., Caldwell, N. D., & Berg, K. (1999). Why ruminators are poor problem solvers: Clues from the phenomenology of dysphoric rumination. *Journal of Personality and Social Psychology, 77,* 1041–1060.

Maccoby, E. E., & Jacklin, C. N. (1974). *The psychology of sex differences.* Stanford, CA: Stanford University Press.

Mineka, S., Watson, D., & Clark, L. A. (1998). Comorbidity of anxiety and unipolar mood disorders. *Annual Review of Psychology, 49,* 377–412.

Nolen-Hoeksema, S. (1998, August). *Contributors to the gender difference in rumination.* Paper presented to the annual meeting of the American Psychological Association, San Francisco.

Nolen-Hoeksema, S. (2000). The role of rumination in depressive disorders and mixed anxiety/depressive symptoms. *Journal of Abnormal Psychology, 109,* 504–511.

Nolen-Hoeksema, S. (2002). Gender differences in depression. In I. H. Gotlib & C. L. Hammen (Eds.), *Handbook of depression* (pp. 492–509). New York: Guilford Press.

Nolen-Hoeksema, S. (2003). The response styles theory. In C. Papageorgiou & A. Wells (Eds.), *Depressive rumination: Nature, theory, and treatment of negative thinking in depression* (pp. 107–123). New York: Wiley.

Nolen-Hoeksema, S., & Davis, C. G. (1999). "Thanks for sharing that": Ruminators and their social support networks. *Journal of Personality and Social Psychology, 77,* 801–814.

Nolen-Hoeksema, S., & Jackson, B. (2001). Mediators of the gender difference in rumination. *Psychology of Women Quarterly, 25,* 37–47.

Nolen-Hoeksema, S., & Larson, J. (1999). *Coping with loss.* Mahwah, NJ: Erlbaum.

Nolen-Hoeksema, S., Larson, J., & Grayson, C. (1999). Explaining the gender difference in depressive symptoms. *Journal of Personality and Social Psychology, 77,* 1061–1072.

Nolen-Hoeksema, S., & Morrow, J. (1991). A prospective study of depression and posttraumatic stress symptoms after a natural disaster: The 1989 Loma Prieta earthquake. *Journal of Personality and Social Psychology, 61,* 115–121.

Nolen-Hoeksema, S., Parker, L. E., & Larson, J. (1994). Ruminative coping with depressed mood following loss. *Journal of Personality and Social Psychology, 67,* 92–104.

Olenick, N., & Chalmers, D. (1991). Gender-specific drinking styles in alcoholics and non-alcoholics. *Journal of Studies on Alcohol, 52,* 325–330.

Peirce, R., Frone, M., Russell, M., & Cooper, M. L. (1994). Relationship of financial strain and psychosocial resources to alcohol use and abuse: The mediating role of negative affect and drinking motives. *Journal of Health and Social Behavior, 35,* 291–308.

Ratliff, K., & Burkhart, B. (1984). Sex differences in motivations for and effects of drinking among college students. *Journal of Studies on Alcohol, 45,* 26–32.

Rubonis, A., Colby, S., Monti, P., Rohsenow D., Gulliver, S., & Sirota, A. (1994). Alcohol cue reactivity and mood induction in male and female alcoholics. *Journal of Studies on Alcohol, 55,* 487–494.

Rusting, C., & Nolen-Hoeksema, S. (1998). Regulating responses to anger: Effects of rumination and distraction on angry mood. *Journal of Personality and Social Psychology, 74,* 790–803.

Substance Abuse and Mental Health Administration/Office of Applied Studies. (1997). Percent reporting alcohol use in the past year by age group and demographic characteristics: NHSDA, 1994–1997. Retrieved December 3, 2002, from *http://www.niaaa.nih.gov/databases*

Sannibale, C., & Hall, W. (2001). Gender-related symptoms and correlates of alcohol dependence among men and women with a lifetime diagnosis of alcohol use disorders. *Drug and Alcohol Review, 20,* 369–383.

Siegel, S. J., & Alloy, L. B. (1990). Interpersonal perceptions and consequences of depressive-significant other relationships: A naturalistic study of college roommates. *Journal of Abnormal Psychology, 99,* 361–373.

Stewart, S. H., Karp, J., Pihl, R. O., & Peterson, R. A. (1997). Anxiety sensitivity and self-reported reasons for drug use. *Journal of Substance Abuse, 9,* 223–240.

Swendsen, J. D., Tennen, H., Carney, M. A., Affleck, G., Willard, A., & Hromi, A. (2000). Mood and alcohol consumption: An experience sampling test of the self-medication hypothesis. *Journal of Abnormal Psychology, 109,* 198–204.

Timmer, S., Veroff, J., & Colten, M. (1985). Life stress, helplessness, and the use of alcohol and drugs to cope: An analysis of national survey data. In S. Shiffman & T. Wills (Eds.), *Coping and substance use* (pp. 171–198). New York: Academic Press.

Ward, A., Lyubomirsky, S., Sousa, L., & Nolen-Hoeksema, S. (2003). Can't quite commit: Rumination and uncertainty. *Personality and Social Psychology Bulletin, 29,* 96–107.

Wilsnack, R., & Wilsnack, S. (Eds.). (1997). *Gender and alcohol: Individual and social perpectives.* New Brunswick, NJ: Rutgers Center of Alcohol Studies.

Windle, M., & Miller, B. (1989). Alcoholism and depressive symptomatology among convicted DWI men and women. *Journal of Studies on Alcohol, 50,* 406–413.

Zahn-Waxler, C. (2000). The development of empathy, guilt, and internalization of distress: Implications for gender differences in internalizing and externalizing problems. In R. Davidson (Ed.), *Wisconsin Symposium on Emotion: Vol. 1. Anxiety, depression, and emotion* (pp. 222–265). Oxford, UK: Oxford University Press.

22

Self-Regulation: Context-Appropriate Balanced Attention

DONAL G. MacCOON
JOHN F. WALLACE
JOSEPH P. NEWMAN

In this chapter, we discuss a broad self-regulatory framework in which self-regulation is defined as the context-appropriate allocation of attentional capacity to dominant and nondominant cues. We use the response modulation hypothesis (RMH; Patterson & Newman, 1993) and neural network language to clarify this definition, to argue that the definition captures essential characteristics of self-regulation, to discuss the neurobiological plausibility of our perspective, and to demonstrate the generalizability and relevance of the perspective by applying it to psychopathy, self-discrepancies, eating disorders, neuroticism and extraversion, and acute alcohol consumption. To distinguish this updated framework from the original RMH, we refer to it as the context-appropriate balanced attention (CABA) framework.

SELF-REGULATION: THE CONTEXT-APPROPRIATE ALLOCATION OF ATTENTIONAL CAPACITY TO DOMINANT AND NONDOMINANT CUES

Our definition of self-regulation views limited-capacity, selective attention as a key self-regulatory mechanism. Consistent with this point of view, many perspectives on self-regulation highlight the role of attention (e.g., Baumeister & Heatherton, 1996; Carver & Scheier, 1981; Cohen, Botvinick, & Carter, 2000; Cohen, Dunbar, & McClelland, 1990; Kanfer & Gaelick, 1986; Logan & Cowan, 1984; Norman & Shallice, 1985; Posner & Rothbart, 2000; Thayer & Lane, 2000). Despite important differences in the regulation of emotion, cognition, and behavior, selective attention represents a common regulatory mechanism for each of these domains. Thus, though often categorized as a cognitive variable, we view attention as a "top–down" self-regulatory mechanism capable of enhancing appropriate cognitions, emotions, or behaviors, and suppressing inappropriate cognitions, emotions, or behaviors. Such a mechanism is consistent with recent neural network models and neuroscientific approaches that emphasize selective attention and cognitive control (e.g., Botvinick, Braver, Barch, Carter, & Cohen, 2001; Cohen et al., 1990; Desimone & Duncan, 1995).

In neural network models, particular cognitions, emotions, and behaviors can be represented as networks of coactivated neurons. These networks are activated automatically in a "bottom–up" manner as responses to particular stimuli. According to this perspective, the most activated network of neurons represents the most dominant or prepotent cognition, emotion, or behavior. These are the most likely responses in a given situation. However, alternative responses also are available in the form of less activated neural networks. These responses can become dominant if their activation levels are enhanced by top–down, selective attention. Thus, according to this perspective, the regulation of a dominant response requires the use of limited-capacity, selective attention to enhance the activation level of a nondominant, but more adaptive, response.

The neural network language fits well into language previously used by the RMH (Patterson & Newman, 1993), according to which failures in self-regulation can occur when individuals fail to shift attention to nondominant cues that suggest an important modification of an individual's current dominant response set. We use the phrase "dominant response set" or "dominant response" to refer to the most dominant networks activated at a given time, whereas the term "response" is used generally to refer not only to behavioral responses but also to cognitive and emotional responses. We refer to dominant or nondominant "cues" to indicate that certain stimuli are associated with, or activate, a dominant or nondominant network. Finally, cues can be external stimuli (e.g., a phone ringing) or internal stimuli (e.g., one thought activates another, related thought). Thus, according to the current form of the RMH, if an individual fails to allocate attention to nondominant cues, the responses associated with these cues will fail to achieve a level of activation necessary to compete successfully with a dominant network. Thus, the dominant response set remains unmodified by nondominant cues. This will lead to dysregulation if these nondominant cues are associated with a more adaptive response than the dominant response set.

A classic example of a failure to modify a dominant response is provided by Hamilton, who reports that "Archimedes . . . was so absorbed in geometrical meditation that he was first made aware of the storming of Syracuse by his own death-wound" (as cited by James, 1890, p. 419). In the language of RMH, Archimedes allocated so much attention to his dominant set (thoughts of geometry, geometrical figures on the page, etc.) that he failed to allocate sufficient attention to nondominant cues (e.g., the sound of a battle) that could have saved his life.

The allocation of attention is central to self-regulation in our framework. If too much capacity is allocated to dominant cues, individuals may fail to moderate their dominant behavior by accommodating important information suggested by nondominant cues (e.g., Archimedes). This is the classic case emphasized by the RMH. On the other hand, if too little capacity is allocated to dominant cues, nondominant cues can become dominant and hijack behavior. In such a case, individuals may be distracted from engaging in their most adaptive response, because attention is hijacked by a less adaptive response. The addition of this second case extends and generalizes the RMH by emphasizing the need for context-appropriate attention allocation to dominant and nondominant cues.

The appropriate balance of allocation to dominant and nondominant cues depends on the particular context. For example, if students need to concentrate on studying for a geometry exam, it is adaptive to focus more attention on studying (their dominant response) and less attention on distracting, nondominant cues. In this case, dysregulation might occur if the students fail to maintain enough attention to their studies and become distracted by irrelevant cues. On the other hand, undivided attention to study was not appropriate for Archimedes, who successfully allocated attention to accomplish his goal (e.g., understanding a geometric principle) but failed to accommodate cues that should have suggested a more context-appropriate goal (e.g., saving his own life). Thus, dysregulation can occur when attention is allocated inappropriately for a given context. In the first case, nondominant cues can disrupt an important goal and lead to dysregulated behavior. In the second case, nondominant cues fail to disrupt an important goal and lead to dysregulation. In either case, understanding how attention is allocated is critical to self-regulation.

How Is Attention Allocated?

It is seductive to say that "I" allocate attention to an important goal or a salient cue. The language conveys the idea of a free agent choosing where attention should be placed. However, this explanation is homuncular: How do "I" allocate attention? Also tempting is to propose that attention is allocated according to a current goal: "I adopt a particular goal and then allocate my attention to cues that will help me meet this goal." This is satisfying, because one can define effective self-regulation as anything that furthers one's goal, and dysregulation as anything that disrupts it. However, this answer also invokes a hidden homunculus: Who is adopting the goal? Furthermore, relying on goals in this manner leaves outside the discussion the case in which an individual successfully meets the wrong goal, as in Archimedes' case. In our view, this is important territory to include in a discussion of self-regulation.

Answering the question about how attention is allocated in a nonhomuncular manner is a daunting task, but one that seems tractable if we use the logic of neural networks (see Botvinick, Braver, Carter, Barch, & Cohen, 1998; Botvinick, Nystrom, Fissell, Carter, & Cohen, 1999; Botvinick et al., 2001). Indeed, one primary reason for the attractiveness of neural network models is the promise they hold for a nonhomuncular understanding of human behavior. The answer we present is not complete, but it does push us toward a nonhomuncular understanding of this critical question.

To answer the question, we first propose a tentative, nonhomuncular principle of attention allocation and present evidence for its plausibility. We suggest that selective attention is attracted to the currently most activated network and will activate nondominant networks as capacity allows. Thus, less activated networks will be processed only if capacity is available after processing more activated networks. Recent research on inattentional blindness suggests that this perspective is plausible. In a series of studies, Lavie (1995) manipulated perceptual load and found that as load on the primary task increased, attention to irrelevant distractors decreased. In the language of the CABA framework, when more capacity is allocated to dominant cues, less capacity is allocated to nondominant cues. Thus, as load is increased, attention to nondominant cues decreases.[1]

Finally, there is evidence that even highly salient emotional stimuli are not processed if attentional capacity is not available. Pessoa, McKenna, Gutierrez, and Ungerleider (2002) presented to participants fearful, happy, or neutral faces in the center of a computer screen, with bars in the left and right corners of the screen. After 200 msec, the bars were masked and the face was replaced with an "r", indicating that participants should respond. In the low attentional load condition, participants were instructed to attend to the face and indicate its gender. In the high attentional load condition, participants were instructed to attend to the bars and indicate whether bars were of similar (e.g., both horizontal) or different orientations. The activations of a variety of brain areas were measured with the use of fMRI. The results showed that all brain regions that indicated more activation to emotional faces than to neutral faces demonstrated this differential activation in the low load condition only. In the high load condition, each of these brain areas failed to show differential activation levels to emotional versus neutral faces. This suggests that the emotionality of the faces was not processed when top–down attentional resources were allocated to a demanding task. In CABA terms, the dominant cue in the low load condition was the face, whereas in the high load condition, the dominant cues were the bars. Thus, similar to the logic outlined by Lavie (1995), in the high load condition, the nondominant cues (i.e., the faces) were not processed when the dominant cues (i.e., the bars) required full processing capacity.

Given the importance of dominance within the CABA framework, it is worth noting again that dominance is viewed on a continuum; that is, we believe that a cue's relevance to a dominant response set is continuous rather than dichotomous. This is consistent with feature-based models of attention (e.g., Most et al., 2001), in which a dominant response set consists of attended dimensions or features (spatial location, luminance, shape, etc.). A cue will be very related to the dominant set if it shares all relevant dimensions, and it will be dissimilar to the degree that its characteristics do not overlap with all the relevant attributes specified by the dominant set. A series of experiments conducted by Most and colleagues (2001) provides evidence that this is the case. In Experiment 1, participants were asked to focus on the number of times L's and T's bounced off the edge of a computer screen. Half the participants were told to focus on white L's and T's, and the other half were told to focus on black L's and T's. On a critical trial, a cross took 5 sec to move horizontally across the screen, past the fixation point, and off the left side of the screen. The number of participants who noticed this unexpected stimulus was a dependent measure. Critically, the luminance of the unexpected cross varied across subjects from white to light-gray to dark-gray to black. Thus, the similarity of the cross to a participant's dominant set was manipulated. For example, for participants focusing on black L's and T's, a black cross overlapped on the luminance dimension with this dominant response set. Results demonstrated that the more overlap present between the cross and the participant's dominant set, the more likely the participant was to notice the presence of this unexpected stimulus. In a separate experiment, Most, Simons, Scholl, and Chabris (2000) found that when an unexpected cue (which did not overlap with any participant's dominant set) was presented in the same spatial location as targets, less than half the participants noticed its presence, if they were required to allocate attention to counting targets. However, when attentional capacity was available (participants were not required to count), every participant noticed the unexpected cue. These data are consistent with the idea that nondominant cues differ from dominant cues on a continuum, and that attention will be attracted to such cues to the extent that attentional capacity is available.

Taken together, these studies suggest that an individual's dominant set impacts what nondominant cues will receive attention. Furthermore, if more capacity is dedicated to dominant cues, there appears to be less attention available to attend to nondominant cues. This may be true even when nondominant cues are well-learned, and this apparently extends to emotional cues as well. Thus, when substantial capacity is required for the processing of a dominant set, an individual may lack the capacity to attend to nondominant cues. However, the flip side of this coin is that attention can be hijacked by a nondominant cue, if capacity is available.

Another way that attention can be allocated to a nondominant network is if a dominant and nondominant network compete. If two (or more) networks suggesting incompatible responses achieve about the same level of activation, this conflict must be resolved by top–down attention. Otherwise, there is no clear response available. In the language of the RMH, if a nondominant cue indicates a problem with the current dominant response set, this conflict emits a "call for processing." This call must be answered by top–down attention for effective self-regulation to occur. For example, in an incongruent trial of a classic Stroop task (Stroop, 1935), individuals must choose between a word-related and a color-related response. If the word "red" appears in blue ink, for instance, one response network indicates "red" as an answer, whereas the other indicates "blue" as the answer (see Cohen & Huston, 1992). Top–down attention can resolve this conflict by activating the appropriate response.

Another important type of conflict is the conflict between expected or goal-consistent cues and unexpected cues, between expectations and reality. As with a response conflict, this type of conflict emits a call for processing that must be answered by top–down attention. In this case, attention is necessary to process the incongruent cue, to determine whether it represents valuable information that indicates current behavior must be changed or modified.

Does Our Definition Capture Self-Regulation?

Before describing specific applications of the CABA framework, we consider whether the current definition of "self-regulation" captures what is normally meant by self-regulation. In an overview of self-regulation failure, Baumeister and Heatherton (1996) specify three main ingredients of self-regulation, as suggested by feedback-loop models of self-regulation (e.g., Carver & Scheier, 1998): (1) standards and goals, (2) monitoring, and (3) correction. In this scheme, a failure in self-regulation can occur because of a lack of standards or goals, standards or goals that are too high or too low, or the presence of incompatible/conflicting standards or goals. Dysregulation also can occur as a result of a failure to monitor existing states, thereby failing to register a discrepancy between an individual's standards and actual state. Finally, it is possible that an individual has appropriate goals, is aware that current responses need to be corrected, but lacks the ability to do so.

The CABA framework captures each of these possibilities. From our point of view, standards or goals are conceived as networks (see MacCoon & Newman, in press). Though neither a goal nor a standard need be conscious, both could be established by directing top–down attention to a network or group of networks that, together, represent a current goal or standard. The lack of a goal would be represented as the lack of a coherent set of networks suggesting a clear response to a particular situation. If a network representing the actual state of affairs conflicts with a dominant response, or current goals and expectations, this discrepancy would represent a call for processing. Answering this call for processing will depend on the allocation of attentional capacity. Consistent with the literature reviewed on inattentional blindness, an individual may not recognize the existence of conflicting nondominant cues without available capacity. Correcting a maladaptive response depends on whether enough capacity is available to activate a nondominant network above the current dominant network. Thus, the reasons for dysregulation suggested by Baumeister and Heatherton (1996) can be translated into the neural network terms used by the CABA framework. Furthermore, the current emphasis on the limited capacity of top–down attention, and the important role it plays in self-regulation, is consistent with Baumeister and Heatherton's similar emphasis.

Neurobiological Plausibility

Using a neural network approach to the RMH allows our model of self-regulation to dovetail with modern cognitive neuroscience. At a minimum, we believe that the mechanisms proposed by a self-regulatory perspective should be biologically plausible. Accordingly, we briefly discuss the neurobiological plausibility of our framework. At a general level, neural network approaches highlight the important interaction of "top–down" cognitive control and "bottom–up" automatic influences (e.g., Cohen & Huston, 1992; Cohen et al., 1990; Desimone & Duncan, 1995). Top–down control corresponds to our use of selective attention, whereas sensitivities or biases correspond to bottom–up influences. Cognitive neuroscience is attempting to map top–down control and bottom–up biases to specific neural circuitry. For example, the prefrontal cortex (PFC) has been associated with top–down control (e.g., Cohen et al., 2000) and the maintenance of a current attentional set in the face of distractors (Miller & Cohen, 2001). In our language, the activation of dominant cues is likely to be maintained, in part, by the neurons in the PFC. How information is "gated in" to the PFC is a critical issue that may be illuminated by neuroscientific advances. For example, phasic activity of the locus coeruleus–norepinephrine (LC-NA) system has been associated with increased signal-to-noise ratios and coincides with attentional orienting and superior selective attention (Aston-Jones, Rajkowski, & Cohen, 1999; Usher, Cohen, Servan-Schreiber, Rajkowski, & Aston-Jones, 1999). Dopamine (DA) may also play a critical role in changes in cortical acetylcholine, which appear to mediate allocation of attentional resources (Sarter, Bruno, Turchi, & Nadasdy, 1999; Turchi & Sarter, 1997), and possibly mediate narrowed attention (Dunne & Hartley, 1985). Both systems provide potential neurobiological mechanisms for attentional allocation to dominant and nondominant cues.

The amygdala also is likely to play a role in attentional allocation. The amygdala is best known for its role in the acquisition and expression of fear (e.g., Armony & LeDoux, 2000). However, the amygdala also responds to reward cues (Gallagher, Graham, & Holland, 1990; Hatfield, Han, Conley, Gallagher, & Holland, 1996; Rolls, 2000; Roozendaal, Oldenburger, Strubbe, Koolhaas, & Bohus, 1990) and is involved in processing stimuli that signal a change in reinforcement (e.g., Hatfield et al., 1996). These and other data (e.g., Whalen, 1998) have led to a broader view of the amygdala as a structure that processes ambiguous stimuli that are important for current learning. Particular nuclei of the amygdala are thought to play specific roles in this processing, with the central nucleus in particular being well-suited to increase the allocation of top–down attention to the processing of contextual (in our words, nondominant) cues (Whalen, 1998; Whalen et al., 2001).

The functions of the anterior cingulate cortex (AC) are consistent with a call for processing that results from response conflict. Specifically, activation of the AC may be associated with evaluating response conflicts and indicating the need for top–down control (Carter et al., 2000). Consistent with this proposal, Carter and colleagues (2000) used fMRI to measure AC activation in response to different conditions of a Stroop task. When participants expected a high degree of conflict (in blocks with 80% incongruent and 20% congruent trials) and were thus likely to exert top–down control to minimize response conflict, the AC was relatively inactive on incongruent trials. However, when participants expected a low degree of conflict (in blocks with 20% incongruent and 80% congruent trials), and thus were unlikely to exert top–down control to minimize response conflict, the AC was relatively active on incongruent trials. In other words, the activation of the AC appears to correspond to those trials in which response conflict is high and top–down control is low, a pattern consistent with the view that the AC recognizes conflict and calls for the top–down control necessary to resolve it.

The functions of the hippocampus may be consistent with a call for processing emitted by a conflict between expected or goal-consistent cues and unexpected cues. The hippocampus, a structure that has been a focus for the RMH since the model's inception, responds differentially to cues and secondary goals that are not adequately represented in the current top–down set (Gray & McNaughton, 2000); that is, the hippocampus may boost the activation level of nondominant cues that may be important for moderating the dominant set. For example, rats with a lesioned hippocampus showed fear conditioning to a tone associated with shock but did not show fear conditioning to contextual cues (Kim & Fanselow, 1992), whereas rats with a lesioned amygdala showed no conditioning to the tone but did show conditioning to the context (see also Kim, Rison, & Fanselow, 1993; Phillips & LeDoux, 1992).

We have associated various brain regions (e.g., the PFC, amygdala, and hippocampus) and systems (e.g., the LC-NA and DA systems) with particular aspects of our framework. Bottom–up cues are not likely to be represented by any region in particular; instead, bottom–up processes are likely to be represented throughout the brain. For example, visual stimuli are represented in visual cortices, whereas auditory aspects of stimuli are represented in the auditory cortex. Further research will determine what cognitive concepts can be mapped onto particular brain circuitry, but the RMH view of self-regulation is well-poised both to inform this search and to benefit from its progress.

Summary

We have defined "self-regulation" as the context-appropriate allocation of attentional capacity to dominant and nondominant cues. We have described how a given cognition, emotion, or behavior can be represented as the most activated neural network at a particular moment, and have discussed how this dominant network may be moderated by the influence of other, nondominant networks through attentional allocation. If capacity is available, attention can increase the activation of nondominant networks, thereby increasing their moderating influence on the current dominant response. We have specified a continuous relationship between dominant and nondominant cues, suggesting that a cue is nondominant to the extent its features are dissimilar to features of the dominant set. Put another way, a cue is nondominant to the extent its features do not overlap with the features of the currently dominant cues. Finally, we have proposed that top–down attention is allocated automatically from the most to the least dominant cues, as capacity allows. If two networks achieve similar levels of activation, this conflict attracts attention and is resolved by top–down attention.

Together, these points suggest that regulation is necessary when there is a conflict that, if resolved correctly, will lead to a more adaptive response. Regulation is advisable when a nondominant network represents a more adaptive response. Regulation will fail if there is a context-inappropriate allocation of attention, a situation that can occur for a variety of reasons: (1) if an adaptive network does not achieve the level of bottom–up activation necessary to compete effectively with dominant networks; (2) if an adaptive network achieves enough activation to compete with a dominant response but the conflict is not registered; and (3) if a conflict is registered but there is no allocation of top–down resources to respond to the conflict.

THREE MECHANISMS

In the sections that follow, we use the CABA framework to describe three distinct mechanisms for a failure to allocate necessary top–down resources. First, we argue that psychopathic individuals have a deficit in automatically allocating top–down resources to nondominant cues. We discuss this mechanism in relation to psychopathy, because much of the research done with the RMH has been applied to psychopathic individuals, and much of the available laboratory data can be explained by a deficit in automatically allocating top–down attention. It is this research with psychopathic individuals that best supports the existence of this mechanism and its importance for self-regulation. The mechanism may be overlooked by many self-regulatory theorists, however, because it may be relatively specific to low-anxious, psychopathic individuals. In contrast, the second mechanism may represent a more widely applicable mechanism for self-regulatory problems. The mechanism involves individual emotional biases that prevent a context-appropriate allocation of top–down attention. We explore this mechanism in reference to a variety of psychopathologies and temperaments (e.g., extraversion and neuroticism). Finally, we review theoretical and empirical work suggesting that acute alcohol consumption leads to dysregulation by reducing the amount of capacity available to allocate.

Psychopathy: A Deficit in Automatically Allocating Top–Down Attention

Consider a scene inspired by the movie *Kalifornia* (Bigelow & Sena, 1993). On a rainy night, a bored young man named Early comes across a large rock. Seeing a bridge nearby and an approaching car, he casually decides to see what would happen if he dropped the rock on the car. Early watches as the rock he has dropped from the bridge lands on the windshield of the car, cracking it. He watches as the driver loses control, the car flips over, and both people in the car die. Thirty minutes later, Early enjoys his girlfriend's appreciation as she receives his gift to her, a pair of red pumps worn by the female passenger in the car.

Such a series of acts is a dramatic example of behavior that might be carried out by a psychopathic individual. It is also an example of behavior that some would call "evil," carried out by a "monster" with no regard for human life. We argue that the callous, antisocial behavior and impulsive violence characteristic of psychopathic individuals occur because such individuals fail to interrupt their current dominant set and shift their attention automatically to nondominant cues that suggest a more adaptive response (Wallace & Newman, in press; Wallace, Schmitt, Vitale, & Newman, 2000). We review laboratory evidence supporting this hypothesis, evidence that also argues against other possible mechanisms, such as low intelligence, inadequate motivation, increased sensitivity to reward, or decreased sensitivity to punishment (i.e., fearlessness; for more complete reviews, see Newman, 1998; Newman & Lorenz, 2003).

Our attentional hypothesis suggests that regulating a violent response requires that networks associated with a nonviolent response be activated enough to attract attention, and that attention is allocated to these networks. The RMH suggests that the latter mechanism is deficient in psychopaths. Thus, if a violent behavior becomes dominant, psychopaths are less likely than others to allocate capacity to process nondominant networks associated with a nonviolent response.

Passive avoidance tasks are ideal for testing this hypothesis. RMH predicts that psychopaths will show poor passive avoidance compared to controls. When a psychopath is focused on "go" behavior and cues suggesting inhibition of this behavior are non-dominant, he or she will "go," whereas nonpsychopaths will inhibit this response.

In a classic passive avoidance experiment by Lykken (1957), individuals were required to navigate a mental maze by pressing one of four levers. At each point in the maze, pressing one of the incorrect levers resulted in electric shock. The dominant task was to learn to navigate the maze as quickly as possible. Because shock was incidental to learning the maze, our perspective suggests that the nondominant task was to avoid electric shock. Psychopaths and controls did not differ on the dominant task: Both learned to navigate the maze with equal speed. However, whereas controls showed decreasing numbers of shocks as they learned the maze, psychopaths committed the same number of punished errors throughout, apparently not trying to avoid the shocks at all. This experiment led to the hypothesis that psychopaths are insensitive to punishment (i.e., fearless).

This intuitively appealing hypothesis predicts that psychopaths will differ from controls when punishment cues are present, but will not differ from controls when reward or neutral cues are the only stimuli present in a task. However, this clear prediction has been proved false. We review studies demonstrating that psychopaths' deficit is more general (e.g., the two groups differ in experiments that use only neutral cues) and more specific (e.g., the two groups do not differ in when punishment cues are the only cues present in a task). Instead of supporting a fear deficit, this evidence supports the idea that psychopaths fail to attend to nondominant cues when their attention is engaged already in another, dominant task. Furthermore, because psychopathic and nonpsychopathic participants were well matched on intelligence in each of the studies we review, this does not present a likely explanation for group differences. Several of the studies also argue against the hypothesis that psychopaths are less motivated to perform well than controls.

Newman and Kosson (1986; see also Thornquist & Zuckerman, 1995) used a passive avoidance task to test whether psychopaths were insensitive to punishment, or whether their insensitivity was dependent on an attentional shift. In one condition, participants received money for correctly responding to "good" numbers and lost money for responding to "bad" numbers. Another condition was identical to the first except that the reward contingency was eliminated—only punishment or avoidance of punishment was possible. Because the first condition involves shifting attentional focus between reward and punishment and the second does not involve a shift of focus, the RMH predicts that psychopaths will fail to inhibit their "go" response in the reward–punishment condition but not in the punishment-only condition. In contrast, the low-fear hypothesis predicts passive avoidance deficits in both conditions. Consistent with the RMH, psychopaths showed poorer passive avoidance only when a shift of attention was required (in the reward–punishment condition). Note that because psychopaths' performance was comparable to that of controls in the punishment-only condition of the task, low motivation is not a plausible explanation for the results.

Thus, it appears that psychopaths are responsive to punishment cues when these are the only cues available. However, the RMH makes a more specific prediction: Psychopaths should attend to punishment cues even in a combined reward–punishment task if the task does not require automatic attentional shifts. Newman, Patterson, and Howland (1990) tested this prediction by using a passive avoidance task in which participants were forced to allocate top–down attention to both reward and punishment cues from the outset of the task. In this way, both types of cues were dominant, obviating the need to reallocate attention to nondominant cues during the execution of the task itself. Under these conditions, psychopaths and controls performed similarly.

Results from a gambling task (Newman, Patterson, & Kosson, 1987; Siegel, 1978) also support the attentional hypothesis. In the Newman and colleagues (1987) study, participants won money if a face card was dealt by the computer and lost money if a nonface card was dealt. Because face cards occurred frequently in early blocks and were gradually reduced as play continued, players started the task by winning frequently, gradually won less money as the task continued, and ultimately began losing money. Participants were told that they could stop playing at any time. This decision required modifying the dominant set of playing and winning by using information about the increasing probability of losing (a nondominant cue). Participants played the game in one of three conditions: The computer screen showed no record of cards played, showed a cumulative record of cards displayed on the top of the computer screen in 10-trial blocks, or showed a cumulative record and interrupted play for 5 sec after each trial. In the first condition, nondominant cues of changing probabilities were less salient than in the second condition. In the third condition, participants were forced to interrupt their dominant set, and they were provided with salient, nondominant cues. The authors predicted and found poor performance in psychopaths compared to controls in all but the last condition. Thus, only when their dominant response was interrupted were psychopaths able to allocate attention to nondominant cues, process the fact that contingencies were changing, and modify their card playing behavior as a result. In addition to supporting the RMH, this task makes it clear that psychopaths' deficit can result in harm to themselves, thus emphasizing the self-regulatory nature of their problem.

If it is true that attentional allocation, rather than reward or punishment sensitivities, accounts for psychopaths' dysregulated behavior, psychopaths should fail to attend to any nondominant cue, even when emotion is not involved at all. This is exactly what was found by Newman, Schmitt, and Voss (1997), who used a computer task with emotionally neutral dominant and nondominant cues. In this task, participants viewed pictures with words printed on them. If the dominant cue was a picture, a "P" preceded the trial, if the dominant cue was a word, a "W" preceded the trial. Participants performed better on the task when they were able to focus on the dominant cue and ignore the other, nondominant cue. In this case, psychopaths' deficits should help them perform well on the task, because they fail to shift attention to nondominant cues, whereas controls should do so automatically. Results were consistent with this prediction: The irrelevant, nondominant cue interfered less with the performance of psychopaths than with that of controls. Importantly, these results have been replicated (Hiatt, Schmitt, & Newman, in press).

Finally, it is important to note that the RMH *does* predict that psychopaths will have difficulty using emotion. In this way, the theory is consistent with other theories that emphasize emotion as a deficit in psychopathic individuals (e.g., Blair, 1995; Lykken, 1957, 1995). In keeping with the passive avoidance findings, the RMH predicts that psychopaths will show poor processing of emotion when emotional cues are nondominant and attention is focused on another, dominant cue. To test this prediction, Lorenz and Newman (2002) used a lexical decision task adapted from Williamson, Harpur, and Hare (1991), with positive, negative, and neutral words. Based on a constellation of findings, the authors suggested that psychopaths' failure to process emotion cues is better construed as a failure in response modulation.

The studies described are consistent with the idea that psychopaths fail to allocate attention to nondominant cues when their attention is already allocated to dominant cues. Whereas controls can use nondominant cues automatically, psychopaths appear to have difficulty doing so (see Newman, 1998). This deficit explains why psychopaths can look fearless, but it specifies the conditions under which this will be the case. It also successfully predicts situations in which psychopaths will not look fearless or appear insensitive to punishment cues. The deficit is also consistent with the idea that psychopaths can be emotionless, but, again, it specifies the particular conditions in which this is likely to be the case.

We have been interested in the boundary conditions of the psychopathic deficit. For example, what are the precise conditions under which a psychopath will be able to use a nondominant cue? What role does capacity play? The RMH proposes that psychopaths can allocate attention to cues that are highly related to the dominant response set or that have been made explicitly the object of attention as part of task instructions (in this sense, they become dominant cues). However, when nondominant cues minimally overlap with the dominant set, allocating attention to these cues may be more effortful in psychopaths than in controls and, thus, require more capacity. There is some evidence that psychopaths can make moment-to-moment shifts of attention between one set of cues and another, such as in a divided attention task, but will have to allocate more capacity than controls to the superordinate task of managing a "joint allocation policy" (Kosson & Newman, 1986). For example, Kosson and Newman (1986) used a visual search task and a go/no-go probe-reaction time task with psychopaths and controls in two conditions. In the focused attention condition, participants were told that the visual search task was their primary task, whereas in the divided attention condition, instructions emphasized that performance on both tasks was important. There were no baseline differences between psychopaths and controls, and both groups performed equally well in the focused attention condition, in which switching attention to the nondominant task was not required. However, in the divided attention condition, psychopaths performed more poorly than controls on the visual search task, indicating that they had less capacity available for the search. The authors concluded that the most likely explanation was that psychopaths required more capacity to manage the allocation of their attention between the two tasks; that is, psychopathic individuals must use more capacity to reallocate attention from their top–down set to nondominant cues. Put slightly differently, controls can rely on a more automatic allocation of attention than can psychopaths. Thus, the RMH hypothesis predicts that manipulations meant to reduce limited-capacity resources (e.g., memory load) would not result in performance differences between psychopathic individuals and controls, unless a psychopath is required to manage attention shifts effortfully (which takes capacity) and controls accomplish those shifts relatively automatically.

The CABA perspective makes unique predictions regarding psychopathic information processing. If cue overlap is important, as we have suggested, we would expect such overlap to have a significant effect on whether psychopathic individuals can process information automatically. Recent evidence presented by Hiatt and colleagues (in press) suggests that this is the case. In Experiment 1, which used a color–word Stroop task, psychopaths and controls showed similar interference, indicating similar processing of irrelevant word meaning. In Experiment 3, however, the Stroop task was modified so that the color and word did not overlap spatially. This was accomplished by having white-colored words appear in the center of a colored rectangle (e.g., the word "blue" appeared in the center of a red rectangle). In this way, participants could focus their attention on the spatially distinct colored rectangle, ignoring the irrelevant word displayed in the center of the rectangle. Controls, but not psychopaths, showed significant Stroop interference on this task, which suggests that psychopaths did not process incongruent words. However, psychopaths and controls showed comparable facilitation on trials in which the word and rectangle color matched (e.g., the word "blue" appeared in the center of a blue rectangle).

Although, for these trials, the cues obviously remain spatially separated, note that word meaning and color overlap semantically—they are the same color. Consistent with the current perspective, this suggests that psychopathic individuals do process information automatically when cues overlap, but they fail to do so when overlap is minimized.

In a different experiment (Newman, MacCoon, & Vaughn, 2003, Study 3), psychopaths and controls were compared in their processing of nondominant cues under conditions of low and high load. If psychopathic individuals have difficulty processing secondary information automatically, their failure to process secondary information should exist, regardless of load manipulations. Results were consistent with this perspective.

Several features of the scene from *Kalifornia* described earlier deserve mention. First, consistent with clinical descriptions of psychopathic individuals (e.g., Cleckley, 1976), Early's decision to throw the rock was poorly motivated. In *Kalifornia*, the narrator reminds us that many people have had fleeting thoughts of dropping a penny from the top of a high building. Most of us, however, also attend to a variety of other thoughts (e.g., "Someone will be hurt badly, perhaps a child"; "I might get in trouble for causing injury to someone"; "I can use the penny in the gumball machine instead"; etc.) that cause us to dismiss the idea. According to our account, Early does not shift his attention to nondominant cues such as these; therefore, he does not dismiss the idea. Without attention to these nondominant thoughts, a casual idea is converted into action. Second, Early shows little or no compassion for his victims. Instead of running away from the scene, or exhibiting horror or remorse at what he has done, Early steals a victim's shoes. According to our attentional hypothesis, Early simply focuses his attention on the shoes and does not shift his attention from this dominant cue to other cues associated with compassion, horror, remorse, or fear. Indeed, given a lifetime of nonshifting, it is unlikely that Early will have learned to associate emotional responses with his behavior. Finally, Early gives the stolen shoes to his girlfriend. This is noteworthy for three reasons. First, the fact that Early's girlfriend's birthday falls on that same evening emphasizes the fact that Early did not plan the gift ahead of time: His gift was a spontaneous convenience, much as the thought of throwing the rock was inspired by its coincidental presence. Second, this "evil" man is doing something nice for his girlfriend for her birthday. According to the RMH, the reason Early is doing something nice is much the same as the reason that he picked up a rock and killed two people: Seeing the shoes activated a network associated with his girlfriend's birthday. After Early's attention was focused on this goal, it became his new dominant response. Third, Early shows no apparent discomfort when giving the shoes to his girlfriend. It is as though Early has divorced himself completely from the act that led to his acquisition. Indeed, the ability to achieve such complete separation is consistent with a failure to shift attention to anything unrelated to the current dominant response.

Finally, whereas psychopathy, as diagnosed by the Psychopathy Checklist—Revised (Hare, 1991), includes criminal or antisocial behavior in several of its items, the attentional mechanism we propose should be present in persons without an antisocial background; that is, the form that dysregulated behavior takes should depend on the learning history of the individual: A person with an antisocial background is more likely to have a violent response become activated in a particular situation than is a person without such a background. Thus, a corporate executive with the same attentional deficit would exhibit dysregulated behavior consistent with his background. For example, he might be more likely to harass an employee sexually than to assault that employee. How would this work according to the current framework? Suppose a particular executive's dominant response upon seeing a beautiful woman is to make sexual advances toward her. He likes the challenge and has enjoyed a fair amount of success. When he sees a beautiful employee, his dominant response may be the same. However, because he is less likely than a nonpsychopathic executive to attend to nondominant networks (e.g., "Sexual advances are unethical"; "Sexual advances may ruin our working relationship"; "Sexual advances toward another woman would anger my wife," etc.), the psychopathic executive is more likely to harass his employee sexually. Thus, compared to an executive without the attentional deficit (but with the same background), he is more likely to exhibit a dysregulated dominant response.

Emotion-Driven Narrowed Attention

Whereas the psychopath's deficit is unrelated to the emotionality of a given situation, dysregulation in other forms of psychopathology is related to emotion. Newman and Wallace (1993) proposed three pathways to dysregulated behavior, all of which emphasize the importance of dominant and nondominant cues. The psychopath's deficit in shifting attention represents one pathway. The other two pathways emphasize the role of emotion in causing dysregulation. The principle is that individuals with a bias to a particular type of emotional cue will tend to focus more of their attentional capacity on that cue, thus having less capacity available to attend to nondominant cues that might otherwise moderate their behavior. Thus, like the psychopathic pathway, the emotion pathways emphasize the importance of attending to dominant and nondominant cues in a context-appropriate balance. Unlike that of a psychopath, the deficit specified for the emotion pathway is specific to a situation involving an individual's emotional bias.

Consider a person with an eating disorder. In one situation, a room is relatively free of cues related to weight or eating; in another situation, the room is the same except for the presence of a scale. In the first situation, this individual will be able to attend to networks representing multiple response options and choose the best—or most adaptive—response as a result. In the second situation, a network associated with the individual's concern over weight will become highly activated, and the individual will focus more of his or her attention on this network, leaving less capacity to activate (and thus consider) the other response options. Thus, the individual in this situation is less likely to choose the most adaptive response.

This hypothesis was tested in a study conducted by Newman and colleagues (1993, Study 3). Controls and participants from an eating disorders clinic were asked to respond to letter or number strings presented centrally (75% of the time) or peripherally (25% of the time) on a computer monitor. The high probability of centrally presented stimuli established a dominant attentional set. To signal the start of each trial, a word appeared centrally. The word was either related to body concerns (e.g., "scale"), an emotional word unrelated to body concerns (e.g., "sad"), or a neutral word (e.g., "pattern"). The authors predicted that participants from the eating disorders clinic would make slower letter–number decisions to peripheral strings than controls when words related to their bias were presented as a warning stimulus, because these words would attract attention and slow the processing of the nondominant peripheral cues. Results supported these predictions.

A similar study (Experiment 1) used a modified version of the task with non-clinically anxious and nonanxious participants. Warning words consisted of physical threat words (e.g., "injury"), social threat words (e.g., "ridiculed") or safety words (e.g., "friend"). Anxious individuals were slower to respond to targets when the central word was related to their bias (i.e., a threatening word), a result consistent with the idea that when individuals are presented with a cue related to their bias, attention focuses on this cue and reduces the processing of nondominant cues.

Given the importance of self-discrepancies in the initiation of self-regulation (e.g., Carver, 1979; Carver & Scheier, 1998; Higgins, 1987), the authors tested whether warning words related to a self-discrepancy also would reveal a similar pattern (Newman et al., 1993, Experiment 2). Self-discrepancy theory (Higgins, 1987) proposes that individuals are motivated to reduce any discrepancy between their actual self (qualities that the individual believes she or he possesses) and their ought self (qualities that the individual or significant others believe she or he should possess). Controls were individuals who had low discrepancies of any kind, and the experimental group had high actual–ought discrepancies. Participants were given words that were either relevant or irrelevant to their discrepancies. Results were consistent with prediction. When members of the high-discrepancy experimental group were presented with words related to their discrepancies in the center of the computer screen, they responded more slowly to peripheral cues relative to trials in which irrelevant words were presented centrally. These and the other results reviewed are consistent with the idea that emotionally relevant cues can disrupt the processing of nondominant cues and cause poorer performance on a laboratory task in anxious individuals, individuals with eating disorders, or nonpathological individuals presented with self-discrepant cues.

These three studies suggest the generalizability of emotion-mediated narrowing of attention and suggest its applicability to self-regulation. The framework also has been used to understand the role of neuroticism in dysregulation. Neuroticism, an important variable in self-regulation, is associated with negative affect (e.g., Costa & McCrae, 1980; Eaves, Eysenck, & Martin, 1989; Larsen & Ketelaar, 1989; Tellegen, 1985; Watson & Clark, 1984) and various forms of psychopathology, including anxiety (Gray, 1981; Wallace, Bachorowski, & Newman, 1991), depression (Enns & Cox, 1997; Scott, Williams, Brittleband, & Ferrier, 1995), alcoholism (Sher & Trull, 1994), and personality disorders (Widiger & Costa, 1994). Based on past work from our laboratory (Wallace & Newman, 1997; Wallace et al., 1991), we view extraversion as a bias to allocate attention preferentially to reward cues, and introversion as a bias to allocate attention preferentially to punishment cues. Neuroticism is associated with overallocating attention to an individual's particular bias (i.e., cues with high degrees of bottom–up activation). Thus, we typically investigate the effect of neuroticism on self-regulation by testing the effects of reward on extraverts, and the effects of punishment on introverts. We often compare stable (i.e., non-neurotic) extraverts to neurotic introverts, for example, because we expect the largest differences between these groups. This is because neurotic introverts have a punishment bias that is likely to be magnified by their neuroticism, whereas stable extraverts do not have such a bias and are not neurotic. Use of this approach has yielded results consistent with the proposal that neuroticism leads to dysregulation by increasing the allocation of attention to dominant cues.

For example, Wallace and Newman (1990) asked participants to trace a circle as slowly as possible, a task that requires the regulation of motor responses and has been used as a measure of executive function (e.g., Giancola & Parker, 2001). Wallace and Newman predicted that failures in self-regulation would occur if participants were required to perform the task in the presence of bias-related cues. According to the current perspective, bias-related cues can lead to dysregulated circle tracing as a result of several processing stages. First, such cues will activate networks incompatible with slow circle tracing. Second, these networks will attract more attention by virtue of their greater levels of activation, leaving less capacity available to regulate a motor response in accordance with task demands. Third, bias-related cues should increase nonspecific arousal in participants, especially in neurotic individuals. This increased arousal will increase the attention allocated to bias-related cues, further decreasing the capacity available to regulate motor responses. This perspective predicts that, in the presence of reward cues, neurotic extraverts will trace faster than controls (stable introverts), and that in the presence of punishment cues, neurotic introverts will show dysregulated (in this case, faster) motor responses. Results were consistent with these predictions and have been replicated (e.g., Bachorowski & Newman, 1990; Nichols & Newman, 1986), indicating a failure to regulate responses. These variables also have been applied to passive avoidance deficits, considered fundamental to maladaptive impulsivity (e.g., Patterson, Kosson, & Newman, 1987, Segarra, Molto, & Torrubia, 2000).

Newman, Schmitt, and colleagues (1997) conducted a two-phase study that provides better evidence for the current perspective. In the first phase, participants were told to press a button when letter strings appeared on the computer screen, unless the string contained the letter "Q." In this case, responses were punished. Thus, in phase 1, participants were trained to have an attention bias to a previously neutral stimulus. In phase 2, participants were told to respond to strings on the computer screen, unless they contained a number. Though the letter "Q" is irrelevant for phase 2, it should moderate responses to the degree it was attended to and processed as a punishment cue in phase 1. Thus, according to the current framework, an introvert with a preexisting bias to attend to punishment cues would be more likely to allocate capacity to processing the "Q." This tendency would be magnified in a neurotic introvert, because increased arousal should increase the amount of capacity allocated to punishment cues. Results were consistent with this perspective. Compared to stable extraverts, neurotic introverts responded more slowly to "Q"-present trials relative to "Q"-absent trials in phase 2, indicating that the bias acquired in phase 1 was difficult to regulate in phase 2. The performance of high- and low-anxious participants as defined by the State–Trait Anxiety Inventory (STAI; Spielberger, Gorsuch, Lushene, & Vagg, 1977) mirrored that of the neurotic introverts and stable extraverts, respectively. In this task, it is most adaptive to attend to the "Q" in phase 1, but allocate no special attention to it in phase 2. As predicted, however, anxious individuals who have a bias to process punishment cues have difficulty allocating their attention appropriately when the context changes in phase 2. As a result, they are more likely than controls to attend to an irrelevant stimulus, and their response times suffer.

The CABA framework's emphasis on the role of capacity in self-regulation makes unique predictions about information processing. For example, the framework predicts that as capacity decreases, individuals will continue to process bias-related cues (their priority) at the expense of processing cues unrelated to this bias. According to this perspective, anxious individuals should process neutral and bias-related (e.g., threatening or novel cues) cues alike, when capacity is available, but should process threat cues differentially as capacity decreases.

To illustrate the applicability of this situation to a nonlaboratory situation, imagine an anxious person, who is afraid of public speaking, standing in front of a large audience. Her task is to deliver her speech fluently, something she has done in practice when her attention was allocated completely to the task. However, in a room full of people, her bias is to attend to negative (or potentially negative) cues. Her speech will proceed smoothly to the extent that she can maintain her attention on her primary task without overallocating capacity to negative cues. At the beginning of the speech, networks associated with fluent speaking may be dominant. However, a bias toward negative cues means that such cues easily activate other networks that might include increased heart rate, sweating, and the urge to escape the situation. If cues associated with this network begin to capture attentional capacity, the activation level of these negative networks—and thus, their influence on behavior—will increase. Furthermore, as capacity is allocated increasingly to these negative networks, less capacity exists to activate a network consistent with a fluent delivery of the speech. As the allocation of attention changes, the likelihood that the anxious presenter will make an error increases. Unfortunately, a stutter, a long pause, or a mispronounced word are likely to increase the activation of negative networks and the amount of attention allocated to such networks, thus deepening the dysregulatory cycle.

In summary, emotional bias can cause a context-inappropriate allocation of attention by increasing an individual's allocation of attention to bias-related cues. This may negatively impact self-regulation either because affected individuals fail to attend to nondominant cues that might suggest a more adaptive response, or because bias-related cues distract individuals from the appropriate focus. We have presented evidence consistent with this type of mechanism in individuals with eating disorders, anxious individuals, individuals presented with self-discrepancies, and neurotic individuals with either reward- or punishment-related biases.

Alcohol-Induced Narrowed Attention

Giancola (2000) documents the positive relationship between acute alcohol consumption and impulsive aggression, and reviews several theories advanced to account for this relationship, including his own executive functioning framework. As Giancola's discussion makes clear, many theories emphasize concepts related to the dominant–nondominant dimension we are highlighting. Furthermore, these theories emphasize the role that alcohol plays in narrowing attention to dominant cues, the same mechanism advocated in the current framework. Pernanen (1976) proposed that alcohol reduces the ability to attend to and process environmental or internal cues that would moderate an aggressive response. Taylor and Leonard (1983) also proposed that alcohol reduces the number of cues to which an individual can attend: As the number of attended cues decreases, the likelihood of attending to inhibitory cues also decreases, thus making aggression more likely. Steele and Josephs (1990) proposed that alcohol impairs an individual's ability to allocate attention to nonsalient cues. As a result, processing and behavior are dominated by the most salient cues in the current context. If these dominant cues suggest an aggressive response and less dominant cues suggest an inhibitory response, aggression is made more likely.

Giancola's own framework (2000) emphasizes four skills that can inhibit impulsive aggression, each of which involves attending to and processing nondominant cues: (1) attending to and appraising situational information; (2) taking the perspective of others; (3) considering the consequences of one's actions; and (4) defusing a hostile situation. The first skill requires attending to multiple aspects of the environment; the second requires shifting attention from cues of personal relevance to cues representing another person's perspective; the third involves attending to nondominant cues that may suggest the inhibition of aggression; and the fourth requires scanning the environment to plan, monitor, and modify attempts to reduce hostility in an opponent. In short, inhibiting impulsive aggression may require the consideration of an alternative response. Finally, in integrating empirical work on alcohol's effects on emotion, Lang, Patrick, and Stritzke (1999) argue that alcohol affects emotion by disrupting higher brain functions, such as selective attention, that modulate affective brain systems.

The elements highlighted in each theory are consistent with our view of self-regulation. Specifically, they suggest that alcohol increases dysregulation by limiting the processing of nondominant cues through a reduction in top–down capacity. This perspective has been supported by recent studies that have used fear-potentiated startle. For example, in a study by Curtin, Lang, Patrick, and Stritzke (1998), participants who were served alcoholic or nonalcoholic drinks viewed gray backgrounds (low load) or pleasant slides (high load) either under threat of shock or in a safety condition. The authors found robust fear-potentiated startle in the threatening versus safe condition regardless of load in the nonalcohol group. Intoxicated participants also showed fear-potentiated startle in the low-load condition; however, when concurrent processing was required (i.e., high load), intoxicated participants did not show significant fear-potentiated startle.

These findings were replicated conceptually and extended by Curtin, Patrick, Lang, Cacioppo, and Birbaumer (2001) in a study that measured fear-potentiated startle, P3 event-related potentials, and response inhibition. In this paradigm, participants viewed animal or body part words on a computer screen. Shock was predicted by words of a particular category (e.g., animals), and the trial ended with the presentation of a blue square. In the low-load condition, participants simply viewed the words and were thus free to focus their attention on the threatening aspect of the word. In the divided attention condition, participants were required to hit a button when the blue square appeared, if the word had been presented in the color green, and to inhibit this response, if the word had been colored red. Thus, in this condition, participants were required to divide their attention between task instructions and the threatening aspect of the word. As predicted, when attentional capacity was divided, intoxicated participants showed reduced processing of threat (as indexed by reduced P3 differentiation between threat and safe words), reduced fear-potentiated startle, and reduced response inhibition.

Impulsive aggression is one form of dysregulation increased by alcohol. However, the emphasis on dominant and nondominant cues suggests that alcohol-related aggression is part of a more general self-regulatory problem: By reducing the amount of attention to nondominant cues, alcohol increases the likelihood that behavior will reflect only the dominant cues in a given context. Thus, if the dominant cues suggest an aggressive response, aggression is more likely. However, if the dominant cues suggest a nonaggressive response, nonaggression is more likely.

In a recent study, Casbon, Curtin, Lang, and Patrick (2003) manipulated memory load and dominant responses in alcohol-intoxicated or nonintoxicated students (for a review of alcohol, self-awareness, and self-regulation failure, see Hull & Sloane, Chapter 24, this volume). The experiment used an *n*-back task, in which letters are presented successively on the screen, and participants respond by pressing a button if the current letter matches the letter presented one screen before (the low-load, 1-back condition) or two screens before (the high-load, 2-back condition). The memory load condition was manipulated within-subject across blocks. In addition, the frequency of responding was manipulated by instructing participants to respond to targets on some blocks and respond to nontargets on others (targets were present on 20% of trials). The authors predicted that relative to nonintoxicated controls, intoxicated participants would fail to use changing contingencies to moderate their dominant response in the high-load condition. Consistent with this prediction, intoxicated participants in the high-load condition committed errors specific to the response made most dominant by the task: In 20% response blocks, these participants committed more omission errors than did controls; in 80% response blocks, they committed more errors of commission than did controls. Groups did not differ in the low-load condition or in overall task performance. These data suggest that when capacity is limited by the use of alcohol and then taxed by a demanding task, individuals are unable to use attentional capacity to modify their dominant response.

SUMMARY

We have defined self-regulation as the context-appropriate allocation of attention to dominant and nondominant cues. We suggest that for any given context, there is an ideal balance in the allocation of top–down attention, such that an individual's goals are met but can be flexibly modified by new information. We identified neural circuitry that might underlie the mechanisms we hypothesize. We have discussed how the allocation of attention to dominant and nondominant cues provides a useful perspective for understanding the callous and violent behavior that characterizes incarcerated psychopaths. Specifically, we have argued that psychopathic individuals fail to allocate their attention automatically from dominant to nondominant networks. We also have discussed one way that emotional biases can hijack top–down attention, thus disrupting context-appropriate allocation of attention. We have illustrated this point by highlighting neuroticism and extraversion as individual difference variables that play a prominent role in impulsivity and anxiety. Finally, we have reviewed theoretical and empirical work suggesting that alcohol acts as yet another way in which attention to nondominant cues can be reduced. As we have seen, the narrowed attention that accompanies acute alcohol consumption can lead to impulsive aggression and other dysregulated responses. Thus, it appears that, across several domains, self-regulation can be conceptualized as the context-appropriate allocation of attention to dominant and nondominant cues. In addition to offering a broadly applicable conceptualization of self-regulation, the CABA framework also suggests specific self-regulatory mechanisms that can be tested empirically. Finally, the perspective suggests particular individual-difference variables that can be used to understand these mechanisms and the consequences of poor self-regulation.

NOTE

1. If conscious awareness of stimuli depends on the activation level of a particular network, top–down attention focused on a network will increase awareness of that network. In a recent functional magnetic resonance imaging (fMRI) study, Rees, Frith, and Driver (1999) found that when attention was occupied with pictures, brain activation indicated no distinction between words and random letter strings, even when these stimuli were viewed directly. The authors concluded that "visual recognition wholly depends on attention even for highly familiar and meaningful stimuli at the center of gaze" (p. 2504); that is, when an individual's dominant set included only pictures, fMRI indicated no processing of nondominant words and letter strings. Similarly, in a study using event-related brain potentials, Bentin, Kutas, and Hillyard (1995) concluded that both attended and unattended words in a dichotic listening task activated semantic representations, but that attended words were more likely than unattended words to achieve the activation level necessary for conscious accessibility.

REFERENCES

Armony, J. L., & LeDoux, J. E. (2000). How danger is encoded: Toward a systems, cellular, and computational understanding of cognitive-emotional interactions in fear. In M. S. Gazzaniga

(Ed.), *The new cognitive neurosciences* (2nd ed., pp. 1067–1079). Cambridge, MA: MIT Press.

Aston-Jones, G., Rajkowski, J., & Cohen, J. (1999). Role of locus coeruleus in attention and behavioral flexibility. *Biological Psychiatry, 46,* 1309–1320.

Bachorowski, J. A., & Newman, J. P. (1990). Impulsive motor behavior: Effects of personality and goal salience. *Journal of Personality and Social Psychology, 58*(3), 512–518.

Baumeister, R. F., & Heatherton, T. F. (1996). Self-regulation failure: An overview. *Psychological Inquiry, 7*(1), 1–15.

Bentin, S., Kutas, M., & Hillyard, S. A. (1995). Semantic processing and memory for attended and unattended words in dichotic listening: Behavioral and electrophysiological evidence. *Journal of Experimental Psychology: Human Perception and Performance, 21*(1), 54–67.

Blair, R. J. R. (1995). A cognitive developmental approach to morality: Investigating the psychopath. *Cognition, 57*(1), 1–29.

Bigelow, L. (Producer), & Sena, D. (Director). (1993). *Kalifornia* [Motion picture]. United States: Metro-Goldwyn-Mayer.

Botvinick, M., Nystrom, L. E., Fissell, K., Carter, C. S., & Cohen, J. D. (1999). Conflict monitoring versus selection-for-action in anterior cingulate cortex. *Nature, 402,* 179–181.

Botvinick, M. M., Braver, T. S., Barch, D. M., Carter, C. S., & Cohen, J. D. (2001). Conflict monitoring and cognitive control. *Psychological Review, 108*(3), 624–652.

Botvinick, M. M., Braver, T. S., Carter, C. S., Barch, D. M., & Cohen, J. D. (1998). *Toward a nonhomuncular account of control: Cognitive neuroscientific evidence for crosstalk monitoring.* (Report No. TR 001-98). Pittsburgh, PA: Center for the Neural Basis of Cognition.

Carter, C. S., MacDonald, A. M., Botvinick, M., Ross, L., Stenger, V. A., & Noll, D. C. J. (2000). Parsing exectuve processes: Strategic vs. evaluative functions of the anterior cingulate cortex. *Proceedings of the National Academy of Sciences, USA, 97*(4), 1944–1948.

Carver, C., & Scheier, M. (1981). *Attention and self-regulation.* New York: Springer-Verlag.

Carver, C. S. (1979). A cybernetic model of self-attention processes. *Journal of Personality and Social Psychology, 37,* 1251–1281.

Carver, C. S., & Scheier, M. F. (1998). *On the self-regulation of Behavior.* Cambridge, UK: Cambridge University Press.

Casbon, T. S., Curtin, J. J., Lang, A. R., & Patrick, C. J. (2003). Deleterious effects of alcohol intoxication: Diminished cognitive control and its behavioral consequences. *Journal of Abnormal Psychology, 112*(3), 476–487.

Cleckley, H. (1976). *The mask of sanity* (5th ed.). St. Louis, MO: Mosby.

Cohen, J. D., Botvinick, M., & Carter, C. S. (2000). Anterior cingulate and prefrontal cortex: Who's in control? *Nature Neuroscience, 3*(5), 421–423.

Cohen, J. D., Dunbar, K., & McClelland, J. L. (1990). On the control of automatic processes: A parallel distribution processing account of the Stroop effect. *Psychological Review, 97*(3), 332–361.

Cohen, J. D., & Huston, T. A. (1992). Progress in the use of interactive models for understanding attention and performance. In C. Umilta & M. Moscovitch (Eds.), *Attention and performance: XV. Conscious and nonconscious information processing* (pp. 453–476). Cambridge, MA: MIT Press.

Costa, P. T., & McCrae, R. R. (1980). Influence of extraversion and neuroticism on subjective well-being: Happy and unhappy people. *Journal of Personality and Social Psychology, 38*(4), 668–678.

Curtin, J. J., Lang, A. R., Patrick, C. J., & Stritzke, W. G. K. (1998). Alcohol and fear-potentiated startle: The role of competing cognitive demands in the stress-reducing effects of intoxication. *Journal of Abnormal Psychology, 107*(4), 547–557.

Curtin, J. J., Patrick, C. J., Lang, A. R., Cacioppo, J. T., & Birbaumer, N. (2001). Alcohol affects emotion through cognition. *Psychological Science, 12*(6), 527–531.

Desimone, R., & Duncan, J. (1995). Neural mechanisms of selective visual attention. *Annual Review of Neuroscience, 18,* 193–222.

Dunne, M. P., & Hartley, L. R. (1985). The effects of scopolamine upon verbal memory: Evidence for an attentional hypothesis. *Acta Psychologia, 58*(3), 205–217.

Eaves, L. J., Eysenck, H. J., & Martin, N. G. (1989). *Genes, culture and personality: An empirical approach.* San Diego, CA: Academic Press.

Enns, M. W., & Cox, B. J. (1997). Personality dimensions and depression: Review and commentary. *Canadian Journal of Psychiatry, 42*(3), 274–284.

Gallagher, M., Graham, P. W., & Holland, P. C. (1990). The amygdala central nucleus and appetitive Pavlovian conditioning: Lesions impair one class of conditioned performance. *Journal of Neuroscience, 10,* 1906–1911.

Giancola, P. R. (2000). Executive functioning: A conceptual framework for alcohol-related aggression. *Experimental and Clinical Psychopharmacology, 8*(4), 576–597.

Giancola, P. R., & Parker, A. M. (2001). A six-year prospective study of pathways toward drug use in adolescent boys with and without a family history of a substance abuse disorder. *Journal of Studies on Alcohol, 62,* 166–178.

Gray, J. A. (1981). A critique of Eysenck's theory of personality. In H. J. Eysenck (Ed.), *A model for personality* (pp. 246–276). Berlin: Springer-Verlag.

Gray, J., & McNaughton, N. (2000). *The neuropsychology of anxiety: An enquiry into the functions of the septo-hippocampal system* (2nd ed). Oxford, UK: Oxford University Press.

Hare, R. D. (1991). *The Hare Psychopathy Checklist—Revised.* Toronto: Multi-Health Systems.

Hatfield, T., Han, J.-S., Conley, M., Gallagher, M., & Holland, P. (1996). Neurotoxic lesions of the basolateral, but not central, amygdala interfere with Pavlovian second-order conditioning and reinforcer-devaluation effects. *Journal of Neuroscience, 16,* 5256–5265.

Hiatt, K. D., Schmitt, W. A., & Newman, J. P. (in press). Stroop tasks reveal abnormal selective attention among psychopathic offenders. *Neuropsychology.*

Higgins, E. T. (1987). Self-discrepancy: A theory relating self and affect. *Psychological Review, 94,* 319–340.

James, W. (1890). *The principles of psychology.* New York: Dover.

Kanfer, F. H., & Gaelick, L. (1986). Self-management models. In F. H. Kanfer & A. P. Goldstein (Eds.), *Helping people change: A textbook of methods* (3rd ed., pp. 283–345). New York: Pergamon Press.

Kim, J. J., & Fanselow, M. S. (1992). Modality specific retrograde amnesia of fear following hippocampal lesions. *Science, 256,* 675–677.

Kim, J. J., Rison, R. A., & Fanselow, M. S. (1993). Effects of amygdala, hippocampus, and periaqueductal gray lesions on short- and long-term contextual fear. *Behavioral Neuroscience, 107*(6), 1093–1098.

Kosson, D. S., & Newman, J. P. (1986). Psychopathy and the allocation of attentional capacity in a divided-attention situation. *Journal of Abnormal Psychology, 95*(3), 257–263.

Lang, A. R., Patrick, C. J., & Stritzke, W. G. K. (1999). Alcohol and emotional response: A multidimensional–multilevel analysis. In K. E. Leonard & H. T. Blane (Eds.), *Psychological theories of drinking and alcoholism* (2nd ed., pp. 328–371). New York: Guilford Press.

Larsen, R. J., & Ketelaar, T. (1989). Extraversion, neuroticism and susceptibility to positive and negative mood induction procedures. *Personality and Individual Differences, 10*(12), 1221–1228.

Lavie, N. (1995). Perceptual load as a necessary condition for selective attention. *Journal of Experimental Psychology: Human Perception and Performance, 21*(3), 451–468.

Logan, G. D., & Cowan, W. B. (1984). On the ability to inhibit thought and action: A theory of an act of control. *Psychological Review, 91,* 295–327.

Lorenz, A. R., & Newman, J. P. (2002). Deficient response modulation and emotion processing in low-anxious Caucasian psychopathic offenders: Results from a lexical decision task. *Emotion, 2*(2), 91–104.

Lykken, D. T. (1957). A study of anxiety in the sociopathic personality. *Journal of Abnormal and Social Psychology, 55,* 6–10.

Lykken, D. T. (1995). *The antisocial personalities.* Hillsdale, NJ: Erlbaum.

MacCoon, D. G., & Newman, J. P. (in press). Content meets process: Using attributions and standards to inform cognitive vulnerability in psychopathy, antisocial personality disorder, and depression. *Journal of Social and Clinical Psychology.*

Miller, E. K., & Cohen, J. D. (2001). An integrative theory of prefrontal cortex function. *Annual Review of Neuroscience, 24,* 167–202.

Most, S. B., Simons, D. J., Scholl, B. J., & Chabris, C. F. (2000). Sustained inattentional blindness: The role of location in the detection of unexpected dynamic events. *Psyche, 6*(14). Retrieved September 23, 2003, from *http://psyche.cs.monash.edu.au/v6/psyche-6–14–most.html*

Most, S. B., Simons, D. J., Scholl, B. J., Jimenez, R., Clifford, E., & Chabris, C. F. (2001). How not to be seen: The contribution of similarity and selective ignoring to sustained inattentional blindness. *Psychological Science, 12*(1), 9–17.

Newman, J. P. (1998). Psychopathic behavior: An information processing perspective. In D. J. Cooke, R. D. Hare, & A. Forth. (Eds.), *Psychopathy: Theory, research and implications for society* (pp. 81–104). Netherlands: Kluwer Academic.

Newman, J. P., & Kosson, D. S. (1986). Passive avoidance learning in psychopathic and nonpsychopathic offenders. *Journal of Abnormal Psychology, 95,* 257–263.

Newman, J. P., & Lorenz, A. R. (2003). Response modulation and emotion processing: Implications for psychopathy and other dysregulatory psychopathology. In R. J. Davidson, K. Scherer, & H. H. Goldsmith (Eds.), *Handbook of affective sciences* (pp. 1043–1067). Oxford, UK: Oxford University Press.

Newman, J. P., MacCoon, D. G., & Vaughn, L. J. (2003). *Identifying Primary and secondary psychopaths: Low fear or general anxiety?* Manuscript submitted for publication.

Newman, J. P., Patterson, C. M., Howland, E. W., & Nichols, S. L. (1990). Passive avoidance in psychopaths: The effects of reward. *Personality and Individual Differences, 11*(11), 1101–1114.

Newman, J. P., Patterson, C. M., & Kosson, D. S. (1987). Response perseveration in psychopaths. *Journal of Abnormal Psychology, 96,* 145–148.

Newman, J. P., Schmitt, W. A., & Voss, W. D. (1997). The impact of motivationally neutral cues on psychopathic individuals: Assessing the generality of the response modulation hypothesis. *Journal of Abnormal Psychology, 106*(4), 563–575.

Newman, J. P., & Wallace, J. F. (1993). Diverse pathways to deficient self-regulation: Implications for disinhibitory psychopathology in children. *Clinical Psychology Review, 13,* 699–720.

Newman, J. P., Wallace, J. F., Schmitt, W. A., & Arnett, P. A. (1997). Behavioral inhibition system functioning in anxious, impulsive and psychopathic individuals. *Personality and Individual Differences, 23*(4), 583–592.

Newman, J. P., Wallace, J. F., Strauman, T. J., Skolaski, R. L., Oreland, K. M., Mattek, P. W., et al. (1993). Effects of motivationally significant stimuli on the regulation of dominant responses. *Journal of Personality and Social Psychology, 65*(1), 165–175.

Nichols, S. L., & Newman, J. P. (1986). Effects of punishment on response latency in extraverts. *Journal of Personality and Social Psychology, 50*(3), 624–630.

Norman, D. A., & Shallice, T. (1985). Attention to action: Willed and automatic control of behaviour. In R. J. Davidson, G. E. Schwartz, & D. Shapiro (Eds.), *Consciousness and self-regulation: Advances in research* (Vol. 4, pp. 1–18). New York: Plenum Press.

Patterson, C. M., & Newman, J. P. (1993). Reflectivity and learning from aversive events: Toward a psychological mechanism for the syndromes of disinhibition. *Psychological Review, 100*(4), 716–736.

Patterson, C. M., Kosson, D. S., & Newman, J. P. (1987). Reaction to punishment, reflectivity, and passive avoidance in extraverts. *Journal of Personality and Social Psychology, 52*(3), 565–575.

Pernanen, K. (1976). Alcohol and crimes of violence. In B. Kissin & H. Begleiter (Eds.), *The biology of alcoholism: Social aspects of alcoholism* (Vol. 4, pp. 351–444). New York: Plenum Press.

Pessoa, L., McKenna, M., Gutierrez, E., & Ungerleider, L. G. (2002). Neural processing of emotional faces requires attention. *Proceedings of the National Academy of Sciences, USA,* 99(17), 11458–11463.

Phillips, R. G., & LeDoux, J. E. (1992). Differential contribution of amygdala and hippocampus to cued and contextual fear conditioning. *Behavioral Neuroscience, 106,* 274–285.

Posner, M. I., & Rothbart, M. K. (2000). Developing mechanisms of self-regulation. *Development and Psychopathology, 12,* 427–441.

Rees, G., Russell, C., Frith, C., & Driver, J. (1999). Inattentional blindness versus inattentional amnesia for fixated but ignored words. *Science, 286,* 2504–2507.

Rolls, E. T. (2000). Memory systems in the brain. *Annual Review of Psychology, 51,* 599–630.

Roozendaal, B., Oldenburger, W. P., Strubbe, J. H., Koolhaus, J. M., & Bohus, B. (1990). The central amygdala is involved in the conditioned but not in the meal-induced cephalic insulin response in the rat. *Neuroscience Letters, 116,* 210–215.

Sarter, M., Bruno, J. P., Turchi, J., & Nadasdy, Z. (1999). Basal forebrain afferent projections modulating cortical acetylcholine, attention, and implications for neuropsychiatric disorders. In J. F. McGinty (Ed.), *Advancing from the ventral striatum to the extended amygdala: Implications for neuropsychiatry and drug use: In honor of Lennart Heimer* (Vol. 877, pp. 368–382). New York: New York Academy of Sciences.

Scott, J., Williams, J. M., Brittleband, A., & Ferrier, I. N. (1995). The relationship between premorbid neuroticism, cognitive dysfunction and persistence of depression: A 1-year follow-up. *Journal of Affective Disorders, 33*(3), 167–172.

Segarra, P., Molto, J., & Torrubia, R. (2000). Passive avoidance learning in extraverted females. *Personality and Individual Differences, 29,* 239–254.

Sher, K. J., & Trull, T. J. (1994). Personality and disinhibitory psychopathology: Alcoholism and antisocial personality disorder. *Journal of Abnormal Psychology, 103*(1), 92–102.

Siegel, R. A. (1978). Probability of punishment and suppression of behavior in psychopathic and nonpsychopathic offenders. *Journal of Abnormal Psychology, 87,* 514–522.

Spielberger, C. D., Gorsuch, R. L., Lushene, R., Vagg, P. R., & Jacobs, G. A. (1977). *Manual for the State–Trait Anxiety Inventory (Form Y).* Palo Alto, CA: Consulting Psychologists Press.

Steele, C. M., & Josephs, R. A. (1990). Alcohol myopia: Its prized and dangerous effects. *American Psychologist, 45*(8), 921–933.

Stroop, J. R. (1935). Studies of interference in serial verbal reactions. *Journal of Experimental Psychology, 18,* 643–662.

Taylor, S., & Leonard, K. (1983). Alcohol and human physical aggression. In R. Green & E. Donnerstein (Eds.), *Aggression: Theoretical and empirical reviews* (Vol. 2, pp. 77–101). New York: Academic Press.

Tellegen, A. (1985). Structures of mood and personality and their relevance to assessing anxiety, with an emphasis on self-report. In A. H. Tuma & J. Maser (Eds.), *Anxiety and the anxiety disorders* (pp. 681–706). Hillsdale, NJ: Erlbaum.

Thayer, J. F., & Lane, R. D. (2000). A model of neurovisceral integration in emotion regulation and dysregulation. *Journal of Affective Disorders, 61,* 201–216.

Thornquist, M. H., & Zuckerman, M. (1995). Psychopathy, passive-avoidance learning and basic dimensions of personality. *Personality and Individual Differences, 19,* 525–534.

Turchi, J., & Sarter, M. (1997). Cortical acetylcholine and processing capacity: Effects of cortical cholinergic deafferentation on crossmodal divided attention in rats. *Cognitive Brain Research, 6*(2), 147–158.

Usher, M., Cohen, J. D., Servan-Schreiber, D., Rajkowski, J., & Aston-Jones, G. (1999). The role of the locus coeruleus in the regulation of cognitive performance. *Science, 283,* 549–554.

Wallace, J. F., Bachorowski, J. A., & Newman, J. P. (1991). Failures of response modulaton: Impulsive behavior in anxious and impulsive individuals. *Journal of Research in Personality, 25*(1), 23–44.

Wallace, J. F., & Newman, J. P. (1990). Differential effects of reward and punishment cues on response speed in anxious and impulsive individuals. *Personality and Individual Differences, 11*(10), 999–1009.

Wallace, J. F., & Newman, J. P. (1997). Neuroticism and the attentional mediation of dysregulatory psychopathology. *Cognitive Therapy and Research*, *21*(2), 135–156.

Wallace, J. F., & Newman, J. P. (in press). A theory-based treatment model for psychopathy. *Cognitive and Behavioral Practice*.

Wallace, J. F., Schmitt, W. A., Vitale, J. E., & Newman, J. P. (2000). Experimental investigations of information-processing deficiencies in psychopaths: Implications for diagnosis and treatment. In C. B. Gacono (Ed.), *The clinical and forensic assessment of psychopathy: A practitioner's guide* (pp. 87–109). Mahwah, NJ: Erlbaum.

Watson, D., & Clark, L. A. (1984). Negative affectivity: The disposition to experience aversive emotional states. *Psychological Bulletin*, *96*, 465–490.

Whalen, P. J. (1998). Fear, vigilance, and ambiguity: Initial neuroimaging studies of the human amygdala. *Current Directions in Psychological Science*, *7*(6), 177–188.

Whalen, P. J., Shin, L. M., McInerney, S. C., Fischer, H., Wright, C. I., & Rauch, S. L. (2001). A functional MRI study of human amygdala responses to facial expressions of fear versus anger. *Emotion*, *1*(1), 70–83.

Widiger, T. A., & Costa, P. T. (1994). Personality and personality disorders. *Journal of Abnormal Psychology*, *103*(1), 78–91.

Williamson, S., Harpur, T. J., & Hare, R. D. (1991). Abnormal processing of affective words by psychopaths. *Psychophysiology*, *28*(3), 260–273.

VI

Everyday Problems with Self-Regulation

23

Self-Regulatory Failure and Addiction

MICHAEL A. SAYETTE

Since the publication of *Losing Control: How and Why People Fail at Self-Regulation* (Baumeister, Heatherton, & Tice, 1994), there has been a proliferation of research examining self-regulatory processes and addiction. "Self-regulation," a term sometimes used interchangeably with "self-control" or "self-management," refers generally to any effort by a human being to alter its own responses (Baumeister et al., 1994). With respect to addiction, self-regulation often refers to an attempt to override a well-learned drug use behavior or habit to realize a positive, long-term outcome. As outlined by Baumeister and colleagues, the constituent actions required for drug use (e.g., asking a friend for a cigarette, holding it, lighting it, inhaling) are voluntary behaviors that can be controlled. Accordingly, drug use is a particularly interesting domain for examining self-regulation failure.

Self-regulation failure can be subdivided into failures of *underregulation* and *misregulation*. The former refers to a failure to exert control over oneself, whereas the latter refers to exerting control in a way that fails to bring about the desired result (Baumeister et al., 1994). Both misregulation and underregulation likely contribute to addictive behavior and are addressed herein.

This chapter focuses on nicotine addiction (more specifically, cigarette smoking). There are several reasons why smoking presents an ideal model for considering the relation between self-regulation and addiction. First, although millions of Americans try to quit smoking each year, 81% of these attempts will fail within the first month (Hughes et al., 1992), suggesting that nicotine is an especially good drug to consider when examining self-regulatory failure. Second, the public health implications of nicotine dependence dwarf those of all other drugs (U.S. Department of Health and Human Services, 1989), highlighting the importance of studying self-regulatory processes related to smoking. Third, compared to other substances, such as alcohol, nicotine is an especially addictive drug, and the majority of regular users become dependent. Fourth, because withdrawal states can be induced via robust deprivation manipulations in a medically safe manner, a substantial amount of research has examined smoking motivation and self-regulatory processes.

Smokers may require self-regulation under two different circumstances. During periods of abstinence–avoidance, one desires to smoke but cigarettes are unavailable (e.g., while watching a film in a theater). Self-regulation here may reflect a need to override temporary urges. In contrast, during periods of abstinence seeking, one wishes to abstain. As noted by Tiffany (1990), in either case, a smoker may experience cravings. Effective self-regulation typically requires overriding the craving to smoke. Accordingly, research protocols that provoke cigarette cravings provide a suitable environment for investigating self-regulation.

Research interest in craving has intensified in recent years (e.g., see special issue of *Addiction* [Vol. 95, 2000] devoted to craving). Craving, often used interchangeably with urge, is provoked by a variety of manipulations, including drug deprivation, drug use imagery, and drug cue exposure (Niaura et al., 1988; Sayette et al., 2000; Tiffany, 1992). This chapter addresses research examining self-regulation difficulties faced by smokers who have already developed the habit. (Readers interested in the role of self-regulation in the initiation of smoking are referred elsewhere; e.g., Baumeister et al., 1994.) Misregulation failures are discussed first, followed by an analysis of the role of underregulation in smoking.

MISREGULATION

Most discussion of self-regulation failure and addiction has centered on underregulation. Many problems linked to addiction, however, also can be conceived of as failures of misregulation. Rather than assuming that a person who experiences a smoking lapse (i.e., an initial violation of abstinence) does so as a result of a breakdown in impulse control, it is possible that the act of smoking represents an attempt, albeit misguided, to address a critical problem for the smoker.

Baumeister and colleagues (1994) suggest that one example of misregulation among smokers is the belief that quitting smoking will lead to weight gain. Although quitting often is linked to an increase of 5 or 10 pounds, there is overwhelming evidence that the harmful effects of continuing to smoke override this short-term weight gain (Baumeister et al., 1994). Thus, smoking is mistakenly viewed as a "reasonable" method for controlling weight.

A second example of misregulation is the use of cigarettes to improve mood. A fundamental question regarding nicotine addiction concerns why a smoker who appears to be committed to quitting will suffer a smoking lapse. It often is assumed that such a lapse is an indication of a breakdown in impulse control. Alternatively, a lapse may represent a strategic attempt to regulate affect. Tice, Bratslavsky, and Baumeister (2001) found that, following a negative affect induction, impulsive behaviors—such as eating fattening, tasty snacks—occurred only when participants believed that their mood was modifiable. When they believed that their negative affective state was "frozen," participants' desire to engage in impulsive behaviors was not enhanced. Tice and colleagues concluded that regardless of the ultimate success of these actions, the "impulsive" behavior may be viewed as a rational attempt to address a pressing concern.

The research by Tice and colleagues (2001) suggests that a former smoker who is under stress may lapse, because the short-term need to alleviate negative affect becomes particularly salient. This begs a question that has interested addiction researchers for years: Just how often does a lapse or relapse occur during moments of distress? Early models of addiction articulated by Wikler (1948) and Conger (1956), for example, posited that drugs and alcohol were consumed by addicts to alleviate negative affective states. These initial negative reinforcement models have been challenged (see Tiffany, 1990). It has been suggested, for instance, that smokers who lapse or relapse often do not report experiencing negative affect (Shiffman, Gwaltney, et al., 2002), and that many "absent-minded lapses" seem to occur outside of awareness (Tiffany, 1990).

Nevertheless, updated versions of negative reinforcement models assert that the chief component of the withdrawal response is negative affect, and that with some modifications to original formulations, "escape and avoidance of negative affect is the prepotent motive for addictive drug use" (Baker, Piper, McCarthy, Majeskie, & Fiore, in press). These authors examined a diverse set of animal and human studies to address many of the criticisms levied against negative reinforcement models. Their review suggests that, construed broadly, negative affect can motivate some, if not most, lapses (see also Brownell, Marlatt, Lichtenstein, & Wilson, 1986; Piasecki et al., 2000).

If smoking a cigarette is viewed as an attempt to improve mood, then treatments that focus on mood regulation may prove effective. Consistent with this position is the success of the antidepressant buproprion (e.g., Jorenby et al., 1999). In addition, as argued by Baker and colleagues (in press), even nicotine replacement products suppress negative affect. From a psychological perspective, smoking cessation treatments that ignore concerns related to negative affect are unlikely to succeed.

UNDERREGULATION

As noted earlier, much of the smoking research on self-regulation failure has emphasized underregulation. Baumeister and colleagues (1994) discuss three basic features of self-regulation that may fail and lead to underregulation: (1) setting proper standards; (2) monitoring oneself in relation to these standards, and (3) altering one's responses to conform to these standards. Though not all the findings I address later fit cleanly into just one of these categories, to retain this structure is nevertheless heuristic.

Setting Standards

Difficulty setting proper standards may interfere with smoking cessation. Most smokers believe that smoking is a bad habit, and one that they would like to break (Baumeister et al., 1994). Yet smokers may hold distorted standards related to smoking and health (Kunda, 1990). In a prospective study of smokers attempting to quit, Gibbons and Eggleston (1996) found that a smoker's perception of the "typical smoker" at the outset of treatment was a reliable predictor of relapse. Specifically, those vulnerable to relapse were more likely to view typical smokers in a positive light than were those who successfully quit. Thus, continuing smokers may construct a standard of what it means to be a smoker that protects them from feeling irrational for maintaining their habit. Research from a social learning perspective may shed light on how such standards may develop (Marlatt & Gordon, 1985).

Rather than viewing standards solely as stable character traits, it may be useful to consider them as being subject to momentary fluctuations. Specifically, when smokers are craving a cigarette, the way that they think about smoking may change. In her theory of motivated reasoning, Kunda (1990) suggested that motivation could bias how one generates and evaluates information related to the topic of interest. The degree of change in the generation and evaluation of information may be a function of one's momentary level of smoking motivation (Sayette, 1999).

One study that tested the effects of craving on the generation of smoking-related information required smokers to attend two (counterbalanced) laboratory sessions held within 10 days of each other (Sayette & Hufford, 1997). Prior to one session, participants were asked to abstain from smoking for 12 hours, whereas they were allowed to smoke normally before the other session. During the abstinence session, each participant held a lit cigarette without smoking, which led to elevated urge ratings. In contrast, during the nonabstinent session, each participant simply held a control cue (roll of tape) in his or her hand, which led to low urge ratings. While in these high and low urge states, smokers were given 90 sec to list as many positive characteristics of smoking, then 90 sec to list as many negative characteristics as they could. During the high-urge session, smokers generated significantly more positive items about smoking than they did during the low-urge assessment. Although craving increased generation of positive, smoking-related information, it did not have this effect on negative information. Indeed, craving led to a nonsignificant drop in the generation of negative, smoking-related information. Thus, while craving, smokers generated a list of smoking characteristics that was positively biased compared to when they were not craving.

Craving also may be associated with the way that smoking-related information is evaluated. Sayette, Martin, Wertz, Shiffman, and Perrott (2001) examined the effects of craving on the evaluation of smoking consequences. While holding a lit cigarette, abstinent and nonabstinent smokers were asked to rate (on a 10-point scale ranging from "not at all likely" to "extremely likely"), the probability that a list of smoking consequences would occur. Twenty-four items (e.g., "By smoking I risk heart disease and lung cancer"; "Smoking calms me down when I feel nervous") were selected from the Smoking Consequences Questionnaire developed by Copeland, Brandon, and Quinn (1995). Abstinent smokers, compared to nonabstinent smokers, tended to judge positive consequences to be more probable than negative ones. As suggested by Marlatt (1985), craving may distort outcome expectancies, such that positive outcomes appear more likely than negative ones.

These studies suggest that standards related to smoking may be viewed differently when one is in a craving as opposed to a neutral state (Sayette, 1999). Consequently, measuring one's views about smoking may require careful consideration of the assessment context. A clinician who learns that a smoker holds a negative view of smoking, and is motivated to quit, may be surprised to learn of a quick relapse. Had these standards been assessed while the smoker was in a craving state, the obtained information might have revealed that the smoker was ambivalent about giving up the habit. After all, it takes only a single moment of weakness during a high-risk situation for a committed quitter to reconsider and smoke a cigarette.

In addition to appreciating the importance of momentary shifts in attitudes, another complicating factor when considering standards is that smokers may simultaneously hold conflicting standards. For instance, they may not only believe that it is foolish to risk their health by continuing to smoke but also that, because life is uncertain, they might as well enjoy the moment. Which of these standards predominates may switch from moment to moment, and when a person is craving, a standard that promotes smoking may emerge.

In summary, there are myriad ways that one's standards regarding smoking may contribute to underregulation. The concept of smoking, or of being a smoker, may shift over time as a smoker becomes more committed to the habit. Furthermore, at particular moments, such as when motivation to smoke is high, one's standards may tilt even more toward a position that promotes smoking.

Monitoring

Research also has focused on the adverse consequences of failing to monitor one's thoughts, feelings, and actions with respect to one's standards. Even if one holds standards that promote smoking cessation, it remains important to monitor oneself in relation to these standards. The need to monitor oneself vigilantly is thought to be instrumental in preventing relapse (Brownell et al., 1986).

Attention plays a critical role in monitoring. Baumeister and colleagues (1994) argue that managing attention may be the most effective approach to self-regulation. An individual can exercise self-regulation by attending to information that reaches beyond the immediate stimulus environment, what Baumeister and colleagues label "transcendence." Rather than merely focusing on the immediate object of desire, one engages in high-level thinking that recognizes the standards that promote self-regulation. Such a perspective is needed to override impulses. In contrast, transcendence failure occurs when an individual attends only to the immediate present and does not monitor discrepancies between current interests and long-term goals.

Monitoring requires self-awareness, which is often compromised during high-risk moments. Social cues (e.g., social celebrations) have been implicated in smoking relapse (Brownell et al., 1986). Presumably these situations do not provide fertile ground for self-reflection and monitoring. Similarly, monitoring may prove difficult during highly emotional states. Baumeister and colleagues (1994) posit that affectively charged moments may focus attention on immediate stimuli, while leaving little attention available for self-reflection.

It also is likely that monitoring of standards related to smoking will be inhibited following alcohol consumption. There is evidence that drinking alcohol increases smoking behavior (e.g., Griffiths, Bigelow, & Liebson, 1976; Nil, Buzzi, & Bättig, 1984). Moreover, relapse to smoking occurs more often after drinking alcohol than after any other identified situational variable (Shiffman & Balabanis, 1995). Several models of the effects of alcohol suggest that drinking impairs cognitive processes (see also Hull & Slone, Chapter 24, this volume; Sayette, 1999). Whether due to an impaired ability to encode information in terms of self-relevance (Hull, 1987), or a reduced capacity to focus on information other than immediate smoking cues (Steele & Josephs, 1990), alcohol intoxication may impede self-regulation by compromising the ability to monitor performance relative to standards (Baumeister et al., 1994). (If cues that inhibit smoking are salient, however, then intoxication might even support self-regulation (MacDonald, Fong, Zanna, & Martineau, 2000). Research that addresses directly the effects of alcohol on the monitoring of standards and norms would be useful.

One final danger related to monitoring is that smokers may have developed unrealistic expectations about the impact of quitting. Smokers may assume, for example, that quitting will influence all aspects of their life. Although quitting is likely to improve health, it may not substantially affect one's personality. When cessation fails to produce such global change, monitoring may have the unfortunate effect of revealing a substandard outcome and may precipitate a relapse. This process has been referred to as the "false hope syndrome" (Polivy, 2000; see also Rothman, Baldwin, & Hertel, Chapter 7, this volume, for a review of behavioral health change models and possible reasons for relapse).

Altering Responses

Smokers may recognize that smoking conflicts with their standards, and they may be able to monitor a discrepancy between their smoking behavior and their standards, yet still experience a lapse. Indeed, the bulk of research on self-regulation failure centers on an inability to exercise the necessary control or discipline to resist a temptation to smoke. Baumeister and colleagues (1994) have conceived of this control in terms of *strength*. From this perspective, a smoker requires sufficient "muscle" to resist the impulse to smoke (see Muraven & Baumeister, 2000). Baumeister and colleagues propose that repeated encounters with high-risk situations over a particular time interval may deplete muscle strength, leaving an individual vulnerable for a lapse.

The concept of self-regulation strength has been examined from three perspectives. The first relates to stable individual differences. Certain people may be "weak" and may lack the inhibition necessary to resist succumbing to temptation. This person-level analysis of smoking is likely to yield important individual-difference markers for relapse risk (Shiffman & Balabanis, 1995).

A second approach to examining strength involves situational constraints that deplete the limited capacity resources needed to resist a temptation to smoke (Baumeister et al., 1994). This capacity view of self-regulation is consistent with Tiffany's (1990) cognitive model of drug urge. With repeated use, the act of smoking becomes increasingly well learned, and smoking becomes automatized. For the heavy smoker, who has performed this action sequence countless times, the act of smoking may require virtually no cognitive effort. Moreover, the stimulus-bound nature of automatized behaviors suggests that once the sequence is initiated, it will move to completion, without reliance on limited-capacity, nonautomatic processes (Tiffany, 1990).

Unlike the automatized behavior associated with habitual smoking, cravings are defined as a collection of verbal, somatovisceral, and behavioral responses supported by limited-capacity, nonautomatic processes (Tiffany, 1990). Craving only occurs when execution of a well-learned pattern of responses culminating in drug use is blocked. Under conditions in which the smoking routine has been triggered (by internal or environmental cues) but is not completed, limited-capacity processing resources are mobilized either to support (abstinence avoidance) or to prevent (abstinence seeking) the completion of this action sequence.

Given the effort required to override a temptation to smoke, factors that undermine limited-capacity processing resources should hamper self-regulation. For instance, fatigue may prevent effective self-regulatory behavior in the face of a smoking urge. Accordingly, Baumeister and colleagues (1994) suggest that smokers attempt smoking cessation at a time when other demands requiring self-control are relatively low (see also Vohs & Heatherton, 2000). Similarly, while under stress, a person may be too exhausted to combat a strong urge to smoke. Stressors that threaten one's self-concept, or that require self-monitoring, may be especially exhausting.

Related to stress is tobacco withdrawal. It has been suggested that subtle effects of tobacco withdrawal can begin to occur even after very brief periods of abstinence (Hughes, 1991; Sayette, Martin, et al., 2001). Furthermore, Baker and colleagues (in press) have argued that the cardinal feature of withdrawal is negative affect, or stress.

They review animal and human data suggesting that either stress or withdrawal is sufficient to motivate drug use. From a self-regulatory strength perspective, people may smoke when distressed because they are unable to cope simultaneously with the stressors and their desire to smoke. This would be consistent with the view that self-control is a limited resource (Baumeister et al., 1994).

Because alcohol demands limited-capacity, nonautomatic resources (Josephs & Steele, 1990), it is likely that there would be insufficient cognitive capacity to override a well-learned smoking routine during intoxication (Sayette, 2002a; Tiffany, 1990). Moreover, because alcohol is often a cue for smoking, drinking may initiate automatized smoking behavior (Burton & Tiffany, 1997). Thus, like fatigue and stress, alcohol consumption is likely to compromise one's ability to alter responses in the service of self-regulation.

The third approach to examining strength involves temporary states influenced by appetitive cues. Smokers may lack the strength to resist an urge not only because of a weakness—whether it be chronic or temporary—but also because of powerful appetitive stimuli. According to Baumeister and colleagues (1994), even a "strong" individual with well-developed self-regulatory skills can become overwhelmed by external factors. As I discussed earlier, the intense emotional context of many high-risk situations may draw all available resources toward the object of desire, leaving a person fewer resources to monitor the big picture, or to enact coping responses necessary for resisting the temptation.

Recent studies reveal that craving disrupts limited-capacity processes (see Sayette, 1999; Tiffany 1995). Exposure to smoking cues, for example, led smokers to respond more slowly during a secondary-response time probe than during exposure to control cues, suggesting that limited-capacity, nonautomatic processing resources were diverted during the craving manipulation (Cepeda-Benito & Tiffany, 1996; Juliano & Brandon, 1998; Sayette & Hufford, 1994; Sayette, Martin, et al., 2001). These performance deficits suggest a demand on processing resources during craving.

If smoking does represent a well-learned routine, then it is likely that it will take considerable effort requiring limited-capacity, nonautomatic resources to refrain from completing the smoking action sequence once it has been initiated (Tiffany, 1990). Indeed, the ability to override a well-learned habitual behavior is the central feature of self-regulation (Baumeister et al., 1994). Baumeister et al. also suggest that the further one is into the routine, the more difficult (i.e., the more cognitive resources will be required) it is to terminate. Thus, it is far easier to resist smoking when one first sees a friend smoking than after lighting and holding the cigarette that is offered, a process they label "psychological inertia."

After a smoking routine is activated, limited-capacity cognitive resources are likely directed toward several other functions, in addition to the struggle to resist completing the routine (Sayette, Martin, Hull, Wertz, & Perrott, 2003). Resources may be directed toward monitoring: the level of motivation or desire to use the drug (e.g., "I really want a cigarette"); the drug cues themselves (e.g., thoughts of how the cigarette will feel in one's hand); anticipated positive effects of smoking (e.g., "If I smoke this cigarette, then I will feel better"); feelings associated with the event (e.g., frustration that a friend lit a cigarette in one's presence); as well as problem-solving cognitions associated with completing the smoking action plan (e.g., "How can I hide this cigarette from my spouse?"). Resources directed toward any of these cognitions leave fewer resources available for the successful self-regulation involved in maintaining abstinence.

Addiction researchers have used measures other than secondary-response time probes to examine shifts in attention and cognitive processing during high-risk situations

(Sayette, 1999). An increasingly popular measure of attentional bias is the color-naming task, also called the emotional Stroop task (Williams, Mathews, & MacLeod, 1996), in which participants name the color of words, while ignoring word content. When words are personally or emotionally relevant, individuals are thought to be automatically drawn to them, and the latency to name the color of the word generally increases. Patients with phobias, for instance, take longer to color-name words describing phobic material, and this attentional bias has been found across a range of disorders (Williams et al., 1996). In some cases, color naming has predicted emotional distress better than have self-report measures (e.g., MacLeod & Hagan, 1992), though the exact mechanism underlying the color-naming effect remains unclear (cf. de Ruiter & Brosschot, 1994; Waters, Sayette, & Wertz, 2003; Williams et al., 1996).

A number of emotional Stroop studies have shown that smokers display greater response interference when presented with smoking-related words during withdrawal than when they were permitted to smoke normally (Gross, Jarvik, & Rosenblatt, 1993; Waters & Feyerabend, 2000; Wertz & Sayette, 2001a). These data are consistent with models of addiction emphasizing shifts in the incentive salience of drug cues, such that these cues "grab attention" and cue the addict to engage in further drug use (Robinson & Berridge, 1993, p. 261).

Recently, we found that performance on a version of the emotional Stroop task on quit day predicted subsequent relapse, even after controlling for self-reported urge (Waters, Shiffman, et al., 2003). Thus, during moments of temptation, attention appears to be biased toward smoking-related stimuli. Such a drift may hamper the ability to produce altering responses, also known as "coping responses."

The issue of coping is particularly important in discussions of self-regulation. Smokers who relapse often fail to use coping skills (Shiffman, 1982). Perhaps not surprisingly, Brandon, Tiffany, Obremski, and Baker (1990) reported that among smokers entering treatment, who had quit smoking but subsequently relapsed, 71% failed to use any of the coping skills successfully gained during treatment. These data suggest that, in many cases, relapsers fail despite having obtained relevant coping skills. Additional support for the notion that drug urge is entwined with coping skills stems from a study of alcohol-dependent individuals (Abrams et al., 1991). During hypothetical role-play encounters, patients manifested deficient coping skills in high-risk (alcohol-specific) situations, but not in general situations requiring socially competent responses. These investigators also found that when alcohol-dependent patients were exposed to alcohol cues, their coping skills were impaired (Binkoff et al., 1984). Taken together, these studies suggest a direct connection between temptation and the ability to cope with temptation, such that high-urge situations are associated with weak coping responses.

As cravings emerge, coping resources may become inaccessible (Sayette, 1999). Alternatively, coping resources may remain accessible, but smokers may just choose not to engage them (Loewenstein, 1999). In either case, the motivation to smoke may fundamentally influence the way coping-related information is processed. Thus, we might expect a smoker to generate and employ an impressive array of coping resources while experiencing a mild urge but to fail to do so during a strong urge (Sayette, 1999). From this perspective, it may be wiser to teach coping skills in a high-urge environment than in a sterile, low-urge context.

Related to coping is Bandura's (1997) concept of self-efficacy, which has been applied to a range of addictive behaviors (for a review of self-regulation and self-efficacy, see Cervone, Mor, Orom, Shadel, & Scott, Chapter 10, this volume). The most prominent conceptualization of self-efficacy in the smoking literature involves abstinence self-efficacy, or the confidence in one's ability to abstain from smoking (Gwaltney et al., 2001). Individuals with greater confidence in their ability to abstain should be more likely to maintain abstinence (Marlatt & Gordon, 1985; Niaura et al., 1988). Pretreatment abstinence self-efficacy judgments, however, do not always predict relapse (e.g., Baer & Lichenstein, 1988; Gwaltney et al., 2001). Furthermore, abstinence self-efficacy does not appear to mediate the effect of concurrent smoking on future smoking (Baer, Holt, & Lichtenstein, 1986; Shiffman et al., 2000). One reason may be that initial efficacy judgments usually are made in a neutral state, whereas the temptation periods that one must overcome to remain abstinent are typically affectively charged.

Persons in an affectively neutral, "cold" state often underestimate the impact of being in an affectively charged, "hot" state on their own future behavior, referred to by Loewenstein (1999) as the "cold-to-hot empathy gap." Consistent with this proposition, a recent review finds that a disproportionate number of subjects inaccurately report maximum self-efficacy scores (Forsyth & Carey, 1998). Similarly, O'Brien and colleagues (1988) reported that recovering cocaine addicts often return home, after a period of brief treatment, with an unrealistic confidence that they will not resume drug use. (These findings also are in accord with studies showing that people lose confidence in their prospects for success the closer they are to the critical moment [Gilovich, Kerr, & Husted-Medvec, 1993].) Were initial self-efficacy perceptions recorded in a craving state, which more closely approximates high-risk situations, they might prove more accurate than they typically are in predicting cessation. Experimental manipulation of alcohol craving reveals that, during cue exposure, alcoholics reported a decreased self-efficacy to resist future drinking (Cooney, Gillespie, Baker, & Kaplan, 1987).

To test the relation between abstinence self-efficacy and cigarette craving, we recently used Ecological Momentary Assessment in a sample of smokers who participated in a smoking cessation treatment (Gwaltney, Shiffman, & Sayette, 2003). Smokers reported their urge to smoke and abstinence self-efficacy, using palm-top computers during multiple temptation and nontemptation periods. When smokers reported high urges, they tended to report less abstinence self-efficacy than when reporting weaker craving states. Thus, both laboratory and field research support the notion that smokers' ability, and confidence in their ability, to cope with temptation diminishes during the precise moments that they are most needed. In summary, converging evidence indicates that cravings brought about by nicotine deprivation, smoking cue exposure, or both, may alter cognitive processes, such that the ability to resist smoking may be compromised.

ACQUIESCENCE

A strength model implies that self-regulation will fail only when an individual lacks sufficient strength and is "powerless" to exert self-control. A provocative issue raised by Baumeister and colleagues (1994) was "whether people actually acquiesce in their own self-regulation failures" (p. 29). The idea is that people may sometimes, perhaps unconsciously, cooperate in their failure to self-regulate. These authors suggest that acquiescence may be common, and that few impulsive behaviors are truly involuntary. MacAndrew and Edgerton (1969), in their cross-cultural analysis of drinking behavior, posited that most societies need periods of time-out from typical standards of conduct, and that drinking alcohol implicitly permits group members to relax their behavioral norms. Similarly, Baumeister and colleagues suggest that there are times when individuals may want to loosen up and relax their level of self-awareness, which is likely to reduce further the monitoring necessary for successful self-regulation.

Although the notion that smokers may indulge their cravings has rarely been studied, indirect evidence suggests that people may sometimes acquiesce to their urges. Data across multiple, substance-abusing samples indicate that exposure to drug cues leads to elevated urge ratings (see Carter & Tiffany, 1999). What is surprising, however, is the variability in the magnitude of this effect. In a recent review of this literature, we tested the hypothesis that addicts who perceived an opportunity to consume the drug would report stronger urges than would those who did not perceive the opportunity to use (Wertz & Sayette, 2001b). We used the term "perceived drug use opportunity" rather than "drug availability," because sometimes a drug may be physically present, but the person may not perceive an opportunity to use it (e.g., due to religious customs). Schachter, Silverstein, and Perlick (1977), for example, observed that Orthodox Jewish smokers, who are forbidden to smoke on the Sabbath, reported little difficulty in abstaining.

Addicts who are conflicted about drug use may experience their urges in a variety of ways. If they attempt to exert self-control in the situation, then they would likely be motivated to suppress their urge. In contrast, were addicts at some level inclined to acquiesce and consume their drug, they would no longer be motivated to suppress their urge. Indeed, they might even wish to embellish their urge to justify drug use: "I had no real choice but to smoke. Anyone with a craving as strong as mine would have smoked." Consistent with this position, in a review of cue exposure studies, we found that across substances, participants who perceived an opportunity to use reported significantly higher urges then did those who did not anticipate use (Wertz & Sayette, 2001b).

All of the smoking cue exposure studies included in Wertz and Sayette (2001b) recruited smokers who were not at that time interested in quitting. Because these participants were still active smokers, they presumably could cope with urges by simply smoking a cigarette. Accordingly, they would be expected to report strong cigarette urges during cue exposure. Consistent with this hypothesis, these studies reveal that participants report high levels of craving (about 74% of maximum value on scales; see Table 1 in Wertz & Sayette, 2001b). In contrast, when smokers are attempting cessation, they may be motivated to cope with urges by suppressing rather than indulging them. Accordingly, smokers undergoing a cue exposure assessment at the beginning of a quit attempt ought to report relatively low urges. Recently, a smoking cue exposure study examined smokers interested in quitting who were beginning a smoking cessation program (Shiffman, Shadel, et al., 2003). When these smokers were exposed to potent smoking cues, which included holding a lit cigarette, their urges were quite modest (about 43% of maximum value on scale). The urges reported in this study with smokers interested in quitting look quite similar to urges reported by addicts interested in quitting other drugs, which averaged about 37% of maximum value on scale (see Table 2 in Wertz & Sayette, 2001b).

In addition to influencing the magnitude of craving, acquiescence may affect the emotional valence of a craving experience. Typically, the affect associated with craving is assumed to be negative (Tiffany, 1992). When a smoker expects to satisfy an urge rather than resist it, however, he or she may actually experience positive affect. The moments just prior to use, and even the beginning of consumption, may be particularly positive. It is often difficult, however, to capture brief experiences of positive affect in the laboratory. Often, studies have relied on self-report instruments, which are not ideally suited to the task (see Baker et al., in press). Self-report measures are poorly equipped to assess moment-to-moment fluctuations in emotion response that occur over time. Instead, when participants complete self-report measures, they aggregate their experience over time. Moreover, after their responses are filtered through consciousness, they must impose language on what may be a nonverbal experience (Nisbett & Wilson, 1977; Stone et al., 2000).

Analysis of expressive behavior may provide a more direct measure of emotional response than autonomic arousal or self-report (Barlow, 1988), and may prove to be a nice complement to more traditional measures (Sayette et al., 2000). Facial coding analysis of expressive behavior, which can be conducted unobtrusively, can capture affect in real time (e.g., Ekman, Friesen, & Ancoli, 1980). The most sophisticated and established system for assessing facial expression, the Facial Action Coding System (FACS; Ekman & Friesen, 1978), is an anatomically based system derived from 7,000 different expressions, decomposed into 44 action units (AUs) that can be combined to describe all possible visible movements of the face. FACS has proven to be reliable and provides accurate, specific information across a range of emotional experiences (Ekman & Rosenberg, 1997; Sayette, Cohn, Wertz, Perrott, & Parrott, 2001). Although facial expressions can serve a variety of purposes, it is clear that many are related to subjective affective experience, with particular AUs differentially reflecting affective valence (Ekman & Rosenberg, 1997). Because FACS can reliably code rapid changes in expressions, it may be particularly sensitive for examining perceived drug use opportunity during cue exposure.

Studies using FACS indicate that manipulating instructions (i.e., informing smokers that they will or will not be able to smoke a lit cigarette) influences the probability of evincing AUs associated with either positive or negative affect (Sayette & Hufford, 1995; Sayette, Wertz, et al., 2003); that is, under certain conditions, craving may even be linked to positive affect (see also Carter & Tiffany, 2001). Similarly, Zinser, Fiore, Davidson, and Baker (1999) used an electrophysiological assessment that suggested a pattern of activation associated with approach motivation during craving. Together, these data suggest that some of the perceived reward generally associated with drug use may actually precede drug consumption. Such a proposition is consistent with recent neurobiological evidence indicating that dopamine is released during presentations of cues predictive of drug, food, and alcohol use (see Weiss et al., 2000). For instance, using Wistar rats, Weiss and colleagues (2000) found that anticipation of cocaine use increased dopamine efflux in the nucleus accumbens and amygdyla, structures implicated in reward. Thus, craving itself may be rewarding, particularly to those who anticipate using the drug very soon.

Anticipation of drug use may be rewarding when considered from an economic perspective. Loewenstein (1987) has described *savoring* as the "positive utility derived from anticipation of future consumption" (p. 667). Children who horde their stash of Halloween candy rather than eating it, for example, may prefer savoring their candy to actually consuming it. In summary, under certain conditions, smokers may in fact acquiesce or indulge their cravings.

One further implication of acquiesence is that poor coping may not cause lapses; rather, it may be a reflection of an intended lapse; that is, once individuals decide, perhaps unconsciously, that they are going to indulge their craving, then it stands to reason that they will fail to employ coping skills, even those skills they have mastered. This proposition is at odds with most models of temptation and coping, which, as noted earlier, imply that poor coping causes temptations to become lapses. Alternatively, coping may be a reflection of urges, such that mild urges provide opportunities for coping responses to be employed, whereas strong urges, or at least urges associated with an intention to use, may to some extent preclude coping.

This alternative resembles Lazarus and Folkman's (1984) conception of stress and coping. Their three-stage appraisal model holds that an experience of stress reflects a primary appraisal of loss, threat, or harm, coupled with a secondary appraisal of coping resources available to counter the stressor. A third "reappraisal" stage, which takes into account both the primary and secondary appraisals, ultimately determines the degree of stress response. Importantly, these three appraisal processes blend together seamlessly.

In the context of craving, this model suggests that, in an instant, an "urge appraisal" can emerge that actually is a function of (1) a primary appraisal of a desire to smoke; (2) a secondary appraisal regarding whether one will acquiesce or attempt to resist the desire; and (3) an urge reappraisal that may reveal a strong urge, along with weak efforts to cope, or less intense urges accompanied by strong attempts to cope. Future research is needed to determine the utility of this conceptualization of urges and coping, and to explore more generally the possible role of acquiescence in self-regulation failure.

CONCLUSIONS AND FUTURE DIRECTIONS

This chapter has considered several aspects of self-regulation failure in smokers. The self-regulation framework proposed by Baumeister and colleagues (1994) provides a useful structure for examining a diverse set of findings related to smoking urges and lapse. Studies suggest that misregulation may play a critical role in understanding smoking motivation. As proposed recently by Baker and colleagues (in press), the possibility that smoking represents an attempt to attenuate, or perhaps ward off negative moods, is a model that still warrants serious attention.

Recognition of the potential role of acquiescence in self-regulation failure highlights the need to develop multiple methods and a wide range of measures to capture processes that may not always be available to conscious awareness (Sayette, 1999). Indeed, Baumeister and colleagues (1994) suggested a decade ago that the distinction between nonautomatic limited-capacity processes and automatic-effortless processes needed to be incorporated into self-regulation theory. Use of implicit cognitive measures may improve understanding of mechanisms underlying self-regulation failure and help generate predictions regarding relapse risk. For instance, the use of the emotional Stroop task to predict relapse highlights the importance of attentional processes in self-regulation (Waters, Shiffman, et al., 2003). Another area of cognition that deserves focus is time perception (Sayette, 1999). Shifts in temporal perception may play a role in self-control and decision-making processes related to addiction (Hoch & Loewenstein, 1991). Recent data suggest that while waiting to smoke, time may seem to pass more rapidly when participants are not craving than when they are in a craving state (Sayette, 2002b). These data are in accord with recent data revealing that the act of self-regulation changes the subjective experience of time, such that time feels longer than it really is, and this state leads to subsequent failures in self-regulation (Vohs & Schmeichel, 2003).

As with cognition, improved understanding of self-regulatory process in addiction requires development of new approaches for assessing affect. The use of observational measures (such as FACS) and electrophysiological measures (such as EEG) (e.g., Zinser et al., 1999) that are conceptually linked to theories of craving and self-regulation may prove especially useful. Studies have revealed that particular facial expressions provide important etiological information regarding schizophrenia, affective disorders, and other forms of psychopathology (see Ekman & Rosenberg, 1997). For instance, the presence of particular expressions at intake predicts length of hospital stay (Ekman, Matsumoto, & Friesen, 1997). It remains to be seen whether particular facial expressions during cue exposure assessment might predict relapse in addiction. Future research also is needed to understand better the link between affect and cognition. More generally, addiction research that accounts for affective and motivational, as well as cognitive changes, will likely prove especially useful.

Many of the studies described in this chapter illustrate that while a person is craving, cognitive processes and decision making related to smoking may change. Perhaps more important is the concern that smokers and other addicts may substantially underestimate the power of these effects (see Loewenstein, 1999). Research in our laboratory currently is focused on testing the hypothesis that smokers in a neutral state will underpredict the motivational force of future cravings, and underrecall the power of past cravings.

Most laboratory research that has focused on self-regulatory failure in addiction has used designs in which subjects participate one at a time. Yet it is clear that many lapses and relapses occur in group settings. Investigations that incorporate theory and methods from social psychology will help to provide an important context for examining self-regulation (Sayette, Kirchner, Moreland, Levine, & Travis, in press). Social comparison (e.g., Wood, 1989), group formation, and peer pressure are just a few examples of the kinds of social processes that may influence self-regulation.

Drug use requires a series of voluntary actions; thus, it is fair to claim that addiction is a failure of self-regulation (Baumeister et al., 1994; Marlatt & Gordon, 1985). Yet the studies examined in this chapter do show that during affectively charged moments, the information available to smokers may shift in a manner that promotes smoking. Given the disappointing relapse rates among smokers attempting cessation, it is imperative that research begin to translate these laboratory observations into clinical interventions that help smokers recognize and undermine these biases.

This chapter has not addressed individual differences that influence self-regulation processes. This area, of great interest from biological, psychological, and social perspectives, relates to initiation of smoking, as well as to maintenance and relapse. Indeed, it is likely that future efforts will cut across these perspectives to provide a richer understanding of self-regulation processes. Clearly, imaging research that is already being conducted is an illustration of such integration (Beauregard, Lévesque, & Bourgouin, 2001; Goldstein & Volkow, 2002; Jentsch & Taylor, 1999). Instead, this chapter has focused primarily on momentary changes that may affect self-regulation. Research examining changes in cognitive processing during cigarette cravings provides insight into the role of underregulation in addiction. Shifts in attentional bias and selective processing of smoking-related information, for example, may affect how one sets and then monitors personal standards and goals (e.g., the goal of remaining abstinent), as well as how one executes attempts to alter impulsive responses. These effects ultimately may promote smoking.

CLINICAL IMPLICATIONS

The research described in this chapter also suggests clinical applications. Cognitive-behavioral therapies emphasize that one's cognitive biases and distortions can contribute fundamentally to a range of psychopathological behaviors. Often, treatment involves helping patients uncover and modify these biases. In the field of addiction, preventing relapse has been the greatest clinical challenge (Brownell et al., 1986; Marlatt & Gordon, 1985). Consider the challenges awaiting smokers who have only recently quit. Data from cognitive studies suggest that when smokers walk down the street, there appears to be much that reminds them of a cigarette. Every cigarette butt that has been dropped on the pavement grabs their attention like a billboard. Even ambiguous cues may remind them of their habit:

> These ambiguous, yet ubiquitous, cues serve to activate well practiced . . . smoking routines. Once initiated, limited cognitive resources must be directed toward resisting the completion of this [smoking] action sequence. In essence, under certain conditions, the world can become one big temptation, requiring a vigilant effort to resist its allure. (Sayette, 1999, pp. 277–278)

In a clinic setting, patients may be warned that they will face these temptations, and will need to dispute rationally the distorted perceptions and judgments that follow. Perhaps writing down the pros and cons of resuming smoking may help them to regain perspective. Yet if this list is generated while craving, it may not resemble one generated in a noncraving state. While craving, the balance of pros and cons may shift, and the reinforcing consequences of drug use might be strengthened. Suddenly, the decision to resume drinking or smoking may not appear to be such a bad idea (Sayette, 1999).

Pavlov's research suggested the potential of cue exposure/response prevention to extinguish previously conditioned appetites. Yet only recently have addiction researchers begun to focus on the clinical implications of this research (see Conklin & Tiffany, 2002). Poulos, Hinson, and Siegel (1981) suggest that treatment programs would fare better if they altered their sterile environments to include the types of drug cues likely to elicit cravings.

In addition to conditioning models, cognitive theories also may account for the utility of cue exposure treatment (e.g., Marlatt, 1985). Treatment should include helping patients prepare to refrain from drinking in the context of the often powerful cognitive shifts that occur outside the clinic. Craving-induction treatments in which smoking is prevented may help patients learn to cope with temptations while they are experiencing them. Coping skills taught in the context of a craving manipulation may be especially effective (e.g., Monti et al., 1993). In addition to developing skills to deal with high-risk situations, patients may enhance their self-efficacy beliefs that they will be able to cope, which may also prove important for preventing relapse (Wilson, 1987).

In summary, this chapter has highlighted the importance of self-regulation in the context of addiction. Using cigarette smoking as a model, I presented data that illustrate the multiple domains in which craving might contribute to self-regulation failure (e.g., underregulation, misregulation, acquiescence). With a self-regulation framework, future work promises to provide both conceptual and clinical advances in the understanding of drug craving.

ACKNOWLEDGMENTS

Preparation of this chapter was supported in part by Grant No. R01 DA10605 from the National Institute on Drug Abuse. I thank William Klein and Stephen Wilson for their comments on an initial draft of this chapter.

REFERENCES

Abrams, D. B., Binkoff, J. A., Zwick, W. R., Liepman, M. R., Nirenberg, T. D., Munroe, S. M., &

Monti, P. M. (1991). Alcohol abusers' and social drinkers' responses to alcohol-relevant and general situations. *Journal of Studies on Alcohol, 52,* 409–414.

Baer, J. S., Holt, C. S., & Lichtenstein, E. (1986). Self-efficacy and smoking reexamined: Construct validity and clinical utility. *Journal of Consulting and Clinical Psychology, 54,* 846–852.

Baer, J., & Lichtenstein, E. (1988). Classification and prediction of smoking relapse episodes: An exploration of individual differences. *Journal of Consulting and Clinical Psychology, 56,* 104–110.

Baker, T. B., Piper, M. E., McCarthy, D. E., Majeskie, M. R., & Fiore, M. C. (in press). Addiction motivation reformulated: An affective processing model of negative reinforcement. *Psychological Review.*

Bandura, A. (1997). *Self-efficacy: The exercise of control.* New York: Freeman.

Barlow, D. H. (1988). *Anxiety and its disorders: The nature and treatment of anxiety and panic.* New York: Guilford Press.

Baumeister, R. F., Heatherton, T. F., & Tice, D. M. (1994). *Losing control: How and why people fail at self-regulation.* San Diego, CA: Academic Press.

Beauregard, M., Lévesque, J., & Bourgouin, P. (2001). Neural correlates of conscious self-regulation of emotion. *Journal of Neuroscience, 21*(RC165), 1–6.

Binkoff, J. A., Abrams, D. B., Collins, R. L., Liepman, M. R., Monti, P. M., Nirenberg, T. D., & Zwick, W. R. (1984, November). *Exposure to alcohol cues.* Paper presented at the annual meeting of the Association for Advancement of Behavior Therapy, Philadelphia.

Brandon, T. H., Tiffany, S. T., Obremski, K. M., & Baker, T. B. (1990). Postcessation cigarette use: The process of relapse. *Addictive Behaviors, 15,* 105–114.

Brownell, K. D., Marlatt, G. A., Lichtenstein, E., & Wilson, G. T. (1986). Understanding and preventing relapse. *American Psychologist, 41,* 765–782.

Burton, S. M., & Tiffany, S. T. (1997). The effect of alcohol consumption on craving to smoke. *Addiction, 92,* 15–26.

Carter, B. L., & Tiffany, S. T. (1999). Meta-analysis of cue reactivity in addiction research. *Addiction, 94,* 327–340.

Carter, B. L., & Tiffany, S. T. (2001). The cue-availability paradigm: Impact of cigarette availability on cue reactivity in smokers. *Experimental and Clinical Psychopharmacology, 9,* 183–190.

Cepeda-Benito, A., & Tiffany, S. T. (1996). The use of a dual-task procedure for the assessment of cognitive effort associated with cigarette craving. *Psychopharmacology, 127,* 155–163.

Conger, J. (1956). Reinforcement theory and the dynamics of alcoholism. *Quarterly Journal of Studies on Alcohol, 17,* 296–305.

Conklin, C. A., & Tiffany, S. T. (2002). Applying extinction research and theory to cue-exposure addiction treatments. *Addiction, 97,* 155–167.

Cooney, N. L., Gillespie, R. A., Baker, L. H., & Kaplan, R. F. (1987). Cognitive changes after alcohol cue exposure. *Journal of Consulting and Clinical Psychology, 55,* 150–155.

Copeland, A. L., Brandon, T. H., & Quinn, E. P. (1995). The Smoking Consequences Questionnaire—Adult: Measurement of smoking outcome expectancies of experienced smokers. *Psychological Assessment, 7,* 484–494.

de Ruiter, C., & Brosschot, J. F. (1994). The emotional Stroop interference effect in anxiety: Attentional bias or cognitive avoidance? *Behaviour Research and Therapy, 32,* 315–319.

Ekman, P., & Friesen, W. V. (1978). *Facial Action Coding System.* Palo Alto, CA: Consulting Psychologists Press.

Ekman, P., Friesen, W. V., & Ancoli, S. (1980). Facial signs of emotional experience. *Journal of Personality and Social Psychology, 39,* 1125–1134.

Ekman, P., Matsumoto, D., & Friesen, W. V. (1997). Facial expression in affective disorders. In E. L. Rosenberg & P. Ekman (Eds.), *What the face reveals: Basic and applied studies of spontaneous expression using the Facial Action Coding System (FACS)* (pp. 331–341). New York: Oxford University Press.

Ekman, P., & Rosenberg, E. L. (Eds.). (1997). *What the face reveals: Basic and applied studies of spontaneous expression using the Facial Action Coding System (FACS).* New York: Oxford University Press.

Forsyth, A., & Carey, M. P. (1998). Measuring self-efficacy in the context of HIV risk reduction: Research challenges and recommendations. *Health Psychology, 17,* 559–568.

Gibbons, F. X., & Eggleston, T. J. (1996). Smoker networks and the "typical smokers": A prospective analysis of smoking cessation. *Health Psychology, 15,* 469–477.

Gilovich, T., Kerr, M., & Husted-Medvec, V. (1993). Effect of temporal perspective on subjective confidence. *Journal of Personality and Social Psychology, 64,* 552–560.

Goldstein, R. Z., & Volkow, N. D. (2002). Drug addiction and its underlying neurobiological basis: Neuroimaging evidence for the involvement of the frontal cortex. *American Journal of Psychiatry, 159,* 1642–1652.

Griffiths, R., Bigelow, G., & Liebson, I. (1976). Facilitation of human tobacco self-administration by ethanol: A behavioral analysis. *Journal of the Experimental Analysis of Behavior, 25,* 279–292.

Gross, T., Jarvik, M., & Rosenblatt, M. (1993). Nicotine abstinence produces content-specific Stroop interference. *Psychopharmacology, 110,* 333–336.

Gwaltney, C. J., Shiffman, S., Norman, G. J., Paty, J. A., Kassel, J. D., & Gnys, M. (2001). Does smoking abstinence self-efficacy vary across situations?: Identifying context-specificity within the Relapse Situation Efficacy Questionnaire. *Journal of Consulting and Clinical Psychology, 69,* 516–527.

Gwaltney, C. J., Shiffman, S. & Sayette, M. A. (2003, February). *Situational correlates of abstinence self-efficacy.* Poster presented at annual meeting of Society for Research on Nicotine and Tobacco, New Orleans, LA.

Hoch, S. J., & Loewenstein, G. F. (1991). Time-inconsistent preferences and consumer self-control. *Journal of Consumer Research, 17,* 492–507.

Hughes, J. R. (1991). Distinguishing withdrawal relief and direct effects of smoking. *Psychopharmacology, 104,* 409–410.

Hughes, J. R., Gulliver, S. B., Fenwick, J. W., Valliere, W. A., Cruser, K., Pepper, S., Shea, P., Solomon, L. J., & Flynn, B. S. (1992). Smoking cessation among self-quitters. *Health Psychology, 11,* 331–334.

Hull, J. G. (1987). Self-awareness model. In H. T. Blane & K. E. Leonard (Eds.), *Psychological theories of drinking and alcoholism* (pp. 272–304). New York: Guilford Press.

Jentsch, J. D., & Taylor, J. R. (1999). Impulsivity resulting from frontostriatal dysfunction in drug abuse: Implications for the control of behavior by reward-related stimuli. *Psychopharmacology, 146,* 373–390.

Jorenby, D. E., Leischow, S. J., Nides, M. A., Rennard, S. I., Johnston, J. A., Hughes, A. R., Smith, S. S., Muramoto, M. L., Daughton, D. M., Doan, K., Fiore, M. C., & Baker, T. B. (1999). A controlled trial of sustained-release bupropion, a nicotine patch, or both for smoking cessation. *New England Journal of Medicine, 340,* 685–691.

Josephs, R. A., & Steele, C. M. (1990). The two faces of alcohol myopia: Attentional mediation of psychological stress. *Journal of Abnormal Psychology, 99,* 115–126.

Juliano, L. M., & Brandon, T. H. (1998). Reactivity to instructed smoking availability and environmental cues: Evidence with urge and reaction time. *Experimental and Clinical Psychopharmacology, 6,* 45–53.

Kunda, Z. (1990). The case for motivated reasoning. *Psychological Bulletin, 108,* 480–498.

Lazarus, R. S., & Folkman, S. (1984). *Stress, appraisal, and coping.* New York: Springer.

Loewenstein, G. (1987). Anticipation and the valuation of delayed consumption. *Economic Journal, 97,* 666–684.

Loewenstein, G. (1999). A visceral account of addiction. In J. Elster & O. J. Skog (Eds.), *Getting hooked: Rationality and addiction* (pp. 235–264). Cambridge, UK: Cambridge University Press.

MacAndrew, C., & Edgerton, R. B. (1969). *Drunken comportment: A social explanation.* Chicago: Aldine.

MacDonald, T., Fong, G. T., Zanna, M. P., & Martineau, A. M. (2000). Alcohol myopia and condom use: Can alcohol intoxication be associated with more prudent behavior? *Journal of Personality and Social Psychology, 78,* 605–619.

MacLeod, C., & Hagan, R. (1992). Individual differences in the selective processing of threatening information, and emotional responses to a stressful life event. *Behaviour Research and Therapy, 30,* 151–161.

Marlatt, G. A. (1985). Cognitive factors in the relapse process. In G. A. Marlatt & J. R. Gordon (Eds.), *Relapse prevention: Maintenance strategies in the treatment of addictive behaviors* (pp. 128–200). New York: Guilford Press.

Marlatt, G. A., & Gordon, J. R. (Eds.). (1985). *Relapse prevention: Maintenance strategies in the treatment of addictive behaviors.* New York: Guilford Press.

Monti, P. M., Rohsenow, D. J., Rubonis, A. V., Niaura, R. S., Sirota, A. D., Colby, S. M., Goddard, P., & Abrams, D. B. (1993). Cue exposure with coping skills treatment for male alcoholics: A preliminary investigation. *Journal of Consulting and Clinical Psychology, 61,* 1011–1019.

Muraven, M., & Baumeister, R. F. (2000). Self-regulation and depletion of limited resources: Does self-control resemble a muscle? *Psychological Bulletin, 126,* 247–259.

Niaura, R. S., Rohsenow, D. J., Binkoff, J. A., Monti, P. M., Pedraza, M., & Abrams, D. B. (1988). Relevance of cue reactivity to understanding alcohol and smoking relapse. *Journal of Abnormal Psychology, 97,* 133–152.

Nil, R., Buzzi, R., & Bättig, K. (1984). Effects of single doses of alcohol and caffeine on cigarette smoke puffing behavior. *Pharmacology, Biochemistry, and Behavior, 20,* 583–590.

Nisbett, R., & Wilson, T. D. (1977). Telling more than we know: Verbal reports on mental processes. *Psychological Review, 84,* 231–259.

O'Brien, C. P., Childress, A. R., Arndt, I. O., McLellan, A. T., Woody, G. E. & Maany, I. (1988). Pharmacological and behavioral treatments of cocaine dependence: controlled studies. *Journal of Clinical Psychiatry, 49,* 17–22.

Piasecki, T. M., Niaura, R., Shadel, W. G., Abrams, D., Goldstein, M., Fiore, M. C., et al. (2000) Smoking withdrawal dynamics in unaided quitters. *Journal of Abnormal Psychology, 109,* 74–86.

Polivy, J. (2000). The false hope syndrome: Unfulfilled expectations of self-change. *Current Directions in Psychological Science, 9,* 128–131.

Poulos, C. X., Hinson, R. E., & Siegel, S. (1981). The role of Pavlovian processes in drug tolerance and dependence: Implications for treatment. *Addictive Behaviors, 6,* 205–211.

Robinson, T. E., & Berridge, K. C. (1993). The neural basis of drug craving: An incentive–sensitization theory of addiction. *Brain Research Reviews, 18,* 247–291.

Sayette, M. A. (1999). Cognitive theory and research. In K. E. Leonard & H. T. Blane (Eds.), *Psychological theories of drinking and alcoholism* (2nd ed., pp. 247–291). New York: Guilford Press.

Sayette, M. A. (2002a). The effects of alcohol on cigarette craving. *Alcoholism: Clinical and Experimental Research, 26,* 1925–1927.

Sayette, M. A. (2002b, February). *What laboratory research can teach us about relapse.* Paper presented at National Institute on Drug Abuse meeting, "Novel Approaches to Drug Relapse," Bethesda, MD.

Sayette, M. A., Cohn, J. F., Wertz, J. M., Perrott, M. A., & Parrott, D. J. (2001). A psychometric evaluation of the Facial Action Coding System for assessing spontaneous expression. *Journal of Nonverbal Behavior, 25,* 167–186.

Sayette, M. A., & Hufford, M. R. (1994). Effects of cue exposure and deprivation on cognitive resources in smokers. *Journal of Abnormal Psychology, 103,* 812–818.

Sayette, M. A., & Hufford, M. R. (1995). Urge and affect: A facial coding analysis of smokers. *Experimental and Clinical Psychopharmacology, 3,* 417–423.

Sayette, M. A., & Hufford, M. R. (1997). Effects of smoking urge on generation of smoking-related information. *Journal of Applied Social Psychology, 27,* 1395–1405.

Sayette, M. A., Kirchner, T. R., Moreland, R. L., Levine, J. M., & Travis, T. (in press). The effects of alcohol on risk-seeking behavior: A group-level analysis. *Psychology of Addictive Behaviors.*

Sayette, M. A., Martin, C. S., Hull, J. G., Wertz, J. M., & Perrott, M. A. (2003). The effects of nicotine deprivation on craving response covariation in smokers. *Journal of Abnormal Psychology, 112,* 110–118.

Sayette, M. A., Martin, C. S., Wertz, J. M., Shiffman, S., & Perrott, M. A. (2001). A multidimensional analysis of cue-elicited craving in heavy smokers and tobacco chippers. *Addiction, 96,* 1419–1432.

Sayette, M. A., Shiffman, S., Tiffany, S. T., Niaura, R. S., Martin, C. S., & Shadel, W. G. (2000). The measurement of drug craving. *Addiction, 95,* S189–S210.

Sayette, M. A., Wertz, J. M., Martin, C. S., Cohn, J. F., Perrott, M. A., & Hobel, J. (2003). Effects of smoking opportunity on cue-elicited urge: A facial coding analysis. *Experimental and Clinical Psychopharmacology, 11,* 218–227.

Schachter, S., Silverstein, B., & Perlick, D. (1977). Psychological and pharmacological explanations of smoking under stress. *Journal of Experimental Psychology: General, 106,* 31–40.

Shiffman, S. (1982). Relapse following smoking cessation: A situational analysis. *Journal of Consulting and Clinical Psychology, 50,* 71–86.

Shiffman, S., & Balabanis, M. (1995). Associations between alcohol and tobacco. In J. B. Fertig & J. P. Allen (Eds.), *Alcohol and tobacco: From basic science to clinical practice* (Research Monograph No. 30). Bethesda, MD: National Institute on Alcohol Abuse and Alcoholism.

Shiffman, S., Balabanis, M. H., Paty, J. A., Engberg, J., Gwaltney, C. J., Liu, K., Gnys, M., Hickcox, M., & Paton, S. M. (2000). Dynamic effects of self-efficacy on smoking lapse and relapse. *Health Psychology, 19,* 315–323.

Shiffman, S., Gwaltney, C. J., Balabanis, M. K., Liu, K. S., Paty, J. A., Kassel, J. D., Hickcox, M., & Gnys, M. (2003). Immediate antecedents of cigarette smoking: An analysis from ecological momentary assessment. *Journal of Abnormal Psychology, 111,* 531–545.

Shiffman, S., Shadel, W. G., Niaura, R., Khayrallah, M. A., Jorenby, D. E., Ryan, C. F., & Ferguson, C. L. (2003). Efficacy of acute administration of nicotine gum in relief of cue-provoked cigarette craving. *Psychopharmacology, 166,* 344–350.

Steele, C. M., & Josephs, R. A. (1990). Alcohol myopia: Its prized and dangerous effects. *American Psychologist, 45,* 921–933.

Stone, A. A., Turkkan, J. S., Bachrach, C. A., Jobe, J. B., Kurtzman, H. S., & Cain, V. S. (Eds.). (2000). *The science of self-report: Implications for research and practice.* Mahwah, NJ: Erlbaum.

Tice, D. M., Bratslavsky, E., & Baumeister, R. F. (2001). Emotional distress regulation takes precedence over impulse control: If you feel bad, do it! *Journal of Personality and Social Psychology, 80,* 53–67.

Tiffany, S. T. (1990). A cognitive model of drug urges and drug-use behavior: Role of automatic and nonautomatic processes. *Psychological Review, 97,* 147–168.

Tiffany, S. T. (1992). A critique of contemporary urge and craving research: Methodological, psychometric, and theoretical issues. *Advances in Behaviour Research and Therapy, 14,* 123–139.

Tiffany, S. T. (1995). The role of cognitive factors in reactivity to drug urges. In D. C. Drummond, S. T. Tiffany, S. Glautier, & B. Remington (Eds.), *Addictive behaviour: Cue exposure theory and practice* (pp. 137–165). London: Wiley

U.S. Department of Health and Human Services. (1989). *Reducing the health consequences of smoking: 25 years of progress: A report of the Surgeon General.* Rockville, MD: Public Health Service, Office on Smoking and Health.

Vohs, K. D., & Heatherton, T. F. (2000). Self-regulatory failure: A resource-depletion approach. *Psychological Science, 11,* 249–254.

Vohs, K. D., & Schmeichel, B. J. (2003). Self-regulation and the extended now: Controlling the self alters the subjective experience of time. *Journal of Personality and Social Psychology, 85,* 217–230.

Waters, A. J., & Feyerabend, C. (2000). Determinants and effects of attentional bias in smokers. *Psychology of Addictive Behaviors, 14*(2), 111–120.

Waters, A. J., Sayette, M. A., & Wertz, J. M. (2003). Carry-over effects can modulate emotional Stroop effects. *Cognition and Emotion, 17*, 501–509.

Waters, A. J., Shiffman, S., Sayette, M. A., Paty, J., Gwaltney, C., & Balabanis, M. (2003.) Attentional bias predicts outcome in smoking cessation. *Health Psychology, 22*, 378–387.

Weiss, F., Maldonado-Vlaar, C. S., Parsons, L. H., Kerr, T. M., Smith, D. L., & Ben-Shahar, O. (2000). Control of cocaine-seeking behavior by drug associated stimuli in rats: Effects on recovery of extinguished operant-responding and extracellular dopamine levels in amygdala and nucleus accumbens. *Proceedings of the National Academy of Sciences, 97*, 4321–4326.

Wertz, J. M., & Sayette, M. A. (2001a). Effects of smoking opportunity on attentional bias in smokers. *Psychology of Addictive Behaviors, 15*, 268–271.

Wertz, J. M., & Sayette, M. A. (2001b). A review of the effects of perceived drug use opportunity on self-reported urge. *Experimental and Clinical Psychopharmacology, 9*, 3–13.

Wikler, A. (1948). Recent progress in research on the neurophysiological basis of morphine addiction. *American Journal of Psychiatry, 105*, 329–338.

Williams, J. M. G., Mathews, A., & MacLeod, C. (1996). The emotional Stroop task and psychopathology. *Psychological Bulletin, 120*, 3–24.

Wilson, G. T. (1987). Cognitive processes in addiction. *British Journal of Addiction, 82*, 343–353.

Wood, J. V. (1989). Theory and research concerning social comparisons of personal attributes. *Psychological Bulletin, 106*, 231–248.

Zinser, M. C., Fiore, M. C., Davidson, R. J., & Baker, T. B. (1999). Manipulating smoking motivation: Impact on an electrophysiological index of approach motivation. *Journal of Abnormal Psychology, 108*, 240–254.

24

Alcohol and Self-Regulation

JAY G. HULL
LAURIE B. SLONE

O God, that men should put an enemy
In their mouths to steal away their brains!
—CASSIO TO IAGO (*Othello*, Act II, scene iii)

The substance of which Cassio speaks is alcohol. As he notes, alcohol is often conceived as an enemy: hazardous to oneself and to others. Indeed, alcohol is associated with greater personal risks for a variety of health problems, including cirrhosis, cancer, stroke, and physical injury (Corrao, Bagnardi, Zambon, & Arico, 1999). Increased risk to others includes both accidents and (as in the case of Cassio) assaults. Hingson, Heern, Zakocs, Kopstein, and Wechsler (2002) reported that, in 1998, over 500,000 college students were unintentionally injured under the influence of alcohol, a slightly larger number were hit or assaulted by an intoxicated student, and over 1,400 students died from alcohol-related injuries, including motor vehicle accidents. According to one large survey of adults 18 years and older, alcohol is involved in two thirds of incidents involving physical aggression (Wells, Graham, & West, 2000). Despite such grim consequences, Cassio also notes that alcohol is *voluntarily* consumed. Why? What do people gain, or hope to gain, by consuming alcohol, and what do they lose? Perhaps the answer lies in Cassio's final observation: They lose their brains, and sometimes this is a gain.

In keeping with the theme of this handbook, we adopt a self-regulatory perspective on the causes and consequences of alcohol use (cf. Baumeister, 1991; Baumeister, Heatherton, & Tice, 1994). We begin by briefly reviewing recent research on self-regulatory factors associated with alcohol consumption. Two broad hypotheses subsume much of this literature: (1) Individuals with low self-regulatory skills are less able to control their drinking; and (2) individuals attempt to regulate their social and affective experiences by consuming alcohol. We then turn to a consideration of self-regulatory factors associated with the behavioral consequences of intoxication. One hypothesis underlying much of this research is that intoxication impairs cognitive processes central to self-regulation. After briefly reviewing recent research on the consequences of intoxication for selected social behaviors, we turn to a consideration of the specific mechanisms responsible for these effects. We conclude by suggesting avenues for future research.

THE EFFECT OF SELF-REGULATION
ON ALCOHOL CONSUMPTION

As noted, two hypotheses based on self-regulation are often offered to explain differences in alcohol consumption: Individuals with low self-regulatory skills are less able to control their drinking, and individuals attempt to regulate their affect by consuming alcohol. Each hypothesis has received considerable support.

Alcohol Consumption and Self-Control

Studies using a variety of methodologies suggest that individuals with weak self-regulatory skills consume larger amounts of alcohol than do individuals with strong self-regulatory skills. With respect to general personality variables, studies implicate low conscientiousness (Kubicka, Matejcek, Dytrych, & Roth, 2001), typically understood to include low self-control, as associated with increased alcohol use. More specific to self-regulation, numerous studies associate increased alcohol consumption with individual differences in (lack of) self-control (e.g., Adalbjarnardottir & Rafnsson, 2001; Wills, DuHamel, & Vaccaro, 1995), behavioral undercontrol (Martin, Lynch, Pollock, & Clark, 2000; Slutske et al., 2002), and susceptibility to temptation (Collins, Koutsky, & Izzo, 2000; Palfai, 2001; Wulfert, Block, Ana, Rodriguez, & Colsman, 2002). Furthermore, generalized self-control appears to mediate the influence of a variety of temperament variables in early substance use (e.g., Wills & Stoolmiller, 2002).

With respect to individual differences specific to alcohol use, perceptions of inability to control drinking have been used to predict future consumption, particularly among individuals who have experienced alcohol dependence. According to the Marlatt and Gordon (1985) model of relapse prevention, following interventions to reduce drinking, those who perceive a lower efficacy to refuse alcohol across a variety of situations are more likely to experience relapse. This analysis has been supported using a variety of measures of self-efficacy (e.g., Allsop, Saunders, & Phillips, 2000; Goldbeck, Myatt, & Aitchison, 1997; Lee, Oei, & Greeley, 1999; Maisto, Connors, & Zywiak, 2000; Wells-Parker, Kenne, Spratke, & Williams, 2000).

Situationally, the feeling that one has reduced control may be experienced as "craving," defined as the "subjective desire or urge to take a drug or feel its effects" (de Wit, 2000; p. S165). Among drinkers, increased craving is typically hypothesized to be primed by the presence of drug-related cues, such that the perceived opportunity to use the drug increases urge ratings (e.g., Wertz & Sayette, 2001) and, presumably, decreases ability to exert self-control. Although controversy exists as to the proper measurement of craving (Tiffany, Carter, & Singleton, 2000) and its utility as a predictor of alcoholic relapse (Drummond, Litten, Lowman, & Hunt, 2000), there is little doubt that the presence of alcohol can serve as a cue that primes drinking among some individuals. Indeed, following exposure to an alcohol cue, social drinkers (Chutuape, Mitchell, & de Wit, 1994), heavy drinkers (Kambouropoulos & Staiger, 2001), and inpatient alcoholics (Cooney, Litt, Morse, Bauer, & Gaupp, 1997; Hussong, Hicks, Levy, & Curran, 2001; Jansma, Breteler, Schippers, De Jong, & Van der Staak, 2000) all report greater urges to drink. Furthermore, when these individuals are given preloads of various amounts, alcohol dose dependently increases subjective reports of drug liking and desire to consume more alcohol (Kirk & de Wit, 2000).

Although situations can function to increase alcohol use by reducing perceptions of self-control, it is also true that environments that foster self-control (close parental monitoring, clearly defined rules for behavior, appropriate parental rewards for good behavior, high refusal skills, and a strong belief in moral order; Guo, Hawkins, Hill, & Abbott, 2001) are associated with lower risk for alcohol dependence and abuse. Likewise, restrictive environments tend to decrease alcohol abuse (Wechsler, Lee, Gledhill-Hoyt, & Nelson, 2001), and permissive drinking environments appear to foster such abuse (e.g., Knight et al., 2002).

On the basis of these studies, it is reasonable to conclude that individuals who are generally low in self-control, low in efficacy to avoid consumption, or situationally induced to experience a lack of control are likely to consume more alcohol.

Alcohol Consumption and Affect Regulation

According to the foregoing discussion, higher amounts of alcohol consumption may reflect a lack of self-control. This implies that increased alcohol consumption is the unintentional consequence of self-regulatory failure. It is also possible, however, that alcohol consumption is intentionally adopted as a means of regulating social and affective experiences. Specifically, individuals may drink to avoid negative affect and enhance positive experiences (see Larsen & Prizmic, Chapter 3, this volume). The most popular form of this analysis links drinking to tension reduction (Conger, 1951, 1956) or, more generally, to relief from negative affect. In terms of general personality variables, studies indicate that high neuroticism or negative affectivity (e.g., negative emotionality, Martin et al., 2000; loneliness and depression, Bonin, McCreary, & Sadava, 2000) is associated with increased alcohol use. Likewise, nervousness predicts increased alcohol consumption later in the course of the day (Swendsen et al., 2000); anticipation of giving a stressful speech is associated with increased alcohol consumption, particularly among individuals high in social anxiety (Kidorf & Lang, 1999), and negative affective imagery leads to increased subjective reporting of desire to drink among alcoholics (Cooney et al., 1997).

A number of studies have implicated negative affect in response to interpersonal difficulties as especially motivating of alcohol consumption. Using daily diaries, Mohr and colleagues (2001) found that participants engaged in more solitary drinking on days with more negative interpersonal experiences (particularly individuals high in neuroticism). Similarly, negative interpersonal status, such as being held in low esteem by one's roommate (Joiner, Vohs, & Schmidt, 2000) or abused at work (Richman, Shinsako, Rospenda, Flaherty, & Freels, 2002), is associated with increased alcohol use. At the same time, there appear to be some gender differences in this regard (see Nolen-Hoeksema & Corte, Chapter 21, this volume). In a study by Hodgins, el-Guebaly, and Armstrong (1995), the most frequent precipitant of major relapses among alcohol-dependent individuals was negative emotional states; however, interpersonal determinants were more influential among females, and intrapersonal determinants were more influential among males. Frank, Jacobson, and Tuer (1990) found that, for women, excessive drinking to reduce emotional distress was predicted by problems with intimacy, whereas among men, it was predicted by poor conflict resolution skills and less adult work statuses.

Workplace problems appear to predict increased alcohol consumption in part because they increase distress (Richman et al., 2002) and the length of time to unwind (Delaney, Grube, Greiner, Fisher, & Ragland, 2002). Such stress-motivated drinking seems to be more prevalent in early than in late adulthood. In later years, it appears to be associated with more problematic drinking (Perkins, 1999) rather than greater alcohol use per se (see also McCreary & Sadava, 1998, 2000). Finally, there is some evidence of a reciprocal relationship between drinking and negative affect, such that increased sadness and hostility in the context of few intimate and supportive friendships lead to greater drinking, which in turn predicts subsequent increases in sadness and hostility (Hussong et al., 2001).

Whereas it would appear that alcohol is sometimes consumed in an attempt to reduce negative states (i.e., to serve as a negative reinforcer by reducing states such as tension), it also seems to be the case that alcohol is consumed to achieve a variety of positive states (i.e., to serve as a positive reinforcer by enhancing states such as self-confidence). Although this issue is explored in greater detail in a subsequent section, we note here that high extraversion (e.g., Flory, Lynam, Milich, Leukefeld, & Clayton, 2002; Gotham, Sher, & Wood, 1997; Kubicka et al., 2001) and high openness to experience (e.g., Gotham et al., 1997); and low rigidity (Koppes, Twisk, Snel, De Vente, & Kemper, 2001) are associated with increased drinking, suggesting that people may drink both to achieve positive experiences (e.g., increased sociability, novelty) and to avoid negative experiences.

In summary, this literature suggests that alcohol is consumed in part as a means of escaping negative affective states and achieving positive states. Negative states that are a consequence of interpersonal difficulties appear to be especially likely to motivate alcohol consumption, particularly among women.

Alcohol Consumption and Expectancies

Although individuals may drink to improve their mood state, this effect is mediated in part by individuals' cognitive expectations regarding the psychological consequences of alcohol. Thus, it is logical that only individuals who *expect* alcohol to have the effect of improving their mood would *choose* to consume alcohol when they experience a relevant mood state. It is therefore important to understand the nature of these cognitive associations or expectancies regarding the effects of alcohol: their origins, consequences for behavior, and susceptibility to change.

The Nature of Expectancies Regarding the Effects of Alcohol

Alcohol intoxication is generally expected to be associated with a variety of positive and negative psychological effects (see Brown, Goldman, Inn, & Anderson, 1980; Goldman, Del Boca, & Darkes, 1999). With respect to positive effects, it is expected to (1) reduce tension, (2) improve mood, (3) increase sociability and facilitate social interactions, (4) boost assertiveness and feelings of power, (5) improve sexual functioning and experiences, and (6) create pleasant physical sensations. With respect to negative effects, alcohol is expected to (1) impair cognitive performance, (2) decrease self-control, (3) increase aggressiveness, (4) increase the likelihood of injuries, and (5) at high levels, create unpleasant physical sensations.

Although alcohol is typically associated with positive and negative consequences, such as those listed here, variation exists among individuals in the extent to which they hold these expectancies. Differences in expectancies exist as a function of variables such as (1) drinking status (e.g., problem drinkers, Lewis & O'Neill, 2000; heavy drinkers, Orford et al., 2002); (2) cultural background (Lindman, Sjoeholm, & Lang, 2000; Velez-Blasini, 1997); (3) gender (Wall, Hinson, & McKee, 1998); (4) age (e.g., Dunn & Goldman, 1996, 1998; Lundahl, Davis, Adesso, & Lukas, 1997); (5) family history of alcoholism (e.g., Lundahl et al., 1997), and (6) exposure to advertising (e.g., Dunn & Yniguez, 1999). More psychologically based individual differences may also be associated with differences in the expected effects of alcohol. For example, individuals with lower self-efficacy expect greater psychological benefits from drinking (e.g., improved social skills, less depression and tension; Skutle, 1999). In addition to affecting the actual expectancies individuals hold, individual differences also exist that moderate the strength of the link between expectancies and alcohol use (e.g., private self-consciousness; Bartholow, Sher, & Strathman, 2000), and between expectancies and alcohol-related problems (e.g., Johnson & Glassman, 1999).

Association of Expectancies with Consumption

Much of the research on the behavioral effects of alcohol expectancies concerns its link to consumption. As noted earlier, positive expectancies are generally associated with increased consumption, and negative expectancies with decreased consumption. Such effects have been shown for different types of drinkers (e.g., social drinkers, Oei, Fergusson, & Lee, 1998; alcoholics, Connors, Tarbox, & Faillace, 1993) and age groups (e.g., elementary school children, Miller, Smith, & Goldman, 1990; adolescents, Simons-Morton et al., 1999; Wiers, Hoogeveen, Sergeant, & Gunning, 1997; older adults, Cooper, Russell, Skinner, & Windle, 1992). Not only are these expectancies correlated with use, but positive expectancies are also predictive of future drinking (e.g., Aas, Leigh, Anderssen, & Jakobsen, 1998) and persistent alcohol dependence (e.g., Kilbey, Downey, & Breslau, 1998). On the other hand, negative expectancies appear to increase readiness to change drinking behavior (e.g., Ramsey et al., 2000), and persons who expect negative consequences may drink less as a consequence (Sharkansky & Finn, 1998). Furthermore, interventions that alter expectancies have been shown to decrease subsequent alcohol use (e.g., Darkes & Goldman, 1998; Dunn, Lau, & Cruz, 2000; for a review, see Jones, Corbin, & Fromme, 2001). Although positive and negative expectancies are typically viewed as contributing independently and linearly to alcohol use, some research suggests that they may predict different aspects of consumption (e.g., quantity vs. frequency of consumption; Lee, Greeley, & Oei, 1999) and may interactively combine to predict consumption (e.g., Grube & Agostinelli, 1999).

Beyond the effects of expectancies on consumption, expectancies have also been linked to a variety of other alcohol-related behaviors. Some of these effects are independent of the pharmacological effects of the drug, such that individuals act in a manner consistent with their expectancies whenever they *think* that they have consumed alcohol (regardless of the alcoholic content of the beverage they consumed; see Hull & Bond, 1986). Alcohol expectancies have also been observed to interact with the pharmacological effects of the drug, although these effects have been inconsistent. Thus, some researchers find that alcohol has its most detrimental effects among those who expect impairment (e.g., Fillmore, Carscadden, & Vogel-Sprott, 1998; Fillmore & Vogel-Sprott, 1998), whereas others suggest that expected impairment leads to compensation (e.g., Fillmore & Blackburn, 2002). In a meta-analysis of research that included both alcohol consumption and expectancy manipulations, Hull and Bond (1986) concluded that these variables interact no more frequently than would be expected by chance.

The Dynamic Function of Expectancies

One way to conceptualize the effects of expectancies is that they function as nodes in a cognitive network (e.g., Goldman, 1999). Repeated use of alcohol (e.g., Leigh & Stacy, 1998; Rather & Goldman, 1994; Stacy, Leigh & Weingardt, 1994) or encountering environments in which alcohol is used (Brown, Tate, Vik, Haas, & Aarons, 1999) strengthens the associations between alcohol consumption and observed positive and negative outcomes. The resultant expectancy nodes can be differentially activated by situational cues (e.g., Wall, McKee, & Hinson, 2000; Wall, Hinson, McKee, & Goldstein, 2001). The specific nature of the activated expectancy varies as a function of the differential salience of particular situational cues (e.g., MacLatchy-Gaudet & Stewart, 2001). Differences in the accessibility and strength of expectancies in turn predict differences in alcohol use (e.g., Palfai & Wood, 2001; Stacy & Newcomb, 1998). Consumption is increased when positive expectancies are activated (Carter, McNair, Corbin, & Black, 1998; Roehrich & Goldman, 1995; Stein, Goldman, & Del Boca, 2000) and decreased when negative expectancies are activated (Carter et al., 1998). For example, men who anticipate that alcohol creates a sense of carelessness drink more on stressful than on nonstressful days compared to those who did not have this expectancy (Armeli, Carney, Tennen, Affleck, & O'Neil, 2000), and men who expect alcohol to increase their assertiveness drink more when anticipating the delivery of a stressful speech than during a baseline control session (Kidorf & Lang, 1999).

In addition to external situational cues, alcohol cues and the intoxicated state itself may differentially activate expectancies. Thus, alcohol-related information is more accessible after exposure to alcohol cues (e.g., Glautier & Spencer, 1999), and expectancies (e.g., regarding the tension reducing effects of alcohol) are most likely to be reported when individuals are at the peak of intoxication relative to periods during which the effects of the drug are diminished or have worn off (Kushner et al., 2000). Similarly, Jones and Schulze (2000) found that words depicting the positive consequences of alcohol consumption were more accessible than words depicting negative consequences in a group primed with an alcohol drink than in a group primed with a nonalcohol drink. As would be expected from the fact that individuals differ in their expectancies, the particular associations activated by intoxication vary (e.g., Kramer & Goldman, 2003). For example, heavy drinkers are most likely to activate positive expectancies on the ascending limb of the blood alcohol curve, whereas light drinkers are most likely to activate negative expectancies on the descending limb of the blood alcohol curve (Dunn & Earleywine, 2001).

Expectancies as Mediators

Given a direct link between expectancies and consumption, numerous variables have been theorized to have indirect effects on consumption via their effects on expectancy. Among others, these include (1) peer alcohol use and attitudes (Ouellette, Gerrard, Gibbons, & Reis-Bergan, 1999; Scheier & Botvin, 1997), (2) parental influence (e.g., Ouellette et al., 1999), (3) individual differences in excitement seeking (Finn, Sharkansky, Brandt, & Turcotte, 2000), (4) individual differences in disinhibition (McCarthy, Kroll, & Smith, 2001; McCarthy, Miller, Smith, & Smith, 2001), and (5) imitation or social modeling (Wood, Read, Palfai, & Stevenson, 2001). According to these analyses, more distal variables (e.g., peer alcohol use) affect alcohol consumption because they affect more proximal positive or negative expectancies. The result is a "mediational" model of consumption, in which personality variables, environmental history, and situational cues indirectly increase consumption because they affect expectancies regarding the psychological consequences of the drug.

Although a pure mediational model suggests a simple, albeit indirect, relationship between distal variables and alcohol consumption via expectancies, a slightly more complicated model proposes that this relationship will hold true for some individuals and not others. According to one form of this "moderated mediation" model (Baron & Kenny, 1986), expectancies should *only* mediate increased consumption for individuals motivated to achieve a particular psychological state. We have already seen examples of such moderated mediation: Men who anticipate that alcohol creates a sense of carelessness drink more *on stressful than on nonstressful days* compared to those who do not have this expectancy (Armeli et al., 2000), and men who expect alcohol to increase their assertiveness drink more *when anticipating the delivery of a stressful speech* than during a baseline control session (Kidorf & Lang, 1999). Thus, it is not the case that expectancies increase consumption per se; rather, they increase consumption when individuals are motivated to achieve the psychological state they expect alcohol to be able to produce (e.g., tension reduction). This notion of "moderated mediation" returns us to the issue of consumption as motivated self-regulation. In this case, however, such motivations include but extend well beyond tension reduction and affect enhancement.

Motives to Drink

Even if expectancies were uniform regarding alcohol's effects, people would undoubtedly drink for different reasons. Major dimensions of such motivations include drinking for (1) social motives (Labouvie & Bates, 2002; MacLean & Lecci, 2000); (2) enhancement motives (Comeau, Stewart, & Loba, 2001; MacLean & Lecci, 2000), such as reducing negative affect and enhancing enjoyment (Carpenter & Hasin, 1998); (3) coping motives (Comeau et al., 2001; Labouvie & Bates, 2002; MacLean & Lecci, 2000), such as reducing self-dissatisfaction (Downey, Rosengen, & Donovan, 2000); (4) conformity motives (Comeau et al., 2001; MacLean & Lecci, 2000), including self-presentation (Sharp & Getz, 1996); and (5) disinhibition motives (Labouvie & Bates, 2002). From a self-regulation perspective, each of these motivations can be conceptualized as reference values that serve to guide the individual's behavior (e.g., see Carver, Chapter 2, this volume; Hull, 2002).

Within the alcohol literature, coping motives play a prominent role. Thus, numerous studies have suggested that drinking at times of stress is motivated by maladaptive coping styles typical of disengagement. Wills, Sandy, Yaeger, Cleary, and Shinar (2001) found that disengagement coping styles were positively related to substance use and growth in use over time, whereas engagement-related coping styles showed the opposite pattern. Furthermore, consistent with the notion of the moderating influences of self-regulatory motives, Wills and colleagues found that the effects of coping were significantly greater at times of stress (see also Tyssen, Vaglum, Aasland, Gronvold, & Ekeberg, 1998). Other studies have likewise found that avoidant coping styles are predictive of drinking to cope, alcohol use, and alcohol-related problems (e.g., see Laurent, Catanzaro, & Callan, 1997; Simpson & Arroyo, 1998). Finally, research has demonstated the utility of a specific "drinking to cope" measure as a predictor of alcohol consumption and problems (e.g., Holahan, Moos, Holahan, Cronkite, & Randall, 2001, 2003; Park & Levenson, 2002). Once again, consistent with the notion of the moderating influences of motivation, Cooper, Frone, Russell, and Mudar (1995) found that positive expectancies regarding the effects of alcohol are more strongly associated with "drinking to cope" among those higher in (1) negative affect, (2) sensation seeking, and (3) a desire to cope through avoidance.

Summary

As can be seen from this brief review, people have a variety of expectancies regarding the effects of alcohol, and they are more likely to consume alcohol when they are motivated to achieve a state that they expect it to be able to produce. Thus, in addition to alcohol being consumed as a result of self-regulatory failure (lack of self-control), it would also appear that alcohol is consumed as a consequence of an intentional effort to regulate personal experiences.

THE EFFECT OF ALCOHOL CONSUMPTION ON SELF-REGULATION

Whereas self-regulation is related to alcohol consumption in a variety of ways, it is also the case that intoxication affects self-regulation in numerous ways. Generally speaking, alcohol is hypothesized to impair or disrupt self-regulation. On the basis of this logic, alcohol is predicted to increase dysfunctional behavior in situations that require self-control. Three research topics that may reflect dysfunctional self-regulation concern the effects of alcohol intoxication on (1) aggression, (2) risk taking, and (3) indiscriminate sex. Somewhat independent of questions regarding the behavioral consequences of intoxication are those regarding the processes responsible for such effects. Several mechanisms have been proposed, including the effect of alcohol on (1) narrowing attentional focus, (2) impairing the cognitive processing of information to which one attends, (3) decreasing negative affect, (4) decreasing the ability to inhibit responses in situations that provide conflicting cues, and (5) impairing executive functioning generally.

The Social Behavioral Consequences of Intoxication

Although research has examined the effects of intoxication on numerous forms of social behavior, three topics appear especially relevant to the question of alcohol's effects on self-regulation: aggression, risk, and sex.

Alcohol and Aggression

Alcohol is popularly conceived as a major cause of inappropriate aggressive behavior. As noted early in this chapter, alcohol is linked to various forms of aggression and violence (Wells et al., 2000). Accounts of naturally occurring incidents of alcohol-related aggression revolve around (1) cognitive impairment due to alcohol, (2) risk taking due to alcohol, (3) heightened emotionality due to alcohol, (4) a macho subculture, and (5) a permissive environment (e.g., Graham, West, & Wells, 2000). These accounts parallel accounts offered by alcohol researchers involving the pharmacological effects of the drug, expectancies regarding its typical consequences, the societal/cultural framing of intoxication and aggression, and the situational context associated with the event of intoxicated aggression (Graham et al., 1998).

Both cross-sectional and longitudinal studies have associated alcohol consumption and heavy drinking with increased likelihood of acting violent, as well as increased likelihood of being a victim of violence (e.g., Giancola, 2002a; Scott, Schafer, & Greenfield, 1999; White & Chen, 2002). Some studies have suggested that quantity of alcohol consumption is more predictive of violence-related injuries than frequency of drinking (Borges, Cherpitel, & Rosovsky, 1998). This suggests that high levels of intoxication are especially likely to be associated with aggressive responses. Furthermore, being a victim of intimate partner violence has been shown to increase the likelihood of subsequent heavy drinking, with a resulting cycle of alcohol use and violence (e.g., Kilpatrick, Acierno, Resnick, Saunders, & Best, 1997). In instances of intimate partner violence, alcohol is typically associated with male physical aggression against a female partner (e.g., Leonard & Quigley, 1999; Scott et al., 1999), although Leonard and Roberts (1998) found that alcohol led to increased negativity of both husbands and wives in marital interactions.

Laboratory research on the effects of alcohol on aggression has a rich history. Indeed, sufficient research exists that over the years, multiple meta-analyses have supported the conclusion that alcohol increases aggression in the laboratory, although this effect is subject to multiple qualifications (cf. Bushman & Cooper, 1990; Hull & Bond, 1986; Ito, Miller, & Pollock, 1996). Much of this research has been conducted with use of a paradigm in which participants experience various levels of provocation during a competitive task and can retaliate by administering different levels and durations of electric shock (the Taylor Aggression Paradigm; Taylor, 1967). Within this paradigm, the effect of alcohol on increasing electric shock aggression appears to be qualified by a variety of factors, including the level of threat (e.g., alcohol appears to have minimal or no effects in low-threat situations; Taylor, Gammon, & Capasso, 1976), participants' gender (e.g., men, but not women, typically show effects of alcohol; Giancola et al., 2002), personality traits (e.g., participants with moderate levels of trait anger show the greatest effects of alcohol on increasing aggression, Parrott & Zeichner, 2002; as do those with moderate and high aggressive dispositions, Bailey & Taylor, 1991; Giancola, 2002b), drinking experience (e.g., participants with low levels of drinking experience show the greatest effects of alcohol on increasing aggression; Laplace, Chermack, & Taylor, 1994), and the blood alcohol curve (alcohol has an effect of increasing aggression during the ascending limb, and little or no effect during the descending limb; Giancola & Zeichner, 1997).

Alcohol and Risky Behavior

Although there is no doubt that individuals engage in risky behavior when intoxicated (e.g., driving under the influence), it is not clear to what extent intoxication is responsible for increasing their willingness to accept risk and, if so, by what mechanism (see Leigh, 1999). It is quite possible that individuals who engage in a variety of risky behaviors also engage in excessive alcohol consumption. Perhaps both types of behavior have common causes (e.g., Barnes, Welte, Hoffman, & Dintcheff, 1999), such as an underlying "problem behavior syndrome" (Donovan & Jessor, 1985; Donovan, Jessor, & Costa, 1999). As noted by Leigh (1999), experimental studies that have directly examined the effects of alcohol on risk taking have used a variety of paradigms, including gambling, choice dilemma questionnaires, driving simulators, card games, visuomotor tasks, and video games. The effects of alcohol in these paradigms are best characterized as inconsistent. With respect to gambling, many researchers have noted that problem gambling and problem drinking appear to go hand in hand, and some have found that alcohol impairs gambling decisions (e.g., Fromme, Katz, & D'Amico, 1997; Kyngdon & Dickerson, 1999). However, most experimental studies have found no association between intoxication and gambling choices or outcomes (Breslin, Sobell, Cappell, Vakili, & Poulos, 1999; Meier, Brigham, Ward, Myers, & Warren, 1996; Sjöberg, 1969, Experiment 1; see also Wilde, Trimpop, & Joly, 1989), or effects that were qualified in unexpected ways by dose (Sjöberg, 1969, Experiment 2) or individual differences (e.g., Cutter, Green, & Harford, 1973). As a consequence, we are forced to agree with Leigh's observation: "Given the limitations of available methods, we are far from being able to make statements about the causal nature of the relationship between alcohol use and risk taking" (1999, p. 377).

Alcohol and Sexual Behavior

A third line of alcohol research relevant to self-regulation concerns the association of intoxication with risky sexual behavior. If alcohol impairs self-regulation, one might well expect intoxicated individuals to be less discriminating with respect to their choice of partner, and, once again, to be less risk averse. Consistent with such reasoning, many authors have noted that heavy episodic drinking is associated with "indiscriminate sex," typically defined as sex with multiple partners in the past month (e.g., Graves, 1995; Wechsler, Dowdall, Davenport, & Castillo, 1995). Furthermore, intoxicated participants perceive lower levels of risk and see fewer negative consequences from unsafe sex than do sober participants (Fromme, D'Amico, & Katz, 1999). Women are more likely to have sex with partners they just met when the encounter involves alcohol (Testa & Collins, 1997), to anticipate less risk and more benefit from actions that increase sexual vulnerability (Testa, Livingston, & Collins, 2000), and to see less risk and higher relationship potential for attractive, sexually risky partners (Murphy, Monahan, & Miller, 1998). Whereas much of this research implicates the pharmacological properties of the drug as being responsible for impaired self-control, other studies have found that alcohol use is especially likely to be associated with greater sexual risk taking (e.g., Dermen, Cooper, & Agocha, 1998) and judged likelihood of sexual risk taking (Fromme et al., 1999) among those who *expect* alcohol to lead to risky sexual behavior (see also George, Stoner, Norris, Lopez, & Lehman, 2000).

In addition to moderating perception of risk, alcohol also appears to bias the perception of the other as sexually receptive. Thus, intoxicated individuals appear to exaggerate the meaning of dating availability cues, and ignore the meaning of ambiguous cues, when making sexual judgments (e.g., Abbey, Zawacki, & McAuslan, 2000). More ominously, intoxicated men are slower to recognize the inappropriateness of a man's behavior in a date rape vignette and more likely to perceive the woman as experiencing higher levels of sexual arousal (Gross, Bennett, Sloan, Marx, & Juergens, 2001; see also Abbey, McAuslan, & Ross, 1998). Consistent with the implications of this research, numerous studies have linked alcohol with sexual assault (Abbey, 2002; Brecklin & Ullman, 2002).

Given this general pattern, Cooper (2002) concluded that 10 years of published studies suggest that alcohol consumption is related to the decision to have sex, and to engage in indiscriminate forms of sex (e.g., having multiple or casual sex partners). Despite the fact that alcohol seems to be associated with lower risk perception, and more risky perceptions and decisions regarding sexual partners, however, it does not appear to increase the probability of unprotected sex (e.g., Testa & Collins, 1997; see also Cooper, 2002; Morris & Albery, 2001). Cooper attributes the inability of researchers to observe a strong association between these variables to their failure to take into account the nature of the relationship between partners and the meaning of the sex act for the individuals. Thus, in a study by Cooper and Orcutt (2000), drinking and condom use were both more common with casual than with serious sexual partners, and the relationship between alcohol use and condom use only became significant and negative after controlling for the seriousness of the relationship.

Summary

As can be seen from this brief review of recent research, alcohol (1) is associated with increased aggression, (2) is inconsistently related to general risk taking, and (3) is associated with various forms of indiscriminate sexual behavior, perception, and judgment. In each of these cases, the effects of alcohol appear to be qualified by characteristics of the person and the situation. This suggests that the effects of alcohol do not follow as a consequence of the drug per se, but rather from the effect of the drug on psychological processes that are more likely to be involved in particular situations, and among certain individuals. Such findings beg the question as to the exact mechanisms whereby alcohol is having its effects.

Self-Regulatory Mechanisms Impaired by Intoxication

As noted at the beginning of this chapter, one hypothesis underlying much of the research on the behavioral consequences of intoxication holds that alcohol impairs psychological processes central to self-regulation. At the same time, multiple accounts have been offered of the particular processes that are proposed to be impaired, including attention, cognition, affect, and reactions to conflicting cues, as well as processes that best fall under the umbrella of executive function. We briefly consider several influential accounts.

Attention

Research using a variety of paradigms suggests that alcohol impairs attentional processes related to self-regulation (e.g., Fillmore, Dixon, & Schweizer, 2000). In accounting for the effects of alcohol on aggressive behavior, Pernanen (1976) argued for a mechanism that involves a "narrowing of the perceptual field," that effectively reduces the number of cues available to the intoxicated person. Similarly, Taylor and Leonard (1983) argued that the intoxicated person focuses on the most salient aspects of the situation. When cues that instigate aggression are dominant, an intoxicated person is more likely than a sober person to react aggressively. When such cues are minimal, intoxicated individuals are predicted to be no more aggressive than are sober individuals (see also Zeichner & Pihl, 1979).

Cognition

Distinct from an attentional account, other researchers have argued that alcohol impairs cognitive information processes (e.g., Birnbaum, Johnson, Hartley, & Taylor, 1980; Birnbaum & Parker, 1977; Hashtroudi, Parker, DeLisi, & Wyatt, 1983). Controlled, effortful processing appears to be particularly susceptible to alcohol impairment (e.g., Fillmore, Vogel-Sprott, & Gavrilescu, 1999; Tracy & Bates, 1999).

With respect to the implications of such findings for self-regulation, Hull (1981) proposed that alcohol interferes with higher order encoding and elaboration strategies that are fundamental to self-awareness (Hull, Levenson, Young, & Sher, 1983). As a consequence of such deficits, alcohol was proposed to decrease self-regulation with respect to personal and situational standards of conduct (e.g., Bailey, Leonard, Cranston, & Taylor, 1983). Given that alcohol decreases the tendency of intoxicated individuals to use higher order cognitive strategies but does not interfere with their ability to benefit from such strategies when they are explicitly provided by the experimenter (e.g., Birnbaum, et al., 1980), Hull and Van Treuren (1986) proposed that alcohol will have its greatest effects on behavior when the link between situational cues and appropriate standards of conduct is implicit as opposed to explicit (e.g., Leonard, 1989).

Affect

According to a third account, the effect of alcohol on behavior is mediated by its impact on affect. Thus, Conger (1951, 1956) argued that alcohol decreases anxiety and, as a consequence, may disinhibit responses such as aggression in response to threat. Although Conger proposed a direct effect of alcohol on affect, others have proposed an indirect effect via the impact of alcohol on attention and cognition (e.g., Curtin, Patrick, Lang, Cacioppo, & Birbaumer, 2001). Indeed, elsewhere, we have argued that individuals may be motivated to achieve affective relief by consuming alcohol to disrupt processing of personally painful information (e.g., feedback regarding personal failures; Hull & Young, 1983; Hull, Young, & Jouriles, 1986).

With respect to these accounts, several authors have noted that intoxication is not always associated with decreases in negative affect, and may in fact be associated with increases in negative affect (e.g., Sayette, 1999; Steele & Josephs, 1990). According to Sayette (1993), the key to determining when alcohol has the effect of decreasing versus increasing anxiety involves whether a cue has been sufficiently appraised to yield a perception of threat. If the cue has not been appraised, then intoxicated individuals will be less anxious than sober individuals when the threatening stimulus appears, because alcohol disrupts the cognitive appraisal process itself (e.g., Sayette, Smith, Breiner, & Wilson, 1992). On the other hand, if the threat cue has been sufficiently appraised, then subsequent intoxication will be less effective in decreasing, and may actually increase, anxiety (e,.g., Sayette, Martin, Perrott, Wertz, & Hufford, 2001). Research by Steele and Josephs (1988; Josephs & Steele, 1990; Steele, Southwick, & Pagano, 1986) suggests that even in conditions in which alcohol increases anxiety, the effect can be reversed if alcohol is combined with a distractor, presumably because of the synergistic effect of alcohol and distraction on impairment of cognitive processes. Note that these accounts, once again, implicate the effects of alcohol on attention and cognition as key mediators of its ultimate impact on behavior.

Inhibitory Conflict

Although attentional and cognitive mechanisms of the effects of alcohol are distinct, most researchers endorse both accounts. Steele and Josephs (1990) characterized the resultant impaired state as "alcohol myopia." More importantly from a theoretical perspective, Steele and his colleagues (1986) elaborate this account to identify situations in which alcohol is most likely to have its effects. Specifically, they argue that because (1) alcohol interferes with attention and cognition, and (2) inhibiting cues are less likely to be in focal attention than are instigating cues, and more likely to require additional cognitive processing to extract their meaning, (3) the behavior of the intoxicated individual is more likely than that of the sober individual to be under the control of instigating as opposed to inhibiting cues. As a consequence, alcohol is especially likely to affect behavior when instigating and inhibiting cues are both strong and relatively equal, a condition that Steele and Southwick (1985) characterize as high in inhibitory conflict.

Steele and his colleagues provide both a meta-analysis (Steele & Southwick, 1985) and original research in support of this analysis (e.g., Banaji & Steele, 1989; Steele, Critchlow, & Liu, 1985). More recently, the notions of alcohol myopia and inhibitory conflict have been used to account for the effects of alcohol on attribution (e.g., Herzog, 1999) and attitudes toward drunk driving (MacDonald, Zanna, & Fong, 1996). The most extensive application involves the effects of alcohol on sexual risk taking. Consistent with the notion of alcohol myopia, it has been found that (1) when sexually instigatory cues are present, intoxicated people report greater intentions to have unprotected sex than do sober people, whereas when strong inhibiting cues are present, they report more prudent intentions than sober people (MacDonald, Fong, Zanna, & Martineua, 2000); (2) in situations containing both male attractiveness cues and sexual assault cues, intoxicated women rate the man more positively and anticipate less risk from behaviors likely to increase sexual vulnerability than do sober women (Testa et al., 2000); (3) when focused on a romantic conflict, intoxicated individuals report more negative emotion and more negative perceptions of their partner's feelings than do sober individuals (MacDonald, Zanna, & Holmes, 2000). Consistent with the notion of inhibitory conflict, it has been found that (1) self-reported quantity of alcohol consumed was significantly negatively associated with condom use at first intercourse *only* among individuals who were highly conflicted about using a condom (Dermen & Cooper, 2000), and (2) in dating couples, the effects of alcohol on intercourse were found primarily among males who were highly conflicted about having intercourse (although a similar effect was not found among highly conflicted females; Cooper & Orcutt, 1997).

Conflict and Inhibition: Go/No-Go and Stop

The notion that alcohol is likely to be associated with disinhibition under conditions of conflict has a relatively long history (e.g., Conger, 1956; Masserman & Yum, 1946). The mechanisms behind such effects are less clear. As noted, Steele and his colleagues attribute the effect to attentional and cognitive impairment that differentially affects processing of instigatory and inhibitory cues. In this regard, their model is very similar to the Taylor and Leonard (1983) analysis of the effects of alcohol on processing dominant and nondominant cues and the Hull and Van Treuren (1986) account of its effects on processing of implicit and explicit cues. Nonetheless, many of the studies that offer support for the inhibitory conflict model do so by identifying situations in which (or individuals for whom) alcohol has its greatest effects, and are not designed to investigate the specific mechanisms whereby alcohol has its effects.

Recently studies have begun to investigate systematically the effects of alcohol on disinhibition in conflictual situations, using a paradigm originally developed to study cognitive self-control (Logan, Cowan, & Davis, 1984). According to Logan and Cowan (1984), self-control involves the ability to inhibit thought and action. Inhibitory control involves a race between two independent and competitive cognitive processes: activating "go" processes and inhibiting "stop" processes. When both signals are present, the conflicting processes race against each other. If the activating process is completed first, the response is executed; if the inhibiting process is completed first, the response is withheld. The prototypical "go–stop" paradigm usually involves presentations of cues (e.g., letters) that require responses and, hence, act as "go signals." Other cues (e.g., sounds) are occasionally presented that require inhibition of the response and, hence, act as "stop signals." Inhibitory control is measured by the ability of the individual to inhibit responses to go signals after stop signals appear.

Using such a paradigm, it has been demonstrated that a moderate dose of alcohol reduces inhibitions to stop signals, without affecting the responses to go signals (Mulvihill, Skilling, & Vogel-Sprott, 1997). Subsequent research has demonstrated that this effect depends on the existence of cognitive conflict. Thus, an effect of alcohol occurs if rewards are offered for *both* acting (quickly responding to the go signal) *and* inhibiting (successful nonresponding following a stop signal). However, if the conflict is resolved by rewarding *either* acting *or* inhibiting, alcohol has no effects (Fillmore & Vogel-Sprott, 1999, 2000). Futhermore, these effects appear to be due to cognitive rather than motivational conflict insofar as alcohol has the same disinhibitory properties when (1) neither response was rewarded as when (2) both responses were rewarded (Fillmore & Vogel-Sprott, 2000). In other words, it is the equivalence of the consequences for responding and inhibiting that determines alcohol's impact on inhibitory control (see also Easdon & Vogel-Sprott, 2000).

A study by Marinkovic, Halgren, Klopp, and Maltzman (2000) may provide a key insight into why alcohol has these effects. These authors assessed brain activity in sober and intoxicated individuals in a "go/no-go" study. Participants were to respond when presented with one type of cue (a word that had been previously memorized) but not when presented with a different type of cue (an unlearned word). Measures of brain activity suggested that sober individuals waited to prepare to respond until after they processed the go signal. In contrast, the same measure suggested that intoxicated individuals prepared to respond *before* they processed the signal, then terminated their response if the signal they received was not in fact a go signal (see also Marczinski & Fillmore, 2003). In our minds, this study provides a potentially important insight into intoxicated disinhibition and a qualification of attentional–cognitive accounts of such behavior. Thus, it may well be that alcohol impairs attention to and processing of cues that one should not act, but this combines with an effect of alcohol on the operation of behavioral scripts. To use a military analogy: Given a plan, intoxicated individuals seem to be set on a "hair trigger," such that they are prepared to execute the plan unless told to "stand down," whereas sober individuals do not prepare to respond until told to "mobilize."

Impaired Executive Functioning

Beyond these specific processes, a variety of additional processes with direct relevance to self-regulation appear to be impaired by alcohol and may serve to mediate its effects on some behaviors. Following Giancola (2000), we include these under an umbrella term, "impaired executive functioning." Thus, Peterson, Roghfleisch, Zelazo, and Pihl (1990) reported that alcohol impairs cognitive processes such as the planning, the verbal fluency, and the sequencing of behaviors. These effects are attributed to the impact of alcohol on the prefrontal and temporal lobes (see Pihl, Peterson, & Lau, 1993, for an elaborated model of such effects). Similarly, Sayette, Wilson, and Elias (1993) reported that acute alcohol consumption interferes with a range of social information-processing skills, including response generation, anticipation of different consequences, response selection, and coping with obstacles. Indeed, according to Giancola, alcohol affects aggressive responding because of its impact on attentional capacity: "impaired planning, reviewing, abstract reasoning, appraisal, cognitive flexibility, social and self-monitoring, organization, sequencing, hypothesis generation, and working memory skills" (2000, p. 589).

For the most part, it remains to be demonstrated that alcohol affects behavior *because* of its impact on these various processes. Nonetheless, the more general point that researchers should consider a wider variety of cognitive processes as potential mediators of alcohol effects remains valid. Unfortunately, self-regulation is itself a complex process and depends on a numerous, interacting attentional, cognitive, affective, and response-preparatory processes, any or all of which might be affected by intoxication (see Hull, 2002). Despite the large number of studies on the causes and effects of alcohol consumption over the past 20 years, many of these provocative leads have not been subjected to systematic empirical examination.

Overcoming the Effects of Intoxication

Most research on the effects of alcohol on self-regulation demonstrates its tendency to increase socially inappropriate or maladaptive behaviors. A small number of studies have sought to examine ways in which these dysfunctional consequences can be overcome. For example, some researchers suggest that having an expectancy that alcohol leads to a particular effect induces a correction. Thus, among intoxicated individuals in the go–stop paradigm, Fillmore and Blackburn (2002) found that expecting alcohol to impair reaction times resulted in faster responses compared to those who did not hold this expectancy. Likewise, expectancy that alcohol increases aggression has actually been shown to *decrease* intoxicated aggression, presumably because the individual attempts to restrain an anticipated outcome (Quigley & Leonard, 1999). Hoaken, Assaad, and Pihl (1998) found that intoxicated subjects, even though cognitively impaired relative to nonintoxicated subjects, had no difficulty inhibiting aggression to gain a monetary reward. Fillmore and Vogel-Sprott (1997) reported that intoxicated subjects can overcome information-processing deficits when given an immediate monetary consequence that conveys information about the adequacy of performance. Consistent with the implications of such effects, we have argued (Hull, 1981; Hull & Reilly, 1983) that alcohol reduces the propensity of individuals to become self-aware, rather than their ability to become self-aware, such that explicit cues to self-focus may function to overcome the effects of intoxication (see also Bailey et al., 1983; Carey, 1995).

The fact that the effects of alcohol can be reduced by internal or external cues to regulate behavior makes it more difficult to predict the overt behavioral consequences of the drug. Despite this added complexity, it need not obscure the processes responsible for this behavior, if adopted experimental designs allow one to examine the compensatory processes themselves.

CONCLUSIONS

In conclusion, self-regulatory processes appear to play key roles in both the causes and effects of alcohol consumption. Increased alcohol consumption is associated with both failures of self-control and explicit self-regulatory attempts to achieve specific experiences. Conversely, intoxication following consumption of alcohol would appear to affect a wide range of behaviors as a consequence of its effects on attentional, cognitive, affective, and executive processes central to self-regulation. Although clear progress has been made in developing a general understanding of how alcohol affects behavior, additional research is necessary that demonstrates the specific consequences of impairment to particular processes, as well as the circumstances necessary to overcome these effects. Ultimately, the effects of alcohol are much more complicated than the unalloyed evil that Cassio attributes to it. The key is to determine exactly how to adhere to Iago's stipulation:

> CASSIO: Every inordinate cup is unblessed,
>   And the ingredient is a devil.
>
> IAGO: Come, come. Good wine is a good familiar creature,
>   *If it be well used* . . .
>   —*Othello* (Act II, Scene iii; emphasis added)

REFERENCES

Aas, H. N., Leigh, B. C., Anderssen, N., & Jakobsen, R. (1998). Two year longitudinal study of alcohol expectancies and drinking among Norwegian adolescents. *Addiction, 93*, 373–384.

Abbey, A. (2002). Alcohol-related sexual assault: A common problem among college students. *Journal of Studies on Alcohol [Special issue: College drinking, what it is, and what do to about it: Review of the state of the science]*, Suppl. 14, 118–128.

Abbey, A., McAuslan, P., & Ross, L. T. (1998). Sexual assault perpetration by college men: The role of alcohol, misperception of sexual intent, and sexual beliefs and experiences. *Journal of Social and Clinical Psychology, 17*, 167–195.

Abbey, A., Zawacki, T., & McAuslan, P. (2000). Alcohol's effects on sexual perception. *Journal of Studies on Alcohol, 61*, 688–697.

Adalbjarnardottir, S., & Rafnsson, F. D. (2001). Perceived control in adolescent substance use: Concurrent and longitudinal analyses. *Psychology of Addictive Behaviors, 15*, 25–32.

Allsop, S., Saunders, B., & Phillips, M. (2000). The process of relapse in severely dependent male problem drinkers. *Addiction, 95*, 95–106.

Armeli, S., Carney, M. A., Tennen, H., Affleck, G., & O'Neil, T. (2000). Stress and alcohol use: A daily process examination of the stressor–vulnerability model. *Journal of Personality and Social Psychology, 78*, 979–994.

Bailey, D. S., Leonard, K. E., Cranston, J. W., & Taylor, S. P. (1983). Effects of alcohol and self-awareness on human physical aggression. *Personality and Social Psychology Bulletin, 9*, 289–295.

Bailey, D. S., & Taylor, S. P. (1991). Effects of alcohol and aggressive disposition on human physical aggression. *Journal of Research in Personality, 25*, 334–342.

Banaji, M. R., & Steele, C. M. (1989). The social cognition of alcohol use. *Social Cognition, 7*, 137–151.

Barnes, G. M., Welte, J. W., Hoffman, J. H., & Dintcheff, B. A. (1999). Gambling and alcohol use among youth: Influences of demographic, socialization, and individual factors. *Addictive Behaviors [Special issue: Addictions in special populations], 24*, 749–767.

Baron, R. M., & Kenny, D. A. (1986). The moderator-mediator variable distinction in social psychological research: Conceptual, strategic, and statistical considerations. *Journal of Personality and Social Psychology, 51*, 1173–1182.

Bartholow, B. D., Sher, K. J., & Strathman, A. (2000). Moderation of the expectancy–alcohol use relation by private self-consciousness: Data from a longitudinal study. *Personality and Social Psychology Bulletin, 26*, 1409–1420.

Baumeiser, R. F. (1991). *Escaping the self: Alcoholism, spirituality, masochism, and other flights from the burden of selfhood*. New York: Basic Books.

Baumeister, R. F., Heatherton, T. F., & Tice, D. M. (1994). *Losing control: How and why people fail at self-regulation*. San Diego, CA: Academic Press.

Birnbaum, I. M., Johnson, M. K., Hartley, J. T., & Taylor, T. H. (1980). Alcohol and elaborative schemas for sentences. *Journal of Experimental Psychology: Human Learning and Memory, 6*, 293–300.

Birnbaum, I. M., & Parker, E. S. (1997). *Alcohol and human memory*. Hillsdale, NJ: Erlbaum.

Bonin, M. F., McCreary, D. R., & Sadava, S. W. (2000). Problem drinking behavior in two community-based samples of adults: Influence of gender, coping, loneliness, and depression. *Psychology of Addictive Behaviors 14*, 151–161.

Borges, G., Cherpitel, C. J., & Rosovsky, H. (1998). Male drinking and violence-related injury in the emergency room. *Addiction, 93*, 103–112.

Brecklin, L. R., & Ullman, S. E. (2002). The roles of victim and offender alcohol use in sexual assaults: Results from the National Violence Against Women Survey. *Journal of Studies on Alcohol, 63*, 57–63.

Breslin, F. C., Sobell, M. B., Cappell, H., Vakili, S., & Poulos, C. X. (1999). The effects of alcohol, gender, and sensation seeking on the gambling choices of social drinkers. *Psychology of Addictive Behaviors, 13*, 243–252.

Brown, S. A., Goldman, M. S., Inn, A., & Anderson, L. R. (1980). Expectations of reinforcement from alcohol: Their domain and relation to drinking patterns. *Journal of Consulting and Clinical Psychology, 48*, 419–426.

Brown, S. A., Tate, S. R., Vik, P. W., Haas, A. L., & Aarons, G. A. (1999). Modeling of alcohol use mediates the effect of family history of alcoholism on adolescent alcohol expectancies. *Experimental and Clinical Psychopharmacology, 7*, 20–27.

Bushman, B. J., & Cooper, H. M. (1990). Effects of alcohol on human aggression: An integrative research review. *Psychological Bulletin, 107*, 341–354.

Carey, K. B. (1995). Effects of alcohol intoxication on self-focused attention. *Journal of Studies on Alcohol, 56*, 248–252.

Carpenter, K. M., & Hasin, D. S. (1998). Reasons for drinking alcohol: Relationships with DSM-IV alcohol diagnoses and alcohol consumption in a community sample. *Psychology of Addictive Behaviors, 12*, 168–184.

Carter, J. A., McNair, L. D., Corbin, W. R., & Black, D. H. (1998). Effects of priming positive and negative outcomes on drinking responses. *Experimental and Clinical Psychopharmacology, 6*, 399–405.

Chutuape, M. A. D., Mitchell, S. H., & de Wit, H. (1994). Ethanol preloads increase ethanol preference under concurrent random-ratio schedules in social drinkers. *Experimental and Clinical Psychopharmacology, 2*, 310–318.

Collins, R. L., Koutsky, J. R., & Izzo, C. V. (2000). Temptation, restriction, and the regulation of alcohol intake: Validity and utility of the Temptation and Restraint Inventory. *Journal of Studies on Alcohol, 61*, 766–773.

Comeau, N., Stewart, S. H., & Loba, P. (2001). The relations of trait anxiety, anxiety sensitivity and sensation seeking to adolescents' motivations for alcohol, cigarette and marijuana use. *Addictive Behaviors, 26*, 803–825.

Conger, J. J. (1951). The effects of alcohol on conflict behavior in the albino rat. *Quarterly Journal of Studies on Alcohol, 12*, 1–29.

Conger, J. J. (1956). Alcoholism: Theory, problem, and challenge: II. Reinforcement theory and the dynamics of alcoholism. *Quarterly Journal of Studies on Alcohol, 17*, 296–305.

Connors, G. J., Tarbox, A. R., & Faillace, L. A. (1993) Changes in alcohol expectancies and drinking behavior among treated problem drinkers. *Journal of Studies on Alcohol, 53*, 676–683.

Cooney, N. L., Litt, M. D., Morse, P. A., Bauer, L. O., & Gaupp, L. (1997). Alcohol cue reactivity, negative-mood reactivity, and relapse in treated alcoholic men. *Journal of Abnormal Psychology, 106*, 243–250.

Cooper, M. L. (2002). Alcohol use and risky sexual behavior among college students and youth: Evaluating the evidence. *Journal of Studies on Alcohol [Special issue: College drinking, what it is, and what do to about it: Review of the state of the science]*, Suppl. 14, 101–117.

Cooper, M. L., Frone, M. R., Russell, M., & Mudar, P. (1995). Drinking to regulate positive and negative emotions: A motivational model of alcohol use. *Journal of Personality and Social Psychology, 69*, 990–1005.

Cooper, M. L., & Orcutt, H. K. (1997). Drinking and sexual experience on first dates among adolescents. *Journal of Abnormal Psychology, 106*, 191–202.

Cooper, M. L., & Orcutt, H. K. (2000). Alcohol use, condom use and partner type among heterosexual adolescents and young adults. *Journal of Studies on Alcohol, 61*, 413–419.

Cooper, M. L., Russell, M., Skinner, J. B., & Windle, M. (1992). Development and validation of a three dimensional measure of drinking motives. *Psychological Assessment, 4*, 123–132.

Corrao, G., Bagnardi, V., Zambon, A., & Arico, S. (1999). Exploring the dose–response relationship between alcohol consumption and the risk of several alcohol-related conditions: A meta-analysis. *Source Addiction, 94*(10), 1551–1573.

Curtin, J. J., Patrick, C. J., Lang, A. R., Cacioppo, J. T., & Birbaumer, N. (2001). Alcohol affects emotion through cognition. *Psychological Science, 12*, 527–531.

Cutter, H. S., Green, L. R., & Harford, T. C. (1973). Levels of risk taken by extraverted and introverted alcoholics as a function of drinking whisky. *British Journal of Social and Clinical Psychology*, *12*, 83–89.

Darkes, J., & Goldman, M. S. (1998). Expectancy challenge and drinking reduction: Process and structure in the alcohol expectancy network. *Experimental and Clinical Psychopharmacology*, *6*, 64–76.

Delaney, W. P., Grube, J. W., Greiner, B., Fisher, J. M., & Ragland, D. R. (2002). Job stress, unwinding and drinking in transit operators. *Journal of Studies on Alcohol*, *63*(4), 420–429.

Dermen, K. H., & Cooper, M. L. (2000). Inhibition conflict and alcohol expectancy as moderators of alcohol's relationship to condom use. *Experimental and Clinical Psychopharmacology*, *8*, 198–206.

Dermen, K. H., Cooper, M. L., & Agocha, V. B. (1998). Sex-related alcohol expectancies as moderators of the relationship between alcohol use and risky sex in adolescents. *Journal of Studies on Alcohol*, *59*, 71–77.

de Wit, H. (2000). Laboratory-based assessment of alcohol craving in social drinkers. *Addiction*, *95*, S165–S169.

Donovan, J. E., & Jessor, R. (1985). Structure of problem behavior in adolescence and young adulthood. *Journal of Consulting and Clinical Psychology*, *53*, 6890–6904.

Donovan, J. E., Jessor, R., & Costa, F. M. (1999). Adolescent problem drinking: Stability of psychosocial and behavioral correlates across a generation. *Source Journal of Studies on Alcohol*, *60*, 352–361.

Downey, L., Rosengren, D. B., & Donovan, D. M. (2000). To thine own self be true: Self-concept and motivation for abstinence among substance abusers. *Addictive Behaviors*, *25*, 743–757.

Drummond, D. C., Litten, R. Z., Lowman, C., & Hunt, W. A. (2000). Craving research: Future directions. *Addiction*, *95*, S247–S255.

Dunn, M. E., & Earleywine, M. (2001). Activation of alcohol expectancies in memory in relation to limb of the blood alcohol curve. *Psychology of Addictive Behaviors*, *15*, 18–24.

Dunn, M. E., & Goldman, M. S. (1996). Empirical modeling of an alcohol expectancy memory network in elementary school children as a function of grade. *Experimental and Clinical Psychopharmacology*, *4*, 209–217.

Dunn, M. E., & Goldman, M. S. (1998). Age and drinking-related differences in the memory organization of alcohol expectancies in 3rd-, 6th-, 9th-, and 12th-grade children. *Journal of Consulting and Clinical Psychology*, *66*, 579–585.

Dunn, M. E., Lau, H. C., & Cruz, I. Y. (2000). Changes in activation of alcohol expectancies in memory in relation to changes in alcohol use after participation in an expectancy challenge program. *Experimental and Clinical Psychopharmacology*, *8*, 566–575.

Dunn, M. E., & Yniguez, R. M. (1999). Experimental demonstration of the influence of alcohol advertising on the activation of alcohol expectancies in memory among fourth-and fifth-grade children. *Experimental and Clinical Psychopharmacology*, *7*, 473–483.

Easdon, C. M., & Vogel-Sprott, M. (2000). Alcohol and behavioral control: Impaired response inhibition and flexibility in social drinkers. *Experimental and Clinical Psychopharmacology*, *8*, 387–394.

Fillmore, M. T., & Blackburn, J. (2002). Compensating for alcohol-induced impairment: Alcohol expectancies and behavioral disinhibition. *Journal of Studies on Alcohol*, *63*, 237–246.

Fillmore, M. T., Carscadden, J. L., & Vogel-Sprott, M. (1998). Alcohol, cognitive impairment and expectancies. *Journal of Studies on Alcohol*, *59*, 174–179.

Fillmore, M. T., Dixon, M. J., & Schweizer, T. A. (2000). Alcohol affects processing of ignored stimuli in a negative priming paradigm. *Journal of Studies on Alcohol*, *61*, 571–578.

Fillmore, M. T., & Vogel-Sprott, M. (1997). Resistance to cognitive impairment under alcohol: The role of environmental consequences. *Experimental and Clinical Psychopharmacology*, *5*, 251–255.

Fillmore, M. T., & Vogel-Sprott, M. (1998). Behavioral impairment under alcohol: Cognitive and pharmacokinetic factors. *Alcoholism: Clinical and Experimental Research*, *22*, 1476–1482.

Fillmore, M. T., & Vogel-Sprott, M. (1999). An alcohol model of impaired inhibitory control and its treatment in humans. *Experimental and Clinical Psychopharmacology, 7,* 49–55.

Fillmore, M. T., & Vogel-Sprott, M. (2000). Response inhibition under alcohol: Effects of cognitive and motivational conflict. *Journal of Studies on Alcohol, 61,* 239–246.

Fillmore, M. T., Vogel-Sprott, M., & Gavrilescu, D. (1999). Alcohol effects on intentional behavior: Dissociating controlled and automatic influences. *Experimental and Clinical Psychopharmacology, 7,* 372–378.

Finn, P. R., Sharkansky, E. J., Brandt, K. M., & Turcotte, N. (2000). The effects of familial risk, personality, and expectancies on alcohol use and abuse. *Journal of Abnormal Psychology, 109,* 122–133.

Flory, K., Lynam, D., Milich, R., Leukefeld, C., & Clayton, R. (2002). The relations among personality, symptoms of alcohol and marijuana abuse, and symptoms of comorbid psychopathology: Results from a community sample. *Experimental and Clinical Psychopharmacology, 10,* 425–434.

Frank, S. J., Jacobson, S., & Tuer, M. (1990). Psychological predictors of young adults' drinking behaviors. *Journal of Personality and Social Psychology, 59,* 770–780.

Fromme, K., D'Amico, E. J., & Katz, E. C. (1999). Intoxicated sexual risk taking: An expectancy or cognitive impairment explanation? *Journal of Studies on Alcohol, 60,* 54–63.

Fromme, K., Katz, E., & D'Amico, E. (1997). Effects of alcohol intoxication on the perceived consequences of risk taking. *Experimental and Clinical Psychopharmacology, 5,* 14–23.

George, W. H., Stoner, S. A., Norris, J., Lopez, P. A., & Lehman, G. L. (2000). Alcohol expectancies and sexuality: A self-fulfilling prophecy analysis of dyadic perceptions and behavior. *Journal of Studies on Alcohol, 61,* 168–176.

Giancola, P. R. (2000). Executive functioning: A conceptual framework for alcohol-related aggression. *Experimental and Clinical Psychopharmacology, 8,* 576–597.

Giancola, P. R. (2002a). Alcohol-related aggression during the college years: Theories, risk factors, and policy implications. *Journal of Studies on Alcohol [Special issue: College drinking, what it is, and what do to about it: Review of the state of the science],* Suppl. 14, 129–139.

Giancola, P. R. (2002b). Alcohol-related aggression in men and women: The influence of dispositional aggressivity. *Journal of Studies on Alcohol, 63,* 696–708.

Giancola, P. R., Helton, E. L., Osborne, A. B., Terry, M. K., Fuss, A. M., & Westerfield, J. A. (2002). The effects of alcohol and provocation on aggressive behavior in men and women. *Journal of Studies on Alcohol, 63,* 64–73.

Giancola, P. R., & Zeichner, A. (1997). The biphasic effects of alcohol on human physical aggression. *Journal of Abnormal Psychology, 106,* 598–607.

Glautier, S., & Spencer, K. (1999). Activation of alcohol-related associative networks by recent alcohol consumption and alcohol-related cues. *Addiction, 94,* 1033–1041.

Goldbeck, R., Myatt, P., & Aitchison, T. (1997). End-of-treatment self-efficacy: A predictor of abstinence. *Addiction, 92,* 313–324.

Goldman, M. S. (1999). Risk for substance abuse: Memory as a common etiological pathway. *Psychological Science, 10,* 196–198.

Goldman, M. S., Del Boca, F. K., & Darkes, J. (1999). Alcohol expectancy theory: The application of cognitive neuroscience. In K. E. Leonard & H. T. Blane (Eds.), *Psychological theories of drinking and alcoholism* (2nd ed., pp. 203–246). New York: Guilford Press.

Gotham, H. J., Sher, K. J., & Wood, P. K. (1997). Predicting stability and change in frequency of intoxication from the college years to beyond: Individual-difference and role transition variables. *Journal of Abnormal Psychology, 106,* 619–629.

Graham, K., Leonard, K. E., Room, R., Wild, T. C., Pihl, R. O., Bois, C., & Single, E. (1998). Current directions in research on understanding and preventing intoxicated aggression. *Addiction, 93,* 659–676.

Graham, K., West, P., & Wells, S. (2000). Evaluating theories of alcohol-related aggression using observations of young adults in bars. *Addiction, 95,* 847–863.

Graves, K. L. (1995). Risky sexual behavior and alcohol use among young adults: Results from a national survey. *American Journal of Health Promotion, 10*, 27–36.

Gross, A. M., Bennett, T., Sloan, L., Marx, B. P., & Juergens, J. (2001). The impact of alcohol and alcohol expectancies on male perception of female sexual arousal in a date rape analog. *Experimental and Clinical Psychopharmacology, 9*, 380–388.

Grube, J. W., & Agostinelli, G. E. (1999). Perceived consequences and adolescent drinking: Nonlinear and interactive models of alcohol expectancies. *Psychology of Addictive Behaviors, 13*, 303–312.

Guo, J., Hawkins, J. D., Hill, K. G., & Abbott, R. D. (2001). Childhood and adolescent predictors of alcohol abuse and dependence in young adulthood. *Journal of Studies on Alcohol, 62*, 754–762.

Hashtroudi, S., Parker, E. S., DeLisi, L. E., & Wyatt, R. J. (1983). On elaboration and alcohol. *Journal of Verbal Learning and Verbal Behavior, 22*, 164–173.

Herzog, T. A. (1999). Effects of alcohol intoxication on social inferences. *Experimental and Clinical Psychopharmacology, 7*, 448–453.

Hingson, R. W., Heeren, T., Zakocs, R. C., Kopstein, A., & Wechsler, H. (2002). Magnitude of alcohol-related mortality and morbidity among U.S. college students ages 18–24. *Journal of Studies on Alcohol, 63*, 136–144.

Hoaken, P. N. S., Assaad, J.-M., & Pihl, R. O. (1998). Cognitive functioning and the inhibition of alcohol-induced aggression. *Journal of Studies on Alcohol, 59*, 599–607.

Hodgins, D. C., el-Guebaly, N., & Armstrong, S. (1995). Prospective and retrospective reports of mood states before relapse to substance use. *Journal of Consulting and Clinical Psychology, 63*, 400–407.

Holahan, C. J., Moos, R. H., Holahan, C. K., Cronkite, R. C., & Randall, P. K. (2001). Drinking to cope, emotional distress and alcohol use and abuse: A ten-year model. *Journal of Studies on Alcohol, 62*, 190–198.

Holahan, C. J., Moos, R. H., Holahan, C. K., Cronkite, R. C., & Randall, P. K. (2003). Drinking to cope and alcohol use and abuse in unipolar depression: A 10-year model. *Journal of Abnormal Psychology, 112*, 159–165.

Hull, J. G. (1981). A self-awareness model of the causes and effects of alcohol consumption. *Journal of Abnormal Psychology, 90*, 586–600.

Hull, J. G. (2002). Modeling the structure of self-knowledge and the dynamics of self-regulation. In A. Tesser, D. Stapel, & J. Wood (Eds.), *Self and motivation: Emerging psychological perspectives* (Vol. 2, pp. 173–203). Washington, DC: American Psychological Association.

Hull, J. G., & Bond, C. F. (1986). Social and behavioral consequences of alcohol consumption and expectancy: A meta-analysis. *Psychological Bulletin, 99*, 347–360.

Hull, J. G., Levenson, R. W., Young, R. D., & Sher, K. J. (1983). Self-awareness reducing effects of alcohol consumption. *Journal of Personality and Social Psychology, 44*, 461–473.

Hull, J. G., & Reilly, N. P. (1983). Self-awareness, self-regulation, and alcohol: A reply to Wilson. *Journal of Abnormal Psychology, 92*, 514–519.

Hull, J. G., & Van Treuren, R. R. (1986). Experimental social psychology and the causes and effects of alcohol consumption. In H. D. Cappell, F. B. Glaser, Y. Israel, H. Kalant, W. Schmidt, E. M. Sellers, & R. S. Smart (Eds.), *Research advances in alcohol and drug problems* (pp. 211–243). New York: Plenum Press.

Hull, J. G., & Young, R. D. (1983). Self-consciousness, self-esteem, and success–failure as determinants of alcohol consumption in male social drinkers. *Journal of Personality and Social Psychology, 44*, 1097–1109.

Hull, J. G., Young, R. D., & Jouriles, E. (1986). Applications of the self-awareness model of alcohol consumption: Predicting patterns of use and abuse. *Journal of Personality and Social Psychology, 51*, 790–796.

Hussong, A. M., Hicks, R. E., Levy, S. A., & Curran, P. J. (2001). Specifying the relations between affect and heavy alcohol use among young adults. *Journal of Abnormal Psychology, 110*, 449–461.

Ito, T. A., Miller, N., & Pollock, V. E. (1996). Alcohol and aggression: A meta-analysis on the moderating effects of inhibitory cues, triggering events, and self-focused attention. *Psychological Bulletin, 120,* 60–82.

Jansma, A., Breteler, M. H. M., Schippers, G. M., De Jong, C. A. J., & Van der Staak, C. P. F. (2000). No effect of negative mood on the alcohol cue reactivity on in-patient alcoholics. *Addictive Behaviors, 25,* 619–624.

Johnson, P. B., & Glassman, M. (1999). The moderating effects of gender and ethnicity on the relationship between effect expectancies and alcohol problems. *Journal of Studies on Alcohol, 60,* 64–69.

Joiner, T. E. J., Vohs, K. D., & Schmidt, N. B. (2000). Social appraisal as correlate, antecedent and consequence of mental and physical health outcomes. *Journal of Social and Clinical Psychology, 19,* 336–351.

Jones, B. T., Corbin, W., & Fromme, K. (2001). A review of expectancy theory and alcohol consumption. *Addiction, 96,* 57–72.

Jones, B. T., & Schulze, D. (2000). Alcohol-related words of positive affect are more accessible in social drinkers' memory than are other words when sip-primed by alcohol. *Addiction Research, 8,* 221–232.

Josephs, R. A., & Steele, C. M. (1990). The two faces of alcohol myopia: Attentional mediation of psychological stress. *Journal of Abnormal Psychology, 99,* 115–126.

Kambouropoulos, N., & Staiger, P. K. (2001). The influence of sensitivity to reward on reactivity to alcohol-related cues. *Addiction, 96,* 1175–1185.

Kidorf, M., & Lang, A. R. (1999). Effects of social anxiety and alcohol expectancies on stress-induced drinking. *Psychology of Addictive Behaviors, 13,* 134–142.

Kilbey, M. M., Downey, K., & Breslau, N. (1998). Predicting the emergence and persistence of alcohol dependence in young adults: The role of expectancy and other risk factors. *Experimental and Clinical Psychopharmacology, 6,* 149–156.

Kilpatrick, D. G., Acierno, R., Resnick, H. S., Saunders, B. E., & Best, C. L. (1997). A 2-year longitudinal analysis of the relationships between violent assault and substance use in women. *Journal of Consulting and Clinical Psychology, 65,* 834–847.

Kirk, J. M., & de Wit, H. (2000). Individual differences in the priming effect of ethanol in social drinkers. *Journal of Studies on Alcohol, 61,* 64–71.

Knight, J. R., Wechsler, H., Kuo, M., Seibring, M., Weitzman, E. R., & Schuckit, M. A. (2002). Alcohol abuse and dependence among U.S. college students. *Journal of Studies on Alcohol, 63,* 263–270.

Koppes, L. L. J., Twisk, J. W. R., Snel, J., De Vente, W., & Kemper, H. C. G. (2001). Personality characteristics and alcohol consumption: Longitudinal analyses in men and women followed from ages 13 to 32. *Journal of Studies on Alcohol, 62,* 494–500.

Kramer, D. A., & Goldman, M. S. (2003). Using a modified Stroop task to implicitly discern the cognitive organization of alcohol expectancies. *Journal of Abnormal Psychology, 112,* 171–175.

Kubicka, L., Matejcek, Z., Dytrych, Z., & Roth, Z. (2001). IQ and personality traits assessed in childhood as predictors of drinking and smoking behaviour in middle-aged adults: A 24-year follow-up study. *Addiction, 96,* 1615–1628.

Kushner, M. G., Thuras, P., Kaminski, J., Anderson, N., Neumeyer, B., & Mackenzie, T. (2000). Expectancies for alcohol to affect tension and anxiety as a function of time. *Addictive Behaviors, 25,* 93–98.

Kyngdon, A., & Dickerson, M. (1999). An experimental study of the effect of prior alcohol consumption on a simulated gambling activity. *Addiction, 94,* 697–707.

Labouvie, E., & Bates, M. E. (2002). Reasons for alcohol use in young adulthood: Validation of a three-dimensional measure. *Journal of Studies on Alcohol, 63,* 145–155.

Laplace, A. C., Chermack, S. T., & Taylor, S. P. (1994). Effects of alcohol and drinking experience on human physical aggression. *Personality and Social Psychology Bulletin, 20,* 439–444.

Laurent, J., Catanzaro, S. J., & Callan, M. K. (1997). Stress, alcohol-related expectancies and coping preferences: A replication with adolescents of the Cooper et al. (1992) model. *Journal of Studies on Alcohol, 58*, 644–651.

Lee, N. K., Greeley, J., & Oei, T. P. S. (1999). The relationship of positive and negative alcohol expectancies to patterns of consumption of alcohol in social drinkers. *Addictive Behaviors, 24*, 359–369.

Lee, N. K., Oei, T. P. S., & Greeley, J. D. (1999). The interaction of alcohol expectancies and drinking refusal self-efficacy in high and low risk drinkers. *Addiction Research, 7*, 91–102.

Leigh, B. C. (1999). Peril, chance, adventure: Concepts of risk, alcohol use and risky behavior in young adults. *Addiction, 94*, 371–383.

Leigh, B. C., & Stacy, A. W. (1998). Individual differences in memory associations involving the positive and negative outcomes of alcohol use. *Psychology of Addictive Behaviors, 12*, 39–46.

Leonard, K. E. (1989). The impact of explicit aggressive and implicit nonaggressive cues on aggression in intoxicated and sober males. *Personality and Social Psychology Bulletin, 15*, 390–400.

Leonard, K. E., & Quigley, B. M. (1999). Drinking and marital aggression in newlyweds: An event-based analysis of drinking and the occurrence of husband marital aggression. *Journal of Studies on Alcohol, 60*, 537–545.

Leonard, K. E., & Roberts, L. J. (1998). The effects of alcohol on the marital interactions of aggressive and nonaggressive husbands and their wives. *Journal of Abnormal Psychology, 107*, 602–615.

Lewis, B. A., & O'Neill, H. K. (2000). Alcohol expectancies and social deficits relating to problem drinking among college students. *Addictive Behaviors, 25*, 295–299.

Lindman, R. E., Sjoeholm, B. A., & Lang, A. R. (2000). Expectations of alcohol-induced positive affect: A cross-cultural comparison. *Journal of Studies on Alcohol, 61*, 681–687.

Logan, G. D., & Cowan, W. B. (1984). On the ability to inhibit thought and action: A theory of an act of control. *Psychological Review, 91*, 295–327.

Logan, G. D., Cowan, W. B., & Davis, K. A. (1984). On the ability to inhibit simple and choice reaction time responses: A model and a method. *Journal of Experimental Psychology: Human Perception and Performance, 10*, 276–291.

Lundahl, L. H., Davis, T. M., Adesso, V. J., & Lukas, S. E. (1997). Alcohol expectancies: Effects of gender, age, and family history of alcoholism. *Addictive Behaviors, 22*, 115–125.

MacDonald, G., Zanna, M. P., & Holmes, J. G. (2000). An experimental test of the role of alcohol in relationship conflict. *Journal of Experimental Social Psychology, 36*, 182–193.

MacDonald, T. K, Fong, G. T., Zanna, M. P., & Martineau, A. M. (2000). Alcohol myopia and condom use: Can alcohol intoxication be associated with more prudent behavior? *Journal of Personality and Social Psychology, 78*, 605–619.

MacDonald, T. K., Zanna, M. P., & Fong, G. T. (1996). Why common sense goes out the window: Effects of alcohol on intentions to use condoms. *Personality and Social Psychology Bulletin, 22*, 763–775.

MacLatchy-Gaudet, H. A., & Stewart, S. H. (2001). The context-specific positive alcohol outcome expectancies of university women. *Addictive Behaviors, 26*, 31–49.

MacLean, M. G., & Lecci, L. (2000). A comparison of models of drinking motives in a university sample. *Psychology of Addictive Behaviors, 14*, 83–87.

Maisto, S. A., Connors, G. J., & Zywiak, W. H. (2000). Alcohol treatment changes in coping skills, self-efficacy, and levels of alcohol use and related problems 1 year following treatment initiation. *Psychology of Addictive Behaviors, 14*, 257–266.

Marczinski, C. A., & Fillmore, M. T. (2003). Preresponse cues reduce the impairing effects of alcohol on the execution and suppression of responses. *Experimental and Clinical Psychopharmacology, 11*, 110–117.

Marinkovic, K., Halgren, E., Klopp, J., & Maltzman, I. (2000). Alcohol effects on movement-related potentials: A measure of impulsivity? *Journal of Studies on Alcohol, 61*, 24–31.

Marlatt, G. A., & Gordon, J. R. (1985). *Relapse prevention: Maintenance strategies in the treatment of addictive behaviors*. New York: Guilford Press.

Martin, C. S., Lynch, K. G., Pollock, N. K., & Clark, D. B. (2000). Gender differences and similarities in the personality correlates of adolescent alcohol problems. *Psychology of Addictive Behaviors*, *14*, 121–133.

Masserman, J. H., & Yum, K. S. (1946). An analysis of the influence of alcohol on experimental neuroses in cats. *Psychosomatic Medicine*, *8*, 36–52.

McCarthy, D. M., Kroll, L. S., & Smith, G. T. (2001). Integrating disinhibition and learning risk for alcohol use. *Experimental and Clinical Psychopharmacology*, *9*, 389–398.

McCarthy, D. M., Miller, T. L., Smith, G. T., & Smith, J. A. (2001). Disinhibition and expectancy in risk for alcohol use: Comparing black and white college samples. *Journal of Studies on Alcohol*, *62*, 313–321.

McCreary, D. R., & Sadava, S. W. (1998). Stress, drinking, and the adverse consequences of drinking in two samples of young adults. *Psychology of Addictive Behaviors*, *12*, 247–261.

McCreary, D. R., & Sadava, S. W. (2000). Stress, alcohol use and alcohol-related problems: The influence of negative and positive affect in two cohorts of young adults. *Journal of Studies on Alcohol*, *61*, 466–474.

Meier, S. E., Brigham, T. A., Ward, D. A., Myers, F., & Warren, L. (1996). Effects of blood alcohol concentrations on negative punishment: Implications for decision making. *Journal of Studies on Alcohol*, *57*, 85–96.

Miller, P. M., Smith, G. T., & Goldman, M. S. (1990). Emergence of alcohol expectancies in childhood: A possible critical period. *Journal of Studies on Alcohol*, *51*, 343–349.

Mohr, C. D., Armeli, S., Tennen, H., Carney, M. A., Affleck, G., & Hromi, A. (2001). Daily interpersonal experiences, context, and alcohol consumption: Crying in your beer and toasting good times. *Journal of Personality and Social Psychology*, *80*, 489–500.

Morris, A. B., & Albery, I. P. (2001). Alcohol consumption and HIV risk behaviours: Integrating the theories of alcohol myopia and outcome-expectancies. *Addiction Research and Theory*, *9*, 73–86.

Mulvihill, L. E., Skilling, T. A., & Vogel-Sprott, M. (1997). Alcohol and the ability to inhibit behavior in men and women. *Journal of Studies on Alcohol*, *58*, 600–605.

Murphy, S. T., Monahan, J. L., & Miller, L. C. (1998). Inference under the influence: The impact of alcohol and inhibition conflict on women's sexual decision making. *Personality and Social Psychology Bulletin*, *24*, 517–528.

Oei, T. P. S., Fergusson, S., & Lee, N. K. (1998). The differential role of alcohol expectancies and drinking refusal self-efficacy in problem and nonproblem drinkers. *Journal of Studies on Alcohol*, *59*, 704–711.

Orford, J., Dalton, S., Hartney, E., Ferrins-Brown, M., Kerr, C., & Maslin, J. (2002). How is excessive drinking maintained?: Untreated heavy drinkers' experiences of the personal benefits and drawbacks of their drinking. *Addiction Research and Theory*, *10*, 347–372.

Ouellette, J. A., Gerrard, M., Gibbons, F. X., & Reis-Bergan, M. (1999). Parents, peers, and prototypes: Antecedents of adolescent alcohol expectancies, alcohol consumption, and alcohol-related life problems in rural youth. *Psychology of Addictive Behaviors*, *13*, 183–197.

Palfai, T., & Wood, M. D. (2001). Positive alcohol expectancies and drinking behavior: The influence of expectancy strength and memory accessibility. *Psychology of Addictive Behaviors*, *15*, 60–67.

Palfai, T. P. (2001). Individual differences in temptation and responses to alcohol cues. *Journal of Studies on Alcohol*, *62*, 657–666.

Park, C. L., & Levenson, M. R. (2002). Drinking to cope among college students: Prevalence, problems and coping processes. *Journal of Studies on Alcohol*, *63*, 486–497.

Parrott, D. J., & Zeichner, A. (2002). Effects of alcohol and trait anger on physical aggression in men. *Journal of Studies on Alcohol*, *63*, 196–204.

Perkins, H. W. (1999). Stress-motivated drinking in collegiate and postcollegiate youn adulthood: Life course and gender patterns. *Journal of Studies on Alcohol*, *60*, 219–227.

Pernanen, K. (1976). Alcohol and crimes of violence: In B. Kissin & H. Begleiter (Eds.), *The biology of alcoholism: Vol. 4. Social aspects of alcoholism* (pp. 351–444). New York: Plenum Press.

Peterson, J. B., Roghfleisch, J., Zelazo, P. D., & Pihl, R. O. (1990). Acute alcohol intoxication and cognitive functioning. *Journal of Studies on Alcohol, 51*, 114–122.

Pihl, R., Peterson, J., & Lau, M. (1993, September). A biosocial model of the alcohol–aggression relationship. *Journal of Studies on Alcohol* (Suppl. 11), 128–139.

Quigley, B. M., & Leonard, K. E. (1999). Husband alcohol expectancies, drinking, and marital-conflict styles as predictors of severe marital violence among newlywed couples. *Psychology of Addictive Behaviors, 13*, 49–59.

Ramsey, S. E., Gogineni, A., Nirenberg, T. D., Sparadeo, F., Longabaugh, R., Woolard, R., Becker, B. M., Clifford, P. R., & Minugh, P. A. (2000). Alcohol expectancies as a mediator of the relationship between injury and readiness to change drinking behavior. *Psychology of Addictive Behaviors, 14*, 185–191.

Rather, B. C., & Goldman, M. S. (1994). Drinking-related differences in the memory organization of alcohol expectancies. *Experimental and Clinical Psychopharmacology, 2*, 167–183.

Richman, J. A., Shinsako, S. A., Rospenda, K. M., Flaherty, J. A., & Freels, S. (2002). Workplace harassment/abuse and alcohol-related outcomes: The mediating role of psychological distress. *Journal of Studies on Alcohol, 63*, 412–419.

Roehrich, L., & Goldman, M. S. (1995). Implicit priming of alcohol expectancy memory processes and subsequent drinking behavior. *Experimental and Clinical Psychopharmacology, 3*, 402–410.

Sayette, M. A. (1993). An appraisal–disruption model of alcohol's effects on stress responses in social drinkers. *Psychological Bulletin, 114*, 459–476.

Sayette, M. A. (1999). Cognitive theory and research. In K. E. Leonard & H. T. Blane (Eds.), *Psychological theories of drinking and alcoholism* (2nd ed., pp. 247–291). New York: Guilford Press.

Sayette, M. A., Martin, C. S., Perrott, M. A., Wertz, J. M., & Hufford, M. R. (2001). A test of the appraisal–disruption model of alcohol and stress. *Journal of Studies on Alcohol, 62*, 247–256.

Sayette, M. A., Smith, D. W., Breiner, M. J., & Wilson, G. T. (1992). The effect of alcohol on emotional response to a social stressor. *Journal of Studies on Alcohol, 53*, 541–545.

Sayette, M., Wilson, G., & Elias, M. (1993). Alcohol and aggression: A social information processing analysis. *Journal of Studies on Alcohol, 54*, 399–407.

Scheier, L. M., & Botvin, G. J. (1997). Expectancies as mediators of the effects of social influences and alcohol knowledge on adolescent alcohol use: A prospective analysis. *Psychology of Addictive Behaviors, 11*, 48–64.

Scott, K. D., Schafer, J., & Greenfield, T. K. (1999). The role of alcohol in physical assault perpetration and victimization. *Journal of Studies on Alcohol, 60*, 528–536.

Sharkansky, E. J., & Finn, P. R. (1998). Effects of outcome expectancies and disinhibition on ad lib alcohol consumption. *Journal of Studies on Alcohol, 59*, 198–206.

Sharp, M. J., & Getz, J. G. (1996). Substance use as impression management. *Personality and Social Psychology Bulletin, 22*, 60–67.

Simons-Morton, B., Haynie, D. L., Crump, A. D., Saylor, K. E., Eitel, P., & Yu, K. (1999). Expectancies and other psychosocial factors associated with alcohol use among early adolescent boys and girls. *Addictive Behaviors, 24*, 229–238.

Simpson, T., & Arroyo, J. A. (1998). Coping patterns associated with alcohol-related negative consequences among college women. *Journal of Social and Clinical Psychology, 17*, 150–166.

Sjoberg, L. (1969). Alcohol and gambling. *Psychopharmacologia, 14*, 284–298.

Skutle, A. (1999). The relationship among self-efficacy expectancies, severity of alcohol abuse, and psychological benefits from drinking. *Addictive Behaviors, 24*, 87–98.

Slutske, W. S., Heath, A. C., Madden, P. A. F., Bucholz, K. K., Statham, D. J., & Martin, N. G. (2002). Personality and the genetic risk for alcohol dependence. *Journal of Abnormal Psychology, 111*, 124–133.

Stacy, A. W., Leigh, B. C., & Weingardt, K. R. (1994). Memory accessibility and association of alcohol use and its positive outcomes. *Experimental and Clinical Psychopharmacology, 2*, 269–282.

Stacy, A. W., & Newcomb, M. D. (1998). Memory association and personality as predictors of alcohol use: Mediation and moderator effects. *Experimental and Clinical Psychopharmacology*, 6, 280–291.

Steele, C. M., Critchlow, B., & Liu, T. J. (1985). Alcohol and social behavior: 2. The helpful drunkard. *Journal of Personality and Social Psychology*, 48, 35–46.

Steele, C. M., & Josephs, R. A. (1988). Drinking your troubles away: II. An attention-allocation model of alcohol's effect on psychological stress. *Journal of Abnormal Psychology [Special issue: Models of addiction]*, 97, 196–205.

Steele, C. M., & Josephs, R. A. (1990). Alcohol myopia: Its prized and dangerous effects. *American Psychologist*, 45, 921–933.

Steele, C. M., & Southwick, L. (1985). Alcohol and social behavior: I. The psychology of drunken excess. *Journal of Personality and Social Psychology*, 48, 18–34.

Steele, C. M., Southwick, L., & Pagano, R. (1986). Drinking your troubles away: The role of activity in mediating alcohol's reduction of psychological stress. *Journal of Abnormal Psychology*, 95, 173–180.

Stein, K. D., Goldman, M. S., & Del Boca, F. K. (2000). The influence of alcohol expectancy priming and mood manipulation on subsequent alcohol consumption. *Journal of Abnormal Psychology*, 109, 106–115.

Swendsen, J. D., Tennen, H., Carney, M. A., Affleck, G., Willard, A., & Hromi, A. (2000). Mood and alcohol consumption: An experience sampling test of the self-medication hypothesis. *Journal of Abnormal Psychology*, 109, 198–204.

Taylor, S. P. (1967). Aggressive behavior and physiological arousal as a function of provocation and the tendency to inhibit aggression. *Journal of Personality*, 35, 297–310.

Taylor, S. P., Gammon, C. B., & Capasso, D. R. (1976). Aggression as a function of the interaction of alcohol and threat. *Journal of Personality and Social Psychology*, 34, 938–941.

Taylor, S. P., & Leonard, K. E. (1983). Alcohol and human aggression. In R. G. Geen & E. I. Donnerstein (Eds.), *Aggression: Theoretical and empirical reviews* (pp. 77–102). New York: Academic Press.

Testa, M., & Collins, R. L. (1997). Alcohol and risky sexual behavior: Event-based analyses among a sample of high-risk women. *Psychology of Addictive Behaviors*, 11, 190–201.

Testa, M., Livingston, J. A., & Collins, R. L. (2000). The role of women's alcohol consumption in evaluation of vulnerability to sexual aggression. *Experimental and Clinical Psychopharmacology*, 8, 185–191.

Tiffany, S. T., Carter, B. L., & Singleton, E. G. (2000). Challenges in the manipulation, assessment and interpretation of craving relevant variables. *Addiction*, 95, S177–S187.

Tracy, J. I., & Bates, M. (1999). The selective effects of alcohol on automatic and effortful memory processes. *Neuropsychology*, 13, 282–290.

Tyssen, R., Vaglum, P., Aasland, O. G., Gronvold, N. T., & Ekeberg, O. (1998). Use of alcohol to cope with tension, and its relation to gender, years in medical school and hazardous drinking: A study of two nation-wide Norwegian samples of medical students. *Addiction*, 93, 1341–1349.

Velez-Blasini, C. J. (1997). A cross-cultural comparison of alcohol expectancies in Puerto Rico and the United States. *Psychology of Addictive Behaviors*, 11, 124–141.

Wall, A. M., Hinson, R. E., & McKee, S. A. (1998). Alcohol outcome expectancies, attitudes toward drinking and the theory of planned behavior. *Journal of Studies on Alcohol*, 59, 409–419.

Wall, A. M., Hinson, R. E., McKee, S. A., & Goldstein, A. (2001). Examining alcohol outcome expectancies in laboratory and naturalistic bar settings: A within-subject experimental analysis. *Psychology of Addictive Behaviors*, 15, 219–226.

Wall, A. M., McKee, S. A., & Hinson, R. E. (2000). Assessing variation in alcohol outcome expectancies across environmental context: An examination of the situational-specificity hypothesis. *Psychology of Addictive Behaviors*, 14, 367–375.

Wechsler, H., Dowdall, G. W., Davenport, A., & Castillo, S. (1995). Correlates of college student binge drinking. *American Journal of Public Health, 85,* 921–926.

Wechsler, H., Lee, J. E., Gledhill-Hoyt, J., & Nelson, T. F. (2001). Alcohol use and problems at colleges banning alcohol: Results of a national survey. *Journal of Studies on Alcohol, 62,* 133–141.

Wells, S., Graham, K., & West, P. (2000). Alcohol-related aggression in the general population. *Journal of Studies on Alcohol, 61,* 626–632.

Wells-Parker, E., Kenne, D. R., Spratke, K. L., & Williams, M. T. (2000). Self-efficacy and motivation for controlling drinking and drinking/driving: An investigation of changes across a driving under the influence (DUI) intervention program and of recidivism prediction. *Addictive Behaviors, 25,* 229–238.

Wertz, J. M., & Sayette, M. A. (2001). A review of the effects of perceived drug use opportunity on self-reported urge. *Experimental and Clinical Psychopharmacology, 9,* 3–13.

White, H. R., & Chen, P.-H. (2002). Problem drinking and intimate partner violence. *Journal of Studies on Alcohol, 63,* 205–214.

Wiers, R. W., Hoogeveen, K.-J., Sergeant, J. A., & Gunning, W. B. (1997). High- and low-dose alcohol-related expectancies and the differential associations with drinking in male and female adolescents and young adults. *Addiction, 92,* 871–888.

Wilde, G. J. S., Trimpop, R. M., & Joly, R. (1989). The effects of various amounts of ethanol upon risktaking tendency and confidence in task performance. *Proceedings of the 11th International Conference on Alcohol, Drugs, and Traffic Safety, T89,* 494–499.

Wills, T. A., DuHamel, K., & Vaccaro, D. (1995). Activity and mood temperament as predictors of adolescent substance use: Test of a self-regulation mediational model. *Journal of Personality and Social Psychology, 68,* 901–916.

Wills, T. A., Sandy, J. M., Yaeger, A. M., Cleary, S. D., & Shinar, O. (2001). Coping dimensions, life stress, and adolescent substance use: A latent growth analysis. *Journal of Abnormal Psychology, 110,* 309–323.

Wills, T. A., & Stoolmiller, M. (2002). The role of self-control in early escalation of substance use: A time-varying analysis. *Journal of Consulting and Clinical Psychology, 70,* 986–997.

Wood, M. D., Read, J. P., Palfai, T. P., & Stevenson, J. F. (2001). Social influence processes and college student drinking: The mediational role of alcohol outcome expectations. *Journal of Studies on Alcohol, 62,* 32–43.

Wulfert, E., Block, J. A., Ana, E. S., Rodriguez, M. L., & Colsman, M. (2002). Delay of gratification: Impulsive choices and problem behaviors in early and late adolescence. *Journal of Personality, 70,* 533–552.

Zeichner, A., & Pihl, R. O. (1979). Effects of alcohol and behavior contingencies on human aggression. *Journal of Abnormal Psychology, 88,* 153–160.

25

The Self-Regulation of Eating

Theoretical and Practical Problems

C. PETER HERMAN
JANET POLIVY

In this chapter, we attempt to impose a self-regulatory framework on eating. Eating is normally regarded as a highly regulated activity, as it must be if it is to serve its biological function. Of course, closer examination reveals that eating is not as well-regulated as one might imagine. Moreover, it turns out that the regulation of eating is often opposed by the self-regulation of eating, which naturally creates all sorts of personal and theoretical problems. In this chapter, we consider the extent to which eating (and its cousin, weight) are regulated, and how that regulation is achieved. The bulk of the chapter is devoted to self-regulation, successful and unsuccessful, including a survey of the empirical evidence and a consideration of various models of self-regulation and self-regulation failure. We conclude that there is still much to be learned.

REGULATION OF EATING

Because eating is essential to life, it is not surprising that it is part of a well-regulated system. Before they can do almost anything else, infants cry to express their hunger and cease crying when they are fed. For infants, regulation requires the assistance of another person, who provides the food; but as we get older, the principle remains the same: We feel hunger; we seek out and consume food; we experience a satisfying satiation; and eventually, as nutrients are depleted over time, we once again feel hunger and the cycle recurs.

This rendition of the regulatory cycle is drastically oversimplified; moreover, it obscures several difficult questions about how elements of the cycle work. For instance, what is the hunger signal, and how is it conveyed from the periphery to the brain (not to mention to consciousness)? Do we eat only enough to eliminate our current hunger, or enough to forestall anticipated hunger? Why do we occasionally overeat? What is the satiety signal, and how does it operate? Why does it not always operate reliably? How vulnerable is the regulatory system to perturbations such as emotional and social influences on intake? In short, how well-regulated is the system, and how does the regulation occur?

Bruch (1961) argued that even in infants, the regulatory system may become seriously deranged through the mother's mismanagement of feeding. For instance, if the mother misinterprets the infant's pain cry as a hunger cry (or vice versa), she may feed the infant inappropriately. Not only will such inappropriate feeding perturb normal caloric regulation, but it may lead to long-term misreading of hunger signals by the developing child and eventuate in obesity or eating disorders.

In a more familiar example of misregulation, the social facilitation of eating (de Castro & de Castro, 1989; see Herman, Roth, & Polivy, 2003, for a review), people tend to eat considerably more in groups than when alone. We do not have adequate space to explore the various explanations that have been offered for this phenomenon; suffice it to say, none of them postulate that people in groups face an increased caloric demand. In short, the additional food consumed in groups is truly excessive and violates basic regulatory principles; either that, or people eating alone eat insufficiently, again violating basic regulatory principles.

Whether or not the regulatory system operates smoothly, in most cases it operates fairly automatically. We do not mean to suggest that eating is a reflex; rather, eating normally starts and stops in response to hunger and satiety cues. When our eating is affected by social or emotional factors, the influence again is relatively spontaneous. We do not deliberate much about whether to eat more in groups or less when we are depressed; we just do it, often without even being aware that we are doing it. To this extent, all eating is regulated, albeit not necessarily consciously, and not always in a nice, neat, negative-feedback loop.

REGULATION VERSUS SELF-REGULATION OF EATING

Self-regulation opposes regulation. Self-regulation is undertaken when our normal or typical regulatory processes do not accomplish what we want. When we cannot count on automatic regulation to get us where we want to go, we must deliberately alter the regulatory landscape, introducing new interventions designed to remedy the situation. Just as we do not normally think about our breathing, unless it poses a problem for us, we also do not normally think about our eating, unless it becomes problematic. Self-regulation represents our attempts to solve that problem, whatever it may be.

SELF-REGULATION *QUA* WEIGHT LOSS

Where is it that we want to go in terms of food intake? Why not just let our intake follow its natural course and rely on hunger to let us know when to start and stop eating? Reliance on natural regulation is problematic for several reasons.

As we have already implied, hunger and satiety do not operate as efficiently as one might imagine. Consider hunger. We may count on hunger signals to let us know when we need food, but such signals may arise at an inopportune time, either when food is not immediately available, or when eating is not an option. This problem is exacerbated by the fact that eating a relatively small amount of food is often sufficient to eliminate hunger. If we were to eat only when under the direct influence acute hunger signals, and stop when such signals ceased, then we would eat relatively small meals, because these small meals would eliminate hunger signals, at least for a while. But we would then find ourselves experiencing hunger repeatedly throughout the day; the amount of food required to eliminate hunger signals is considerably less than is that required to prevent the onset of hunger signals for an appreciable period of time (allowing us to spend our time doing things other than eating every hour or so). So we must eat more than is necessary simply to stave off acute hunger. But how much more? We might eat until we felt full, which would maximize the time between meals. The problem with eating until we are full is that for many of us, that much food is more than we are willing to eat, for one reason or another. Plus, it takes some time for the gut to feed information back to the brain that satiety has been reached; by the time we experience clear satiety signals, we may already have eaten too much, to the point where the feedback, when it eventually arrives, is aversive.

The discomfort of a distended stomach aside, why might we be "unwilling" to eat in a way that maximizes the intermeal interval? One practical reason is that our mealtimes are dictated by factors other than hunger and satiety. Mealtimes, in fact, tend to be coordinated to a schedule that is more responsive to social and work requirements than to strictly nutritional considerations. Thus, there is no point in eating enough breakfast to forestall hunger for 7 or 8 hours if we are going to have lunch in 4 or 5 hours anyway. Another reason for not maximizing our intake at a given meal—a reason that for many people supersedes all others—is that we believe (probably with some justification) that eating maximally is not conducive to slenderness. This is a different kind of reason than the previous ones we have considered, because it introduces a truly extraneous element into the calculations. Rather than accepting the demands of our bodies, but trying to make minor adjustments to maximize physiological comfort and mundane convenience, we may oppose the demands of our bodies, because they conflict with some other personal agenda. In a nutshell, our bodies are concerned about (1) short-term regulation of energy and (2) maintaining a reserve of energy for emergencies. We, however, may be intensely concerned about our appearance. A slim physique may be unachievable if we eat all that our bodies demand, so we may deliberately eat less, even though our bodies demand more. For the most part, the self-regulation of eating is tantamount to dieting, just as "weight control" is a euphemism for weight loss. Some people are unconcerned about losing weight; indeed, there are even some people—mostly scrawny teenage boys—who want to gain weight, if the added weight takes the shape of muscles. Still, for the vast majority, self-regulation of eating means eating in an unnatural, mindful way designed to achieve (or perhaps maintain) weight loss.

Deliberately eating less than what the body demands has several consequences. For one thing, it means that one may become chronically hungry. Although even a diet meal will satisfy immediate hunger, it will not do so for long, so hunger is likely to reappear sooner. This situation is parallel to the one discussed earlier, in which the eater eats only enough to satisfy immediate hunger. The difference is that the dieter does not allow herself to eat whenever hunger arises; rather, she must wait until the next scheduled (and inadequate) meal. Even if the dieter adheres to the diet, things do not always go as planned. Weight loss induces in the body various defensive reactions designed to counteract the attempt to reduce weight. Such defenses—most notably, changes in metabolism—make it increasingly difficult to continue to lose weight, even with the same spartan diet that initially produced weight loss. Some of the defensive changes experienced by dieters are more subtle: fatigue makes it more difficult to maintain one's customary activity level; changes in taste make certain high-calorie foods more attractive (e.g., "negative alliesthesia," a process whereby eating a meal reduces the hedonic value of sweets, is suppressed by weight loss, so that for dieters, postmeal sweets remain sweeter). These defensive adjustments, then, occur at both physiological and behavioral levels. In either case, they force the dieter to impose an even tighter self-regulatory regimen if further weight loss is to be accomplished.

It is worth remembering that self-regulation of intake is a means to the end of self-regulation of weight. People rarely worry about regulation of intake for its own sake. It is usually a matter of appearance, or health, or some other goal beyond intake itself. Still, the means can sometimes become an end in itself. In order to lose (i.e., down-regulate) weight, one must eat less (i.e., down-regulate intake). (Of course, one could try to lose weight by other means [acupuncture, food combining, exercise, drugs, etc.], but the most frequently used method is caloric restriction. Indeed, many of these "alternative" methods are really just other ways of making it easier for one to eat less.)

DIETING AS A SELF-REGULATORY STRATEGY

How exactly do people who are eager to achieve slimness by means of caloric restriction organize their attempt? A reduction in caloric intake, after all, might be achieved in all sorts of ways. For instance, one might set a target for a certain (reduced) number of calories per day, as seen in many diets. But obviously that is not the only way that one might achieve a caloric reduction. Instead of reducing one's daily caloric quota by, say, 15%, one might simply eat normally for 6 days of the week and fast on the seventh. From a purely psychological point of view, perhaps it is easier to eat nothing at all than to eat sparingly. After all, to eat sparingly entails exposure to appetite-stimulating food cues, whereas fasting allows one to avoid food cues, which may make restriction easier. Most diets do not involve fasting, but as a self-regulatory issue, why exactly is fasting not more popular?

Even if we rule out fasting, there are all sorts of self-regulatory choices to be made. The typical diet prescribes a daily caloric quota, but why is the quota specified on a daily basis? Why not weekly, monthly, or yearly? There are good psychological reasons for adopting a daily quota (see Herman & Polivy, 2003, for an extended discussion), but a daily quota also presents problems for successful self-regulation, as we see later when we discuss self-regulatory failure.

Taking this issue to the other extreme, might it not be easier to regulate intake if we were to manage intake in a more microscopic way, say, by specifying an hourly intake quota? Such a quota does not map easily onto the typical meal pattern in our (or any other) culture, so perhaps it is unrealistic. But there is clearly an option of partitioning the daily quota among the (three?) meals that most people eat. Still, do we want the calories to be apportioned equally across the meals? Many people prefer a smaller breakfast and/ or lunch, which allows them to eat more later in the day (and spend the day looking forward to eating more). Self-regulatory problems may arise in this scenario as well, as indeed is the case for all scenarios. Our point here is simply that usually more than one self-regulatory strategy is available to reach any particular goal. The choice of strategy is often made without a great deal of thought about its implications for self-regulatory success.

Although many diets specify (daily) caloric quotas, other weight-loss diets do not demand an explicit caloric sacrifice. These "all-you-can-eat" diets operate on alleged "secret," or at least arcane, nutritional principles. You can eat all you want as long as you stay away from (certain) carbohydrates; or you can eat all you want as long as you load up on (certain) carbohydrates. Some foods (e.g., fruits) can be eaten without limit and/or other foods (e.g., potatoes, chocolate) must be avoided at all costs. We are not critiquing the nutritional merits of these various diets (other than to point out that insofar as they are successful, it is usually because they indirectly induce dieters to consume fewer calories than they otherwise would). Our major concern here is to consider the implications of such restrictive–permissive diets for self-regulatory success.

Obviously, being allowed to eat all you want has great appeal for veterans of explicit caloric-restriction diets. Having to stop eating after consuming a certain number of calories may be terribly frustrating. Still, the all-you-can-eat diets are not quite as permissive as they appear at first glance. The emphasis is on eating all you want, but close behind comes the condition that certain foods—even entire categories of foods—are forbidden, even in small amounts. How frustrating is that, empirically? We revisit this issue when we review the literature on self-regulatory failure—more specifically, diet breaking.

SOCIAL NORMS AND SELF-REGULATION

One can set self-regulatory goals by reference to calories or to specific foods; such goals are matters for the individual to decide, either in isolation or in consultation with a diet coach, book, or some other authority. In practice, however, the particular intake choices that one makes may depend less on the rules prescribed by authorities than on the behavior of one's eating companions. Our analysis of social influences on eating (Herman et al., 2003) indicates, first, that social influences are extremely powerful, often overriding other influences on eating, including one's prior intentions or goals. Second, the influence exerted by one's eating companions is of a specifically regulatory sort; that is, people appear to use the intake of their eating companions as a regulatory guide. Studies of modeling, in which an experimental confederate eats more or less and the naive participant eats correspondingly more or less, suggest that we regulate our intake with reference to the intake of others. Note that using the behavior of others as a guide for regulating one's intake does not make much sense in terms of satisfying one's own specific physiological needs; nor does it make much sense for dieters to abandon their caloric or other regulatory scheme and simply follow the example of others. Yet people, dieters and nondieters alike, do follow the example of others.

Although people do follow others' example, they tend to follow at a slight distance. The modeling that occurs is not simply a matter of matching one's intake to that of the companion; closer examination suggests that the naive participant often tends to eat slightly less than does the confederate. It is as if the goal of the eater is to eat less than the other person; accomplishing this goal may be all that is required to convince the eater that he or she has consumed an appropriate amount. Herman and colleagues (2003) suggest that, for some people, the real (regulatory) goal is to avoid excessive intake, and that "excessive" is defined situationally as "more than the companion eats." Eating less than (or no more than) the confederate eats, therefore, serves as a socially based regulatory strategy. Another group of people, according to Herman and colleagues, aim not to avoid excess but to eat minimally, with "minimal" (like excessive) eating defined socially. Eating less than the companion thus qualifies as minimal eating. Distinguishing between the goal of avoiding excessive eating and the goal of eating minimally cannot be accomplished in experimental situations involving a single confederate; multiple confederates who eat different amounts are required. Still, both goals use a situation-specific social definition of appropriate eating, based on the companion's intake. Insufficient attention has been paid to the behavior of other people as the basis for regulation of eating, possibly because it makes so little biological sense—either for dieters or for normal eaters—to allow others to dictate their intake. Our view of the regulation of eating has long been confined to models in which people regulate on the basis of either their internal physiological signals or their own cognitive calculations of appropriate foods (or amounts of foods) to eat. We must expand our view to include the role of others' intake as a regulatory force and recognize that self-regulation may be tantamount to regulation by others.

Before leaving this topic, we should add that using the intake of others as a standard may "regulate" our intake not just by providing intake guidelines. Extensive research (see Herman et al., 2003, for a review) suggests that when we eat in the presence of noneating observers, our intake is suppressed (e.g., Polivy, Herman, Hackett, & Kuleshnyk, 1986). Obviously, we cannot eat less than someone who is not eating at all, but we certainly do "down-regulate." In one interesting, apparent exception to this generalization, Herman, Polivy, and Silver (1979) found that dieters did not eat minimally in the presence of a noneating observer; rather, they ate "sensibly," in that they ate more after a large preload than after a small preload. This "sensible" pattern, which, as we shall see, is uncharacteristic of dieters, was probably due to one additional feature of this study: Participants were instructed to fill themselves up, which precluded minimal eating. Instead, dieters and nondieters alike ate in accordance with what they considered to be appropriate intake norms, enforced by the presence of the observer.

SELF-REGULATORY FAILURE

The seeds of conflict have already been sown. If we consider the models of self-regulation of intake that we have already introduced, it is evident that the goals implicit in the various models may not coincide. The demands of the formal diet, for instance, may not coincide with the intake norms of our eating companions. If we stick to our diet, we may offend our companion. (Remember, the more we eat, the more our companion can eat without eating excessively, so we are likely to be pressured by our companion to "just have a little more.") But if we adhere to the social norm, then the limits imposed by the weight-loss diet may well be exceeded. Only in the case of "dieters" whose diets consist of eating no more than do their eating companions can these two self-regulatory principles be reconciled satisfactorily.

Although the potential exists for conflict between competing self-regulatory principles, the most common and well-appreciated threat to self-regulation arises when a single self-regulatory principle is challenged and defeated by circumstances. Our research program over the past three decades has documented the difficulties of dieting (see Polivy & Herman, 2002). As we have seen, some of the difficulties of dieting occur even when the dieter manages to adhere to a self-regulatory regimen; the development of anabolism (i.e., a more conservative metabolism) as weight loss progresses represents the most well-known hindrance to achieving the ultimate weight-loss goal. It is important, however, to distinguish between this anabolic threat to diet success—a threat that emerges even as, and precisely because, self-regulation succeeds—and self-regulatory failure. Self-regulatory failure destroys the diet not by counteracting its physiological effects but by defeating the attempt to cut back on calories in the first place.

Our very first study of dieters (Herman & Mack, 1975) forced us to start thinking in terms of self-regulation and self-regulatory failure. We had not begun with the intention of studying these phenomena; we had been looking for parallels between the behavior of normal-weight sorority girls and the obese males whom Schachter had been studying (see Schachter & Rodin, 1974, for a review). Schachter had demonstrated that whereas normal-weight individuals were responsive to preload size (i.e., eating more after a small preload and less after a large preload), obese individuals were relatively unresponsive to preload size and seemingly oblivious to this "internal cue." When we tested the effects of preloading experimental participants with 0, 1, or 2 milkshakes (7.5-ounces each), we found that whereas many of them "regulated," subsequently eating in inverse proportion to preload size, others (who eventually came to be known as "restrained eaters") ate more after the 1- or 2-milkshake preload than after no preload at all. This result did not conform to our expectation, namely, that this latter group (like the obese group) would display an absence of regulation by not responding differentially to preload size. Instead, we had uncovered a new pattern, "counterregulation," that demanded a new interpretation. Eventually, we concluded that members of this anomalous group must have been attempting to inhibit their intake (hence the label "restrained eaters"), and that the forced milkshake consumption had disrupted this attempt.

We argued at the time that the forced preload had undermined the restrained eaters' motivation to diet. The rich milkshake had exceeded their caloric quota for the day, and once the diet was ruined, further attempts to restrict intake served no purpose. (We called it the "what-the-hell" effect.) In short, our interpretation of self-regulatory failure was motivational: We assumed that the restrained eaters could have continued (i.e., maintained the ability) to exert self-control when confronted with palatable food, but after the forced preload, there was no point in doing so. Only much later (see later discussion) did we begin to entertain other interpretations.

Note some of the perplexities raised by our interpretation, even accepting a motivational perspective. For one thing, it is absurd to argue that once one's diet has been broken, there is no point in exercising further self-control. Even if one's caloric quota for the day has been exceeded, does it not make sense to compensate for this excess rather than abandon all self-control? If a person exceeds her quota by 200 calories, is that not better than exceeding it by 2,000 calories? According to the perverse logic of the dieter, apparently not. The dieter tends to think in all-or-none terms: Once the diet is broken, it matters little whether one has exceeded it by a lot or a little. At least in part, this irrational calculation stems from the fact that dieters are aware of how much they should eat to satisfy the diet, but they do not have a self-regulatory plan for what happens if and when the diet is broken. A single self-regulatory failure could, in principle, trigger a secondary or "backup" self-regulatory plan, but dieters are generally so invested in the initial plan that no contingency plans are ever developed.

A second perplexity, related to the first, is raised by the assumption that diets should operate diurnally. As we saw earlier, diurnal self-regulation appears to be the norm for dieting (as for many other self-regulatory human activities), but ultimately, it is arbitrary. Excess calories consumed today still "count" tomorrow, in the sense that they contribute to one's continuing weight problem. As long as one has not achieved one's weight-loss goal, one should remain motivated toward it. Why does a milkshake undermine that motivation, especially when everyone knows that the diet will be resumed tomorrow morning, and the consequences of today's postmilkshake binge must be "tacked on" to the diet, probably extending the need to diet for several days? We conclude that if dieters act as if their motivation to diet has been undermined, it may be more than the milkshake per se that contributes to this undermining.

Finally, and again related to the foregoing issues, the milkshake preload, rich as it may be, does not necessarily exceed the caloric quota for the day. An 8-ounce milkshake does not contain *that* many calories, and if it is consumed early in the day, it is quite likely that it is still mathematically possible, by restricting one's subsequent intake, to adhere to the daily allowance. Maybe something else is going on, in addition to quota-busting.

VARIATIONS ON THE THEME OF SELF-REGULATORY FAILURE

Preload Studies

Much of our research has been devoted to exploring various other experimental conditions that lead restrained eaters to (temporarily) abandon their restraint. Some of these variations are extensions of the preloading paradigm; others attack restraint from entirely different angles.

The first preload-variation study (Polivy, 1976) demonstrated that it was not the actual number of calories in the preload that determined whether dieters would "lose control"; rather, it was what they *believed* about the richness of the preload. Participants' beliefs about whether the preload (in this case, pudding) was high or low in calories were manipulated orthogonally to the actual caloric content of the pudding. Perceived calories exerted more control than did actual calories, and restrained eaters who believed that they had consumed a high-calorie preload were more likely to become disinhibited, whether or not that belief was correct. This finding, which has been replicated (Knight & Boland, 1989; Spencer & Fremouw, 1979; Woody, Costanzo, Leifer, & Conger, 1981), indicates that the preload operates through a cognitive (not physiological) mechanism; the dieter is making a calculation pertaining to calories.

We speculated that a rich preload produces disinhibition and subsequent overeating because the preload precludes success at adhering to the daily diet requirements. In most of the studies, that failure is induced by a prior forced preload. If the forced preload were merely anticipated, rather than already consumed, how might that affect the dieter? If the dieter were assured that the impending preload would sabotage the diet before the day was done, then the chances of dietary success would be as negligible as if the preload were already ingested. And indeed, such appears to be the case. Some studies (Ruderman, Belzer, & Halperin, 1985; Tomarken & Kirschenbaum, 1984) have found that anticipating a preload later in the day produces disinhibition and overeating in restrained eaters.

The vulnerability of dietary restraint to disruption by caloric considerations seems to know no bounds. Urbszat, Herman, and Polivy (2002) demonstrated that anticipation of a weeklong diet, starting first thing tomorrow, leads dieters to overeat today. In this case, these researchers argued, the anticipated deprivation may "justify" the prediet overindulgence; another possibility is that, among dieters, the connection between overindulgence today and compensatory deprivation planned for tomorrow is so strong that it may operate reciprocally, with deprivation planned for tomorrow triggering (compensatory) overindulgence today.

Yet another variation on the disinhibitory power of the preload is evident in situations in which the preload is merely encountered rather than consumed. When dieters are exposed to rich, palatable food, but not required (or even allowed) to eat it, and when this exposure to attractive food cues (including smell and indulgent thoughts) extends for several minutes, dieters become more likely to overeat when subsequently given access to palatable food. These studies (Fedoroff, Polivy, & Herman, 1997, 2003) are typically interpreted as evidence of craving as a precipitant of disinhibition. It is not that the diet has been (or will necessarily be) broken; rather, the urge to eat, stimulated by focused concentration on food cues, becomes overwhelming. Note that, in this case, exposure to the preload does not ruin the diet by exceeding the caloric quota for the day; rather, this exposure undermines the diet by making the prospect of eating more attractive than the prospect of not eating. Normally, the dieter's self-regulatory inhibitions are enough to allow her to resist temptation; but sometimes, either because of the sustained power of the tempting food cues, or because of cue-induced cravings at the physiological level, or both, self-regulatory inhibitions fail. Later, we consider more systematically how these various interpretations map onto various models of how self-regulation works in dieters.

Recently, we asked another question about preloads, namely, what is the smallest preload that will produce disinhibited eating? In two studies (Herman, Reisz, & Polivy, 2003), we found that a rich milkshake preload as small as 1 ounce will disinhibit dieters' subsequent eating as effectively as will a preload of 10 or 15 ounces. This finding challenges the notion that it is an accumulation of excessive calories that undermines the diet and renders further restraint during the same day useless. Instead, it may be that a very small amount of a forbidden food will suffice to break a diet. This diet-breaking hinges on the (somewhat magical) notion that some foods, in any quantity, are intolerable. If a diet does not allow a certain type of food, then any amount of that food ruins the diet, and disinhibition will ensue.

Finally, it is important to recognize that when self-regulation failure induces disinhibited eating, this disinhibited eating may proceed in a fashion devoid of self-regulation, but it is not necessarily immune to other (more reliable) regulatory influences. Herman, Polivy, and Esses (1987) showed that whereas a large, rich preload disinhibited eating in restrained eaters, an extralarge preload (twice as large as the large preloads used in prior studies) did not cause restrained eaters to eat any more than they did in the control (no-preload) condition. We believe that in the extralarge-preload condition, restrained eaters were disinhibited, in the sense that they were no longer adhering to their original self-regulatory plans, but because the preload was so huge, they were near the limit of physical capacity and literally could not eat much more. Physical capacity, of course, is a "natural" regulator of intake and should not be confused with self-regulation, which is an "unnatural" regulator not grounded in—and usually opposed to—one's automatic physiological processes.

Whether natural regulators invariably kick in eventually to constrain disinhibited eating is arguable. For instance, some anecdotal evidence indicates that individuals displaying bulimia nervosa occasionally disregard even the physical-capacity regulator and end up eating beyond capacity, to the point where their stomachs literally burst. Another natural regulator is the palatability of the available food. Even when disinhibited, people should be responsive to the taste of food. Nevertheless, some reports (see Herman & Polivy, 1996, for a discussion) indicate that bulimics binge on food universally regarded as unpalatable; in their eating frenzy, some bulimics appear to disregard palatability considerations. This unnatural disregard for palatability may not characterize all bulimics, but it is worth remembering. Moreover, disregard for palatability is not necessarily confined to bulimics. Polivy, Herman, and McFarlane (1994) found that disinhibited dieters were insensitive to a manipulation of palatability of available food. Although the disinhibition in this study was not induced by preloading, and the manipulation of palatability was not extreme (no truly "inedible" food, such as bulimics are occasionally reputed to eat, was offered), at least some tentative evidence indicates that natural regulatory (along with self-regulatory) influences may be disrupted following disinhibition. The dynamics and the factors (if any) that control eating once disinhibition has occurred have only begun to be explored.

Other Studies

As mentioned earlier, Polivy and colleagues (1994) induced disinhibition in restrained eaters using a trigger other than preloading—in this case, anxiety. Several studies have explored the role of emotional arousal as a disrupter of dietary restraint. (Interestingly, just as preloading suppresses eating in unrestrained eaters, while disinhibiting eating in restrained eaters, distress suppresses eating in unrestrained eaters, while disinhibiting eating in restrained eaters.) Distress has been manipulated in many ways, most often in the form of fear (e.g., McKenna, 1972) or anxiety (e.g., Herman, Polivy, Lank, & Heatherton, 1987), but also in the form of acute depression (e.g., Baucom & Aiken, 1981). Anxiety obviously does not exert its effect on self-regulation by ruining the diet; the anxious dieter has not eaten any more than has the nonanxious dieter before encountering whatever food is available for subsequent overeating. From the beginning, we (Herman & Polivy, 1975) assumed that anxiety undermines the diet through a different mechanism, that the anxious dieter rearranges her priorities, so that whereas adhering to the diet successfully remains calorically possible, the dieter no longer cares so much about dietary success; coping with distress is more important, and eating is one way to cope with distress. The notion that emotion regulation is the basis for overeating is nicely captured by Tice, Bratslavsky, and Baumeister (2001), who demonstrated that overeating can be prevented if one is convinced that eating will not improve one's emotional state. Nevertheless, it remains possible that distress may induce disinhibited eating without engaging distress-management mechanisms (see later discussion). Also, the phenomenon has been refined empirically (Heatherton, Herman, & Polivy, 1991), with the discovery that certain types of distress (e.g., ego threat) are more effective in inducing disinhibition than are others (e.g., physical threat). Whatever the underlying mechanism may be, distress does interfere with self-regulation, just as preloading does; these disrupters of self-regulation can substitute for each other, such that if the dieter is preloaded, then anxiety does not produce any additional overeating, and if the dieter is anxious, preloading does not produce any additional overeating (Herman, Polivy, Lank, & Heatherton, 1987).

Finally, we have found that alcohol, at least under certain circumstances, can produce self-regulatory failure (Polivy & Herman, 1976a, 1976b). It will come as no surprise to the reader that alcohol leads to disinhibition (see Hull & Sloane, Chapter 24, this volume), but the precise mechanism underlying the effect remains in dispute, despite millennia of human experience of the phenomenon.

Intoxicants, emotional distress, and diet-threatening preloads all interfere with the self-regulation on which the dieter depends. Empirically, the disruption of self-control by exposure to these conditions or situations is well established, with only some minor details unresolved. What remains to be established, however, is precisely how these experimental (or natural) manipulations exert their effects. We have casually alluded to some interpretations of how these disrupters undermine and often defeat self-regulatory strategies. We now focus on this question more systematically.

MODELS OF SELF-REGULATION
AND SELF-REGULATION FAILURE

Attempts to impose self-regulation on eating, which in most cases amount to attempts to restrict intake, can be understood most simply as the exercise of self-control. We have argued (Herman & Polivy, 1980) that the advent of research on restrained eating represents a significant change in our understanding of controls on eating. Prior research focused on "internal" (physiological) and "external" (environmental) controls but ignored self-control. Obviously, restrained eaters, insofar as they are successful, are resisting both internal and external cues promoting intake; even if they are not successful, or are successful only for a while, dieters are attempting to exercise self-control. Our introduction of self-control as an oppositional force in eating, however, was intuitive and did not specify exactly how self-control operated.

General Self-Regulatory Models

Formal models of self-regulation (e.g., Carver & Scheier, 1982; see Carver, Chapter 2, this volume) specify the goal, assessment of progress toward the goal, and adjustments implemented when progress toward the goal is inadequate. Such models help to explain how dieters approach the long-term goal of weight loss (or possibly weight maintenance), but they are not very helpful when it comes to the more proximate goal of intake regulation in the short term. For one thing, the short-term goal of the dieter tends to be negative: The objective is to avoid eating certain amounts or certain foods. Assessing progress toward a negative goal is difficult, if not impossible, for there really is no progress. One either commits the error or succeeds in avoiding it, with little or no grey area. Feedback that one is succeeding—that one has not (yet) failed—is difficult to act on, especially when the behavior being shaped is a nonbehavior (i.e., not eating). Perhaps because of the negative orientation of the dieter's intake goals, it is especially difficult to sustain success. Moreover, after failure occurs, there is no provision for how to behave. One cannot "make a correction" for having broken one's diet. The reader might argue that dieters certainly can make a correction for their errors by compensating (undereating) for the remainder of the day. As we have seen, however, this compensatory option does not appear to be available to most dieters, who seem to regard dietary success on a given day in the same way that they would regard defending their virginity; it cannot be repaired once it is lost. (Dieters have an advantage over virgins in that they can start over fresh the next day.)

If a model such as that of Carver and Scheier were pursued in the interpretation of short-term dietary restraint, we would be forced to specify more precisely exactly what behaviors the dieter is exhibiting when resisting temptation. This resistance—often conceptualized as an effort of will—is difficult to conceptualize in behavioral terms. Also, one would have to specify the sorts of useful feedback the dieter obtains while pursuing his or her restrictive goal; at the moment, we do not have a clear notion of what feedback the dieter receives or uses. Nor do we have a clear sense of the dieter making adjustments in his or her behavior as a means of more closely approaching the goal. The only feedback of which we, as researchers, are aware is that the diet has been broken, in which case, it is too late to expect to observe compensatory adjustments. We do not mean to suggest that mapping the dieter's goal-directed behavior onto an act–test–adjust model of regulatory control is inappropriate, but, simply, that for the time being it is difficult; doing so would require a much more subtle analysis of what the dieter is doing when resisting temptation or not eating.

Delay of Gratification

Another approach to self-control—one that appears to map quite directly onto the dieter's situation—is represented by Mischel's work on delay of gratification (Mischel, Cantor, & Feldman, 1996; see Mischel & Ayduk, Chapter 6, this volume). Mischel's research appears to be especially pertinent in that it is concerned with acute influences on consummatory behavior. Obviously, we all (try to) delay gratification in the service of long-term goals, but the gratifications that we deny ourselves present themselves in the here and now, and the task boils down to a series of proximate challenges. In Mischel's laboratory studies, success (delay) or failure (capitulation to temptation) is a single-episode phenomenon. The fact that the temptation often takes the form of palatable food brings the parallel closer.

Mischel has focused on factors that enhance or impede delay. For instance, we all know that resistance to temptation may be enhanced if the tempting object is rendered less salient; indeed, ancient behavior therapy recommendations for dieting (e.g., Stuart, 1967) have emphasized distancing oneself from the tempting stimulus, either by removing the temptation from one's environment (e.g., keeping tempting snacks out of sight) or removing oneself from the tempting environment (e.g., staying out of the kitchen). A simple extension of this notion is to reduce the temptingness of the stimulus by psychological means, even while staying in close proximity to it. Mischel demonstrates that delay can be enhanced if the object of temptation is construed in such a way as to reduce its sensory allure (Mischel, Shoda, & Rodriguez, 1992). A chocolate bar can be construed as a log (or worse). Such reconstrual appears to be effective, but we have to wonder how long it can be sustained; a chocolate bar, to paraphrase Freud, is sometimes (in fact, always) a chocolate bar. An alternative tactic to enhance resistance to temptation (Herman & Polivy, 1993) does not require denying that a chocolate bar is what it is, nor does it re-quire denying that it would be delicious; it simply requires making salient the equally true proposition that a chocolate bar represents a significant caloric threat: "It tastes good, but it's not good for me." If the dieter can focus on the negative aspects of the stimulus, while perhaps still acknowledging that the stimulus instantiates both positive and nega-tive features, then perhaps the angel on one shoulder will win the argument with the devil on the other, even though the devil has a good argument. The real threat here, we believe, arises when the dieter's ability to attend to the angel's argument ("Watch out for those calories!") is reduced by distraction. If the dieter's mental energy is depleted or devoted to some more urgent task, the devil is likely to win the argument, if only because the argu-ment can then proceed on a noncognitive level. The distracted dieter does not *think* about the food but merely reacts to its sensory properties in an almost decorticate way. At the sensory level, temptation will always triumph. Resistance requires a clear focus on the downside of consuming a desirable treat, and this downside is fairly abstract: The conse-quences of self-regulatory failure are to be found somewhere off in some vague future, whereas the pleasure of capitulation is immediate.

Eating Hijacked by Salient External Cues

The conflict between sensory- and self-control of behavior is articulated clearly in Heatherton and Baumeister's (1991) analysis of binge eating. They postulate that dis-tress—particularly those forms of distress that pose a threat to one's ego or self-esteem—renders self-awareness aversive (because it is aversive to contemplate a besieged self) and prompts the individual to "escape" from self-awareness. Aspects of the "self" that are discarded during this escape include one's long-range goals (e.g., weight loss, in the case of dieters). Not only is the goal of weight loss (temporarily) abandoned, but the escape from self is a flight into the not-self, more specifically, the immediate environment of sen-sory stimuli. It is almost as though the individual descends to a lower level of conscious-ness, devoid of abstract ideals and goals, and dominated by salient cues demanding an unmediated, reflexive response. In the presence of palatable food, and having lost sight of long-range objectives, the distressed dieter is easy prey for forbidden food.

The idea that distress renders the individual more vulnerable to the sensory allure of food was proposed earlier by Slochower (1983). She argued that certain diffuse types of distress make the individual more "external" (responsive to environmental cues). When the distressed eater is in the presence of salient food cues, overeating will ensue. Slochower's prescient analysis was restricted to the obese, however, and she did not focus on distress-induced externality as a threat to self-regulatory control, if only because her analysis retained Schachter's internal–external framework rather than the inhibition–disinhibition framework that is a prerequisite for a fully realized self-regulatory analysis.

Other models pertinent to self-regulation have emphasized conditions under which behavior is "captured" by salient cues. Steele and Josephs (1990) proposed that alcohol narrows the individual's attentional field, so that behavior comes under the control of most salient cues in the immediate environment. Ward and Mann (2000) extended the "alcohol myopia" model and proposed that a cognitive load of any sort will reduce available cognitive resources and have the net effect of focusing attention more narrowly on salient stimuli (e.g., palatable, forbidden food that is enticingly available to dieters). Ward and Mann found that imposition of a memory task led to disinhibition of eating among restrained eaters.

These models emphasizing the narrowing of attention (and behavioral control) to salient stimuli may be quite directly applied to disinhibited eating under conditions of distress and alcohol intoxication. In both instances, the individual's cognitive resources are depleted: In the case of distress, the impairment is created by the need to devote a certain proportion of resources to coping with the distress; in the case of alcohol, the loss of cognitive resources may be a direct pharmacological effect. In either case, it is not difficult to explain disinhibition of eating in dieters. Whether these models can account for the disinhibition that occurs in response to a forced preload is more debatable. Conceivably, being forced to consume a rich preload is a disturbing experience for the dieter, and we can reconstrue the preload manipulation as a distress manipulation. Still, no direct evidence indicates that preloading has a negative emotional impact on dieters. (We might even argue that a forced preload is a positive event; one gets to eat a fondly desired, forbidden food, while avoiding blame for the episode, because one has no choice in the matter.)

Self-Regulatory Strength

A somewhat different rendition of the impairment of self-regulatory ability is the self-regulatory strength model (Baumeister, Bratslavsky, Muraven, & Tice, 1998; Baumeister & Vohs, 2002; Muraven, Tice, & Baumeister, 1998), which proposes that effective self-regulation demands a certain degree of self-regulatory strength. Like muscular strength, self-regulatory strength can be depleted in the short term by exertions of self-control, although in the long term, repeated exertions of self-control (like regular exercise) supposedly increase one's self-regulatory strength. This metaphor can explain why having to exert self-control in one situation may impair self-regulation in another immediately thereafter. Some evidence (Kahan, Polivy, & Herman, 2003; Vohs & Heatherton, 2000) suggests that such may be the case for restrained eaters: Exertions of self-control, whether or not they are related to inhibiting eating, may make it more difficult to inhibit eating immediately thereafter. Whether repeated efforts over time to resist tempting food strengthen one's self-regulatory abilities (with respect to food or other temptations) remains an unanswered question. Although the details of this model are vague, it has some intuitive explanatory appeal, once again emphasizing threats to self-regulatory capacity.

Desire

Most of the attempts to account for self-regulatory failure in dieters that we have examined locate the main source of the problem in the dieter's impaired capacity to resist temptation. Owing to a lapse in motivation, attention, or self-regulatory strength (willpower) and/or perhaps to temporarily losing sight of long-range goals, the dieter can no longer summon the resources necessary to fend off the desire for palatable food. This analysis of the problem seems reasonable, as far as it goes; but we must remember that there is more than one element in the equation that predicts successful resistance to temptation. Obviously, the fewer the resources that one brings to the resistance effort, the less likely it is to succeed, but, by the same token, not all temptations demand the same amount of resistance. Some temptations are more tempting than others, and the prediction of self-regulatory success should take that fact into consideration. Loewenstein's analysis of self-control (e.g., Hoch & Loewenstein, 1991; Loewenstein, 1996) emphasizes fluctuations in desire, with the probability of self-control success varying inversely with the intensity of desire at the visceral level. If the hungry individual displays less resistance to forbidden food, is it because hunger depletes the resources necessary for resistance, or because hunger renders the forbidden food even sweeter? It may be that the "resistance resources" remain constant but the temptation to be resisted becomes more desirable, overwhelming the resources that formerly were capable of sustaining resistance to less intense temptations. A rich dessert is easier to resist when it is merely described verbally on the menu than when it is glistening right in front of you on your plate. This analysis finds empirical support in the previously described studies by Fedoroff and colleagues (1997, 2003).

CONCLUSIONS

Consideration of the magnitude or intensity of temptation simply reminds us that resistance to temptation is a dynamic process, and that success at a task depends both on our ability and on the difficulty of the task, either of which can in principle be manipulated independently. This perspective, although obvious in a way, also makes clear how far we are from a truly comprehensive analysis of self-regulatory success and failure. The final model will have to include both the state of the dieter and the power of the tempting stimulus. Neither factor is easy to measure independently; most models assume that the "other" factor is held constant, while the factor of interest is varied. Until we achieve much more systematic (and noncircular) assessments of both the ability to resist and the power of the temptation, we will be unable to escape the charge that our manipulations affect both factors, and that assuming only one factor to be crucial amounts to scientific negligence. Furthermore, it may turn out that these "independent" factors mutually influence each other, as well as independently affecting the outcome of the resistance effort.

We have come a long way in understanding self-regulation in the past few decades, although one cannot help thinking that some ancient Greek philosophers must have known all of this, but we clearly have a long way to go in terms of establishing the relative merits of the competing theories (or even the extent to which the competing theories are not just saying the same thing in different words). Eating provides a nice crucible for testing models of self-regulation and self-regulatory failure. As our survey indicates, several intriguing models have been developed specifically in the context of eating, whereas others have been developed elsewhere and imported into the domain of eating. The next step, we believe, will be to identify and articulate more clearly the empirically testable differences among these models and begin to do the sort of research that will help us to decide which models best account for the data.

REFERENCES

Baucom, D. H., & Aiken, P. A. (1981). Effect of depressed mood on eating among obese and nonobese dieting and nondieting persons. *Journal of Personality and Social Psychology, 41*, 577–585.

Baumeister, R. F., Bratslavsky, E., Muraven, M., & Tice, D. M. (1998). Ego depletion: Is the active self a limited resource? *Journal of Personality and Social Psychology, 74*, 1252–1265.

Baumeister, R. F., & Vohs, K. D. (2002). Willpower. In G. Loewenstein, D. Read, & R. F. Baumeister (Eds.), *Time and decision: Economic and psychological perspectives on intertemporal choice* (pp. 201–216). New York: Russell Sage Foundation.

Bruch, H. (1961). Transformation of oral impulses in eating disorders: A conceptual approach. *Psychiatric Quarterly, 35*, 458–481.

Carver, C. S., & Scheier, M. F. (1982). Control theory: A useful conceptual framework for personality—social, clinical, and health psychology. *Psychological Bulletin, 92*, 111–135.

de Castro, J. M., & de Castro, E. S. (1989). Spontaneous meal patterns of humans: Influence of the presence of other people. *American Journal of Clinical Nutrition, 50*, 237–247.

Fedoroff, I. C., Polivy, J., & Herman, C. P. (1997). The effect of pre-exposure to food cues on the eating behavior of restrained and unrestrained eaters. *Appetite, 28*, 33–47.

Fedoroff, I., Polivy, J., & Herman, C. P. (2003). The specificity of restrained versus unrestrained eaters' responses to food cues: General desire to eat, or craving for the cued food? *Appetite, 41*, 7–13.

Heatherton, T. F., & Baumeister, R. F. (1991). Binge eating as escape from self-awareness. *Psychological Bulletin, 110*, 86–108.

Heatherton, T. F., Herman, C. P., & Polivy, J. (1991). Effects of physical threat and ego threat on eating behavior. *Journal of Personality and Social Psychology, 60*, 138–143.

Herman, C. P., & Mack, D. (1975). Restrained and unrestrained eating. *Journal of Personality, 43*, 647–660.

Herman, C. P., & Polivy, J. (1975). Anxiety, restraint, and eating behavior. *Journal of Abnormal Psychology, 84*, 666–672.

Herman, C. P., & Polivy, J. (1980). Restrained eating. In A. J. Stunkard (Ed.), *Obesity* (pp. 208–225). Philadelphia: Saunders.

Herman, C. P., & Polivy, J. (1993). Mental control of eating: Excitatory and inhibitory food thoughts. In D. M. Wegner & J. W. Pennebaker (Eds.), *Handbook of mental control* (pp. 491–505). Englewood Cliffs, NJ: Prentice-Hall.

Herman, C. P., & Polivy, J. (1996). What does abnormal eating tell us about normal eating? In H. Meiselman & H. MacFie (Eds.), *Food choice, acceptance, and consumption* (pp. 207–238). London: Blackie Academic & Professional.

Herman, C. P., & Polivy, J. (2003). Dieting as an exercise in behavioral economics. In G. Loewenstein, D. Read, & R. F. Baumeister (Eds.), *Time and decision: Economic and psychological perspectives on intertemporal choice* (pp. 459–490). New York: Russell Sage Foundation.

Herman, C. P., Polivy, J., & Esses, V. M. (1987). The illusion of counter-regulation. *Appetite, 9*, 161–169.

Herman, C. P., Polivy, J., Lank, C., & Heatherton, T. F. (1987). Anxiety, hunger, and eating behavior. *Journal of Abnormal Psychology, 96,* 264–269.

Herman, C. P., Polivy, J., & Silver, R. (1979). Effects of an observer on eating behavior: The induction of "sensible" eating. *Journal of Personality, 47,* 85–99.

Herman, C. P., Reisz, L., & Polivy, J. (2003). *Preload quality or quantity?* Unpublished manuscript, University of Toronto.

Herman, C. P., Roth, D. A., & Polivy, J. (2003). Effects of the presence of others on food intake: A normative interpretation. *Psychological Bulletin, 129,* 873–886.

Hoch, S. J., & Loewenstein, G. F. (1991). Time-inconsistent preferences and consumer self-control. *Journal of Consumer Research, 17,* 492–507.

Kahan, D., Polivy, J., & Herman, C. P. (2003). Conformity and dietary disinhibition: A test of the ego-strength model of self-regulation. *International Journal of Eating Disorders, 33,* 165–171.

Knight, L. J., & Boland, F. J. (1989). Restrained eating: An experimental disentanglement of the disinhibiting variables of perceived calories and food type. *Journal of Abnormal Psychology, 98,* 499–503.

Loewenstein, G. (1996). Out of control: Visceral influences on behavior. *Organizational Behavior and Human Decision Processes, 65,* 272–292.

McKenna, R. J. (1972). Some effects of anxiety level and food cues on the eating behavior of obese and normal subjects: A comparison of the Schachterian and psychosomatic conceptions. *Journal of Personality and Social Psychology, 22,* 311–319.

Mischel, W., Cantor, N., & Feldman, S. (1996). Principles of self-regulation: The nature of willpower and self-control. In E. T. Higgins & A. W. Kruglanski (Eds.) *Social psychology: Handbook of basic principles* (pp. 329–360). New York: Guilford Press.

Mischel, W., Shoda, Y., & Rodriguez, M. L. (1992). Delay of gratification in children. In G. Loewenstein & J. Elster (Eds.), *Choice over time* (pp. 147–164). New York: Russell Sage Foundation.

Muraven, M., Tice, D. M., & Baumeister, R. F. (1998). Self-control as limited resource: Regulatory depletion patterns. *Journal of Personality and Social Psychology, 74,* 774–789.

Polivy, J. (1976). Perception of calories and regulation of intake in restrained and unrestrained subjects. *Addictive Behaviors, 1,* 237–243.

Polivy, J., & Herman, C. P. (1976a). Effects of alcohol on eating behavior: Disinhibition or sedation? *Addictive Behaviors, 1,* 121–125.

Polivy, J., & Herman, C. P. (1976b). Effects of alcohol on eating behavior: Influences of mood and perceived intoxication. *Journal of Abnormal Psychology, 85,* 601–606.

Polivy, J., & Herman, C. P. (2002). If at first you don't succeed: False hopes of self-change. *American Psychologist, 57,* 677–689.

Polivy, J., Herman, C. P., Hackett, R., & Kuleshnyk, I. (1986). The effects of self-attention and public attention on eating in restrained and unrestrained subjects. *Journal of Personality and Social Psychology, 50,* 1253–1260.

Polivy, J., Herman, C. P., & McFarlane, T. (1994). Effects of anxiety on eating: Does palatability moderate distress-induced overeating in dieters? *Journal of Abnormal Psychology, 103,* 505–510.

Ruderman, A. J., Belzer, L. J., & Halperin, A. (1985). Restraint, anticipated consumption, and overeating. *Journal of Abnormal Psychology, 94,* 547–555.

Schachter, S., & Rodin, J. (Eds.). (1974). *Obese humans and rats.* Potomac, MD: Erlbaum.

Slochower, J. A. (1983). *Excessive eating: The role of emotions and environment.* New York: Human Sciences Press.

Spencer, J. A., & Fremouw, W. J. (1979). Binge eating as a function of restraint and weight classification. *Journal of Abnormal Psychology, 88,* 262–267.

Steele, C. M., & Josephs, R. A. (1990). Alcohol myopia: Its prized and dangerous effects. *American Psychologist, 45,* 921–933.

Stuart, R. B. (1967). Behavioral control of overeating. *Behaviour Research and Therapy*, *5*, 357–365.

Tice, D. M., Bratslavsky, E., & Baumeister, R. F. (2001). Emotional distress regulation takes precedence over impulse control: If you feel bad, do it! *Journal of Personality and Social Psychology*, *80*, 53–67.

Tomarken, A. J., & Kirschenbaum, D. S. (1984). Effects of plans for future meals on counter regulatory eating by restrained eaters. *Journal of Abnormal Psychology*, *93*, 458–472.

Urbszat, D., Herman, C. P., & Polivy, J. (2002). Eat, drink and be merry, for tomorrow we diet: Effects of anticipated deprivation on food intake in restrained and unrestrained eaters. *Journal of Abnormal Psychology*, *111*, 396–401.

Vohs, K. D., & Heatherton, T. F. (2000). Self-regulatory failure: A resource–depletion approach. *Psychological Science*, *11*, 249–254.

Ward, A., & Mann, T. (2000). Don't mind if I do: Disinhibited eating under cognitive load. *Journal of Personality and Social Psychology*, *78*, 753–763.

Woody, E. Z., Costanzo, P. R., Liefer, H., & Conger, J. (1981). The effects of taste and caloric perceptions on the eating behavior of restrained and unrestrained subjects. *Cognitive Therapy and Research*, *5*, 381–390.

26

To Buy or Not to Buy?

Self-Control and Self-Regulatory Failure in Purchase Behavior

RONALD J. FABER
KATHLEEN D. VOHS

Controlling the self and managing executive functions are crucial aspects of human life. Researchers are unearthing even more situations in which self-regulation and the executive function serve to guide people in their behavioral choices (Baumeister & Vohs, 2003; Higgins, 1996). One area that has recently begun to receive attention in the self-regulation literature is buying impulses and decisions (Baumeister, 2002). In Western society, we constantly encounter tempting products, goods, or services that we might elect to acquire. Yet, clearly, we cannot have it all. We must abstain from purchasing some items to be able to have others. This conflict between "having now" versus "having later" requires the person to engage in self-regulation.

Self-regulation has been characterized as having three component parts: (1) establishing a goal; (2) engaging in actions that lead to obtaining this goal; and (3) monitoring progress toward the goal (Baumeister & Vohs, 2003). For example, one may set a goal of putting at least $50 a week into savings. To achieve this, the person may need to cut back on spending or purchasing, then monitor the savings that result from these behaviors to see if they meet the $50 goal. If not, further cutbacks are enacted and more assessments are made, until finally the goal of saving $50 a week is reached.

The act of buying itself may also be designed to lead to a desired goal. Here, for example, the goal may be to become healthier, which spurs actions such as buying low-calorie foods or vitamin supplements; thus, spending may contribute to achieving a goal. A different way that purchasing may achieve a goal is to help motivate an action that will lead to a non-purchase related goal. For example, a woman may decide to buy a new dress, if she reaches a desired weight. Thus, the dress serves to help motivate her to engage in actions leading to weight loss.

Unfortunately, however, self-regulation efforts are not always successful. Baumeister and Heatherton (1996) identified three causes of self-control failure: (1) conflicting goals; (2) failing to track one's own behavior; and (3) depleting the resources that permit self-control to operate. From our perspective, purchasing behaviors may not only contribute to our failure to exert self-regulation but also may be a response to such failures.

Certainly, most people have numerous goals or plans that compete for their financial resources. People may save for a house, for their children's education, for retirement, for a vacation, for a particular good, such as a couch or new car, or any of a number of other things. These items often compete with each other, in that acquiring one item may necessitate not obtaining another. For instance, I would like to take a vacation this year, but that may mean that I will not have enough money saved to retire at the age I have chosen. Additionally, more mundane purchases may conflict with our goals. One way to afford the new television I want may be to stop going out to lunch so often, or to give up buying a latte on the way to work. But the latte tastes good, and going out to lunch is a nice break in the day and also a way to socialize with my colleagues. Thus, immediate and more long-term goals often collide in purchase decisions.

Failure to track one's behavior is also evident in the way people engage in spending. People often resolve to make a budget and stick with it, but not many succeed in doing so. Oftentimes it is difficult to monitor one's goal-related behavior, which makes it significantly less likely that spending will be assessed accurately. For instance, it is time-consuming and labor-intensive to record each purchase, then enter it into a spreadsheet or notebook. At the point of making a purchase decision, rarely do we have our monthly spending balance clearly established in our minds. In short, keeping track of where one's money goes is a difficult task at best. Consequently, reaching one's goals with regard to purchasing becomes less likely.

The last factor that influences self-control in purchasing is resource depletion. We have all experienced the difference between going grocery shopping when we are hungry and after we have just eaten. Exerting control over buying food at the grocery store is far more difficult when we are hungry. Although hunger is not exactly analogous to the concept of regulatory resource depletion, the idea is that being low in energy (physical or psychological energy) makes controlled behavior much more laborious and likely to fail. Similar failures due to resource depletion may be related to prior efforts at self-control and other factors.

Our purpose in this chapter is to demonstrate how the literature on three specific types of purchasing fits what is known about self-control. The purchasing behaviors we analyze include self-gifting, impulse buying, and compulsive buying. We attempt to show how these behaviors may be used in support of self-regulatory goals, how other factors can affect the success of purchase-related goals, and how resource depletion can be used to explain these various types of buying behavior.

SELF-GIFTING

We generally think of gifts as things we buy for other people. However, people can also provide gifts for themselves, which has been termed "self-gifting" (Mick & DeMoss, 1990a). Frequently, such gifts serve as rewards for accomplishments or as consolation for disappointments (Mick & DeMoss, 1990a; Tournier, 1966). Mick and DeMoss (1990a, p. 328) have defined "self-gifts" as "(1) personally symbolic self-communication through (2) special indulgences that tend to be (3) premeditated and (4) highly context bound." Just as in society we mark important events and experiences with cards, presents, or other acknowledgments, so too do we recognize similar events for ourselves with special self-gifts. We tend to give such gifts for our birthday, as a reward for an important personal accomplishment, or to cheer ourselves up (Mick & DeMoss, 1990b). Thus, through these gifts, we communicate the significance of these events to ourselves.

To signify the specialness of the occasion, the items we choose as self-gifts tend to differ from items we buy ourselves for other purposes. They tend to be items we consider exceptional or distinctive (Mick & DeMoss, 1990a). Oftentimes they are more expensive brands than we would ordinarily buy (Mick, DeMoss, & Faber, 1992). In this way, self-gifts are goods or services that we might otherwise deny ourselves. Indeed, if such an item is acquired too frequently, it may well lose its specialness (Mick & DeMoss, 1990a).

The decision to engage in self-gifting is typically premeditated. In analyzing consumers' accounts of their self-gifting behaviors, Mick and DeMoss (1990a) reported that prior to buying themselves something special, 83% of these people indicated that they knew why they were doing so. Additionally, their desire for the specific item often occurred well in advance of the purchase situation. Hence, the item was likely something that people had previously denied themselves, which means that self-control played a role in past refusals. The purchase was deemed acceptable now because of the specific situation.

The notion that a self-gift is allowable because of a particular situation points to the fact that these items are context-bound. Self-gifts tend to be purchased under a limited number of circumstances, such as achieving a personal accomplishment or attaining a desired goal, experiencing negative feelings, or in celebration of a specific holiday. Motivations reported for self-gifting are to reward oneself, to cheer oneself up, to be nice to oneself, to celebrate, to relieve stress, and to provide an incentive toward a goal (Mick & DeMoss, 1990b; see Larsen & Prizmic, Chapter 3, this volume). Even more specific determinants may influence self-gifting. For example, a self-gift to cheer oneself up may be appropriate, if the cause of the negative feelings is an external factor (bad luck), but less so, if it is due to an internal cause, such as a lack of effort (Mick & DeMoss, 1990a). Self-gifting can play a number of roles in the self-regulation process. Failing to stay focused on a distal goal can lead to self-regulatory failure (Baumeister, Heatherton & Tice, 1994). Given that temptations are frequently encountered in the immediate environment, the individual needs to transcend these stimuli and stay committed to the abstract goal. One way to achieve this is by enhancing the value of the long-term goal. Promising oneself a desired gift for achieving a goal can help one overcome proximate temptations and stay focused and committed to the distal goal. In this case, the self-gift serves as an additional incentive for achieving the desired objective. For example, a dieter may promise him- or herself a new item of clothing, if a particular level of weight loss is achieved. The desire for the new suit or dress can then serve to help the person overcome the occasional temptations of fattening foods. In this way, the self-gift also takes on a heightened value, because it was achieved through self-sacrifice (Mick & DeMoss, 1990b). In some cases, people may even impose a relationship between the value of the self-gift and the difficulty in maintaining self-control. For example, Mick and DeMoss (1990a) had one respondent who stated that whenever he did something that to him justified a self-reward, he mentally matched the behavior to a predetermined list of items he wanted and bought himself something that corresponded to the value of the action.

The purchase of prior self-rewards can help people to regulate a future action. In a study that used projective stories in response to pictures of a woman buying perfume as a self-gift, several participants indicated that the woman would relive the positive feelings that led to buying the perfume each time she used the perfume (Mick et al., 1992). Use of a self-gift first acquired as a reward may thus inspire the user to self-regulate successfully in a later situation. This may account for why appropriate self-gifts for a reward were seen by participants as possessing qualities such as "inspiring," "memorable," and "lasting" (Mick & DeMoss, 1992).

Self-regulatory failure can also occur when a person is depleted of resources as a result of prior regulatory effort (Baumeister & Vohs, 2003; Baumeister et al., 1994; Vohs & Heatherton, 2000). Thus, anything that can help the person conserve self-regulatory resources should help to maintain self-control. Evidence suggests that people believe that self-gifts can alter their emotional states and improve their sense of control. In relating accounts of self-gifting, participants typically indicated that the result of purchasing a self-gift was indeed to increase positive affect (Mick & DeMoss, 1990a). People rarely cited negative outcomes such as guilt or regret after the purchase of a self-gift. Similarly, in participants' projective stories, 71% ended with the self-gift purchase having a highly positive outcome (Mick et al., 1992). In only 4% of the stories did the self-gift lead to a negative outcome.

Self-gifts can also affect coping abilities, especially when problems occur (Mick & DeMoss, 1990a). A recurring theme of people using self-gifts to escape from problems temporarily was found in a number of recounted stories of self-gifting (Mick & DeMoss, 1990a). Often, the nature of these gifts was diversionary, such as taking a trip to a museum or movie, or going to a calm and relaxing place, such as the beach or a park. Descriptions of the results of these gifts often seem to suggest that people were better able to cope with problems or to self-regulate afterward. For example, people described feeling "renewed," "refreshed," "like a new person," "more rational," "more in control," and able to ward off unpleasant feelings or experiences (Mick & DeMoss, 1990a; Mick et al., 1992). Thus, self-gifts may be a way for people to overcome situations in which their self-regulatory resources are low and to reinstate their ability to exert control.

Although self-gifts can be used for self-regulatory purposes, they also occur as the result of failures to control self-regulation. As mentioned earlier, people have multiple goals at any point in time. Controlling negative emotional states can often take precedence over more distant goals, because emotions are part of our immediate environment (Tice, Bratslavsky, & Baumeister, 2001). As a result, goals such as saving money may become less important compared to the desire to escape unpleasant emotions. In this way, self-gifts designed to cheer ourselves up, or to be nice to ourselves, may actually be the result of self-regulatory failure. We review more direct examples of regulatory failures in the next two sections on impulse buying and compulsive buying.

IMPULSE BUYING

It has been estimated that impulse purchases account for $4.2 billion dollars in store sales (Mogelonsky, 1998). One study concluded that over one third (38.7%) of department store purchases are impulse buys (Bellenger, Robertson, & Hirschman, 1978). With shop-at-home television networks multiplying, direct marketing techniques becoming more ubiquitous, and the proliferation of Internet stores, opportunities to engage in impulse buying will continue to grow. The likelihood that people will succumb to impulsive purchases may in many cases be traced back to temporary failures in exercising self-control.

Early research on "impulse buying" tended to define it as any unplanned purchase (Kollat & Willett, 1969; Stern, 1962). It was generally assumed that this behavior emanated mainly from the characteristics of the product or the store environment

(Applebaum, 1951; Stern, 1962). Therefore, research in the 1960s and 1970s focused on the properties of so-called "impulse products." Researchers began to question this taxonomic approach to impulse purchases in the 1970s, when they recognized that all products could be purchased on impulse (Bellenger et al., 1978; Shapiro, 1973). By the 1980s, researchers began to recognize that people, rather than products or retail environments, should be the focus of studies in impulse buying (Rook & Hoch, 1985).

More recent definitions of impulse buying have stressed that it occurs in response to a strong or overwhelming urge to buy (Beatty & Ferrell, 1998; Rook, 1987), that there is a conflict between affect (desire) and cognition (control) (Hock & Loewenstein, 1991; Weinberg & Gottwald, 1982; Youn & Faber, 2002), that the decision to buy is a relatively rapid one (Kacen & Lee, 2002; Piron, 1991), and that there is a diminished concern for consequences of the action (Beatty & Ferrell, 1998; Rook, 1987). These characteristics can also be seen as basic elements of failed attempts at self-regulation.

Most people attempt to exert self-control to avoid buying everything they desire. Simply put, unless one has an unlimited budget, excessive purchasing will conflict with other goals, such as saving money or buying more desirable items. A serious challenge to the exercise of self-regulation thus occurs when one is faced with an urge to buy. This urge may stem from spotting a desirable brand, or other elements of the store environment, or it may be an internal state experienced by the consumer. For whatever reason, the urge makes it more difficult to maintain self-regulation. These urges, even if they are very powerful, do not always lead to action (Rook & Fisher, 1995). In fact, the urge to buy was found to account for just 20% of the variance in impulse buying (Beatty & Ferrell, 1998).

Some authors have viewed impulse buying as the interaction of emotional activation and cognitive or normative control (Rook & Fisher, 1995; Weinberg & Gottwald, 1982; Youn & Faber, 2002). Therefore, self-regulation can be maintained by strategies that either reduce desire or increase regulatory resources. Conversely, self-regulatory failure (impulse buying) occurs when desire or emotional activation is increased, or cognitive controls are diminished.

Hoch and Lowenstein (1991) hypothesized that proximity increases desire for goods. People who are exposed to a sensory stimulus become adapted to it. As a result, instead of perceiving the acquisition of the item as a gain, failing to have it is seen as a loss. For example, we can think of buying a cookie. Getting the cookie would be a gain. However, once inside the bakery, we can smell the cookies baking, and we begin to salivate. Now, we might feel that *not* buying the cookie is a deprivation. Research in prospect theory has shown that the amount of displeasure associated with a loss is greater than the amount of pleasure associated with a similar gain (Tversky & Kahneman, 1981). Accordingly, a perceived loss increases desire more than does a perceived gain.

Research in self-regulation also points to the role of proximity in producing failures of self-control. Walter Mischel and colleagues (e.g., Mischel & Ebbesen, 1970; see also Mischel & Ayduk, Chapter 6, this volume) for over 30 years, have shown that children seated near a desired object fare significantly worse in their delay of gratification attempts than do children who are not placed close to such objects. Thus, the temptation of inviting products or goods is more difficult to overcome when the desired product is proximal to the person.

Two types of proximity can influence desire (Hoch & Lowenstein, 1991). One is physical proximity, which allows a person to have a sensory experience with an item. For instance, seeing a product in the store may be enough to alter a person's perspective. Touching a cashmere sweater, tasting a free sample at the supermarket, smelling perfume sprayed by a store clerk, or test-driving a car are all ways in which consumers may experience sensory stimuli through physical proximity. A second method of boosting desire for a product is via temporal proximity. The closer in time one is to having a possession, the more difficult it is to delay gratification. In support of this notion, consumers describe impulse buying as an unexpected, immediate, and intense urge to buy (Rook, 1987; Rook & Hoch, 1985). It appears that the initial desire might be the most difficult to control.

The growth of practices, such as direct marketing, that allow people to buy without waiting may serve to increase impulse buying by boosting desire through temporal proximity. Consumers do not need to travel to a store; rather, they can log onto a computer or call a phone number immediately after seeing an item in a catalog, on a home shopping channel, or on the Internet. The ubiquity of credit cards, the abundance of cash machines in malls and stores, and the rapidity of express shipping are other technological changes that have increased temporal proximity in the past half-century. All of these have contributed to the growth of impulse purchasing in recent years.

Although technological changes and marketing strategies may increase desire, consumers can utilize various strategies to decrease desire, thereby reducing the likelihood of impulse buying. Perhaps the most obvious tactic is to avoid tempting situations. Because impulse purchases frequently start with exposure to desirable stimuli, one might simply stay away from such situations. For example, one may avoid the candy isle of a grocery store when on a diet, or avoid bookstores if easily tempted to buy new books. Avoidance strategies work best if one knows there are certain times when temptation is greatest. For example, many people recognize that they should avoid grocery shopping when they feel hungry, or avoid shopping when they feel lonely.

The second factor that influences impulse buying is willpower, which involves utilization of cognitive effort to exert self-control. As with desire, a number of factors can enhance or diminish the ability to exert self-control in buying situations. The most common form of exerting willpower is to focus mentally on the costs involved in making such a purchase (Puri, 1996; Rook & Hoch, 1985). This generally involves considering other uses for the money about to be spent or reminding oneself of the negative impact of buying the specific item (e.g., "The candy bar will make me fat"; "Buying a martini now means I won't go home and work tonight"; "My spouse will be angry if I bring home another new outfit").

Through interviews with consumers, Rook and Hoch (1985) identified a number of additional strategies that can be employed to maintain willpower over an impulse-buying urge, including delay tactics, bargaining with themselves, and guilt. Delay tactics involve efforts to postpone or delay a purchase. For example, consumers may say to themselves that they will postpone a purchase until after they have looked at other items, or that they will wait for some period of time, and if they find that they still want the item, they will come back and buy it.

Bargaining strategies involve promising oneself a small reward, if the immediate desire is denied. Rook and Hoch (1985) cited examples of purchasing flowers instead of a gold chain, and buying chocolates instead of an expensive handbag. These examples may be viewed as a form of self-gifting as a reward for maintaining one's self-control (see our earlier discussion of self-gifting). Finally, consumers may caution themselves that they will feel bad later if they make a purchase now. Because an impulse purchase may conflict with another goal, such as paying a bill or buying something for a child, reminders of these trade-offs and the guilt the desired purchase may cause can help to boost resistance.

Researchers have demonstrated that cognitive considerations do indeed modify impulse-buying behavior (Puri, 1996; Rook & Fisher, 1995). Rook and Fisher, for example, found that normative evaluations of impulse buying moderated the relationship between respondents' own impulsiveness (measured as a personality trait) and what they thought a hypothetical character in a story should do when faced with the desire to make an impulse purchase. For respondents who viewed impulse buying favorably, there was a significant relationship between their own impulsiveness and thinking that the character should buy impulsively. However, for respondents who held a negative evaluation of impulse buying, the relationship between trait impulsiveness and recommendations for others' hypothetical behavior disappeared. A second study of consumers' actual purchasing behavior replicated these relationships. Thus, it would appear that norms affect resistance and influence the likelihood of impulse buying.

Willpower may help to improve self-control over buying impulses, but in some situations, it may be difficult to exert willpower. Several researchers have noted the role of mood as an antecedent of impulse buying (Beatty & Ferrell, 1998; Rook & Gardner, 1993; Weinberg & Gottwald, 1982). Researchers have found that impulse buying occurs more frequently when people feel positively than when they are distressed or in a bad mood (Beatty & Ferrell, 1998; Rook & Gardner, 1993). Rook and Gardner (1993) reported that 85% of their sample indicated a greater likelihood to buy on impulse if in a positive rather than negative mood. The mood state of pleasure was most frequently reported as preceding impulse buying. Not coincidentally, it has been found that a pleasant mood state can bias evaluations and judgments in a positive direction (Gardner, 1985). By making everything look better, feeling pleasure and other positive moods may increase impulse buying by enhancing desire. People in pleasant moods also want to extend this desirable feeling (Rook & Gardner, 1993), and this motivation may also serve to increase the desire to buy.

Although negative mood states less frequently than positive moods lead to impulse buying, the effects of negative emotions are not negligible: over one third of Rook and Gardner's (1993) sample indicated they had made impulsive purchases when in a negative mood. These respondents indicated that they often made impulsive purchases in the hope of alleviating the unpleasant mood. In this situation, consumers may be making a deliberate decision not to exert self-regulation in one area (spending) to achieve another goal (a more positive mood state; see Tice et al., 2001). In this case, the effort to exert control is diminished, and impulse buying results from this change in willpower. This notion that people make a conscious decision to reduce self-control is supported by respondents' reports that they spent less money on impulse purchases in negative than in positive mood states (Rook & Gardner, 1993). This finding may indicate that consumers have made a conscious decision to permit a small lapse in self-control to achieve the greater good of balancing their mood state. Similar findings of reduced self-control during negative mood states have been found for other self-regulatory behaviors (see, e.g., Heatherton & Baumeister, 1996, for a review of binge eating when distressed).

This example may be labeled as a self-regulatory failure that occurred through acquiescence (Baumeister et al., 1994), because the person chose to give up self-regulation. Similar failures due to acquiescence occur when people are tired either from physical exertion or, more directly, from recent use of self-regulatory resources. The ability to command self-regulation successfully has been conceptualized as a finite resource that can be depleted by situational demands (Baumeister, 2002; Vohs & Heatherton, 2000; see also Schmeichel & Baumeister, Chapter 5, and Vohs & Ciarocco, Chapter 20, this volume). Both exerting self-control and making decisions (Vohs, Twenge, Baumeister, Schmeichel, & Tice, 2003) seem to deplete this resource. Thus, if one has to exert self-regulatory resources for a period of time, they should have less ability to maintain self-control as time progresses. This model suggests that impulse buying may be more common at the end of a shopping trip or after a long day of decision making.

One recent series of studies tested the effect of a depletion of self-regulatory resources on impulse buying (Vohs & Faber, 2002). In the first study, participants were randomly assigned to either a resource-depletion or no-depletion condition. In the resource-depletion condition, participants were instructed to watch a silent video but to avoid looking at part of the content on the screen. Control (no-depletion) participants viewed the same tape but with no instructions to avoid attention to any content. This manipulation had previously been found successful in manipulating self-regulatory resources (Schmeichel, Vohs, & Baumeister, 2003).

Following exposure to the video, participants were asked to complete a modified version of the Buying Impulsiveness Scale (Rook & Fisher, 1995). The Buying Impulsiveness Scale was initially designed to assess trait impulse buying; thus, the modification involved rewording the items to pertain to participants' desires, urges, and inhibitions to buy in the current situation. The results of this study indicated that participants in the resource-depletion condition scored significantly higher on the modified (state) Buying Impulsiveness Scale than did the no-depletion participants. Thus, reducing self-regulatory resources seemed to increase the propensity for impulse buying.

In a second study, self-regulatory resources were similarly manipulated with an attention control task, after which participants were shown pictures of 18 high-priced items (e.g., expensive watches, cars). Participants were asked to give prices indicating how much they were willing to pay for each item. The results of this study converged with those of the first study, showing that resource-depletion participants reported that they would pay significantly more for the items than no-depletion participants.

Finally, in a third study, a different manipulation of self-regulatory resources was used to examine actual impulse buying. Depletion-condition participants were asked to read aloud a series of boring historical biographies, while exaggerating their hand gestures, facial expressions, and emotionality. This task required self-control, because it involved amplifying and creating an emotional reaction (which was difficult given the biographies' lack of emotional content), while also directing nonverbal behaviors. Participants in the no-depletion condition read aloud the same information but were not asked to change their reading style. After the manipulation, participants were given the opportunity to buy items commonly found in a college bookstore or a supermarket at discounted prices. Participants who experienced resource depletion chose to buy more items and spend more total dollars than those whose regulatory resources were not depleted. This finding was especially strong for participants high in trait impulsive buying (as measured by the original scale by Rook and Fisher, 1995), suggesting that among people for whom impulsive purchasing is a problem, having few regulatory resources available considerably increases the prospect of spending impulsively. Together, these studies suggest that people are more likely to acquiesce to an impulse-buying urge when self-regulatory resources are diminished.

COMPULSIVE BUYING

Some important theoretical distinctions have been made between different types of self-regulatory failures (Baumeister et al., 1994). One distinction is between an initial violation and a complete breakdown of self-regulation. Initial violations are cases in which there occurs a single instance of failing to maintain a goal-directed behavior, but control can be quickly reestablished afterward. Alternatively, when there is a total breakdown in self-regulation, an initial failure can lead to major bingeing in the prohibited behavior. Baumeister and colleagues (1994) refer to this effect as "snowballing."

A second distinction in different types of failure is based on the underlying cause. Most research in self-regulation failure has focused on underregulation, which is the failure to exert sufficient self-control. An alternative cause, misregulation, occurs when people attempt to exert regulation, but do so using unproductive or counterproductive strategies.

A consideration of these distinctions leads to the idea that impulse buying may represent a type of initial violation failure that results from underregulation. Conversely, compulsive buying may be a snowballing type of failure, attributable more to misregulation.

"Compulsive buying" has been defined as chronic, repetitive purchasing that becomes an overlearned, automatic response to negative feelings (Faber, 2000a; O'Guinn & Faber, 1989). Buying provides short-term gratifications but ultimately causes harm for the individual and/or for others. Thus, unlike impulsive buying, compulsive buying is a continuous failure in self-regulation. Some compulsive buyers feel a strong urge to buy every day, whereas others binge-buy in response to episodic, negative feelings about the self or about life events (Faber 2000a; O'Guinn & Faber, 1989; Schlosser, Black, Repertinger, & Freet, 1994). Many compulsive buyers report buying multiple, similar items in a shopping trip, such as several T-shirts or sweaters, or even raincoats (Christenson et al., 1994; O'Guinn & Faber, 1989). The positive, immediate gratification experienced by compulsive buyers makes it more likely that they will repeat this behavior in similar circumstances. These factors likely contribute to the snowballing effect.

Compulsive buying has been seen as a potential psychiatric disorder involving problems with impulse control (Christenson et al., 1994; Faber, 2003; Kraepelin, 1915). Comorbidity has been reported between compulsive buying and other impulse-control problems, such as alcoholism and substance abuse (Glatt & Cook, 1987; McElroy, Keck, Pope, Smith, & Strakowski, 1994; Schlosser et al., 1994), bulimia (Christenson et al., 1994; Faber, Christenson, de Zwaan, & Mitchell, 1995), and impulse-control disorders not elsewhere classified (Christenson et al., 1994; Schlosser et al., 1994).

Researchers have found that the primary motivation behind compulsive buying is not the actual desire for the object purchased; rather, it is the temporary improvement in mood or self-esteem (Faber, 2000a; O'Guinn & Faber, 1989). Notably, desire for an object as the motivation for purchasing was actually found to be higher among general consumers than among compulsive buyers (O'Guinn & Faber, 1989). In-depth interviews support this notion by demonstrating that many compulsive buyers report that they never used products they purchased. Instead, months or years later, many of these items remain in their original packages, or with sales tags still attached. As one compulsive buyer stated, "It's not that I want it, because sometimes, I'll just buy it and I'll think, 'Ugh, another sweatshirt'" (O'Guinn & Faber, 1989, p. 154).

Rather than buy to obtain a desired item, compulsive buyers are more likely to buy to alter their mood state or arousal level (Elliott, 1994; Faber, 2000b; Faber & Christenson, 1996). Compared to other consumers, compulsive shoppers report negative mood states more often prior to shopping, and positive mood states more frequently during shopping (Faber & Christenson, 1996). Although virtually all compulsive buyers indicated that buying changes their mood state, this was true for only about one-fourth of the comparison (general shopper) sample. Compulsive buyers were also more likely to state that this change in mood is typically in a positive direction.

Changes in arousal level may also be an important motivating factor behind compulsive buying. Jacobs (1989) proposed a general model for addictive behaviors that focuses on arousal as a key element. He believes that each person has a particular range of arousal that he or she finds to be pleasant. Levels of arousal above or below this range are experienced as aversive states. Jacobs also believes that people differ in what they experience as their normal or resting-state level of arousal. If people have a resting-state level of arousal that is not within the range they experience as pleasant, Jacobs suggests that they will engage in behaviors, with the aim of amplifying or lowering their arousal level to achieve a more optimal state. For these people, any activity that can temporarily produce a desirable level of arousal has the potential to become an excessive or addictive behavior.

Applying this notion to compulsive buying, researchers have found that compulsive buyers enjoy activities that increase arousal (Faber, 2000a). They also tend to describe their compulsive buying experiences as producing highly arousing states. These episodes are often characterized by terms such as feeling "high," a "rush," "powerful," "excited," "elated," or "out-of-control" (Faber, 2000a; Faber & Christenson, 1996; McElroy, Keck, & Phillips, 1995). Several compulsive buyers have reported that their buying occurs in response to feeling bored, and when they want something exciting to provide a temporary lift. As one compulsive buyer put it:

> "There's times when I'm depressed or bored or something. I just want something new and I'll just go and feel like buying and it makes me feel good. I feel different, excited, happy, and I'm ready to go on with other boring things." (in Faber, 2000a, p. 41)

The impact of mood and arousal fits with research on self-regulation failure. People attempt to alter or prolong emotional states via affect regulation. Probably the most common attempt at affect regulation is to overcome a bad mood (Baumeister & Vohs, 2003). Consumption behaviors, such as eating (see Herman & Polivy, Chapter 25, this volume), drinking alcohol (see Hull & Slone, Chapter 24, this volume), or taking drugs (see Sayette, Chapter 23, this volume), represent one type of affect regulation strategy. Importantly, people believe that these behaviors have the ability to alter mood states, but in actuality, they often fail to relieve a bad mood and may in fact eventually worsen it (Heatherton & Vohs, 1998; Vohs & Heatherton, 2000). It would appear that buying is also a way to regulate affect. Indeed, phrases such as "When the going gets tough, the tough go shopping" illustrate a societal view that buying can improve one's emotional state. Additionally, people who are focused on affect regulation frequently end up violating other self-regulatory goals (Tice et al., 2001).

For compulsive buyers, attempts at affect regulation through buying may lead to a pattern of misregulation. The consumer may attempt to overcome a negative mood state by engaging in buying, which serves temporarily to improve their mood. However, soon after buying, a feeling of guilt sets in, when the person is reminded that he or she wasted money or failed at the goal of not buying. This negative state can lead to depression and low self-esteem. Consequently, the person's strong need to overcome negative self-evaluations can lead to buying again (to boost positive affect), and so on. Thus, buying becomes a vicious cycle that is increasingly difficult to break.

Compulsive buyers may be particularly susceptible to this pattern of attempting to cure negative affect with buying, because they often experience painful self-awareness. Self-awareness is an important determinant of maintaining self-regulation. To self-regulate, a person must monitor his or her current circumstances, which includes progression through the environment, tracking progress toward or away from the goal, and reevaluating desired outcomes. All of these tasks require a certain degree of self-awareness. Reductions in self-awareness are linked to disinhibition, which in turn leads to self-regulation failure (e.g., Heatherton & Baumeister, 1991; see Carver, Chapter 2, this volume).

The need to avoid self-awareness often starts with the presence of exceptionally high standards or expectations for oneself (Duval & Wicklund, 1972). As a result, the person is bound to, at least occasionally, fail to meet these extreme expectations. This creates feelings of failure that ultimately result in lower self-esteem, as well as anxiety and depression (Heatherton & Baumeister, 1991). All but the most resilient persons experience these feelings as extremely painful.

Compulsive buyers have been reported to be perfectionists (DeSarbo & Edwards, 1996; Faber, 2000a; O'Guinn & Faber, 1989). They often report that they tried hard to please their parents during childhood but generally felt that they failed (Faber & O'Guinn, 1988), as can clearly be seen in a quote from one compulsive buyer:

> "Because you are the oldest you're suppose to be the good little person. I was always trying to win their [parents] approval but couldn't. You know you could have stood on your head and turned blue and it wouldn't matter. I got straight A's and all kinds of honors and it never mattered." (in Faber & O'Guinn, 1988, p. 10)

The perception of being unable to please parents, feelings of inadequacy, and failure to receive recognition for diligent efforts lead many compulsive buyers to develop low self-esteem. Numerous studies have found that compulsive buyers have low self-esteem compared to other consumers (Elliott, 1994; O'Guinn & Faber, 1989; Scherhorn, Reisch, & Raab, 1990). The relationship between low self-esteem and having a high standard of comparison (e.g., being perfectionistic) is particularly apparent in interviews in which compulsive buyers compare themselves with their siblings, as in the following two examples:

> "I have a brother who is now a dentist, who is everything Mother and Dad ever wanted without question. He was bright and he was very engaging and he is very well to do and all of that. And then there is [informant's name] and my mother did my schoolwork ever since I was in fifth grade. She did all of my schoolwork, even my college papers. It's not much to be proud of." (in O'Guinn Faber, 1989, p. 153)
>
> "Right now my brothers are both millionaires. My father's a millionaire. I was not poor, but I was not very rich." (in Faber & O'Guinn, 1988, p. 9)

As mentioned, aversive self-awareness can lead to depression and anxiety (Higgins, 1987). Not surprisingly, compulsive buyers have been shown to have higher than average levels of depression (McElroy et al., 1994; Schlosser et al., 1994) and anxiety (Christenson et al., 1994; Scherhorn et al., 1990). Not only do compulsive buyers experience these negative feelings more often but the depth of feelings they experience may also be more extreme. Studies indicate that between 25 and 50% of compulsive buyers have clinical histories of major depressive disorder (Christenson et al., 1994; McElroy et al., 1994; Schlosser et al., 1994). These negative self-appraisals may impel people to try to escape self-awareness. One way is to focus on an immediate, concrete, low-level task such as shopping or buying. This phenomenon, referred to as "cognitive narrowing," is a form of misregulation that creates disinhibition and prevents consideration of the longer term consequences of an action (Heatherton & Baumeister, 1991). In self-regulation terms, this is referred to as "transcendence failure."

Research on compulsive buying matches the predictions generated from self-regulation and escape theory. If compulsive buying occurs in an effort to cope with adverse self-awareness, it should follow as a direct response to such negative moods. Several studies have shown this to be the case. Compulsive buyers were asked to complete the sentence fragment, "I am most likely to buy myself something when. . . . " Almost three-fourths finished the sentence by including some mention of a negative emotion, such as "I'm depressed," or "I feel bad about myself" (Faber, O'Guinn, & Krych, 1987). In a different study, compulsive buyers were asked to nominate, from a list of over 400 items, which factors were associated with a worsening of their compulsive buying. A factor analysis of commonly mentioned items indicated that the two things that led to compulsive buying urges were shopping-related stimuli (e.g., being around malls or stores; having money or credit cards) and experiencing negative emotions related to the self, such as feeling fat, bored, stressed, depressed, angry, hurt, or irritable. Finally, some compulsive buying informants have stated that the only time they escape from negative feelings is when they are shopping (Elliott, 1994; Friese & Koenig, 1993).

Compulsive buyers may be particularly susceptible to cognitive narrowing when shopping. They frequently mention noticing stimuli such as colors, textures, sounds, and smells while shopping (Schlosser et al., 1994). The concept of "absorption," which is the tendency to become immersed in self-involving experiences triggered by engaging in external stimuli, has been applied to compulsive shoppers. Individuals high in absorption (1) are emotionally responsive and readily captured by engaging sights and sounds, (2) become absorbed in vivid and compelling recollections and imaginings, and (3) experience episodes of altered states. Perhaps not surprisingly, people prone to compulsive buying, compared to other consumers, have been found to score higher on the personality trait of absorption (Faber, Peterson, & Christenson, 1994). This aspect of shopping was captured by one compulsive buyer describing a particular episode:

> "But it was like, it was almost like my heart was palpitating, I couldn't wait to get in to see what was there. It was such a sensation. In the store, the lights, the people; they were playing Christmas music. I was hyperventilating and my hands were starting to sweat, and all of the sudden I was touching sweaters and the whole of it was just beckoning to me." (in O'Guinn & Faber, 1989, p. 154)

The intense level of cognitive narrowing that can accompany compulsive-buying episodes is viewed as desirable by these shoppers. It may well be that this phenomenological experience is why many compulsive buyers consider sales people to be an unwanted intrusion in their shopping, and most prefer to go shopping by themselves rather than with others (Elliott, 1994; Schlosser et al., 1994).

Another consequence of cognitive narrowing is the failure to recognize the implausibility of beliefs, allowing noncritical, irrational thoughts to emerge that produce magical or fanciful thinking (Heatherton & Baumeister, 1991). This is seen with other impulse disorders, such as gambling or bulimia. Gamblers fantasize about making the one big win that will change their life, and people with eating disorders mistakenly believe that changing their bodies will solve all of their problems.

Similar fantasies are common among compulsive buyers. Many report that, during episodes of buying, they imagine themselves as being more powerful or admired. Their buying is accompanied by self-perceptions of being more fashionable, more admired, or part of an exclusive and desirable group (Krueger, 2000; Scherhorn et al., 1990). Some research has indicated that compulsive buyers are more prone to fantasizing than are other consumers (Elliott, 1994; O'Guinn & Faber, 1989).

Cognitive narrowing and fantasizing keep compulsive buyers from focusing their attention on the goal of not spending money. Thus, although the behavior creates a temporary boost in self-esteem, arousal, and mood, it soon turns to feelings of guilt, regret and despair. This creates a lapse-activated pattern of spiraling distress that is common among people suffering from behavioral and impulse-control problems (Baumeister et al., 1994).

CONCLUSIONS

Our understanding of both buying behavior and the self-regulation process can benefit from greater collaboration and cross-fertilization. This chapter has attempted to show how the self-regulation literature can be used to understand buying behaviors such as self-gifting, impulse buying, and compulsive buying better. In doing so, we demonstrated how, when, and why buying may result from self-regulatory failure. Although much of the work in buying behaviors, such as impulse buying and compulsive buying, has focused on personality factors (i.e., trait characteristics) that can help to explain which people are more prone to engage in these behaviors, the self-regulation literature may be particularly beneficial in explaining situational effects (i.e., state effects), such as why a particular episode of impulsive or compulsive buying may take place.

Self-regulatory research also helps to explain how several commonalities found in descriptions of compulsive buyers work together to cause this behavior. Research regarding cognitive narrowing and misregulation is particularly valuable in explaining compulsive buying behavior. Findings about the primacy of emotion regulation over other areas of self-regulation help to explain why compulsive buyers may continue to engage in this behavior despite its serious consequences for them and for their families. The application of self-regulatory failure to other behaviors such as eating disorders, along with compulsive buying, is potentially helpful in explaining the comorbidity among these disorders.

Self-regulation research may also be helpful in distinguishing between different buying behaviors. A good deal of controversy has emerged in the buying behavior literature over whether impulsive and compulsive buying are qualitatively different behaviors or simply differ as a matter of degree. Work on self-regulatory failures helps to identify their similarities, as well as their differences. Regarding similarities, both disorders may be forms of self-regulatory failure. Regarding differences, however, they may represent different types of failure and stem from different underlying causes. Impulse buying is primarily concerned with single instances or initial violations of self-regulation. Generally, people set a goal and purchase mainly what they intended to purchase. From time to time, however, people may experience a violation of this goal. Typically, this type of lapse is due to underregulation caused by resource depletion. Following this temporary lapse, people are again able to establish control over purchasing.

Although compulsive buying also represents a form of self-regulatory failure, it is chronic and consistent rather than occasional. As a result, it leads to a complete breakdown of the self-regulatory system. The cause of this problem may more likely be a problem of conflicting goals or ineffective monitoring rather than one of resource depletion. Repeated buying occurs because emotional goals consistently overpower purchasing goals. Additionally, the binge buying and multiple-item purchases common in compulsive buying may stem primarily from an inability to monitor behavior, resulting from cognitive narrowing. Thus, the problem of compulsive buying is more one of misregulation than of underregulation.

Research in consumer behavior may also help to extend our understanding of the process of self-regulation. For example, research shows that people sometimes use self-gifts that mark a special occasion when they want to reexperience the feelings associated with the gift. Such efforts may help to enhance future self-regulation. Additionally, buying is an everyday activity that offers much opportunity to those interested in the naturalistic study of self-regulation, which is a critical component in purchasing behavior. As a result, research at the intersection of these areas seems to represent a perfect partnership to enhance our knowledge of both domains.

REFERENCES

Applebaum, W. (1951). Studying consumer behavior in retail stores. *Journal of Marketing, 16,* 172–178.

Baumeister, R. F. (2002). Yielding to temptation: Self-control failure, impulsive purchasing, and consumer behavior. *Journal of Consumer Research, 28,* 670–676.

Baumeister, R. F., & Heatherton, T. F. (1996). Self-regulation failure: An overview. *Psychological Inquiry, 7,* 1–15.

Baumeister, R. F., Heatherton, T. F., & Tice, D. M. (1994). *Losing control: How and why people fail at self-regulation.* San Diego, CA: Academic Press.

Baumeister, R. F., & Vohs, K. D. (2003). Self-regulation and the executive function of the self. In M. R. Leary & J. P. Tangney (Eds.), *Handbook of self and identity* (pp. 197–217). New York: Guilford Press.

Beatty, S. E., & Ferrell, M. E. (1998). Impulse buying: Modeling its precursors. *Journal of Retailing, 74,* 169–191.

Bellenger, D. N., Robertson, D. H., & Hirschman, E. C. (1978). Impulse buying varies by product. *Journal of Advertising Research, 18,* 15–18.

Christenson, G. A., Faber, R. J., de Zwaan, M., Raymond, N., Specker, S., Eckert, M. D., Mackenzie, T. B., Crosby, R. D., Crow, S. J., Eckert, E. D., Mussell, M. P., & Mitchell, J. (1994). Compulsive buying: Descriptive characteristics and psychiatric comorbidity. *Journal of Clinical Psychiatry, 55,* 5–11.

DeSarbo, W. S., & Edwards, E. A. (1996). Typologies of compulsive buying behavior: A constrained clusterwise regression approach. *Journal of Consumer Psychology, 5,* 231–262.

Duval, S., & Wicklund, R. A. (1972). *A theory of objective self-awareness.* San Diego, CA: Academic Press.

Elliott, R. (1994). Addictive consumption: Function and fragmentation in postmodernity. *Journal of Consumer Policy, 17,* 159–179.

Faber, R. J. (2000a). A systematic investigation into compulsive buying. In A. L. Benson (Ed.), *I shop, therefore I am: Compulsive buying and the search for self* (pp. 27–54). Northvale, NJ: Jason Aronson.

Faber, R. J. (2000b). The urge to buy: A uses and gratifications perspective. In S. Ratneshwar, D. G. Mick, & C. Huffman (Eds.), *The why of consumption: Contemporary perspectives on consumer motives, goals, and desires* (pp. 177–196). London: Routledge.

Faber, R. J. (2003). Self-control and compulsive buying. In T. Kasser & A. Kanner (Eds.), *Psychology and the culture of consumption* (pp. 169–187). Washington, DC: American Psychological Association.

Faber, R. J., & Christenson, G. A. (1996). In the mood to buy: Differences in the mood states experienced by compulsive buyers and other consumers. *Psychology and Marketing, 13,* 803–820.

Faber, R. J., Christenson, G. A., de Zwaan, M., & Mitchell, J. E. (1995). Two forms of compulsive consumption: Comorbidity of compulsive buying and binge eating. *Journal of Consumer Research, 22,* 296–304.

Faber, R. J., & O'Guinn, T. C. (1988). Dysfunctional consumer socialization: A search for the roots of compulsive buying. In P. Vanden Abeele (Ed.), *Psychology in micro and macro economics* (Vol. 1, pp. 1–15). Leuven, Belgium: International Association for Research in Economic Psychology.

Faber, R. J., O'Guinn, T. C., & Krych, R. (1987). Compulsive consumption. In M. Wallendorf & P. Anderson (Eds.), *Advances in consumer research* (pp. 132–135). Provo, UT: Association for Consumer Research.

Faber, R. J., Peterson, C., & Christenson, G. A. (1994, August). *Characteristics of compulsive buyers: An examination of stress reaction and absorption.* Paper presented at the American Psychological Association Conference, Los Angeles.

Friese, S., & Koenig, H. (1993). Shopping for trouble. *Advancing the Consumer Interest, 5,* 24–29.

Gardner, M. P. (1985). Mood states and consumer behavior: A critical review. *Journal of Consumer Research, 12,* 281–300.

Glatt, M. M., & Cook, C. C. (1987). Pathological spending as a form of psychological dependence. *British Journal of Addiction, 82,* 1257–1258.

Heatherton, T. F., & Baumeister, R. F. (1991). Binge eating as escape from self-awareness. *Psychological Bulletin, 110,* 86–108.

Heatherton, T. F., & Baumeister, R. F. (1996). Self-regulation failure: Past, present, and future. *Psychological Inquiry, 7,* 90–98.

Heatherton, T. F., & Vohs, K. D. (1998). Why is it so difficult to inhibit behavior? *Psychological Inquiry, 9,* 212–215.

Higgins, E. T. (1996). Knowledge and activation: Accessibility, applicability, and salience. In E. T. Higgins & A. W. Kruglanski (Eds.), *Social psychology: Handbook of basic principles* (pp. 133–168). New York: Guildford Press.

Higgins, E. T. (1987). Self-discrepancy: A theory relating self to affect. *Psychological Review, 94,* 319–340.

Hoch, S. J., & Loewenstein, G. F. (1991). Time inconsistent preferences and consumer self-control. *Journal of Consumer Research, 18,* 492–507.

Jacobs, D. F. (1989). A general theory of addictions: Rationale for and evidence supporting a new approach for understanding and treating addictive behaviors. In H. J. Shaffer, S. A. Stein, B. Gambino, & T. N. Cummings (Eds.), *Compulsive gambling: Theory, research and practice.* Lexington, MA: Heath.

Kacen, J. J., & Lee, J. A. (2002). The influence of culture on consumer impulsive buying behavior. *Journal of Consumer Psychology, 12,* 163–176.

Kollat, D. T., & Willett, R. P. (1969). Is impulse purchasing really a useful concept for marketing decisions? *Journal of Marketing, 33,* 79–83.

Kraepelin, E. (1915). *Psychiatrie* (8th ed.). Leipzig: Verlag Von Johann Ambrosius Barth.

Krueger, D. (2000). The use of money as an action symptom. In A. L. Benson (Ed.), *I shop, therefore I am: Compulsive buying and the search for self* (pp. 288–310). Northvale, NJ: Jason Aronson.

McElroy, S. L., Keck, P. E., Jr., & Phillips, K. A. (1995). Kleptomania, compulsive buying and binge-eating disorder. *Journal of Clinical Psychiatry, 56,* 14–26.

McElroy, S. L., Keck, P. E., Jr., Pope, H. J., Jr., Smith, J. M., & Strakowski, S. M. (1994). Compulsive buying: A report of 20 cases. *Journal of Clinical Psychiatry, 55,* 242–248.

Mick, D., & De Moss, M. (1990a). Self-gifts: Phenomenological insights from four contexts. *Journal of Consumer Research, 17,* 322–332.

Mick, D., & De Moss, M. (1990b). To me from me: A descriptive phenomenology of self-gifts. In M. Goldberg, G. Gorn, & R. W. Pollay (Eds.), *Advances in consumer research* (Vol. 17, pp. 677–682). Provo, UT: Association for Consumer Research.

Mick, D., & De Moss, M. (1992). Further insights on self-gifts: Products, qualities, and socioeconomic correlates. In J. F. Sherry & B. Sternthal (Eds.), *Advances in consumer research* (Vol. 19, pp. 140–146). Provo, UT: Association for Consumer Research.

Mick, D., De Moss, M., & Faber, R. J. (1992). A projective study of motivations and meanings of self-gifts: Implications for retail management. *Journal of Retailing, 68,* 122–144.

Mischel, W., & Ebbesen, E. B. (1970). Attention in delay of gratification. *Journal of Personality and Social Psychology, 16*, 329–337.

Mogelonsky, M. (1998). Keep candy in the aisles. *American Demographics*, pp. 20, 32.

O'Guinn, T. C., & Faber, R. J. (1989). Compulsive buying: A phenomenological exploration. *Journal of Consumer Research, 16*, 147–157.

Piron, F. (1991). Defining impulse purchasing. In *Advances in consumer research* (Vol. 18, pp. 509–514). Provo, UT: Association for Consumer Research.

Puri, R. (1996). Measuring and modifying consumer impulsiveness: A cost–benefit accessibility framework. *Journal of Consumer Psychology, 5*, 87–113.

Rook, D. W. (1987). The buying impulse. *Journal of Consumer Research, 14*, 189–199.

Rook, D. W., & Fisher, R. J. (1995). Normative influences on impulsive buying behavior. *Journal of Consumer Research, 22*, 305–313.

Rook, D. W., & Gardner, M. P. (1993). In the mood: Impulse buying's affective antecedents. *Research in Consumer Behavior, 6*, 1–28.

Rook, D. W., & Hoch, S. J. (1985). Consuming impulses. In *Advances in consumer research* (Vol. 12, pp. 23–27). Provo, UT: Association for Consumer Research.

Scherhorn, G., Reisch, L. A., & Raab, G. (1990). Addictive buying in West Germany: An empirical study. *Journal of Consumer Policy, 13*, 355–387.

Schlosser, S., Black, D. W., Repertinger, S., & Freet, D. (1994). Compulsive buying: Demography, phenomenology, and comorbidity in 46 subjects. *General Hospital Psychiatry, 16*, 205–212.

Schmeichel, B. J., Vohs, K. D., & Baumeister, R. F. (2003). Intellectual performance and ego depletion: Role of the self in logical reasoning and other information processing. *Journal of Personality and Social Psychology, 85*, 33–46.

Shapiro, I. J. (1973). *Marketing terms: Definitions, explanations and/or aspects* (3rd ed.). West Long Branch, NJ: S-M-C.

Stern, H. (1962). The significance of impulse buying today. *Journal of Marketing, 26*, 59–62.

Tice, D. M., Bratslavsky, E., & Baumeister, R. F. (2001), Emotional distress regulation takes precedence over impulse control: If you feel bad, do it! *Journal of Personality and Social Psychology, 80*, 53–67.

Tournier, P. (1966). The meaning of gifts (J. S. Gilmour, Trans.). Richmond, VA: John Knox Press.

Tversky, A., & Kahneman, D. (1981). The framing of decisions and the psychology of choice. *Science, 211*, 453–458.

Vohs, K. D., & Faber, R. J. (2002, October). *Self-regulation and impulsive spending patterns*. Paper presented at the annual meeting of the Association for Consumer Research, Atlanta, GA.

Vohs, K. D., & Heatherton, T. F. (2000). Self-regulatory failure: A resource–depletion approach. *Psychological Science, 11*, 249–254.

Vohs, K. D., Twenge, J. M., Baumeister, R. F., Schmeichel, B. J., & Tice, D. M. (2003). *Decision fatigue: Making multiple personal decisions depletes the self's resources*. Unpublished manuscript. University of Utah.

Weinberg, P., & Gottwald, W. (1982). Impulsive consumer buying as a result of emotions. *Journal of Business Research, 10*, 43–57.

Youn, S., & Faber, R. J. (2002). The dimensional structure of consumer buying impulsivity: Measurement and validation. In *Advances in consumer research* (Vol. 29, pp. 280). Provo, UT: Association for Consumer Research.

27

Self-Control and Sexual Behavior

Michael W. Wiederman

An assumption in the sociological study of sexuality is that societies, or at least certain institutions and structures within societies, attempt to control sexual behavior. People are not free to go around doing whatever they care to do sexually. To achieve this societal control, sanctions are put into place, whether they be secular laws or religious ideals, each entailing rewards and punishments that will be administered either now or in the afterlife. The apparent need for social control over individuals' sexual behavior implies that the individuals themselves cannot be counted on to regulate their own sexual conduct for the common good. However, even such societal control rests ultimately on self-control at the individual level. Regardless of the imposed sanctions, sexual behavior (and thereby the regulation of that behavior) occurs among individuals, typically in private.

Tabloids, and sometimes mainstream news outlets, thrive on reporting cases of difficulty in sexual self-control. Contemporary American history is littered with cases in which politicians, religious leaders, celebrities, and sports stars have been undone (or made notorious) by their apparent lack of control over their sexual impulses. Among the rest of us, unknown thousands of times each year, lapses in sexual self-control result in divorce, molestation of children, rape, unwanted pregnancy, and sexually transmitted disease. Presumably, some individuals have problems with too much sexual self-control, in that they inhibit their own sexuality more than they wish. Accordingly, it seems logical that much research effort would be expended to understand how people exert sexual self-control, why it lapses, and how to strengthen and relax such self-control, when appropriate. It is surprising, then, to learn that relatively little such research has been conducted. The focus of this chapter is a necessarily brief discussion of research and theory on the self-control of sexuality, including the probable pitfalls of trying to empirically investigate sexual self-control.

Typically, academic interest in sexual self-control has been focused on problems, particularly problems with a relative lack of suppression of sexual impulses. Perhaps this is due to an aspect of human nature regarding attentional focus on problems rather than health, or perhaps it relates to anxiety in Western cultures over perceived lack of sexual constraint. Individuals with "too much" sexual self-control are rarely the focus of investigation or intervention, unless these individuals themselves ask for assistance with their "problem." In contrast, individuals who are seen as exhibiting too little sexual self-control often do not perceive a problem; it is the society in which they live that seems to have a vested interest in increasing the individuals' sexual self-control.

In contemporary Western societies, when an individual exhibits behavior sufficiently at odds with cultural norms, he or she may be labeled as having a particular disorder. Accordingly, in this chapter, problems with sexual self-control are most frequently discussed in the context of a recognized behavioral or mental disorder. Problems with acting on sexual impulses to the detriment of the individual's well-being are currently labeled "compulsive sexuality" or "sexual addiction."

COMPULSIVE SEXUALITY OR SEXUAL ADDICTION?

For a variety of reasons, compulsive sexuality, or "sexual addiction," has received increasing attention since the 1980s (Gold & Heffner, 1998). In 1983, Patrick Carnes published his book *Out of the Shadows: Understanding Sexual Addiction*, and a plethora of books and articles followed, mainly in the popular press. The concept of "sexual addiction" has been surrounded by controversy since its inception, although the term is frequently used in media intended for the general public, as well as media produced by Carnes and his associates (e.g., Carnes & Adams, 2002).

What is the controversy over sexual addiction? Some professionals and academics are concerned that labeling certain individuals as having a sexual impulse "problem" amounts to nothing more than stigmatizing and attempting to control those individuals who are statistically deviant with regard to rates of sexual activity. For example, Levine and Troiden (1988, p. 351) wrote: "The invention of sexual addiction or compulsion rests on culturally induced perceptions of what constitutes sexual impulse control." These authors asserted that "sexually addicted" individuals do not differ from "normal" people with regard to their internal makeup, simply with regard to their behavior. Is the issue simply that certain people do things sexually of which the rest of the population does not approve, and so these individuals are labeled as having a clinical problem?

Some professionals answer "no," noting that compulsive sexuality involves much more than excessive sexual activity (e.g., Carnes, 1983; Coleman, 1992; Quadland, 1985). In addition to excessive sexual behavior (typically, both masturbation and partnered sexual activity), sexual compulsivity includes a *subjective experience* of a lack of control. Acting on the sexual urges frequently leads to *problems* in the individual's personal relationships and work life, and in some cases leads to arrest for illegal behavior. Still, the individual continues the behavior, apparently *unable to resist*, despite the costs and continued risks. This is the part of the phenomenon that seems to distinguish it from simply a strong sex drive or an exceptionally high rate of sexual activity. An important distinction is made between overt behavior and subjective experience of that behavior as the result of irresistible impulses or psychological dynamics. Table 27.1 contains a description of the phenomenology of sexual addiction, or compulsive sexuality.

Another controversial issue is that the term "sexual addiction" implies a similarity with the phenomenology of substance abuse. Perhaps the similarity prompting the analogy between sexual addiction and substance abuse is the apparent persistence of problematic behavior in the face of negative consequences. Still, there is ongoing controversy over whether the phenomenon is best conceptualized as sexual compulsivity or sexual addiction (Gold & Heffner, 1998). The *Diagnostic and Statistical Manual of Mental Disor-*

TABLE 27.1. The Phenomenology of Compulsive Sexuality or Sexual Addiction

Behavioral manifestations

1. Frequent sexual encounters, often with strangers
2. Compulsive masturbation
3. Engaging in sexual activity despite a lack of physical arousal
4. Frequent and excessive use of pornography
5. Repeated (unsuccessful) attempts to reduce or cease excessive or problematic sexual behavior
6. Legal complications as a result of problematic sexual behavior

Cognitive manifestations

1. Obsessive and intrusive thoughts about sexual activity
2. Rationalization of behavior

Emotional manifestations

1. Sexual indifference toward, or relative lack of interest in, usual sexual partner
2. Depression, low self-esteem, loneliness, boredom, and/or rage
3. Shame and guilt regarding problematic sexual behavior
4. Desire to escape from persistent unpleasant emotions

Note. Compiled from Carnes (1983), Coleman (1992), Gold and Heffner (1998), and Earle and Crow (1990).

ders (DSM-IV; American Psychiatric Association, 1994) provides seven criteria for substance dependence or addiction, three of which must be met to constitute a clinical diagnosis. Several of those seven criteria appear to be applicable to sexual compulsivity: (1) Efforts to stop or reduce the substance abuse have failed; (2) a great deal of time is spent in activities associated with the substance; (3) important activities are abandoned or reduced as a result of the substance abuse; and (4) use of the substance is continued despite knowledge of detrimental effects. So the behavioral manifestations of substance abuse and compulsive sexuality seem to correspond in certain important ways.

The contention among professionals over the terms "sexual compulsivity" and "sexual addiction" seems to revolve around the following issues: whether sexual compulsivity involves biochemical processes similar to substance abuse; whether it is wise to extend the concept of addiction to experiences that do not entail increasing tolerance, and to the existence of physical withdrawal; and whether it is clinically helpful to label sexually compulsive individuals as having an "addiction" (Gold & Heffner, 1998). Some argue, however, that sexual activity does indeed alter neurochemistry, and through classical conditioning certain ritualized behaviors associated with the problematic sexual behavior may themselves alter neurotransmitter levels (e.g., Robertson, 1990). Other professionals argue that compulsive sexuality is more accurately conceived as a variant of the more generic obsessive–compulsive or impulse-control disorders (e.g., Barth & Kinder, 1987; Coleman, 1990). So I next consider problems with a relative lack of sexual self-control in light of obsessive–compulsive disorder.

SEXUAL COMPULSIVITY
AND OBSESSIVE–COMPULSIVE DISORDER

Obsessive–compulsive disorder (OCD) is characterized by the experience of obsessions (intrusive, uncontrollable thoughts) and/or compulsions (uncontrollable behaviors) that the individual recognizes as excessive or unreasonable, and that interfere with daily functioning, typically because they cause distress or are very time-consuming (American Psychiatric Association, 1994). People experiencing compulsive sexuality typically report both obsessions (e.g., over procuring a partner, scheduling sexual activity so as to avoid detection) and compulsions (e.g., to masturbate, to attempt seduction of a new partner) that they recognize as problematic, and that either consume large portions of their waking hours or interfere with their daily lives (e.g., risking detection by a primary relationship partner, coworkers, or the police). However, the DSM-IV (American Psychiatric Association, 1994) stipulates that obsessions and compulsions in OCD *cannot* revolve around pleasurable events or activities. The rebuttal is that although most people experience sexual activity as pleasurable, those experiencing compulsive sexuality frequently report engaging in the problematic sexual behaviors despite a lack of pleasure per se (Gold & Heffner, 1998). One argument, then, is that compulsive sexuality may simply refer to cases of OCD in which, for one reason or another, sexual obsessions and compulsions are the focus of the primary symptoms (Coleman, 1990, 1991).

Because compulsive sexual activity involves failure to resist an impulse to engage in such activity, some researchers have questioned whether the phenomenon is best conceived of as an impulse-control disorder (e.g., Barth & Kinder, 1987). DSM-IV describes the primary symptom of an impulse-control disorder as a "failure to resist an impulse, drive, or temptation to perform an act that is harmful to the person or others" (American Psychiatric Association, 1994, p. 609). Also, there is often an increased sense of tension prior to indulging in the impulse, followed by relief of that tension as a result of acting on the impulse, along with subsequent guilt, regret, or self-condemnation. This cycle of events and experiences seems to characterize individuals experiencing compulsive sexuality (Gold & Heffner, 1998).

Regardless of whether the experience of sexual compulsivity is labeled an addiction or a variant of OCD or impulse-control disorder, to understand the phenomenon, one must consider the *functions* the process serves. Extending application of the OCD model to sexual compulsivity, one current view of the etiology of OCD is that the affected individual's brain malfunctions, sending inaccurate messages that pertain to the perception of threat (Comer, 2002). Specifically, it appears that the orbital region or the caudate nuclei are too active, allowing the breakthrough of signals of impending danger (Berthier, Kulisevsky, Gironell, & Lopez, 2001). The individual frequently experiences tension and anxiety as a result, and the mind focuses on a perceived source of the experienced threat (e.g., germs, risk of fire, unacceptable thoughts). The compulsive behavior is then engaged in as an attempt to reduce the threat and thereby lower the tension and anxiety. The compulsive behavior may result in some temporary or partial reduction in the tension, so the behavior is thereby reinforced through operant conditioning. However, because the source of the problem is faulty functioning in the brain, engaging in the compulsive behavior will not completely resolve the attendant psychological discomfort.

As applied to individuals experiencing compulsive sexuality, a similar behavioral cycle has been identified (Gold & Heffner, 1998). The initial impetus for engaging in the problematic sexual behavior often appears to be reduction of emotional distress. The source of that distress, and the ways in which engaging in the sexually compulsive behavior alleviate it, remain unknown and may vary across individuals. In general, however, private self-focus on negative aspects of the self is related to the experience of depression and anxiety (Mor & Winquist, 2002). At simply a behavioral level, it is easy to imagine how sexual activity, and preoccupation with such activity prior to its enactment, can at least result in distraction from nonsexual sources of anxiety such as negative self-focus. To the extent that the initial distress is at least temporarily reduced, the sexually compulsive behavior is reinforced and thereby more likely in future instances of experienced distress. In this way, sexually compulsive behavior may function similarly to sadomasochistic behavior, in which a primary function appears to be escape from the self, or relief from pressures in nonsexual areas of life (Baumeister, 1989).

Of course, it is possible to have both OCD and sexual compulsivity, or to experience sexual obsessions and compulsions as symptoms of the OCD (Sealy, 2002). To what extent is OCD characterized by sexual obsessions? Well, in one study, more than one-third of outpatients receiving treatment for OCD reported at least one type of sexual obsession (Freund & Steketee, 1989). One question arising from an OCD model for sexual addiction is why these individuals would experience obsessions and compulsions pertaining to sexual behavior, whereas others with OCD would focus exclusively on concerns over germs and cleanliness, checking behaviors, and so forth. An answer may lie in the observation that individuals exhibiting compulsive sexual behavior frequently were the victims of childhood sexual abuse (Carnes, 1983). At the same time, most people who experienced some form of childhood sexual abuse do not exhibit problems with sexual impulse control (Kendall-Tackett, Williams, & Finkelhor, 1993). So perhaps at least for some individuals prone to an anxiety disorder, early experiences of traumatic sexual events increase the likelihood that the anxiety disorder will manifest with sexual symptoms.

Further extending the model for OCD to cases of sexual addiction, why might childhood sexual abuse dispose certain individuals to experience sexual obsessions and compulsions? First, some theorists propose that early developmental trauma, such as sexual abuse, leads to physical changes in the brain, resulting in potentially lifelong sensitivity to anxiety and depression (e.g., Teicher, 2000; Weiss, Longhurst, & Mazure, 1999). For certain individuals who experienced childhood sexual abuse, frequent anxiety may be common, either because of the genes those individuals were coincidentally dealt or as a result of neuroanatomical changes due to the abuse. If such individuals experience the same theorized brain malfunctioning as individuals with OCD, they likely experience frequent anxiety due to overly sensitive neurological triggers for experienced threat (Comer, 2002). In an attempt to make sense out of why they are experiencing anxiety and feelings of threat, individuals with a history of childhood sexual abuse may be relatively more likely to make attributions related to sexuality. Why? Perhaps because of previous associations between anxiety and sexual behavior, or because early developmental experiences in which the individual learned to cope with anxiety involved (abusive) sexual situations.

If accurate, what might these theorized possibilities look like in practice? Suppose that a hypothetical individual with both a history of childhood sexual abuse and a biological propensity toward OCD experiences perceived anxiety and threat without an apparent external trigger. As a result of classical conditioning, this individual may be likely to associate the experienced anxiety with concerns over sexual activity (due to the earlier experiences as a target of sexual abuse). However, the individual is now an adult, and there is no longer in the immediate environment a more powerful person to be feared as the sexual abuser. The anxious individual may still interpret the subjective experience of threat as sexual (due to the earlier classical conditioning), but now, the most logical attribution might be that the threat is sexual deprivation, or a "need" to engage in sexual activity. Similarly, in an attempt to gain control in response to sexual anxiety related to prior abuse, the individual might become the aggressor (Rickards & Laaser, 2002).

Some individuals apparently cope with childhood sexual abuse by engaging in dissociation, or cognitively distancing themselves from their immediate experience (Chu, Frey, Ganzel, & Mathews, 1999; Maynes & Feinauer, 1994). These individuals cope with sexual abuse by "going somewhere else" in their minds, because they are powerless to remove their bodies from the abusive situation. Now, as an adult, our hypothetical individual may attempt to cope with perceived threat by dissociating. Because this coping method was learned in the context of sexual abuse, perhaps it is easiest or most effective when practiced in a sexual situation. In a sense, acting on sexual compulsions, either alone or with a partner, may be the means by which to cope with problematic feelings such as insecurity or rage (Rickards & Laaser, 2002). This scenario fits with the observation that individuals experiencing sexual compulsivity often engage in partnered sexual activity without regard for their partners, or without sexual arousal, and in ways that seem ritualistic and detached (Carnes, 1983; Gold & Heffner, 1998).

Childhood sexual abuse, dissociation, and problems with sexual impulse control are frequently associated with the clinical concept of borderline personality disorder (BPD; American Psychiatric Association, 1994). Among other characteristics, individuals with BPD frequently exhibit multiple impulse control problems. These may involve indiscriminant sexual behavior or "sexually acting out" (Hull, Clarkin, & Yeomans, 1993; Rickards & Laaser, 2002) and sexual obsessions (Hurlbert, Apt, & White, 1992), as well as substance abuse and binge eating (Koepp, Schildbach, Schmager, & Rohner, 1993; Zanarini et al., 1998). BPD has been conceptualized as a long-term reaction to chronic abuse during childhood (Zanarini et al., 1998), which brings us full circle. Throughout this chapter, we have seen the common themes of childhood abuse, generalized impulsivity, and sexual compulsivity. For example, in 36 respondents who self-identified as having "a problem with compulsive sexual behavior," 64% had a history of substance abuse disorders, and depression, anxiety, and obsessive–compulsive personality traits were nearly as common (Black, Kehrberg, Flumerfelt, & Schlosser, 1997). What implications do these findings have for understanding sexual self-control?

For our purposes, it is important to distinguish between self-control of sexual thoughts, feelings, and behavior, and problematic lack of such control. Because the research and clinical attention has been focused on the latter, it is difficult to determine what sexual compulsivity tells us about sexual self-control among individuals who do not experience clinical problems with such self-control. Even among people displaying compulsive sexuality, there is a great degree of diversity (Black et al., 1997). For example, some such individuals report a history of childhood sexual abuse, whereas others do not; some experience compulsions involving non-normative sexual stimuli, whereas others are focused on normative experiences; and although sexual compulsivity affects many more men than women, there are nevertheless women with such problems. Even among individuals with BPD, compulsive sexual behavior may serve different functions (Rickards & Laaser, 2002). Sexual compulsivity is liable to be multidetermined by genetic endowment, early developmental experiences, and current living conditions, among other influences.

Some discussion is devoted to aspects of sexual self-control that might be fruitfully studied and applied to existing topics of research. First, however, I consider the issue of measuring the construct of sexual self-control.

THE MEASUREMENT OF SEXUAL SELF-CONTROL

Further research on sexual self-control depends heavily on the ability of researchers to measure it and related constructs accurately and reliably. Similar to the paucity of research on sexual self-control, few measures have been published. In these cases, sexual self-control has been measured through self-report, which is consistent with the measurement of the vast majority of variables in sexuality research. Many potentially problematic issues are inherent in relying on peoples' self-reported experience related to sexuality. These have been covered in detail elsewhere (e.g., Wiederman, 2002, 2004). The focus here is on introducing the few previously published measures most relevant for the assessment of sexual self-control and the most closely related constructs.

Exner, Meyer-Bahlburg, and Ehrhardt (1992) were interested in examining sexual self-control as related to high-risk sexual behavior among gay men. Recognizing the lack of an available measure, these authors developed short, self-report instruments designed to assess (1) perceived control over one's sex drive and (2) perceived control over engaging in high-risk behavior. The results of factor analysis across two samples of gay men resulted in a four-item measure of self-control over sex drive (e.g., "Once I get sex on my mind, I can't stop or relax until I've scored") and a six-item measure of self-control over sexual risk behavior (e.g., "No matter how aroused I get, I can still say no to risky sex"). The first measure is most relevant to assessing general control over sexual impulses but has limitations for widespread use. In addition to having been developed on, and for use with, gay men, one of the four items has to do with casual sex (i.e., "I've tried to cut down on casual sex, but I just can't do it") and would not be relevant for either men in committed relationships or those who do not engage in partnered sexual activity.

Janssen, Vorst, Finn, and Bancroft (2002) were interested in the theoretical possibility that sexual inhibition and sexual excitation are distinct phenomena rather than opposite ends of a single continuum. Accordingly, they developed separate self-report inventories of each construct for male respondents. Factor analysis of data from samples of male undergraduates and nonstudent males working on the same university campus revealed three factors. The first scale comprised 20 items and had to do with excitation, or the tendency to become easily aroused (e.g., "When I am taking a shower or a bath, I easily become sexually aroused"). The remaining two factors had to do with inhibition. One 14-item scale focused on easily losing sexual arousal (e.g., "When I have a distracting thought, I easily lose my erection") whereas the other, 11-item, scale focused on loss of arousal in the presence of perceived negative consequences (e.g., "If I am masturbating on my own and I realize that someone is likely to come into the room at any moment, I will lose my erection"). It appears that these scales may be useful for studying self-control of sexual arousal, at least as experienced by males (see Hoon, Hoon, & Wincze, 1976, for a similar scale designed for women), but the relevance to self-control of sexual impulses and behavior is indirect at best.

Only one published instrument has been labeled as a measure of "sexual compulsivity." Kalichman and Rompa (1995) developed a 10-item sexual compulsivity scale with data from samples of gay men and low-income, inner-city men and women. Scores on the scale were correlated with sexual experience, risk-reduction behavior, and other constructs. Virtually all of the items comprising the measure refer to experiencing problems with sexual thoughts and behavior. So scores rely on the respondent identifying his or her level of sexual self-control as problematic. Importantly, the items address lack of control over sexual thoughts (e.g., "I think about sex more than I would like to"), sexual desire (e.g., "My sexual appetite has gotten in the way of my relationships"), and sexual behavior (e.g., "I sometimes fail to meet my commitments and responsibilities because of my sexual behaviors").

Other published scales are purported to measure sexual boredom, or the tendency to become easily bored with routine sexual activities and the desire to seek new, exciting sexual stimuli (Watt & Ewing, 1996), as well as sexual preoccupation (Wiederman & Allgeier, 1993), sexual interest or desire (Spector, Carey, & Steinberg, 1996), and sexual sensation seeking (Kalichman & Rompa, 1995). A case can be made that each of these and similar measures are theoretically related to the issue of sexual self-control, in that a greater preoccupation with sexual stimuli, or an increased drive to seek out sexual activity or increased sexual sensations, will make it more difficult to control sexual impulses. However, there is still a need for development of measures specifically having to do with the process and achievement of sexual self-control.

The measures reviewed here reiterate the need to distinguish conceptually between the ability to control sexual desires and impulses versus the strength of such impulses or desires, or the ease with which they are aroused. Logically, there probably is some relationship between these phenomena, because individuals with extremely strong sexual impulses or desires would be expected to have a more difficult time controlling those feelings compared to those with relatively weak sexual drive. Certainly, however, sexual self-control and sexual drive are not the same thing. Even when considering just self-control of sexual impulses or desires, different phenomena are involved: (1) cognitive control, as in being able to keep from obsessing about sexual feelings, regardless of how strong they are; (2) behavioral control, as in not acting on sexual impulses, desires, or obsessions; and (3) emotional control, as in not allowing oneself to experience affective sexual drive that does otherwise exist. Further work is needed to develop measures of these distinct aspects of sexual self-control.

The existent measures are all based on self-reports. However, alternative measures of sexual self-control should be developed. Although these measures would entail their own methodological limitations, ultimately, they may be more valid than self-reports of sexual self-control. What might such an alternative measure look like? There are numerous possibilities, but one involves measurement of behavioral delay under conditions of sexual arousal. During a period of time in which the respondents experience sexual arousal, each could be presented with the opportunity to view sexually explicit media or to engage in self-stimulation, with weak-to-moderate incentives offered for delaying sexual gratification. The length of time delay of gratification could be operationalized as a measure of sexual self-control (behavioral type). Of course, there would be difficulties in creating such an experimental scenario, as well as controlling for individual differences in the strength of the sexual arousal, propensity to act on the arousal regardless of the experimental incentives, and so forth. In the end, any one measure of a construct such as sexual self-control will have inherent limitations. Still, complete reliance on self-reports leaves research on sexual self-control vulnerable to distortion due to the particular method of measurement (see Wiederman, 2002, 2004, for discussion of these issues).

FUTURE DIRECTIONS

It is far easier to point out what needs to be done than it is to actually do it. Discussing directions for future research and theory is no exception. Many important questions about sexual self-control have yet to be answered, or at least investigated more fully:

1. *What exactly is meant by sexual self-control?* Future investigators should distinguish among self-control of sexual feelings, thoughts, and behaviors. The distinction seems obvious, yet the scant research on sexual self-control has frequently focused on one aspect (referring to it as sexual self-control generally) or confused more than one aspect. Similarly, it is important to distinguish between the strength of sexual feelings, thoughts, and behaviors versus the self-control of those experiences of sexuality. All other things being equal, stronger urges are probably more difficult to control than weaker ones, but

all other things are rarely equal. Also, at least with cognition, attempts to control thoughts may in turn strengthen the force of their intrusiveness (e.g., Lane & Wegner, 1995).

Another distinction that may prove important involves the motivation to engage in self-control of sexuality versus the actual performance of such self-control. Does an individual who displays poor control of sexual behavior but is relatively unaffected by the behavior differ in important ways from a person who displays similarly poor self-control but experiences great distress as a result? In other words, self-control of sexual feelings, thoughts, and behavior involves motivation to exercise such self-control. What is the origin of that motivation? What is the relationship between such motivation and distress, or success, or the perceived consequences of sexual self-control?

2. *What are the factors—neurobiological, psychological, and social—underlying the achievement of sexual self-control?* Previous investigation of compulsive sexuality points to the importance of certain factors involved in unsuccessful sexual self-control, at least for some individuals. However, the influences on sexual self-control in normative contexts remains relatively unexplored. Such factors as personality or temperament (e.g., Caspi et al., 1997) and stage of life (e.g., Heckhausen & Schulz, 1995) may be particularly important to consider, but there are others, such as previous experience and situational factors (including relevant stimuli, opportunity, modeling, and perceived consequences).

3. *How might research on sexual self-control be applied to others areas of research on sexual behavior?* Numerous and potentially important are applications of a better understanding of the processes involved in routine sexual self-control. For example, sexual exclusivity is the professed norm in contemporary Western culture (Wiederman, 1997), yet particular individuals may be faced with numerous opportunities to breach such exclusivity. How do individuals resist temptation to act on impulses to have sexual interactions with partners other than the primary one? What factors distinguish those who successfully resist versus those who do not? There has been research on some of the general demographic correlates of extradyadic sex, or "cheating," as well as investigation of certain personality correlates (e.g., Wiederman, 1997; Wiederman & Hurd, 1999). Similarly, it appears well-established that relationship commitment is maintained at least partially through devaluing potential extradyadic partners (e.g., Johnson & Rusbult, 1989; Miller, 1997; Simpson, Gangestad, & Lerman, 1990). Other factors, and the interactions among them, remain potentially fertile ground for future research.

Another potentially important area of application for investigation of sexual self-control is condom use. With the recognition of AIDS, a multitude of empirical studies have been conducted on the correlates of condom use, in an attempt to understand better why people do or do not use condoms when they logically should. As ignorance about sexual risk and condom use became a less plausible explanation for the failure to use condoms, the implication was that such failure represented problems with sexual self-control. Interestingly, the bulk of the large research literature on condom use has been undertaken from a rational, cognitive perspective (Wulfert & Wan, 1995); that is, the question of why people do not use condoms has been posed primarily from the perspective of decision making. Why do people *decide* not to use condoms when they should?

The research literature on the correlates of condom use is large, and adequate review of that research is beyond the scope of this chapter. The connection to sexual self-control is the surprising lack of focus on this construct in trying to account for why people do not use condoms. Common variables of interest in past research on condom use include interpersonal relationship context (e.g., Secco & Rickman, 1996), communication skills and assertiveness (e.g., Wingood & DiClemente, 1998), and attitudes, normative beliefs, intentions, and perceived vulnerability to disease (e.g., DeHart & Birkimer, 1997). These and other variables make sense and, indeed, they have frequently demonstrated statistically significant correlations with self-reported condom use. Some of these correlates, such as perceived vulnerability to disease, might be conceptualized as motivation to engage in sexual self-control. Ultimately, however, we are left with the question of why some individuals achieve what they perceive as appropriate sexual self-control in a particular situation, whereas others do not (assuming that we have accounted for relevant variables related to the interpersonal relationship context). A few studies on condom use have included passing attention to sexual self-control (e.g., Bryan, Schinkeldecker, & Aiken, 2001; Hernandez & DiClemente, 1992), but in-depth application of the construct to condom use is lacking.

4. *Are clinical difficulties with sexual self-control unique or a component of a more general impulse-control deficit?* If problems in sexual self-control are a component of a more general impulse-control deficit, why do some individuals with such a deficit develop sexual compulsivity, whereas others presumably do not? In other words, if sexual self-control problems are simply a variant of more general impulse-control deficits, or OCD, why do these deficits or obsessions and compulsions manifest themselves sexually in some individuals and not others? Exactly what role does early developmental trauma play in compulsive sexuality as an adult? What are the mechanism through which such trauma might exert influence on adult experience? What role does environment play in the development of sexual compulsivity? For example, to what extent has proliferation of the Internet, and thereby easy access to sexually explicit material, affected rates of sexually compulsive behavior (Cooper, 2002; Cooper, Scherer, Boies, & Gordon, 1999)? Unfortunately, like so many topics in Psychology, we still have many more questions than answers.

REFERENCES

American Psychiatric Association. (1994). *Diagnostic and statistical manual of mental disorders* (4th ed.). Washington, DC: Author.

Barth, R. J., & Kinder, B. N. (1987). The mislabeling of sexual impulsivity. *Journal of Sex and Marital Therapy, 13*, 15–23.

Baumeister, R. F. (1989). *Masochism and the self.* Hillsdale, NJ: Erlbaum.

Berthier, M. L., Kulisevsky, J., Gironell, A., & Lopez, O. L. (2001). Obsessive–compulsive disorder and traumatic brain injury: Behavioral, cognitive, and neuroimaging findings. *NeuroPsychiatry, NeuroPsychology, and Behavioral Neurology, 14*, 23–31.

Black, D. W., Kehrberg, L. L. D., Flumerfelt, D. L., & Schlosser, S. S. (1997). Characteristics of 36 subjects reporting compulsive sexual behavior. *American Journal of Psychiatry, 154*, 243–249.

Bryan, A., Schindeldecker, M. S., & Aiken, L. S. (2001). Sexual self-control and male condom-use outcome beliefs: Predicting heterosexual men's condom-use intentions and behaviors. *Journal of Applied Social Psychology, 31*, 1911–1939.

Carnes, P. (1983). *Out of the shadows: Understanding sexual addiction.* Minneapolis, MN: CompCare.

Carnes, P. J., & Adams, K. M. (Eds.). (2002). *Clinical management of sex addiction.* New York: Brunner/Routledge.

Caspi, A., Begg, D., Dickson, N., Harrington, H., Langley, J., Moffitt, T. E., & Silva, P. A. (1997). Personality differences predict health-risk behaviors in young adulthood: Evidence from a longitudinal study. *Journal of Personality and Social Psychology, 73*, 1052–1063.

Chu, J. A., Frey, L. M., Ganzel, B. L., & Mathews, J. A. (1999). Memories of childhood abuse: Dissociation, amnesia, and corroboration. *American Journal of Psychiatry, 156*, 749–755.

Coleman, E. (1990). The obsessive–compulsive model for describing compulsive sexual behavior. *American Journal of Preventive Psychiatry and Neurology, 2(3)*, 9–14.

Coleman, E. (1991). Compulsive sexual behavior: New concepts and treatments. *Journal of Psychology and Human Sexuality, 4(2)*, 37–52.

Coleman, E. (1992). Is your patient suffering from compulsive sexual behavior? *Psychiatric Annals, 22*, 320–325.

Comer, R. J. (2002). *Fundamentals of abnormal psychology* (3rd ed.). New York: Worth.

Cooper, A. (Ed.). (2002). *Sex and the Internet: A guidebook for clinicians.* New York: Brunner/Routledge.

Cooper, A., Schere, C. R., Boies, S. C., & Gordon, B. L. (1999). Sexuality on the Internet: From sexual exploration to pathological expression. *Professional Psychology: Research and Practice, 30*, 154–164.

DeHart, D. D., & Birkimer, J. C. (1997). Trying to practice safer sex: Development of the sexual risks scale. *Journal of Sex Research, 34*, 11–25.

Earle, R. H., & Crow, G. M. (1990). Sexual addiction: Understanding the phenomenon. *Contemporary Family Therapy, 12(2)*, 89–104.

Exner, T. M., Meyer-Bahlburg, H. F. L., & Ehrhardt, A. A. (1992). Sexual self-control as a mediator of high risk sexual behavior in a New York City cohort of HIV+ and HIV- gay men. *Journal of Sex Research, 29*, 389–406.

Freund, B., & Steketee, G. (1989). Sexual history, attitudes and functioning of obsessive–compulsive patients. *Journal of Sex and Marital Therapy, 15*, 31–41.

Gold, S. N., & Heffner, C. L. (1998). Sexual addiction: Many conceptions, minimal data. *Clinical Psychology Review, 18*, 367–381.

Heckhausen, J., & Schulz, R. (1995). A life-span theory of control. *Psychological Review, 102*, 284–304.

Hernandez, J. T., & DiClemente, R. J. (1992). Self-control and ego identity development as predictors of unprotected sex in late adolescent males. *Journal of Adolescence, 15*, 437–447.

Hoon, E. F., Hoon, P. W., & Wincze, J. P. (1976). An inventory for the measurement of female sexual arousability: The SAI. *Archives of Sexual Behavior, 5*, 291–300.

Hull, J. W., Clarkins, J. F., & Yeomans, F. (1993). Borderline personality disorder and impulsive sexual behavior. *Hospital and Community Psychiatry, 44*, 1000–1002.

Hurlbert, D. F., Apt, C., & White, L. C. (1992). An empirical examination into the sexuality of women with borderline personality disorder. *Journal of Sex and Marital Therapy, 18*, 231–242.

Janssen, E., Vorst, H., Finn, P., & Bancroft, J. (2002). The Sexual Inhibition (SIS) and Sexual Excitation (SES) Scales: II. Predicting psychophysiological response patterns. *Journal of Sex Research, 39*, 127–132.

Johnson, D. J., & Rusbult, C. E. (1989). Resisting temptation: Devaluation of alternative partners as a means of maintaining commitment in close relationships. *Journal of Personality and Social Psychology, 57*, 967–980.

Kalichman, S. C., & Rompa, D. (1995). Sexual sensation seeking and sexual compulsivity scales: Reliability, validity, and predicting HIV risk behavior. *Journal of Personality Assessment, 65*, 586–601.

Kendall-Tackett, K. A., Williams, L. M., & Finkelhor, D. (1993). Impact of sexual abuse on children: A review and synthesis of recent empirical studies. *Psychological Bulletin, 113*, 164–180.

Koepp, W., Schildbach, S., Schmager, C., & Rohner, R. (1993). Borderline diagnosis and substance abuse in female patients with eating disorders. *International Journal of Eating Disorders, 14*, 107–110.

Lane, J. D., & Wegner, D. M. (1995). The cognitive consequences of secrecy. *Journal of Personality and Social Psychology, 69*, 237–253.

Levine, M. P., & Troiden, R. R. (1988). The myth of sexual compulsivity. *Journal of Sex Research, 25*, 347–363.

Maynes, L. C., & Feinauer, L. L. (1994). Acute and chronic dissociation and somatized anxiety as related to childhood sexual abuse. *American Journal of Family Therapy, 22,* 165–175.

Miller, R. S. (1997). Inattentive and contented: Relationship commitment and attention to alternatives. *Journal of Personality and Social Psychology, 73,* 758–766.

Mor, N., & Winquist, J. (2002). Self-focused attention and negative affect: A meta-analysis. *Psychological Bulletin, 128,* 638–662.

Quadland, M. C. (1985). Compulsive sexual behavior: Definition of a problem and an approach to treatment. *Journal of Sex and Marital Therapy, 11,* 121–132.

Rickards, S., & Laaser, M. R. (2002). Sexual acting out in borderline women: Impulsive self-destructiveness or sexual addiction/compulsivity? In P. J. Carnes & K. M. Adams (Eds.), *Clinical management of sex addiction* (pp. 271–284). New York: Brunner/Routledge.

Robertson, J. (1990). Sex addiction as a disease: A neurobehavioral model. *American Journal of Preventive Psychiatry and Neurology, 2*(3), 15–18.

Sealy, J. R. (2002). Psychopharmacologic intervention in addictive sexual behavior. In P. J. Carnes & K. M. Adams (Eds.), *Clinical management of sex addiction* (pp. 199–216). New York: Brunner/Routledge.

Secco, W. P., & Rickman, R. L. (1996). AIDS-relevant condom use by gay and bisexual men: The role of person variables and the interpersonal situation. *AIDS Education and Prevention, 8,* 430–443.

Simpson, J. A., Gangestad, S. W., & Lerman, M. (1990). Perception of physical attractiveness: Mechanisms involved in the maintenance of romantic relationships. *Journal of Personality and Social Psychology, 59,* 1192–1201.

Spector, I. P., Carey, M. P., & Steinberg, L. (1996). The Sexual Desire Inventory: Development, factor structure, and evidence of reliability. *Journal of Sex and Marital Therapy, 22,* 175–190.

Teicher, M. (2000). Wounds that time won't heal: The neurobiology of child abuse. *Cerebrum, 2*(4), 50–67.

Watt, J. D., & Ewing, J. E. (1996). Toward the development and validation of a measure of sexual boredom. *Journal of Sex Research, 33,* 57–66.

Weiss, E. L., Longhurst, J. G., & Mazure, C. M. (1999). Childhood sexual abuse as a risk factor for depression in women: Psychosocial and neurobiological correlates. *American Journal of Psychiatry, 156,* 816–828.

Wiederman, M. W. (1997). Extramarital sex: Prevalence and correlates in a national survey. *Journal of Sex Research, 34,* 167–174.

Wiederman, M. W. (2002). Reliability and validity of measurement. In M. W. Wiederman & B. E. Whitley, Jr. (Eds.), *Handbook for conducting research on human sexuality* (pp. 25–50). Mahwah, NJ: Erlbaum.

Wiederman, M. W. (2004). Methodological issues in studying sexuality in close relationships. In J. Harvey, A. Wenzel, & S. Sprecher (Eds.), *The handbook of sexuality in close relationships.* Mahwah, NJ: Erlbaum.

Wiederman, M. W., & Allgeier, E. R. (1993). The measurement of sexual-esteem: Investigation of Snell and Papini's (1989) sexuality scale. *Journal of Research in Personality, 27,* 88–102.

Wiederman, M. W., & Hurd, C. (1999). Extradyadic involvement during dating. *Journal of Social and Personal Relationships, 16,* 267–276.

Wingood, G. M., & DiClemente, R. J. (1998). Gender-related correlates and predictors of consistent condom use among young adult African-American women: A prospective analysis. *International Journal of STD and AIDS, 9*(3), 139–145.

Wulfert, E., & Wan, C. K. (1995). Safer sex intentions and condom use view from a health belief, reasoned action, and social cognitive perspective. *Journal of Sex Research, 32,* 299–311.

Zanarini, M. C., Frankenburg, F. R., Dubo, E. D., Sickel, A. E., Trikha, A., Levin, A., & Reynolds, V. (1998). Axis I comorbidity of borderline personality disorder. *American Journal of Psychiatry, 155,* 1733–1739.

28

Self-Control and Crime

TRAVIS HIRSCHI

The best predictor of crime is prior criminal behavior. Criminals do not specialize in particular crimes. Those committing any one crime are more likely to commit all other crimes—given opportunities to do so. So it follows that there are individual differences in the propensity to commit criminal acts. It follows, too, that crimes have something in common. This "something" is not their illegality. When previously illegal acts become legal, and vice versa, the same people continue to commit them. The general propensity to commit criminal acts peaks in the late teens and early 20s, then declines rapidly and steadily to the end of life. And it appears to do so for everyone. Group and individual differences in crime rates are stable across the life course. The age distribution of crime is invariant across social and demographic groups. The task of theory is to account for these facts. They remain facts regardless of the adequacy of our explanation of them.

The central issues would appear to be the source and nature of stable individual differences in propensity and the common element in the large variety of delinquent, deviant, and criminal acts. We (Gottfredson & Hirschi, 1990) have argued that the relevant individual level trait is best seen as self-control, and the commonality among the acts in question is that each provides immediate benefit at the risk of long-term pain. This combination of "maladaptive" act and trait has been recognized and much discussed by economists, philosophers, biologists, and psychologists. It has received little attention from sociologists, for the simple reason that its core assumptions are anathema to them.[1] There is irony in this. Sociology claims criminology as a subfield, and the more prominent or popular theories of crime have their origins in that discipline. Thus, we have a discipline that is unable to recognize essential elements of crime and criminality telling us what we should think and do about them (e.g., Uggen, 2003).

Actually, this situation is long-standing. The sociological view was formed as a reaction to rational choice or "classical" theory, epitomized by Hobbes's conclusion that "man is a creature civilized by the fear of death" (Oakeshott, 1957, p. xxxvi). Not so, said sociologists: We behave ourselves because we have learned it is the right thing to do; man is a creature civilized by exposure to "a normative system embodying what ought to be" (Davis, 1948, p. 52). What ought to be is defined by the society's culture and passed on to individuals through a process of socialization. Sociologists granted the existence of a factual world and inclinations of individuals potentially at odds with cultural prescriptions but did not see them as potent threats to social stability. Indeed, from the beginning, sociologists tended to see crime and deviance as minor theoretical problems.

When called upon actually to explain deviant behavior, sociologists had two routes open to them. One led to potential discrepancies between the factual and normative orders, to contradictions between "what was" and what a culture said "ought to be." Thus, a culture might say that all people should be granted equal access to economic opportunities, while the actual organization of society denies such opportunities to some of them. The result for those denied access was frustration that could be relieved only by some form of deviant behavior (Merton, 1938; Parsons, 1957). Contemporary versions of this explanatory scheme are called "strain theories."

The second solution relied on potential conflicts or discrepancies within or between cultures. In modern, pluralistic societies, individuals may be exposed to more than one culture. Following the dictates of one culture may put one's behavior at odds with the dictates of another culture. If the second culture has the power to define as "criminal" the behavior in question, conformity is defined as "deviation" (Sutherland, 1939). Those adopting this explanatory scheme paid little attention to the mental states or emotions of individuals, apparently assuming that those caught in situations of culture conflict did not find their situation particularly stressful. Modern versions of this explanatory scheme are called "cultural deviance" or "social learning theories" (Akers, 1998).

Neither explanation leaves room for notions of agency, or "self-control." The individual might be aware of his or her predicament (especially in strain theories), but distinctions between short- and long-term solutions, or between prudent and impulsive acts, were not part of the conceptual scheme. And, of course, neither perspective accepts the facts summarized at the beginning of this chapter.

A uniquely American approach eventually offered what, at first glance, appears to be a compromise between the rational choice and sociological views. Springing from observation of immigrant communities, it argued that societies *differ* in their ability to socialize and control their members. Societies at one extreme offer a clear and consistent culture and a factual system consistent with it, and have very low rates of deviant behavior. Societies at the other extreme possess a limited or inconsistent culture and impoverished, disorganized economic and social systems. In these societies, families, schools, churches, neighborhoods, and economic and political institutions do not present a consistent cultural context, are unable to satisfy the needs of their members, and have limited power over their behavior. Individuals in such societies may be inadequately socialized— unguided by a coherent system of norms and relatively impervious to social or legal sanctions. (In these conditions, crime and deviant behavior become especially difficult practical and theoretical problems. Whereas Hobbes's subjects had reason to guide them out of their predicament, it is not clear what guides are available to "natural" subjects in sociological theory.) The view just described has from the beginning been called social disorganization theory (Kornhauser, 1978). It is the progenitor of two versions of social control theory: social bonding theory (Hirschi, 1969/2002), and informal social control theory (Sampson & Laub, 1993).

SOCIAL CONTROL THEORY

Social control theory attempts to identify the ties that bind individuals to society and thus control their behavior. The ruling proposition of this perspective is that "delinquent acts result when an individual's bond to society is weak or broken" (Hirschi, 1969/2002,

p. 16). My much-researched version of this theory identified four dimensions of the social bond, which I labeled attachment, commitment, involvement, and belief. These concepts embody common understandings in the social and behavioral sciences and, for that matter, in ordinary usage.

Thus, *attachment*, the first dimension, refers to the emotional bond between the individual and conventional people or institutions, to the degree of love or respect for parents, teachers, friends, institutions, or even nonhuman objects outside oneself. The idea is that the more one is attached to such entities, the less likely one is to engage in criminal or delinquent acts—because such acts threaten social and physical ties to the objects in question. Crimes are, by definition, contrary to the wishes and expectations of conventional others, and their consequences may be incompatible with continued contact with them, whatever the emotional reaction of the controlling "object." Thus, in a current local (Tucson, Arizona) case, the murderer of three professors wrote that his one regret was that his subsequent suicide would leave his dog behind.[2]

The second dimension, *commitment*, refers to the individual's aspirations and expectations, to investments in a line of activity, to his or her "stake in conformity" (Toby, 1957). The idea is that we are controlled by what we are, and by what we wish to be. To the degree that one's goals are incompatible with a history of criminal acts or are endangered by reckless behavior, to that degree such acts and behavior will be avoided.

Involvement, the third dimension, is an attempt to capture the idea that criminal acts require time and effort that may be made unavailable by noncriminal pursuits. Thus, those involved in conventional activities, whatever they may be (fishing, hunting, watching television, talking with parents, playing baseball, or working behind the counter at Burger King), are for the period in question deprived of opportunities to commit criminal or delinquent acts.

The role of the fourth dimension of the bond, *belief*, was and remains controversial—partly because it is claimed by otherwise incompatible theories of crime. The traditional sociological view posits a near-perfect connection between beliefs and behavior, with the former causing the latter. Thus, if we know what a person believes, we know how he or she will behave. In the beginning, even deviant acts were thought to result from beliefs that required them.[3] This view was rejected by social control theorists, who argued that no culture can actively promote criminal behavior and hope to survive. And, indeed, research quickly and clearly demonstrated that groups with markedly different crime rates differ little in their condemnation of criminal acts (Wolfgang, Figlio, Tracy, & Singer, 1985). So it appeared that offenders were acting contrary to the beliefs of their own culture. This fact indicated to some that offenders must rationalize their behavior in order to violate rules while maintaining their belief in their validity. Beliefs that condemn criminal behavior are neutralized by beliefs that support it, at least in relevant circumstances (Cressey, 1953; Matza, 1964).

The same fact indicated to others that acceptance of the moral validity of rules must vary at the individual level. Some people believe more than others. Some believe fully; others, not at all. This is the position I take in my version of social control theory, just described. Beliefs matter. Some "are what bind us to the reality beyond our skins" (Gilbert, 1993, p. 64). Others free us to commit criminal and delinquent acts.

Being true to the assumptions of my discipline (sociology), I did not link social control to self-control. On the contrary, I disavowed the significance of the latter concept. Self-control implies *stable differences* over the life course in the tendency to commit or refrain from criminal acts. At the time I wrote my version of social control theory, sociological criminologists took for granted that whereas most offenders eventually lose their tendencies to offend, others do not. For a theory to be consistent with such "facts," the individual had to be controlled by bonds that would in principle allow offenders to desist and nonoffenders to change places with them from time to time over the life course.

INFORMAL SOCIAL CONTROL
AND THE LIFE COURSE PERSPECTIVE

This emphasis on the potential for individuals to change from delinquent to law-abiding, and vice versa, survives in what is now called *informal* social control theory (Sampson & Laub, 1993). This theory retains the idea that the behavior of individuals is a function of the strength of the "societies" to which they belong, and adds to it the idea that individuals may belong to different societies or groups over the life course. Thus, delinquents reared in weak families may become nondelinquent when they make good marriages and participate in families of their own making. Conversely, previously nondelinquent individuals are more likely to commit delinquent acts when their connections to conventional groups or institutions are severed (through, say, divorce or unemployment). This theory falls within, and gains much of its popularity from, the *life course perspective*, with its optimistic celebration of the possibility of change—for the better. Whereas those operating within this perspective might in principle accept individual variation in self-control, in practice, the concept tends to be avoided because of the analytic and empirical complications it brings with it (see Hardwick, 2002). In practice, talk of transitions, turning points, trajectories, age-graded theory, and salient life events is more rewarding—and continues unabated!

SELF-CONTROL THEORY

After examining age distributions of crimes and analogous acts, Gottfredson and I (Gottfredson & Hirschi, 1990) reversed my original position, concluding that these acts are, after all, manifestations of low self-control on the part of the offender. We were forced to this position by our conclusion that the powerful effects of age on criminal and analogous acts are the same in all social and demographic groups, that *differences* in crime rates persist over the life course and are therefore essentially impervious to changes in the social and economic situations of individuals (Hirschi & Gottfredson, 1983, 1986).

This led in turn to an examination of the nature of criminal acts, in which we concluded that they indeed have something in common beyond their illegality: All offer immediate rewards and are easily accomplished, requiring little skill, training, or preparation. At the same time, all entail the risk of long-term costs greatly exceeding their immediate benefits. Seen in this way, crimes practically define failure of self-control as it is usually conceived, bringing to mind a Faustian bargain, a life of misery for a moment's pleasure.

From our examination of age distributions, we concluded that stable differences in crime rates (across groups and individuals) are established before adolescence and persist throughout life. It follows that one's level of self-control is acquired in childhood (or earlier) and that differences in self-control between individuals are unaffected by subsequent experience. A remarkable fact is the range of behaviors influenced by this trait—practically everything that by hypothesis or observation provides short-term benefit at the risk of long-term cost (e.g., Hirschi & Gottfredson, 1994).

Gottfredson and I (1990, pp. 94–107) adopted a "child-rearing model" to account for the origins of (failure to learn) self-control and illustrated its consistency with the results of delinquency research; we also inferred what we call "the elements of self-control" from the nature of criminal acts. The terms in both discussions are familiar to psychologists.

Our child-rearing model owes much to the work of Gerald Patterson (1980), to that of Sheldon and Eleanor Glueck (1950), and to the most general "social control model" (Hechter, 1987), according to which behavior is shaped by monitoring and sanctioning—both of which presuppose caring or interest in the outcome on the part of the responsible party. This model coincides beautifully with the (apparent) results of delinquency research, in which lack of parental supervision, discipline, and affection are found to be major predictors of offending. The idea is that the child is taught "self-control" by parents or other responsible adults at an early age, and that this trait is subsequently highly resistant to extinction.[4]

We then turned to the concept of self-control. Being unhappy with theories that begin with offenders and infer from them the nature of crime, we decided, in a moment of madness, to reverse the process. Our discussion of "the elements of self-control" in large part follows:

> Criminal acts provide immediate gratification of desires. A major characteristic of people with low self-control is therefore a tendency to respond to tangible stimuli in the immediate environment, to have a concrete "here and now" orientation. People with high self-control, in contrast, tend to defer gratification.
>
> Criminal acts provide easy or simple gratification of desires. They provide money without work, sex without courtship, revenge without court delays. People lacking self-control [will therefore] also tend to lack diligence, tenacity, or persistence in a course of action.
>
> Crimes provide few or meager long-term benefits. They are not equivalent to a job or a career. On the contrary, crimes interfere with long-term commitments to jobs, marriages, family, or friends. People with low self-control thus tend to have unstable marriages, friendships, and job profiles. They tend to be little interested in and unprepared for long-term occupational pursuits.
>
> Crimes require little skill or planning. The cognitive requirements for most crimes are minimal. It follows that people lacking self-control need not possess or value cognitive or academic skills. . . .
>
> Crimes often result in pain or discomfort for the victim. Property is lost, bodies are injured, privacy is violated, trust is broken. It follows that people with low self-control tend to be . . . indifferent or insensitive to the suffering and needs of others.
>
> [C]rime involves the pursuit of immediate pleasure. It follows that people lacking self-control will also tend to pursue immediate pleasures that are not criminal: they will tend to smoke, drink, use drugs, gamble, have children out of wedlock, and engage in illicit sex. . . .
>
> The major benefit of many crimes is not pleasure but relief from momentary irritation. The irritation caused by a crying child is often the stimulus for child abuse. That caused by a taunting stranger in a bar is often the stimulus for aggravated assault. It follows that people with low self-control tend to have minimal tolerance for frustration and little ability to respond to conflict through verbal rather than physical means. . . .
>
> In sum, people who lack self-control will tend to be impulsive, insensitive, physical, risk-seeking, short-sighted, and nonverbal. (Gottfredson & Hirschi, 1990, pp. 89–90)

Thus we discovered the Big Five (plus one), introduced a language I did not understand, championed ideas contradicting our theory, and otherwise muddied the waters. But this state of affairs was not immediately recognized. On the contrary, our exercise was seen as a set of directions for constructing measures of self-control, and much research and analysis have flowed from it, beginning largely with Grasmick, Tittle, Bursik, and Arneklev (1993)—see also Gibbs and Giever (1995). Fortunately, in this case at least, truth is indeed the daughter of time, and we can now see the errors introduced by our excursion into psychology *and* by the measures of self-control stemming from it.

For present purposes, the major problems are these:

1. Both suggest differences among offenders in motives for crime, contrary to explicit assumptions of the theory that offenders do not specialize and that motives are irrelevant.

2. Both contradict our explicit assertion (and firm belief) that personality traits (other than self-control) have proved to be of little value in the explanation of crime.

3. Both fail to explain—in a manner consistent with the theory—how self-control operates. Instead, both suggest that offenders act as they do because they are what they are (impulsive, hot-headed, selfish, physical risk takers), whereas nonoffenders are, well, none of these. When measures based on this exercise are interpreted in a manner consistent with self-control theory, they suggest that potential offenders (a) calculate a factor score based on a linear combination of numerous self-characterizations gleaned from a variety of sources and (b) act accordingly.

4. As would be expected from item 3, and most telling, this exercise fails to produce a measure of self-control in which more is better than less, in which the effects of the individual traits on criminal behavior are cumulative. Single traits (impulsivity, risk taking) predict criminal behavior as effectively as does an all-inclusive self-control scale (Longshore, Stein, & Turner, 1998; Piquero & Rosay, 1998).

We actually define "self-control" as "the tendency to avoid acts whose long-term costs exceed their momentary advantages" (Hirschi & Gottfredson, 1994, p. 3). This definition suggests that the best measure of self-control would be a count of the number of different acts with long-term negative consequences committed by the individual in a specified period of time—the fewer the better. Indeed, we have said that this is the "best" measure of (low) self-control. Others (e.g., Marcus, 2003, in press) agree. It is well established that such counts pass tests of stability (persons scoring high at one point in time tend to attain high scores at subsequent times) and various tests of construct validity (see, e.g., Hirschi & Gottfredson, 2000; Marcus, 2003, in press). Their ability to predict subsequent deviant behavior in a variety of realms is impressive, to say the least. For practical purposes (e.g., assembling a crime-free population, guessing what one will find in criminal records), they are hard to beat.

For theoretical purposes, however, they are problematic.[5] According to the theory, criminal and delinquent acts are not self-perpetuating, but are made possible by the absence of an enduring tendency to avoid them. To find the nature of this tendency, we must look behind the acts it forbids.

So, although we have adequate measures of the acts we wish to explain and useful ideas about what they have in common, we do not understand why they are allowed for some people and denied to others. The argument that self-control is acquired early in life may please social learning theorists, but if pushed too far, it undermines the assumption that self-control involves cognitive evaluation of competing interests—an idea central to control theories. The theory requires an explanatory mechanism that retains elements of cognizance and rational choice.

Sociologists comparing social control theory with self-control theory tend to prefer the former. For example,

> My interpretation is that self-control theory rejects important insights from Hirschi's original formulation of social control and is therefore a less adequate explanation. The adoption of the age-invariance thesis and the assumed stability of self-control beyond early childhood imply that individuals do not have the capacity to change over the life course. Thus, self-control theory completely neglects the impact of wider, structural forces on individuals in later life. . . . (Taylor, 2001, p. 384)

This preference sometimes shows itself in the guise of fact:

> The central theme of Sampson and Laub's work is reconciling the tension between two stylized facts: (1) antisocial (prosocial) adults were invariably antisocial (prosocial) children, and (2) most antisocial children do not become antisocial adults. The first stylized fact is powerful evidence of the continuity of human behavior, while the second provides comparably powerful evidence that change in behavior coexists with continuity of behavior. (Nagin & Paternoster, 1994, p. 582)

Stylized facts, apparently, are facts shorn of natural variations and complications, just as the fleur-de-lis is a stylized iris or lily. Theorists should have no qualms about such facts. Indeed, it seems impossible to proceed without them. So we have continuity and change, and reasonable people must agree that theory should acknowledge and attempt to explain both of them. The fact is, however, that the facts in question here, stylized though they may be, cannot both be true. We cannot have the continuity of fact 1 and the change described by fact 2. If some prosocial adults were antisocial children, prosocial adults were not invariably prosocial children.

What to do? One possibility is to reject the assumption of the stability of individual differences central to self-control theory. But we cannot reject what we believe to be true (see the quote from Gilbert, above). Another possibility is to reject the instability assumption of social control theory. I remain convinced that this assumption rests on unsteady ground and that much of its support comes from a conceptual sleight of hand: To say, correctly, that crime declines with age, is not to say that differences in criminality (self-control) are unstable. To say, correctly, that crime declines with age, is not to say that variables other than age must be responsible for the decline.[6] But there is an even better reason for me to abandon the instability assumption of social control theory. The theory is saved by simply assuming that differences in social control are stable, that social control and self-control are the same thing.

This reconciliation requires a shift in the definition of self-control. Redefined, self-control becomes *the tendency to consider the full range of potential costs of a particular act*. This moves the focus from the *long-term* implications of the act to its *broader* and often contemporaneous implications. With this new definition, we need not impute knowledge of distant outcomes to persons in no position to possess such information. Children need not know the health implications of smoking or the income implications of truancy, if these implications are known to those whose opinion they value.

This new definition is consistent with, and gives meaning to the assertion that "the dimensions of self-control are . . . factors affecting calculation of the consequences of one's acts" (Gottfredson & Hirschi, 1990, p. 95). Put another way, self-control is the set of inhibitions one carries with one wherever one happens to go. Their character may be initially described by going to the elements of the bond identified by social control theory:

attachments, commitments, involvements, and beliefs. As before, the delinquent becomes "a person relatively free of the intimate attachments, the aspirations, and moral beliefs that bind most people to a life within the law" (Hirschi, 2002, p. xxi). This encapsulation left out involvement but probably need not do so when the focus is on self-control. Rather than merely making one too busy to commit criminal acts, in this context, it is closely analogous to the idea of self-control as self-imposed physical restraint (àla Ulysses and the Sirens).

The concept of social bonds requires at least two units, and a variety of possible connections between them. With many units, and multiple connections among them, it evokes images of change and flux incompatible with the concept of a stable trait. If hopes fade, relationships sour, beliefs weaken, and jobs disappear; if people graduate, move on, die—they cannot be dependable sources of control. A set of always changing variables cannot account for stable individual differences in criminal and delinquent behavior. But these concerns put too much emphasis on the second party, or on the relationship between the two units, when, as measured and potentially conceptualized, the source and strength of "bonds" is almost exclusively within the person reporting or displaying them. A central argument of my version of social control theory was that "we honor those we admire not by imitation but by adherence to conventional standards" (Hirschi, 2002, p. 152). The argument here is a variant of that idea. There is direct evidence in favor of this approach.

AGE AND CRIME

Arrest statistics show sharp increases in offending up to the middle and late teens. At that point, both arrest statistics and self-reports show precipitous declines in offending to the mid- to late-20s, with gradual declines thereafter to the end of life. Person crimes (violent and aggressive crimes) tend to peak later than do property crimes, but the shapes of the curves are essentially the same for the two types of offenses. Although criminal and delinquent activity declines in all groups, high-rate groups and individuals retain the relatively high rates first observed in their early teens. Because crime and delinquency so defined do not begin until children are 10–12 years of age, it is easy to conclude that differences in self-control are produced before ages 10–12 by the operation of more and less effective sanctioning systems.

But this conclusion is too easy. Differences in criminal and delinquent behavior in the teen years may themselves be predicted *from the very early years of life*, suggesting that differences in self-control are also present at that time. This suggestion poses problems for "child-rearing" or "learning" hypotheses. Indeed, in my view, research on these early differences offers striking evidence of the continuity of self-control and the compatibility of self- and social control notions. The terms used to describe behavior found later to be predictive of delinquency and crime are often indistinguishable from those encountered in control theories thought to be applicable only to adolescents and adults. In the first years of school, future delinquents are far more likely than nondelinquents to manifest "lack of interest in school work," "inattention," and "laziness" (Glueck & Glueck, 1950, p. 150). In nursery school, girls destined to avoid marijuana and hard drugs are notable for being "eager to please" and "neat and orderly." In the same setting, boys destined to avoid marijuana and hard drugs are notable for being "helpful and cooperative" and for "repressing negative feelings" (Block, Block, & Keyes, 1988, pp. 344–345).[7]

With this information, we can look again at social bonds and how they are assessed or measured. Not surprisingly, they are typically self-reported attachments, aspirations, activities, and beliefs bearing on the costs of criminal, delinquent, reckless, or imprudent behavior. Being self-reported, they define the self in terms relevant to crime, a definition that may very well be impervious to change in the environment. Studies of children such as those by the Gluecks (1950) and Block and colleagues (1988) of course rely on observations of behavior rather than self-reports—which is reassuring, because bond-relevant *behavior* turns out to be especially predictive of subsequent criminal activity.

MEASURES OF THE SOCIAL BOND/SELF-CONTROL

Our new definition of self-control, and our experience with prior definitions and measures, suggests that we begin with the concept of inhibitions. Presumably, these are factors that one takes into account in deciding whether to commit a criminal act—factors that may vary in number and salience. What are the features of these facts or factors? Previous argument suggests that they cannot be latent, hidden, or unknown to the actor; nor can they be prior criminal or delinquent acts. Social control theory tells us that a (if not *the*) principal source of control is concern for the opinion of others. "Others" come in a variety of shapes and sizes: parents, teachers, friends, policemen. With this in mind, one question that the potential offender asks is: "Do I care what X thinks of me?" If the answer is "yes," chalk one up for self-control. A second question the potential offender asks is: "Will X know what I have done?" If the answer is "yes" (because I will tell X what I have done), chalk one more up for self-control (Stattin & Kerr, 2000).

To begin to explore this approach, I constructed a self-control scale based on the following nine items (self-control response in parentheses):

1. Do you like or dislike school? (Like it.)
2. How important is getting good grades to you personally? (Very important.)
3. Do you finish your homework? (Always.)
4. Do you care what teachers think of you? (I care a lot.)
5. It is none of the school's business if a student wants to smoke outside of the classroom.* (Strongly disagree.)
6. Does your mother know where you are when you are away from home? (Usually.)
7. Does your mother know who you are with when you are away from home?* (Usually.)
8. Do you share your thoughts and feelings with your mother? (Often.)
9. Would you like to be the kind of person your mother is? (In every way. In most ways.)

In each case, the self-control response was given a value of 1, producing a count ranging from 0–9. Table 28.1 shows the relation between this index and a standard, 6-item, self-report delinquency scale.

Table 28.1 may be read as follows: Of the 136 students reporting no inhibiting factors, 73% reported committing at least two (of a possible six) different delinquent acts. Of the 249 students reporting one inhibiting factor, 62% reported committing at least two delinquent acts. As the number of reported inhibiting factors (self-control responses) increases, the percentage of students reporting two or more delinquent acts steadily declines. Among those 45 students reporting all nine inhibiting factors, only 2% (one stu-

TABLE 28.1. Percent Reporting Two or More Delinquent Acts by Number of Self-Reported Inhibiting Factors, Richmond, California, 1965

					Number of self-reported inhibiting factors					
0	1	2	3	4	5	6	7	8	9	Total
73	62	50	40	34	25	23	15	8	2	34
(136)	(249)	(399)	(523)	(557)	(565)	(420)	(293)	(152)	(45)	(3,339)

Note. Data are from the Richmond Youth Project, a study of junior and senior high school students conducted in Western Contra Costa County, California, in 1965. A description of the sample and details of data collection may be found in Hirschi (1969/2002). Percentages are based on the numbers in parentheses (see text).

dent) have committed two or more delinquent acts. (Tables 28.2 and 28.3 may be read in the same way.)

In my view, these differences in rates of delinquency are impressive, and they belie arguments about the weak power of control theory. But for present purposes, I should emphasize the symmetry between the sophistication of our theory and the sophistication of my statistical analysis. Neither suggests that people base their choices on self-computed, complex factor scores. Rather, both suggest that people add up in an imprecise way the negative consequences of deviant acts and behave accordingly. It seems notable to me that a measure produced by this logic is able to do what more sophisticated measures of self-control have not been able to do (i.e., show cumulative effects for each of its constituent items).

I, of course, knew in advance that these items were correlated with delinquency, but I did not know how they would behave when dichotomized and combined, and I did not modify or tinker with the scale after it was initially constructed. Even so, an independent replication would seem to be in order. Table 28.2 examines seven of the nine items on a questionnaire administered 32 years later, halfway across the country. The same results are obtained. Of those 152 students without inhibitions as measured, 66% are delinquent, whereas none of the 11 students reporting all seven possible inhibitions is delinquent.

To this point, our measure of self-control taps attachment to parents (mother) and the school (teachers), with an element of commitment found in the homework and im-

TABLE 28.2. Percent Reporting Two or More Delinquent Acts by Number of Self-Reported Inhibiting Factors, Fayetteville, Arkansas, 1997

			Number of self-reported inhibiting factors [a]					
0	1	2	3	4	5	6	7	Total
66	57	41	36	28	27	10	0	37
(152)	(201)	(145)	(118)	(65)	(41)	(21)	(11)	(754)

Note. Data are from a sample of 9th-, 10th-, and 11th-grade students described in Schreck (2002).
[a] The two items missing from the Arkansas data (school control of smoking and mothers' knowledge of companions) are denoted by an asterisk in the list on page 545.

portance of grades items. It contains items typically used to measure parental supervision, but this is justified by the clear finding that parental knowledge of the child's whereabouts is largely provided by the child (Stattin & Kerr, 2000). It is negatively related to parental punishment (slapping, grounding, nagging, name calling), as is, or by now should be, expected. It is more strongly related to grade point average (GPA) than to IQ (.29 vs..08), also a common finding, reflecting the effort component in grades that is not found in IQ. It declines with age–grade (mainly because older students are less likely to grant the school control over smoking or to consider grades to be important), but its effect on delinquency is the same in all grades (7–12) and age groups (13–18). As measured, girls have higher levels of self-control than boys (.22). As delinquency is measured, boys are considerably more likely than girls to be delinquent at all levels of self-control. (The analyses reported in this paragraph are based largely on the Richmond, California, data. GPA and IQ data are unavailable for the Fayetteville, Arkansas, sample, and its age–grade range is limited.)

In theoretically oriented delinquency research, as traditionally practiced, bond measures compete with measures of exposure to delinquent peers (Costello & Vowell, 1999; Matsueda, 1982), where peer behavior is assumed to be a "social learning variable" (Akers, 1998, pp. 110–120). The data often show that measures of peer delinquency are more strongly predictive of delinquency than are bond measures, with the latter having reduced impact when the former are controlled (but see Costello & Vowell, 1999). Control theorists have countered by noting that estimates of peer delinquency are usually provided by the respondents themselves, with no effort made to assess their accuracy. As a result, there is reason to think that respondents are merely providing another report of their own delinquency (Gottfredson & Hirschi, 1987). Research confirms that, indeed, there is a large element of "projection" in such measures. When peers report their own delinquency, the relation between self-reported delinquency and peer delinquency is no longer beyond the reach of properly measured "control" variables (Haynie, 2001).

I have already mentioned a traditional causal variable (parental supervision) whose meaning has been altered radically by careful research. Careful research now shows that a good portion of respondent-reported "delinquency of friends" says as much about the respondent as about his or her friends. Measures of the delinquency of friends in data sets available to me are respondent-generated. Therefore, I am justified in treating "delinquency of friends" as another potentially inhibiting factor. Respondents reporting no delinquent friends have (1) defined themselves as nondelinquent and/or (2) tied themselves to the mast, greatly limiting their opportunities for delinquent behavior. Table 28.3 illustrates the power of this added restraint.

TABLE 28.3. Percent Reporting Two or More Delinquent Acts by Number of Self-Reported Inhibiting Factors and Number of Friends Picked Up by the Police, Richmond, California, 1965

	Number of self-reported inhibiting factors									
	0	1	2	3	4	5	6	7	8	9
No friends picked up by police	52	48	37	27	21	18	14	11	8	0
	(21)	(50)	(121)	(195)	(237)	(286)	(237)	(190)	(111)	(38)
One or more friends picked up by police	76	66	56	48	44	34	32	22	7	*
	(113)	(194)	(271)	(310)	(308)	(269)	(177)	(94)	(41)	(6)

Curiously enough, self-control measures that are traceable to our brief but ill-considered effort to infer the "elements" of self-control from the nature of crime have come to stand in the same relation to "bonds" as "peer delinquency," providing a powerful (sometimes too powerful) alternative interpretation of the results of research (Polakowski, 1994; Schreck, 2002). Offhand, it would seem that we could deal with these measures in the same way we dealt with measures of peer delinquency (i.e., make them bond-equivalent and add them to our self-control measures). It turns out, however, that only some of them can be "saved" in this way. A sample of items found in "self-control" scales (all but item 5 are from Grasmick et al., 1993) follows:

1. I lose my temper easily.
2. The easy things bring me the most pleasure.
3. I sometimes take a risk just for the fun of it.
4. I try to get things I want even when I know that it's causing problems for other people.
5. Most things people call delinquency don't really hurt anyone.
6. I don't devote much thought and effort to preparing for the future.

It should come as no surprise that these items are associated with delinquent behavior. Some (items 1, 3, and 4) are, after all, confessions of delinquency. Others (item 5) are beliefs easily construed as bond measures. And still others (items 2 and 6) tap bond elements already introduced. It seems obvious that if we were to pull out the bond items and place them in competition with the confession items, the bond items would lose. But we are not attempting a theory that can compete on even terms with delinquency in predicting delinquency. If, indeed, the best predictor of crime is prior criminal behavior (see the first sentence of this chapter!), such an attempt would be doomed from the beginning. We are, however, usefully reminded that delinquent acts have multiple causes, and that our theory is an attempt to find a stable cause common to all of them.

APPLYING THE SLIGHTLY REVISED VERSION OF THE THEORY

Research support for our original self-control theory has been, in my view, impressive, as has been the level of criticism and controversy it has evoked. I do not believe that the tinkering I have done here detracts from the value of the original theory. Change in conception of the sources of self-control and the cognitive processes it involves should have little effect on the empirical predictions derived from the theory. For example, a central assertion of the theory is that deviant and reckless acts are also explained by (low) self-control. Immediately available data sets show that, among high school students, self-control as measured here consistently predicts *behavior analogous to crime*: truancy, cheating on exams, being sent out of a classroom, driving while drinking, auto accidents, bike–skateboard–rollerblade accidents, broken bones, shooting dice for money, drinking alcohol, smoking tobacco, and smoking marijuana. For all acts or outcomes listed, a six-item, self-report delinquency scale predicts better than our self-control measure (see Table 28.4). We could easily increase the predictive power of the self-control measure by adding moral belief, involvement, and attachment items, but our delinquency scale could be augmented in the same way with the same results. Because we have already conceded the practical superiority of act measures and continue to claim theoretical advantage for bond mea-

TABLE 28.4. Correlations between a 9-Item Self-Control Measure, a 6-Item Self-Reported Delinquency Measure, and Acts Analogous to Crime, Fayetteville, Arkansas, Sample

	Self-control	Self-reported delinquency
Stay away from school (truancy)	−.38	.50
Cheat on exam or quiz	−.29	.40
Sent out of classroom	−.39	.56
Drive while drinking	−.18	.28
Been in auto accident	−.10	.25
Bike, skateboard, or rollerblade accident	−.19	.29
Suffered broken bones	−.08	.16
Shot dice for money	−.22	.46
Drank alcohol (many times)	−.33	.45
Smoked cigarettes (many times)	−.29	.42
Smoked marijuana	−.31	.49

Note. The numbers on which the correlations are based range from 1,047 to 1,106. The two items added to the self-control measure used in Table 28.2 are number of friends picked up by the police (None) and "I try hard in school" (Strongly agree).

sures, there seems little point in pressing this comparison. (It may be worth recalling here that theoretical issues in criminology are too often "resolved" by comparison of the predictive power of measures that are unequal in quality—see Akers, 1998; Haynie, 2001.)

SELF-CONTROL AND ALCOHOL

For some questions, the revised concept of self-control makes life easier. Alcohol is one of them. Discussion of how it causes crime is more easily couched in the terms employed here. Alcohol dissolves the broad view that ordinarily controls us. It narrows the focus of attention to the here and now, to the insulting word, to the memory of an old transgression, to the desire for more alcohol. In sober circumstances, our pleasures and pains do not come to us unalloyed. There are other things to think about. Not so, or not so much so, when we are drunk. Of course, disinhibition is more likely the fewer the inhibitions one has to begin with, and alcohol consumption, like hanging with peers, is itself indicative of low self-control. Analysis shows that self-control, as measured here, does not predict delinquency among students who report consuming alcohol "many times" as well as it does among non- and low-rate users, as previous discussion would lead us to expect. (The same finding among tobacco users—a common problem—suggests complications too advanced to be dealt with here!)

A particular feature of the concept and measure of self-control that I suggest here is that it positively identifies people with strong bonds, thus making them the focus of attention. Focusing on them, we ask what they do to avoid or resist temptation, and what consequences this has for their wider pattern of activities. Because they are controlled, their behavior is predictable. We know that they will show up on time and at least try to do what they said they would do. Taken seriously, this view leaves "natural man" as a residual category. What he or she is like, and what he or she will do, the theory cannot say. We can say that the possible distractions are many, that they may or may not have serious consequences, and may or may not be of interest to the police. This is another way of saying that control theories are theories of conformity, asking not why they do it, but why we do not.

Of course, having said this, most of us, control theorists or not, like the warden's wife, find the desperados and scalawags too interesting to resist. From the perspective of criminology, this is not a bad thing. There is much to be learned by looking directly at the unrestrained offender, as the evolutionary biologists and psychologists have shown (Brannigan, 1997; Ellis, 1998). From the perspective of control theory, however, the dangers of this romance are apparent. Probably it is better to stick with the warden, at least for now.

NOTES

1. A catalog of the devices sociologists use to discredit theories that assume that some acts are maladaptive, and that some people are consistently more likely to engage in them, may be found in Geis (2000).

2. The first time I wrote on this topic, another campus shooting was in the news. The offender shot people from a tower on the University of Texas campus, but only after he had freed himself from an annoying restraint: "I plan to kill my wife after I pick her up from work. I don't want her to have to face the embarrassment that my actions will surely cause her" (Hirschi, 1969/2002, p. 31).

3. Over time, advocates of what is now called "social learning theory" have come to accept the idea that the relevant beliefs may allow, but not require, deviant behavior (see Akers, 1998).

4. In recent work, we have tended to give "natural sanctions" (the risks to life and limb inherent in many deviant acts) a greater role in this process, and to see parents as spending their time protecting the child from them. Because differences in self-control are observed so early, "legal sanctions" appear to be strictly irrelevant.

5. The most common and persistent criticism of our self-control theory has been that it is tautological. Our defense has had a certain lawyerly quality about it. On the one hand, we say, "yes," it is tautological, as it should be. On the other hand we say, "no," it is not tautological, and the critic's argument proves that it is not (Hirschi & Gottfredson, 1994, 2000). I believe that both of our arguments are legitimate, and the present effort should not be construed as an effort to deal with the tautology issue.

6. The empirical resolution to this issue, in which we examine the less than perfect correlation between past and present behavior and divvy up the variance, with the stability people getting the square root of the explained variance and the instability people getting the remainder, is not as simple and straightforward as it sounds. At first glance, it seems to favor the stability argument on the grounds that unexplained variance is not much of a gift. In practice, this solution tends to give instability more than it deserves, with further investigation revealing that even more of the variance can be explained, or that no real change has occurred.

7. Both the Gluecks (1950) and Block and colleagues (1988) have extensive lists of traits that predict delinquency from an early age. The more predictive traits suggest weak ties to others, little concern for the opinion of adults, and little concern for getting ahead, and Block and colleagues actually use the term "ego undercontrol" to summarize their results. The Gluecks, too, are now often described as adhering to a "control" view of delinquency.

REFERENCES

Akers, R. L. (1998). *Social learning and social structure: A general theory of crime and deviance.* Boston: Northeastern University Press.

Block, J., Block, J. H., & Keyes, S. (1988). Longitudinally foretelling drug usage in adolescence: Early childhood personality and environmental precursors. *Child Development, 59,* 336–355.

Brannigan, A. (1997, October). Self control, social control and evolutionary psychology: Towards an integrated perspective on crime. *Canadian Journal of Criminology,* pp. 403–431.

Costello, B. J., & Vowell, P. R. (1999). Testing control theory and differential association: A reanalysis of the Richmond Youth Project data. *Criminology, 37*(4), 815–842.

Cressey, D. (1953). *Other people's money.* New York: Free Press.

Davis, K. (1948). *Human society.* New York: Macmillan.

Ellis, L. (1998). Neo-Darwinian theories of violent criminality and antisocial behavior: Photographic evidence from nonhuman animals and a review of the literature. *Aggression and Violent Behavior, 3*(1), 61–110.

Geis, G. (2000). On the absence of self-control as the basis for a general theory of crime: A critique. *Theoretical Criminology, 4,* 35–53.

Gibbs, J. T., & Giever, D. (1995). Self-control and its manifestations among university students: An empirical test of Gottfredson and Hirschi's general theory. *Justice Quarterly, 2*(2), 231–255.

Gilbert, D. T. (1993). The assent of man: Mental representation and the control of belief. In D. M. Wegner & J. W. Pennebaker (Eds.), *Handbook of mental control* (pp. 57–87). Englewood Cliffs, NJ: Prentice-Hall.

Glueck, S., & Glueck, E. (1950). *Unraveling juvenile delinquency.* Cambridge, MA: Harvard University Press.

Gottfredson, M., & Hirschi, T. (1987). The methodological adequacy of longitudinal research on crime. *Criminology, 25,* 581–614.

Gottfredson, M., & Hirschi, T. (1990). *A general theory of crime.* Stanford, CA: Stanford University Press.

Grasmick, H. G., Tittle, C. R., Bursik, R. J., & Arneklev, B. J. (1993). Testing the core empirical implications of Gottfredson and Hirschi's general theory of crime. *Journal of Research in Crime and Delinquency, 30,* 5–29.

Hardwick, K. H. (2002). *Unraveling "crime in the making": Reexamining the role of informal social control in the genesis and stability of delinquency and crime.* Doctoral dissertation, Department of Sociology, University of Calgary, Canada.

Haynie, D. L. (2001). Delinquent peers revisited: Does network structure matter? *American Journal of Sociology, 106,* 1013–57.

Hechter, M. (1987). *Principles of group solidarity.* Berkeley: University of California Press.

Hirschi, T. (2002). *Causes of delinquency.* New Brunswick, NJ: Transaction. (Original work published 1969)

Hirschi, T., & Gottfredson, M. (2000). In defense of self-control. *Theoretical Criminology, 4*(1), 55–69.

Hirschi, T., & Gottfredson, M. (1994). The generality of deviance. In T. Hirschi & M. Gottfredson (Eds.), *The generality of deviance* (pp. 1–22). New Brunswick, NJ: Transaction.

Hirschi, T., & Gottfredson, M. (1986). The distinction between crime and criminality. In T. F. Hartnagel & R. Silverman (Eds.), *Critique and explanation: Essays in honor of Gwynne Nettler* (pp. 55–69). New Brunswick, NJ: Transaction.

Hirschi, T., & Gottfredson, M. (1983). Age and the explanation of crime. *American Journal of Sociology, 89,* 552–584.

Kornhauser, R. (1978). *Social sources of delinquency.* Chicago: University of Chicago Press.

Longshore, D., Stein, J. A., & Turner, S. (1998). Reliability and validity of a self-control measure. *Criminology, 36,* 175–182.

Marcus, B. (2003). An empirical examination of the construct validity of two alternative self-control measures. *Educational and Psychological Measurement, 63,* 674–706.

Marcus, B. (in press). Self-control in the general theory of crime: Theoretical implications of a measurement problem. *Theoretical Criminology.*

Matsueda, R. (1982). Testing control theory and differential association: A causal modeling approach. *American Sociological Review, 47,* 489–504.

Matza, D. (1964). *Delinquency and drift.* New York: Wiley.

Merton, R. K. (1938). Social structure and anomie. *American Sociological Review, 3,* 672–682.

Nagin, D., & Paternoster, R. (1994). Personal capital and social control: The deterrence implications of a theory of individual differences in criminal offending. *Criminology, 32,* 581–606.

Oakeshott, M. (1957). Introduction. In T. Hobbes, *Leviathan* (pp. vii–lxvi). Oxford, UK: Basil Blackwood.

Parsons, T. (1957). *The social system.* New York: Free Press.

Patterson, G. R. (1980). Children who steal. In T. Hirschi & M. Gottfredson (Eds.), *Understanding crime* (pp. 73–90). Beverly Hills, CA: Sage.

Piquero, A. R., & Rosay, A. B. (1998). The reliability and validity of Grasmick et al.'s self-control scale: A comment on Longshore et al. *Criminology, 36,* 157–173.

Polakowski, M. (1994). Linking self- and social control with deviance: Illuminating the structure underlying a general theory of crime and its relation to deviant activity. *Journal of Quantitative Criminology, 10,* 41–78.

Sampson, R., & Laub, J. (1993). *Crime in the making.* Cambridge, MA: Harvard University Press.

Schreck, C. J. (2002). How do social bonds restrain crime?: A study of the mechanisms. *Journal of Crime and Justice, 25,* 1–21.

Stattin, H., & Kerr, M. (2000). Parental monitoring: A reinterpretation. *Child Development, 71,* 1072–1085.

Sutherland, E. H. (1939). *Principles of criminology.* Philadelphia: Lippincott.

Taylor, C. (2001). The relationship between social and self-control: Tracing Hirschi's criminological career. *Theoretical Criminology, 5,* 369–388.

Toby, J. (1957). Social disorganization and stake in conformity: Complementary factors in the predatory behavior of hoodlums. *Journal of Criminal Law, Criminology, and Police Science, 48,* 12–17.

Uggen, C. (2003). Criminology and the sociology of deviance. *The Criminologist, 28,* 1–5.

Wolfgang, M., Figlio, R. M., Tracy, P. E., & Singer, S. I. (1985). *The National Survey of Crime Severity.* Washington, DC: U.S. Department of Justice.

Author Index

Aarons, G. A., 470
Aarts, H., 158, 159, 160, 161, 212
Aas, H. N., 470
Aasland, O. G., 472
Abbey, A., 475
Abbott, R. D., 468
Aber, J. L., 116, 265, 327, 348, 364
Abrams, D. B., 454
Abramson, L. Y., 222, 413
Achtziger, A., 216
Acierno, R., 473
Ackerman, B. P., 23, 324, 341
Adalbjarnardottir, S., 467
Adams, C. M., 234
Adams, E., 85
Adams, K. M., 526
Adan, A., 49
Adesso, V. J., 416, 469
Adleman, N. E., 69
Adolphs, R., 234
Affleck, G., 46, 117, 471
Agocha, V. B., 475
Agostinelli, G. E., 470
Ahadi, S. A., 259, 260, 267, 270, 289, 342, 350, 360, 361, 365
Ahern, G. L., 237
Ahrens, A. H., 199
Aiken, L. S., 131, 534
Aiken, P. A., 501
Ainslie, G., 108, 304
Ainsworth, M., 328
Aitchison, T., 467
Ajjanagadde, V., 31
Ajzen, I., 130, 131, 132, 137, 211
Akers, R. L., 538, 547, 549, 550

Aksan, N., 347
Akshoomoff, N., 295
Albery, I. P., 475
Alexander, G. E., 71
Alexander, M. P., 62, 67, 72
Allaire, J. C., 193
Allen, A., 100
Allen, J. J. B., 20, 29
Allessandri, S. M., 28
Allgeier, E. R., 531
Alloy, L. B., 222, 415
Allport, D. A., 85
Allsop, S., 467
Aman, C. J., 344
Amso, D., 344
Ana, E. S., 108, 467
Ancoli, S., 457
Andersen, S. M., 157, 201
Anderson, A. K., 234, 245
Anderson, J. R., 189
Anderson, L. R., 469
Anderson, S. W., 62, 67, 287
Anderssen, N., 470
Andrews, C., 234
Aneshensel, C., 416
Antin, S. P., 70
Apospori, E., 382
Applebaum, W., 513
Apt, C., 530
Arico, S., 466
Arkes, H. R., 179, 180
Armeli, S., 471, 472
Armitage, C. J., 132
Armony, J. L., 245, 427
Armor, D. A., 223
Armstrong, S., 468
Arneklev, B. J., 542
Arriaga, X. B., 118
Arroyo, J. A., 472

Artistico, D., 192, 194, 195
Asch, S. E., 16
Aspinwall, L. G., 26, 27
Assaad, J. M., 480
Aston-Jones, G., 427
Atencio, D. J., 301
Atkins, C. J., 106
Atkins, R., 348
Atkinson, J. W., 24, 162, 165, 179, 211
Auerbach, J. G., 295
Austin, J. T., 14
Averill, J. R., 106, 116
Awh, E., 68
Ayduk, O., 101, 102, 105, 107, 110, 111, 114, 116, 118, 119, 121, 123, 269, 364, 383

B

Babinsky, R., 234
Babler, J., 195
Bachorowski, J. A., 435, 436
Baddeley, A. D., 63, 70, 71, 85, 285, 307, 314, 315
Badgaiyan, R., 69, 70
Baer, J. S., 140
Bagnardi, V., 466
Bailey, D. S., 474, 476, 480
Baillargeon, R., 343
Baird, A. A., 247
Baker, L. H., 455
Baker, N., 107, 113, 265
Baker, T. B., 449, 454, 457, 458
Balabanis, M., 451, 452
Baldwin, M. W., 157, 383
Ballantine, H. T., Jr., 66

Baltes, M. M., 193
Baltes, P. B., 193, 199
Banaji, M. R., 152, 477
Bancroft, J., 531
Bancroft, M., 265, 344
Band, P. H., 291
Bandura, A., 89, 105, 123, 131, 132, 133, 140, 141, 151, 164, 188, 190, 191, 192, 193, 195, 197, 198
Barbaranelli, C., 190, 192
Barber, T. X., 117
Barcelo, F., 235
Barch, D. M., 236, 285, 423, 424
Barchas, J. D., 192
Barndollar, K., 156,
Bargh, J. A., 32, 33, 85, 100, 106, 152, 153, 156, 157, 158, 159, 160, 161, 162, 165, 171, 198, 212, 218, 398
Barkley, R. A., 3, 6, 86, 301, 302, 303, 305, 306, 309, 310, 313, 315, 316, 333, 342, 346
Barkow, J. H., 309, 310
Barlow, D. H., 413, 457
Barndollar, K., 85, 156, 198, 218
Barnes, C. L., 66, 67
Barnes, G. M., 474
Barnett, L. W., 131
Baron, R. M., 471
Baron-Cohen, S., 67
Barth, R. J., 527, 528
Bartholow, B. D., 470
Barton, J., 138
Bashore, T. R., 291
Bates, J. E., 260, 262, 263, 270, 272, 283, 333, 342, 346, 347, 348, 351, 357, 359, 361, 362
Bates, M. E., 472, 476
Bättig, K., 451
Baucom, D. H., 501
Bauer, L. O., 467
Bauman, K. E., 138
Baumann, N., 101
Baumeister, R. F., 2, 3, 15, 27, 30, 31, 44, 45, 49, 85, 86, 88, 89, 91, 92, 95, 108, 142, 151, 152, 155, 165, 199, 217, 373, 374, 375, 376, 379, 382, 384, 393, 394, 398, 401, 403, 422, 426, 447, 448, 449, 451, 452, 453, 455, 458, 459, 466, 501, 504, 509, 511,

512, 515, 516, 517, 518, 519, 520, 521, 529
Baxter, D., 64
Bayer, U. C., 160, 213, 214, 217, 219, 221, 222
Bayles, K., 272, 333
Bazerman, M., 176
Beach, S. R. H., 26, 400
Beatty, S. E., 513, 515
Beauregard, M., 235, 236, 237, 244, 287, 459
Bechara, A., 62, 67, 74, 122, 234, 235, 236, 237, 242
Beck, A. T., 358, 413
Beck, J. E., 272, 332
Becker, M. H., 131
Beckmann, J., 222
Bednarski, R., 384
Beer, J. S., 385, 387
Beer, R. D., 16
Bell, B. S., 197
Bell, M. A., 330, 343
Bell, R., 131
Bellenger, D. N., 512, 513
Belsky, J., 270, 347
Belzer, L. J., 499
Bem, D. J., 89, 100, 181
Bench, C. J., 237
Benes, F., 295
Benjamin, J., 295
Bennett, T., 475
Benson, D. F., 65, 66, 67, 70, 302, 304
Bentin, S., 439
Bentler, P. M., 140
Berg, K., 413
Berger, A., 291
Berger, B., 416
Berk, L. E., 301, 307, 315, 349
Berlin, L. J., 350
Berlyne, D., 112
Berns, G. S., 72, 234
Bernstein, S., 201
Berntson, G. G., 19, 183, 261
Berntzen, D., 117
Berridge, K. C., 454
Berry, J. M., 192, 194
Berthier, M. L., 528
Best, C. L., 473
Betz, N. E., 191, 193
Bianco, A. T., 178
Bibby, P. A., 138
Bigelow, G., 451
Bigelow, L., 429
Bilder, R., 70
Birbaumer, N., 438, 477
Birch, D., 24, 162, 165
Birch, H. G., 359
Birkimer, J. C., 534

Birnbaum, I. M., 476
Black, D. H., 471
Black, D. W., 517, 530
Black, J., 343
Black, S., 67
Blackburn, E. K., 265, 344
Blackburn, I., 202
Blackburn, J., 470, 480
Blackmore, S., 313
Blair, R. J. R., 67, 68, 235, 289, 431
Blaskey, L. G., 302
Blehar, M., 328
Bleske, A. L., 309
Bless, H., 41, 217
Blevins, T., 382
Block, J. A., 108, 467
Block, J. H., 342, 544
Block, J., 342, 362, 387, 544, 545
Blumer, C., 179, 180
Blumer, D., 66, 67
Boden, J. M., 384
Bodenhausen, G. V., 219
Bohner, G., 23
Bohus, B., 427
Boies, S. C., 534
Boivin, M., 346
Boland, F. J., 499
Bonanno, G. A., 45, 51, 117
Bond, C. F., 470, 474
Bonin, M. F., 468
Bookheimer, S. Y., 236
Booth, C. L., 333
Borges, G., 473
Borkovec, T., 202
Borkowski, W., 101
Botvin, G. J., 471
Botvinick, M. M., 68, 69, 236, 285, 287, 293, 422, 423, 424
Bourgouin, P., 287, 459
Boutelle, N., 139
Bower, J. E., 51
Bowlby, J., 27, 327, 329, 374
Bowtell, R., 236
Braaten, E. B., 301, 316
Bradbury, T. N., 400
Bradley, M. M., 19
Bradshaw, J. L., 75
Bradvik, B., 304
Brady, K., 415, 418
Branch, L. G., 131
Brandon, T. H., 450, 453, 454
Brandt, K. M., 471
Brandstätter, V., 160, 213, 214, 223
Brandtstädter, J., 199
Brannigan, A., 550

Bratslavsky, E., 2, 15, 44, 88, 142, 152, 448, 501, 504, 512
Braungart, J. M., 324, 325, 327, 330
Braungart-Rieker, J. M., 266
Braver, T. S., 236, 285, 423, 424
Brazzelli, B., 64
Brecklin, L. R., 475
Breen, M. J., 301
Brehm, J. W., 28, 223
Breiner, M. J., 477
Brendl, C. M., 172
Brennan, M., 395
Breslau, N., 470
Breslin, F. C., 474
Breteler, M. H. M., 467
Brewer, W. F., 158
Brickman, P., 50, 199
Bridges, L. J., 324, 343, 347
Brigham, T. A., 474
Briner, R. B., 40
Brittleband, A., 435
Broadbent, D. E., 284
Brockner, J., 176
Brod, M. I., 141
Brodersen, L., 104
Brodner, M., 65
Brody, G. H., 275
Broidy, L. M., 345
Bronfenbrenner, U., 341, 345, 346, 349, 351
Bronik, M. D., 315
Bronowski, J., 303, 306, 314
Bronson, M. B., 283, 325, 326, 363
Brooks-Gunn, J., 341, 342, 348, 349, 350
Brosschot, J. F., 454
Brouillard, M. E., 192
Brown, G. G., 69
Brown, G. W., 28
Brown, J. D., 117, 379, 383, 387
Brown, L. M., 362
Brown, S. A., 469, 470
Brownell, K. D., 136, 449, 451, 459
Bruce, J., 345
Bruch, H., 493
Bruno, J. P., 427
Bryan, A., 534
Buchel, C., 236
Buchtel, H. A., 72
Buck, R., 45
Buhrmeister, D., 301
Bull, R., 85
Bunge, S. A., 75, 232, 238, 287
Burgess, P., 64, 65
Burkhart, B., 416

Burns, D. J., 304
Burrowes, B. D., 275
Bursik, R. J., 542
Burton, S. M., 453
Bush, G., 68, 69, 75, 236, 237, 285, 287, 290, 362
Bush, T., 301, 315
Bushman, B. J., 41, 45, 474
Bushnell, M. C., 287
Buss, D. M., 309, 373
Buss, K. A., 273, 275
Butler, A. C., 386
Butler, J. L., 394
Butler, L. D., 412
Butter, C. M., 237
Buttermore, N., 377
Button, S. B., 197
Buunk, B. P., 16, 383
Buzzi, R., 451
Bystritsky, A., 202

C

Cabeza, R., 235
Cacioppo, J. T., 19, 55, 183, 202, 203, 261, 438, 477
Cahill, L., 234
Cai, X., 346
Caldwell, N. D., 413
Calkins, S. D., 104, 264, 269, 272, 324, 325, 326, 327, 332, 333, 335, 336, 342, 346, 347, 361
Callan, M. K., 472
Callender, G., 346
Camacho, C. J., 179, 182
Cameron, L., 133
Campbell, S. B., 333, 341
Campbell, W. K., 399, 401, 405
Campos, J. J., 230
Canli, T., 234, 236, 246, 357
Cantor, N., 14, 100, 114, 201, 502
Cantwell, D., 302
Capasso, D. R., 474
Cappell, H., 474
Caprara, G. V., 190, 192
Card, J. A., 329, 331
Carey, K. B., 480
Carey, M. P., 455, 531
Carlson, C. L., 301, 316
Carlson, S. M., 271, 285, 290
Carnes, P. J., 526
Carnes, P., 526, 529, 530
Carney, M. A., 471
Carpenter, K. M., 472
Carpenter, P. A., 154
Carrier, B., 287

Carscadden, J. L., 470
Carstensen, L. L., 41, 248
Carter, B. L., 456, 457, 467
Carter, C. S., 65, 68, 69, 236, 285, 287, 292, 293, 422, 423, 424, 427
Carter, J. A., 471
Carter, S. R., 90
Carter, S., III, 117
Caruso, D. R., 54
Carver, C. S., 2, 4, 13, 14, 15, 16, 17, 19, 20, 21, 22, 23, 25, 27, 28, 29, 30, 31, 32, 52, 84, 100, 118, 133, 151, 164, 196, 211, 373, 376, 426, 435, 502
Casbon, T. S., 438
Casey, B. J., 247
Caspi, A., 266, 268, 269, 270, 341, 361, 533
Cassidy, J., 327, 328, 329
Castellanos, F. X., 306
Castillo, S., 475
Catanese, K. R., 403
Catanzaro, S. J., 472
Caul, W. F., 45
Ceci, S., 341, 345, 346
Cepeda-Benito, A., 453
Cervone, D., 188, 189, 191, 192, 195, 197, 198, 199, 200, 201
Chabay, L. A., 301
Chabris, C. F., 425
Chaiken, S. L., 31, 85, 159, 171
Chalmers, D., 416, 418
Chang, H. T., 316
Chao, L. L., 65, 232
Charles, S. T., 248
Chartrand, T. L., 106, 152, 153, 159, 160, 164, 165, 198
Chassin, L., 138, 271, 276
Chasteen, A. L., 214
Chau, P. M., 234, 237
Chaves, J. F., 117
Chen, P. H., 473
Chen, S., 157, 159, 201
Cheng, C. M., 165
Cheng, C., 114
Chermack, S. T., 474
Cherpitel, C. J., 473
Cherry, E. C., 375
Chess, S., 359
Cheung, J. S., 114
Chiba, A. A., 235
Chiu, C. Y., 114
Choi, H. S., 177
Chokel, J. T., 380
Chow, T. W., 65

Christenson, G. A., 517, 518, 519, 520
Chu, J. A., 529
Chua, P., 236, 237
Chutuape, M. A. D., 467
Ciarocco, N. J., 401
Ciarrochi, J. V., 41
Cibelli, C., 334
Cicchetti, D., 324, 333, 335
Cioffi, D., 192
Cipolotti, L., 67, 68
Clark, C., 316
Clark, D. B., 467
Clark, J. J., 284
Clark, L. A., 359, 413, 435
Clark, R. N., 18
Clayton, R., 469
Cleary, S. D., 271, 472
Cleckley, H., 433
Clements, C., 413
Clinton, A., 296
Clohessy, A. B., 288, 363
Clore, G. L., 16, 22, 199, 200
Coates, D., 50
Coffman, S., 202
Cohen, A. R., 223
Cohen, D., 160
Cohen, J. D., 65, 68, 69, 70, 71, 72, 156, 232, 235, 236, 285, 287, 422, 423, 424, 426, 427
Cohen, M., 334, 341
Cohen, S., 140
Cohn, J. F., 345, 457
Coie, J. D., 275, 350
Colder, C. R., 271
Cole, P. M., 261, 342
Coleman, E., 526, 527, 528
Coles, M. G. H., 287, 290
Collins, A., 16
Collins, J. C., 26
Collins, N. L., 401
Collins, P., 290
Collins, P. F., 19, 261, 359
Collins, R. L., 94, 467, 475
Colombo, J., 288
Colsman, M., 108, 467
Colten, M., 416
Colvin, C. R., 387
Comeau, N., 472
Comer, R. J., 528, 529
Compas, B. E., 261
Conger, J. J., 449, 468, 477, 478, 499
Conklin, C. A., 460
Conley, M., 427
Connell, J. P., 343
Conner, M., 131, 132
Conners, C. K., 301

Connors, G. J., 467, 470
Connor-Smith, J. K., 261
Consedine, N. S., 45, 46
Contreras, J., 335
Conway, A. R. A., 71
Cook, C. C., 517
Cook, E. T., 276
Cooney, N. L., 455, 467, 468
Cooper, A., 534
Cooper, H. M., 474
Cooper, L., 415
Cooper, M. L., 416, 470, 472, 475, 478
Cooper, R., 64
Copeland, A. L., 450
Coplan, R. J., 324, 342
Corballis, M. C., 308
Corbetta, M., 69, 71, 73, 284, 286
Corbin, W. R., 470, 471
Cornell, D., 26
Corrao, G., 466
Cosgrove, T., 324
Cosmides, L., 309, 310, 373, 374
Costa, F. M., 474
Costa, P. T., 100, 246, 435
Costanzo, P. R., 499
Costello, B. J., 547
Cottrell, C. A., 375
Coull, J. T., 237
Courchesne, E., 295
Courtney, S. M., 69
Cowan, G. S., 44
Cowan, W. B., 422, 478
Cox, B. J., 435
Coy, K. C., 263, 264, 266, 341, 365
Craik, F. I., M., 237
Crane, M., 201
Cranston, J. W., 476
Crepaz, N., 26
Cressey, D., 539
Critchley, H., 234, 236, 237, 246
Critchlow, B., 477
Crnic, K., 347
Cronkite, R. C., 472
Crosson, B., 235
Crowe, E., 172, 175, 177
Crowne, D. P., 157
Cruttenden, L., 314
Cruz, I. Y., 470
Csikszentmihalyi, M., 192
Cuite, C. L., 141
Cumberland, A., 267, 270
Cummings, E. M., 333
Cummings, J. L., 65
Curran, P. J., 415, 467
Curran, T., 288
Currie, J., 314

Curry, S. J., 131, 144
Curtin, J. J., 438, 477
Cuthbert, B. N., 19
Cutrona, C. E., 192
Cutter, H. S., 474
Cycowicz, Y. M., 73

D

Daffner, K. R., 72, 73
Daleiden, E. L., 270, 362
Damasio, A. R., 62, 63, 66, 67, 68, 74, 122, 234, 236, 287, 306, 308
Damasio, H., 67, 122, 234, 287
D'Amico, E. J., 474, 475
Daneman, M., 154
Danforth, J. S., 301
Darkes, J., 469, 470
Darwin, C., 311, 312
Datta, H., 294
Davenport, A., 475
Davidson, G., 202, 203
Davidson, M. C., 286, 293
Davidson, R. J., 16, 19, 21, 41, 49, 55, 231, 232, 235, 236, 237, 238, 243, 244, 287, 457, 458
Davies, B., 22
Davies, M., 54
Davies, P., 313
Davis, C. G., 46, 412
Davis, E. P., 345
Davis, K., 537
Davis, K. A., 478
Davis, P. W., 349
Davis, T. M., 469
Dawkins, R., 313
Dawson, D., 67
Dawson, G., 347
Deacon, T. W., 307
DeCarli, C., 248
Deci, E. L., 33, 143, 144, 151, 198, 378
DeCoster, J., 31
Dedmon, S. A., 324, 326, 333
Dedmon, S. E., 264, 269, 272, 327
DeFries, J. C., 294
DeHart, D. D., 534
DeHart, T., 48, 54
Deiber, M. P., 237
Deichmann, R., 237
De Jong, C. A. J., 467
DeKlyen, M., 334
Del Boca, F. K., 469, 471
Delaney, W. P., 468
Deldin, P., 74

DeLisi, L. E., 476
Della Sala, S., 64
Delliquadri, E., 334
Delucia, J., 417
Dembo, T., 199
Dempster, F. N., 222, 247
Denburg, N. L., 74
Denckla, M. B., 85, 302, 304, 305
Denham, S. A., 341
Dennehey, D. M., 192
Dennett, D., 304, 309
Dennis, M., 304
Dennis, T. A., 342
Depue, R. A., 19, 261, 359
Dermen, K. H., 475, 478
DeRosier, M. E., 349
Derryberry, D., 116, 121, 259, 261, 262, 265, 345, 357, 358, 360, 361, 362, 364
de Ruiter, C., 454
DeSarbo, W. S., 519
Desimone, R., 284, 423, 427
Desmond, J. E., 232, 234
D'Esposito, M., 65, 248, 304
De Vente, W., 469
Devine, P. G., 404
Devinsky, O., 69, 70
DeVos, J., 343
de Wit, H., 467
de Zwaan, M., 517
Dhawan, M., 295
Diamond, A., 247, 263, 288, 292, 314, 343, 344, 345, 346, 362
Diamond, R., 301
Dias, R., 237, 242
Diaz, R. M., 301, 307
Dickerson, M., 474
DiClemente, C. C., 131, 191
DiClemente, R. J., 534
Diener, E., 31, 41, 49, 240, 248
Diener, M., 331
DiGirolamo, G. J., 69, 260, 261
Dijksterhuis, A. J., 158, 159, 161, 212
Dilorio, C., 190
Dimitrov, M., 66
Ding, Y. C., 295
Dintcheff, B. A., 474
Dionne, G., 346
Dixon, M. J., 476
Dobmeyer, S., 69
Dobson, K. S., 47
Dodge, K. A., 342, 361
Dolan, R. J., 66, 67, 69, 234, 235, 236, 237, 246, 289
Donald, M., 307, 312, 313
Donchin, E., 290

Donovan, J. E., 474
Donovan, W. L., 331
Donzella, B., 104
Douglas, R. M., 72
Douglas, V. I., 301, 302
Dowdall, G. W., 475
Downey, G., 101, 118, 121, 383
Downey, K., 470
Downs, D. L., 373, 374, 375, 376
Drevets, W. C., 237, 285
Driver, J., 245, 286, 439
Dronkers, N. F., 65
Druin, D. P., 346
Drummond, D. C., 467
Duckworth, K. L., 85, 159
Duclos, S. E., 51
Dudokovic, N. M., 75
Dugatkin, L., 312
DuHamel, K., 467
Dumais, S. T., 165
Dunbar, K., 156, 422
Duncan, G. H., 287
Duncan, G. J., 350
Duncan, J., 73, 287, 423, 427
Duncan, T., 384
Dunn, M. A., 155
Dunn, M. E., 469, 470, 471
Dunne, M. P., 427
Dunning, D., 171
Dupree, D. A., 158
Durham, W. H., 307
Duval, S., 519
Dweck, C. S., 14, 106, 192, 197, 201
Dytrych, Z., 467
Dzewaltowski, D. A., 141

E

Earleywine, M., 471
Earls, F., 270
Early, T. S., 295
Easdon, C. M., 479
Easterbrooks, M., 334
Eaves, L. J., 435
Ebbesen, E. B., 107, 111, 513
Ebstein, R., 295
Eddings, S., 384
Edgell, D., 304
Edgerton, R. B., 455
Edwards, E. A., 519
Edwards, G., 302, 315
Eggleston, T. J., 449
Ehrhardt, A. A., 531
Eidelman, A. I., 347
Eimer, M., 286
Eisenberg, N., 41, 116, 121, 260,

261, 263, 264, 265, 267, 268, 269, 270, 271, 274, 275, 276, 324, 335, 341, 365, 366
Ekeberg, O., 472
Ekkekakis, P., 48
Ekman, P., 457, 458
el-Guebaly, N., 468
El-Hag, N., 270
Elias, C. L., 349
Elias, M., 479
Elliot, A. J., 401
Elliott, A. J., 192, 197
Elliott, E. S., 14
Elliott, R., 67, 68, 69, 235, 517, 519, 520
Ellis, L. K., 260, 283, 289, 362, 364, 366, 550
Ellsworth, P. C., 230, 383
Ely, T. D., 234
Emde, R., 345
Emmons, R. A., 14, 50, 197, 384
Endress, H., 218
Endriga, M. C., 334
Engle, R. W., 71
Enns, J. T., 290
Enns, M. W., 435
Epley, N., 161
Epstein, E., 415
Epstein, S., 31, 106, 109, 110
Erber, R., 22, 155, 236
Ericsson, H., 202
Eriksen, B. A., 290
Eriksen, C. W., 290
Ernst, J., 202
Eslinger, P. J., 67, 74
Espy, K. A., 342, 343
Esses, V. M., 500
Essex, M. J., 269
Esso, K., 296
Estes, W. K., 112
Eunson, K., 202
Evans, A. C., 237
Evans, M. E., 93
Ewing, J. E., 531
Ewing, L. J., 341
Exner, T. M., 531
Eysenck, H. J., 246, 358, 359, 435

F

Faber, R. J., 511, 513, 516, 517, 518, 519, 520
Fabes, R. A., 41, 116, 121, 260, 261, 263, 264, 265, 267, 268, 269, 270, 271, 275, 276, 341, 365

Author Index

Faillace, L. A., 470
Fairhurst, S. J., 191
Fallon, A. E., 374
Fan, J., 283, 286, 287, 289, 290, 292, 294
Fanselow, M. S., 428
Faroy, M., 295
Farrell, A., 348
Farrington, D. P., 361
Fazio, R. H., 152
Feather, N. T., 173
Fedoroff, I. C., 499, 505
Fegley, S., 348
Fein, S., 155
Feinauer, L. L., 529
Feingold, A., 51
Feldman Barrett, L., 236
Feldman, P., 203
Feldman, R., 345, 346, 347
Feldman, S., 100, 118, 383, 502
Fencsik, D. E., 69
Ferber, S., 286
Ferguson, E., 138
Ferguson, M. J., 106
Fergusson, S., 470
Ferrell, M. E., 513, 515
Ferrier, I. N., 435
Festinger, L., 16, 181, 199
Feyerabend, C., 454
Fichman, L., 41, 43, 48, 49, 52
Fiedler, K., 217
Field, T., 329
Figlio, R. M., 539
Filipek, P. A., 306
Fillmore, M. T., 470, 476, 479, 480
Fincham, F. D., 400
Fink, G. R., 234, 237
Finkel, E. J., 399, 405
Finkelhor, D., 529
Finkenauer, C., 15, 44
Finlay-Jones, R., 28
Finn, P. R., 470, 471, 531
Fiore, M. C., 449, 457, 458
Fishbach, A., 163, 164
Fishbein, M., 131, 132
Fisher, J. M., 468
Fisher, L. A., 138
Fisher, P., 260, 360
Fisher, R. J., 513, 514, 516
Fissell, K., 68, 236, 424
Fitzsimons, G. M., 157, 158, 159, 160, 165
Flaherty, J. A., 468
Flavell, J. H., 302
Fletcher, K., 315
Floden, D., 72
Flombaum, J. I., 292

Flory, K., 469
Flumerfelt, D. L., 530
Flynn, H. A., 386
Folkman, S., 47, 240
Fonagy, P., 283, 285
Fong, C., 155
Fong, G. T., 171, 451, 477, 478
Fong, G. W., 234
Ford, T. E., 171
Forgas, J. P., 41
Forman, D. R., 265, 345
Forssberg, H., 296
Förster, J., 177, 178, 179, 183, 184
Forsyth, A., 455
Fossella, J., 283, 294, 295
Foster, E. M., 346
Fowler, J. S., 67
Fowles, D. C., 261
Fox, N. A., 104, 324, 325, 327, 329, 330, 331, 332, 333, 335, 336, 342, 343, 361
Fox, P. T., 69
Frackowiak, R. S., 74, 237
Francis, S., 235, 236
Frank, E., 134, 223
Frank, L., 69
Frank, S. J., 468
Frankel, K. A., 333
Frankl, V. I., 229, 248
Fraser, L., 85
Fredrickson, B. L., 22, 41, 48
Fredrikson, M., 236
Freedman, M., 67
Freedman, Z. R., 144
Freels, S., 468
Freeman, W., 66
Freet, D., 517
Freitas, A. L., 118, 178, 181, 183, 184, 383
Fremouw, W. J., 499
Freud, S., 111
Freund, A. M., 199
Freund, B., 529
Frey, K., 45
Frey, L. M., 529
Friedman, D., 73
Friedman, R. S., 19, 163, 172
Friedman, S. L., 270
Friese, S., 520
Friesen, W. V., 457, 458
Frijda, N. H., 16, 17, 22, 23, 29
Frijters, J., 301
Friston, K. J., 74, 236
Frith, C. D., 65, 67, 74, 75, 235, 236, 237, 289, 439
Friz, J. L., 294
Fromme, K., 170, 171, 175

Frone, M. R., 415, 416, 472
Frosch, C., 331
Fry, A. F., 315
Frye, D., 344
Fuligni, A., 350
Fulker, D., 345
Fuster, J. M., 65, 71, 302, 303, 306, 307, 308

G

Gabrieli, J. D. E., 75, 232, 234, 238, 287, 357
Gaelick, L., 422
Gaeta, H., 73
Gagné, F. M., 222, 224
Gagné, M., 198,
Galanter, E., 14
Gallagher, H. L., 237
Gallagher, M., 235, 237, 427
Gammon, C. B., 474
Gangestad, S. W., 533
Ganzel, B. L., 529
Garavan, H., 75
Garber, J., 413
Garcia, M., 85, 159
Gardner, M. P., 515
Gardner, W. L., 19, 55, 261, 393
Garland, H., 197
Garnefski, N., 53
Garner, P. W., 275
Gartstein, M., 360
Gatenby, J. C., 236
Gatz, M., 248
Gaunt, R., 31, 109
Gaupp, L., 467
Gavrilescu, D., 476
Gayan, J., 294
Gazzaniga, M. S., 32
Ge, X., 275
Geen, R. G., 45
Gehring, W. J., 68, 69, 236, 290
Geis, G., 550
Geller, V., 295
Gentzler, A., 335
George, M. S., 246
George, W. H., 475
Gerardi-Caulton, G., 263, 264, 288, 289, 343, 362, 363
Gerrard, M., 471
Gershberg, F. B., 72
Gerstadt, C. L., 344
Gest, S. D., 361
Getz, J. G., 472
Ghatan, P., 71
Giancola, P. R., 435, 437, 473, 474, 479

Giard, M. H., 73
Gibbons, F. X., 16, 449, 471
Gibbs, J. T., 542
Giedd, J. N., 247
Giever, D., 542
Gilbert, D. T., 31, 109, 155, 396, 539, 543
Gilbert, P., 377
Gilchrist, I., 71
Gill, K. L., 264, 272, 326, 327, 333
Gillberg, C., 301
Gillespie, R. A., 455
Gilliom, M., 272, 332, 333, 347
Gilovich, T., 161, 455
Giovanelli, J., 333, 334
Gironell, A., 528
Glasgow, R. E., 131, 141
Glassman, M., 470
Glatt, M. M., 517
Glautier, S., 471
Gledhill-Hoyt, J., 468
Glisky, M. L., 343
Glover, G. H., 69, 232, 234
Glueck, E., 544
Glueck, S., 544
Glynn, S. M., 190
Godefroy, O., 73, 308
Goel, V., 237, 304
Gold, B., 237
Gold, S. N., 526, 527, 528, 530
Goldbeck, R., 467
Goldberg, E., 62, 66, 70
Goldman, B. M., 386
Goldman, M. S., 469, 470, 471
Goldman-Rakic, P. S., 65, 306, 307
Goldsmith, H. H., 273, 275, 325, 361
Goldstein, A., 471
Goldstein, K., 65
Goldstein, R. Z., 459
Gollwitzer, P. M., 85, 100, 115, 122, 132, 133, 136, 151, 152, 153, 156, 158, 159, 160, 162, 163, 164, 197, 198, 211, 212, 213, 214, 215, 216, 217, 218, 219, 221, 222, 225
Gonzales, N., 271
Goodman, G. S., 288
Goodrick, G. K., 190
Gooley, S., 141
Gordon, A. H., 246
Gordon, B. L., 534
Gordon, H. L., 69
Gordon, J. R., 131, 141, 449, 455, 459, 467

Gordon, L., 41
Gore, J. C., 236
Gorsuch, R. L., 436
Gotham, H. J., 469
Gotlib, I. H., 357
Gottfredson, M., 537, 540, 541, 542, 543, 547, 550
Gottfried, A. W., 361
Gottman, J. M., 41, 275
Gottschaldt, K., 212
Gottwald, W., 513, 515
Gow, C. A., 62, 70
Graber, M., 343
Grabowecky, M., 66
Grady, C. L., 294, 295
Grady, D. L., 295
Grafman, J., 65, 67, 304
Grafton, S. T., 234
Graham, K., 466, 473
Graham, P. W., 427
Grant, H., 192, 197, 201
Grant-Pillow, H., 184, 225
Grasmick, H. G., 542, 548
Graves, K. L., 475
Gray, J. A., 19, 109, 261, 359, 361, 428, 435
Grayson, C., 412
Graziano, W. G., 101
Greeley, J. D., 467
Greeley, J., 415, 470
Green, J. D., 201
Green, L., 305
Green, L. R., 474
Greenberg, M. T., 274, 275, 276, 333, 334, 350
Greenfield, T. K., 473
Greenwald, A. G., 152
Greenwood, P. M., 294
Greiner, B., 468
Griesler, P. C., 349
Griffin, D. W., 383
Griffiths, R., 451
Grigorenko, E. L., 104
Grodzinsky, G. M., 301, 316
Grolnick, W. S., 144, 324, 333, 343, 347
Gronvold, N. T., 472
Gross, A. M., 475
Gross, B., 290
Gross, J. J., 40, 41, 45, 46, 52, 53, 116, 117, 154, 155, 230, 231, 232, 238, 240, 246, 247, 248, 287
Gross, T., 454
Grossier, D. B., 315
Grothaus, L. C., 144
Grube, J. W., 468, 470
Gruenewald, T. L., 51

Gschwandtner, L. B., 49
Guerin, D. W., 361
Guitton, D., 72
Gunnar, M. R., 104, 330, 345
Gunning, W. B., 470
Guo, J., 468
Gusnard, D. A., 237
Guthrie, I. K., 41, 116, 121, 260, 263, 267, 269, 270, 271, 365
Gutierrez, E., 424
Gwaltney, C. J., 449, 455

H

Haaga, D. A., F., 199, 202, 203
Haas, A. L., 470
Habib, M., 66
Hackett, G., 191, 193
Hackett, R., 497
Hagan, R., 454
Haith, M. M., 288
Halberstadt, A. G., 275
Hale, S., 315
Halgren, E., 479
Hall, E. E., 48
Hall, S. M., 141
Hall, W., 418
Halperin, A., 499
Hamann, S. B., 234
Hamilton, D. L., 153
Hamlett, K. W., 301
Hammelbeck, J. P., 216
Hammon, D., 384
Han, J. S., 427
Hancock, T. B., 346
Happe, F., 237
Harackiewicz, J. M., 197
Hardwick, K. H., 540
Hare, R. D., 431, 433
Harford, T. C., 474
Hargis, K., 51
Hariri, A. R., 236, 246
Harlan, E. T., 260, 342, 361
Harlow, J. M., 67
Harlow, R., 172
Harman, C., 264, 288, 360
Harmon-Jones, C., 222
Harmon-Jones, E., 20, 21, 29, 222
Harpur, T. J., 431
Harré, R., 188, 189, 204
Harrington, H., 268
Harris, J. D., 267
Harris, M., 104
Harris, P. L., 247

Harris, S. D., 118
Hart, D., 348
Hart, T., 65
Hartje, W., 293
Hartka, E., 417
Hartley, J. T., 476
Hartley, L. R., 427
Haselton, M. G., 309
Hasher, L., 71, 85
Hashtroudi, S., 476
Hasin, D. S., 472
Hassin, R. R., 154, 158
Hastie, R., 153
Hatfield, T., 427
Haupt, A. L., 379, 380, 382
Hawkins, J. D., 468
Haxby, J. V., 69, 294
Hayes-Roth, B., 25
Hayes-Roth, F., 25
Haynie, D. L., 547, 549
Hazan, C., 288
Heatherton, T. F., 30, 31, 69, 72,
    85, 95, 142, 143, 217, 373,
    393, 403, 422, 426, 447,
    452, 466, 501, 503, 504,
    509, 511, 512, 515, 518,
    519, 520
Heaven, P. C., 382
Hebl, M., 114
Hechenbleikner, N., 376
Hechter, M., 541
Heckhausen, H., 162, 221, 222
Heckhausen, J., 533
Heffner, C. L., 526, 527, 528,
    530
Heiby, E. M., 47
Heider, F., 16
Heidrich, A., 293
Heim, C., 414
Helgeson, V. S., 41
Heller, T., 301
Henderson, H. A., 327
Henry, B., 268
Herbsman, C., 302
Herman, C. P., 403, 493, 495,
    496, 497, 499, 500, 501,
    503, 504
Hernandez, J. T., 534
Hernandez, M., 341
Heron, C., 71
Herscovitch, P., 246
Hershey, K. L., 260, 267, 270,
    289, 342, 361, 360
Hertel, A. W., 132
Hertel, G., 161
Hertsgaard, L., 104
Herzig, M. E., 359
Herzog, T. A., 477

Hesselbrock, M., 415, 418
Hesselbrock, V., 415
Hester, P. P., 346
Hetherington, C., 62
Hiatt, K. D., 431, 432
Hickey, K., 51
Hicks, R. E., 415, 467
Higgins, E. T., 14, 17, 19, 20,
    100, 101, 158, 161, 171,
    172, 173, 174, 175, 176,
    177, 178, 179, 180, 181,
    182, 183, 184, 197, 198,
    200, 201, 397, 435, 509,
    519
Hill, A. L., 266
Hill, G. J., 190
Hill, K. G., 468
Hillis, S., 203
Hillyard, S. A., 439
Himmelbach, M., 286
Hingson, R. W., 466
Hinshaw, S. P., 301, 302, 316
Hinson, R. E., 460, 469, 471
Hirschi, T., 8, 537, 538, 540,
    541, 542, 543, 544, 547,
    550
Hirschman, E. C., 512
Hitch, G. J., 307
Hixon, J. G., 155
Hoaken, P. N. S., 480
Hobfoll, S. E., 27
Hoch, S. J., 458, 505, 513, 514
Hock, E., 347
Hodgins, D. C., 468
Hodgkins, S., 214
Hoelscher, T. J., 141
Hofer, M. A., 329
Hoffman, J. H., 474
Hogan, R., 384
Hokanson, J. E., 386
Holahan, C. J., 472
Holahan, C. K., 472
Holen, A., 117
Holgate, S., 382
Holland, P. C., 427
Holmes, D. S., 116
Holmes, J. G., 383, 478
Holroyd, C. B., 287
Holt, C. S., 455
Hommer, D., 69, 234
Hong, Y. J., 114, 344, 350
Hönig, G., 214
Hoogeveen, K. J., 470
Hooker, K., 106
Hoon, E. F., 531
Hoon, P. W., 531
Hooven, C., 41
Hopfinger, J. B., 69

Hornak, J., 67, 234, 235, 237,
    242
Horowitz, M. J., 117
Houk, J. C., 314
Houle, S., 237
Houston, B. K., 116
Howland, E. W., 430
Howse, R., 333
Hozack, N., 69
Hseih, S., 85
Hsieh, J. C., 71, 237
Hsieh, K. H., 270, 347
Huang-Pollock, C. L., 302
Huba, G., 416
Hufford, M. R., 450, 453, 457,
    477
Hughes, C., 271
Hughes, J. E., 70
Hughes, J. R., 447, 452
Hull, C. L., 111, 152
Hull, J. G., 31, 451, 453, 470,
    472, 474, 476, 477, 478,
    479, 480
Hull, J. W., 530
Humphrey, N., 378
Hunt, W. A., 131, 467
Hur, T., 174
Hurd, C., 533
Hurlbert, D. F., 530
Hurley, C. C., 141
Hurt, R. W., 66
Husarek, S. J., 264
Hussong, A. M., 271, 415, 416,
    467, 469
Husted-Medvec, V., 455
Huston, T. A., 426, 427
Hutton, D. G., 382
Hymes, C., 172
Hynd, G. W., 315

I

Iacono, W. G., 359
Idson, L. C., 172, 176, 179, 180,
    181
Ilardi, B., 198
Ingoldsby, E. M., 347
Ingvar, D. H., 304
Ingvar, M., 71, 237
Inn, A., 469
Ippolito, M. F., 273
Irwin, W., 232, 235, 236, 244
Isaac, W., 315
Isaacowitz, D. M., 248
Isen, A. M., 23, 27
Ito, T. A., 474
Iversen, S. D., 237

Ivry, R. B., 32
Izard, C. E., 19, 23, 324, 341
Izzo, C. V., 467

J

Jacklin, C. N., 415
Jackson, B., 413, 415
Jackson, D. C., 41, 238
Jacobs, D. F., 518
Jacobs, J. W., 109, 110
Jacobson, S., 468
Jacques, S., 345
Jacques, T. Y., 285, 365
Jakobsen, R., 470

Janda, L. H., 93
Janicki, D., 41
Janis, I. L., 117
Janoff-Bulman, R., 50, 199
Janowsky, J. S., 304
Jansma, A., 467
Janssen, E., 531
Jarvik, M., 454
Jastrowitz, M., 65
Jaudas, A., 215
Jeffery, R. W., 131, 133, 139
Jelalian, E., 194
Jencius, S., 201
Jentsch, J. D., 459
Jessor, R., 474
Jetten, J., 219
Jiwani, N., 192
Joffe, R., 47
Johannes, S., 70
John, O. P., 41, 53, 188, 246, 247
Johnson, D. J., 533
Johnson, K., 343
Johnson, L., 327
Johnson, M., 202
Johnson, M. C., 272, 326, 327,
    333, 346, 347
Johnson, M. J., 264, 272
Johnson, M. K., 476
Johnson, P. B., 470
Johnstone, T., 230
Joiner, T. E. J., 468
Joly, R., 474
Jones, B. T., 470, 471
Jones, L., 290, 291
Jones, N. A., 330
Jonides, J., 153, 154, 232, 235
Jordan, C. H., 397
Jorenby, D. E., 449
Josephs, R. A., 31, 437, 451,
    453, 477, 504
Josephson, B. R., 48

Jouriles, E., 477
Judge, T., 41
Juergens, J., 475
Juliano, L. M., 453
Jurica, P. J., 72

K

Kacen, J. J., 513
Kadesjo, B., 301
Kagan, J., 261, 361
Kahan, D., 403, 504
Kahn, B. E., 27
Kahneman, D., 179, 513
Kaiser, A. P., 346
Kaiser, E., 69, 234
Kaiser, H. A., 197
Kalichman, S. C., 531
Kalin, N. H., 41
Kalnok, M., 248
Kalodner, C., 417
Kaloupek, D., 74
Kamarck, T., 140
Kambouropoulos, N., 467
Kane, M. J., 71
Kanfer, F. H., 106, 303, 422
Kaplan, H. B., 382
Kaplan, R. F., 455
Kaplan, R. M., 106
Kapur, S., 237
Karbon, M., 324
Karnath, H. O., 286
Karoly, P., 303
Karp, J., 417
Kashy, D. A., 132
Kasimatis, M., 45
Kasri, F., 47
Kastner, S., 245
Katz, D., 72
Katz, E. C., 474, 475
Katz, L. B., 153
Katz, L. F., 41, 275
Kaufer, D. I., 65
Kaufman, J., 26
Kaufman, M., 74
Kaufmann, P. M., 342, 343
Kaus, C. R., 106
Kavanagh, D. J., 141
Kay, A. C., 161
Kearsley, R. B., 314
Keck, P. E., Jr., 517, 518
Keele, S. W., 288
Keenan, K., 324, 333, 334
Keener, J., 418
Kehrberg, L. L. D., 530
Kelley, H. H., 176
Kelley, W. M., 69, 72, 237

Kelly, K. M., 132, 139, 413
Kelso, J. A. S., 32
Keltner, D., 51, 117
Kemeny, M. E., 51
Kemper, H. C. G., 469
Kendall-Tackett, K. A., 529
Kenne, D. R., 467
Kenny, D. A., 471
Kernis, M. H., 386
Kerns, K. A., 296, 335
Kerr, M., 361, 455, 545, 547
Kerr, N. L., 161
Kessler, R., 415
Ketelaar, T. V., 246, 435
Ketter, T. A., 246
Keyes, S., 544
Khattar, N. A., 387
Khouri, H., 118, 383
Kidorf, M., 468, 471, 472
Kiehl, K. A., 69
Kiers, H. A. L., 101
Kihlstrom, J. F., 14, 114
Kilbey, M. M., 470
Kilpatrick, D. G., 473
Kilts, C. D., 234
Kim, J. J., 428
Kim, S. W., 235, 237, 242
Kimble, M., 74
Kinder, B. N., 527, 528
Kindlon, D., 270
King, C., 133, 139
King, G. A., 200, 201
Kinney, R. F., 222
Kinsella, G. J., 316
Kirby, L. D., 234
Kirchner, T. R., 459
Kirk, J. M., 467
Kirkham, N. Z., 344., 345
Kirschenbaum, D. S., 84, 499
Kirscht, J. P., 130
Kjellstrand, C. M., 51
Klebanov, P. K., 350
Klein, P. S., 345, 346
Klein, S. B., 195
Klingberg, T., 296
Klinger, E., 14, 28, 29
Klinnert, M. D., 361
Klopp, J., 479
Klorman, R., 302
Knaack, A., 263, 265, 266, 269,
    273
Knetsch, J. L., 179
Knight, J. R., 468
Knight, L. J., 499
Knight, R. T., 65, 66, 67, 68, 69,
    72, 73, 232, 235, 236
Knowles, E. S., 395, 396, 405
Knutson, B., 69, 234, 235

Koch, E. J., 376, 383
Kochanska, G., 104, 260, 262, 263, 264, 265, 266, 269, 273, 285, 289, 332, 341, 342, 345, 346, 347, 361, 362, 364, 365
Koenig, A. L., 285, 342, 365
Koenig, H., 520
Koepp, W., 530
Koeppe, R. A., 236, 237
Koestner, R., 41
Kokkonen, M., 54
Kollat, D. T., 512
Koolhaus, J. M., 427
Kopp, B., 292
Kopp, C. B., 40, 264, 272, 313, 314, 324, 325, 326, 327, 342, 343, 363
Kopp, D. A., 199
Koppes, L. L. J., 469
Kopstein, A., 466
Koriat, A., 116
Korn, S., 359
Kornblum, S., 237
Kornhauser, R., 538
Kosslyn, S. M., 238, 314
Kosson, D. S., 430, 431, 432, 436
Koutsky, J. R., 467
Kowalski, R. M., 382
Kozlowski, S. W. J., 197
Kraaij, V., 53
Kraepelin, E., 517
Krakow, J. B., 343
Kramer, D. A., 471
Krams, M., 236, 237
Kremen, A. M., 362
Kring, A. M., 246
Kringelbach, M. L., 234
Kroger, J. K., 65
Kroll, L. S., 471
Krueger, D., 520
Krueger, R. F., 266, 270
Kruglanski, A. W., 93, 100, 101, 152, 163, 171, 173, 196, 200
Krull, D. S., 396
Krych, R., 520
Kubicka, L., 467, 469
Kuhl, J., 100, 101
Kuiper, N. A., 51
Kuleshnyk, I., 497
Kulisevsky, J., 528
Kumar, P. A., 153
Kunda, Z., 101, 171, 173, 397, 449, 450
Kuntsi, J., 316
Kupersmidt, J. B., 349
Kurowski, C. O., 347
Kurzban, R., 374

Kusche, C. A., 276
Kushner, M. G., 415, 416, 471
Kutas, M., 439
Kwiatek, P., 195
Kyngdon, A., 474
Kyrios, M., 269, 272

L

Laaser, M. R., 529, 530
LaBar, K. S., 236
Labouvie, E., 472
Lachman, M. E., 194
Laird, J. D., 51
Lalumiere, M. L., 387
Landau, S., 315
Lane, A. M., 48
Lane, J. D., 533
Lane, R. D., 234, 237, 422
Laneri, M., 315
Lang, A. R., 437, 438, 468, 469, 471, 472, 477
Lang, F. R., 193
Lang, P. J., 19
Langenecker, S. A., 75
Langer, E. J., 117
Langston, C. A., 240
Lank, C., 501
Laplace, A. C., 474
Laplane, D., 66
Laplante, D., 346
Larens, K., 69
Larsen, R. J., 41, 42, 43, 44, 45, 47, 49, 52, 53, 54, 435
Larson, C. L., 238, 287
Larson, J., 46, 412, 413
Larson, M., 104
Latham, G. P., 151, 162, 192, 197
Lau, H. C., 470
Lau, M., 479
Laub, J., 538, 540
Laurent, J., 472
Lavie, N., 424, 425
Lawrence, J. W., 15
Lazarus, R. S., 47, 116, 189, 198, 230, 234, 235, 457
Leary, M. R., 373, 374, 375, 376, 377, 378, 379, 380, 381, 382, 383, 384, 393, 394, 398, 401
Leavitt, L. A., 331
Lecci, L., 472
Lecky, P., 16
LeDoux, J. E., 109, 234, 236, 427, 428
Lee, G. P., 122, 234, 308
Lee, J. A., 513

Lee, J. E., 468
Lee, N. K., 467, 470
Lee, V. E., 342, 348
Lee-Chai, A. Y., 157
Lee-Chai, A., 85, 156, 198, 218
LeeTiernen, S., 101
Lefcourt, H. M., 51
Leggett, E., 197
Lehman, G. L., 475
Leigh, B. C., 470, 474
Leirer, V. O., 153
Lem, K. M., 172
Lemery, K. S., 269, 270, 273, 275, 361
Lengfelder, A., 160, 213, 214
Lengua, L. J., 269, 270, 275, 350
Leonard, K. E., 437, 474, 476, 478, 480
Lerman, M., 533
Lerner, C., 43, 53, 54
Lerner, M., 159, 160
Leuenberger, A., 171
Leukefeld, C., 469
Leung, P. W., L., 350
Levenson, M. R., 472
Levenson, R. W., 19, 41, 48, 230, 232, 248, 476
Leventhal, H., 133
Leventhal, T., 349, 350
Lévesque, J., 244, 287, 459
Levin, H. S., 308
Levine, B. D. T., 62, 67, 72
Levine, J. M., 177, 459
Levine, M. P., 526
Levy, S. A., 415, 467
Levy, S. R., 383
Lewin, K., 161, 162, 179, 199
Lewis, B. A., 469
Lewis, D. A., 65
Lewis, M., 28, 331
Lezak, M. D., 70, 305
Lhermitte, F., 64, 71, 72
Liberman, A., 177
Liberman, N., 108, 172, 175, 178, 179, 183
Liberzon, I., 236
Lichtenstein, E., 136, 140, 449, 455
Lichtman, D., 305
Lichtman, R. R., 106
Lichtstein, K. L., 141
Liddle, P. F., 69, 74
Lieberman, M. D., 31, 109, 229, 234, 238
Liebke, A. W., 304
Liebson, I., 451
Liew, J., 275
Lindman, R. E., 469
Linn, J. A., 395

Linn, L., 202
Lipian, M. S., 247
Litt, M. D., 467
Litten, R. Z., 467
Little, B. R., 14
Litvan, I., 65
Liu, C., 162
Liu, T. J., 477
Livesay, J. R., 304, 313, 314
Livesey, D. J., 342, 344, 345
Livingston, J. A., 475
Loba, P., 472
Locke, E. A., 151, 162, 192, 197
Lockwood, P., 47, 397, 405
Loewenstein, G. F., 108, 454,
    455, 457, 458, 459, 505,
    513
Loftus, J., 195
Logan, G. D., 262, 263, 422,
    478
Logue, A. W., 304
Lomax, L. E., 264, 272, 327
Longhurst, J. G., 529
Longshore, D., 542
Lopez, O. L., 528
Lopez, P. A., 475
Lopez, S. J., 50
Lorch, E. P., 301
Lorenz, A. R., 429, 431
Love, J. M., 348
Lowman, C., 467
Lucas, R. E., 51
Lucas, R., 41
Luciana, M., 344
Lugar, L., 182
Lukas, S. E., 469
Lukon, J. L., 272, 332
Lumsden, C. J., 307
Lundahl, L. H., 469
Luria, A. R., 63, 65, 67, 73, 307
Lushene, R., 436
Luthans, F., 192
Luu, P., 68, 236, 285, 290, 362
Lydon, J. E., 222, 224
Lykken, D. T., 387, 430, 431
Lynam, D. R., 270, 469
Lynch, K. G., 467
Lyon, J. E., 141
Lyons-Ruth, K., 334
Lyubomirsky, S., 41, 47, 411,
    413

M

Macaluso, E., 286
MacAndrew, C., 455
Maccoby, E. E., 415
MacCoon, D. G., 426, 433

MacDonald, A. W., 69, 287
MacDonald, G. A., 141, 381,
    383, 478
MacDonald, T. K., 451, 477
Mack, D., 497
MacKay, D. M., 14
MacLatchy-Gaudet, H. A., 471
MacLean, M. G., 472
MacLeod, C., 454
Macrae, C. N., 69, 71, 72, 153,
    219
Maddux, J. E., 131, 132
Maedgen, J. W., 301, 316
Magai, C., 45
Maibach, E., 190
Maisto, S. A., 467
Majeskie, M. R., 449
Major, B., 106
Malatesta, C., 248
Malmstadt, J. R., 238
Maltzman, I., 479
Manderlink, G., 197
Mangels, J. A., 72
Mangione, C., 315
Mangun, G. R., 32
Mann, T., 504
Manzella, L. M., 157
March, C. L., 341
Marchand, J., 347
Marchetti, C., 64
Marcus, B., 542
Marczinski, C. A., 479
Mariani, M., 301
Marinkovic, K., 479
Markowitsch, H. J., 234
Markus, H., 14, 15, 201
Marlatt, G. A., 131, 136, 141,
    203, 449, 450, 455, 459,
    460, 467
Marlowe, D., 157
Marrocco, R. T., 286, 293
Marshall, P. J., 327
Marshall, T. R., 361
Marsiske, M., 193
Martin, C. S., 450, 452, 453,
    467, 468, 477
Martin, L. L., 22
Martin, N. G., 435
Martin, R., 47, 51
Martin, S. E., 342
Martineau, A. M., 451
Martinussen, R., 301
Maruff, P., 314
Marvin, R. S., 333
Marx, B. P., 475
Marzolf, D., 343
Maslin, C. A., 333
Masserman, J. H., 478
Maszk, P., 324

Matejcek, Z., 467
Matheny, A. P., 264
Mathews, A., 454
Mathews, J. A., 529
Mathieu, J. E., 197
Matsueda, R., 547
Matsumoto, D., 458
Mattis, S., 70
Mattler, U., 292
Matza, D., 539
Mauro, J. A., 359
Mavin, G. H., 201
May, C. P., 71
May, D., 101
Mayberg, H. S., 236
Mayer, J. D., 51, 54, 154
Mayer, N., 65
Maynes, L. C., 529
Mayr, U., 248
Mazur, J. E., 305
Mazure, C. M., 529
Mazziotta, J. C., 236
McAuslan, P., 475
McBride, C. M., 131, 144
McCabe, L. A., 341, 342, 348
McCandliss, B. D., 290, 292
McCann, K. L., 131
McCarthy, D. E., 449
McCarthy, D. M., 471
McCarthy, E. M., 301
McCaul, K. D., 131, 132, 141
McClain, T. M., 42
McClelland, J. L., 101, 156, 422
McClure, S. M., 234
McConahay, J. B., 157
McCrae, R. R., 100, 246, 435
McCreary, D. R., 468
McCulloch, K. C., 160
McCullough, M. E., 50
McDermut, W., 203
McDiarmid, M. D., 343
McDonald, A. W., 65, 66
McElroy, S. L., 517, 518, 519
McFarlane, T., 500
McGaugh, J. L., 234
McGee, R. O., 268
McGlone, F., 236
McGrath, J., 67, 235
McHale, J., 331
McKee, S. A., 469, 471
McKenna, M., 424
McKenna, R. J., 501
McLaughlin, K. A., 293
McMenamy, J. M., 347
McNair, L. D., 471
McNaughton, N., 361, 428
Mecca, A. M., 376, 385
Mednick, S. A., 361
Mefford, I. N., 192

Meier, S. E., 474
Melkman, R., 116
Melnick, S. M., 302, 316
Meltzoff, A. N., 312, 313
Mendoza-Denton, R., 114
Menon, V., 69
Mermelstein, R., 140
Merton, R. K., 538
Messinger, D. S., 22
Mesulam, M. M., 237
Metalsky, G. L., 413
Metcalfe, J., 31, 101, 102, 108, 109, 110, 151, 163
Metevia, L., 302, 315
Metzner, R., 105, 108
Meyer, D. E., 290
Meyer, E., 237
Meyer, G. J., 246
Meyer, R., 418
Meyer-Bahlburg, H. F. L., 531
Mezzacappa, E., 270, 344, 347
Michealis, B., 383
Michel, M. K., 261
Mick, D., 510, 511, 512
Midden, C., 212
Miezin, F. M., 69
Mikulincer, M., 28
Milich, R., 469
Miller, B., 417
Miller, E. K., 71, 232, 235, 236, 427
Miller, G. A., 14
Miller, G. E., 29
Miller, L. C., 32, 101, 158, 401, 475
Miller, N., 474
Miller, N. E., 30
Miller, P. M., 470
Miller, R. E., 45
Miller, R. S., 400, 533
Miller, S. M., 106, 117, 331, 413
Miller, T. L., 471
Milne, A. B., 153, 219
Milne, S., 214
Milner, B., 67, 70
Mineka, S., 413
Minoshima, S., 237
Mintun, M. A., 72
Mischel, H. N., 110, 344
Mischel, W., 14, 31, 100, 101, 102, 104, 105, 107, 108, 109, 110, 111, 112, 113, 114, 115, 116, 119, 121, 122, 123, 163, 165, 191, 195, 262, 265, 269, 271, 303, 304, 327, 342, 344, 348, 364, 373, 502, 503, 513

Mishkin, M., 237
Mitchell, J. E., 517
Mitchell, J. P., 71, 72, 153
Mitchell, R. W., 377
Mitchell, S. H., 467
Miyake, A., 154
Mizruchi, M. S., 23
Moffitt, T. E., 266, 268, 270, 341
Mogelonsky, M., 512
Mohr, C. D., 468
Molden, D. C., 171, 172, 173, 175, 181
Molina, S., 202
Molto, J., 436
Monahan, J. L., 475
Montague, P. R., 234
Monteith, M. J., 404, 405
Monti, P. M., 460
Montoya, I. D., 190
Moore, B., 107, 112, 113
Moos, R. H., 472
Mor, N., 197, 528
Mordkoff, J. T., 15
Moreland, R. L., 459
Moretti, M. M., 158
Morf, C. C., 100, 101, 108, 395
Morgan, G. A., 342, 344, 345
Morgan, M. A., 237
Morrell, M. J., 69
Morris, A. B., 475
Morris, A. S., 260, 261
Morris, J. S., 234, 235, 236, 289
Morris, R. D., 304
Morris, W., 40, 42, 49, 52
Morrow, J., 240, 411, 412
Morse, P. A., 467
Moses, L. J., 271, 285, 290
Moskowitz, G. B., 152, 153, 159, 160, 162, 163, 171, 213
Most, S. B., 425, 433
Moyer, D., 24, 324
Mrazek, D. A., 361
Mudar, P., 415, 472
Mulvihill, L. E., 478
Munoz, R. F., 231
Muraven, M., 2, 27, 31, 85, 88, 89, 90, 94, 95, 142, 152, 155, 217, 394, 452, 504
Murphy, B. C., 260, 263, 267, 268, 269, 270, 324, 365
Murphy, K. R., 301, 302, 315
Murphy, S. T., 475
Murray, H. A., 24
Murray, K. T., 263, 266, 285, 341, 342, 361, 365
Murray, S. L., 383

Myatt, P., 467
Mycielska, K., 63
Myers, F., 474

N

Nachmias, M., 330, 331
Nadasdy, Z., 427
Nagin, D. S., 347, 543
Nauta, W. J. H., 67
Navarick, D. J., 304
Neisser, U., 153
Nelson, C. A., 344
Nelson, G. M., 400
Nelson, T. F., 468
Nerenz, D. R., 133
Nesse, R. M., 29
Nesselroade, J. R., 248
Neter, E., 26
Newcomb, M. D., 140, 471
Newman, D. L., 268, 341
Newman, J. P., 261, 422, 423, 426, 429, 430, 431, 432, 433, 434, 435, 436
Newman, J. R., 42
Newman, M. G., 51
Nezlek, J. B., 382
Nezu, A. M., 131
Niaura, R. S., 448
Nichols, S. L., 436
Nicki, R. M., 141
Nicolich, M., 139
Niedenthal, P. M., 15
Niederhoffer, K. G., 46
Nielsen, K. H., 296
Nielsen-Bohlman, L., 235
Nielson, K. A., 75
Nienhaus, K., 94
Nigg, J. T., 302, 315, 316
Nil, R., 451
Nisbett, R., 90, 457
Noble, J. M., 141
Nobler, M. S., 70
Nobre, A. C., 237
Nolen-Hoeksema, S., 44, 46, 240, 411, 412, 413, 415
Norcross, J. C., 131
Noriega, V., 118
Norman, D. A., 63, 64, 65, 66, 69, 70, 72, 85, 422
Norman, P., 131, 132
Norris, J., 475
Nouwen, A., 198
Novacek, J., 384
Nowak, A., 30, 31, 32, 101
Nurius, P., 14, 15
Nyborg, L., 235
Nystrom, L. E., 68, 236, 424

O

Oakeshott, M., 537
Oberklaid, F., 361
O'Boyle, C. G., 264, 325
Obremski, K. M., 454
O'Brien, C. P., 455
Ochsner, K. N., 229, 232, 234, 235, 236, 238, 241, 287
Ockene, J. K., 131
O'Doherty, J., 234, 235, 236, 237, 242, 246
Oei, T. P. S., 415, 467, 470
Oettingen, G., 190, 211, 214, 225
Ogilvie, D. M., 15
O'Guinn, T. C., 517, 519, 520
Ohman, A., 234, 377
Okun, M. A., 267
Oldenburger, W. P., 427
O'Leary, A., 190
Olenick, N., 416, 418
Oliver, L. M., 237
Olson, K., 345
Olson, R. K., 294
Olson, S. L., 269, 270, 272
O'Neil, T., 471
O'Neill, H. K., 131, 469
Ongur, D., 235, 237
Oosterlaan, J., 262, 270, 316
Orbell, S., 214
Orcutt, H. K., 475, 478
O'Regan, J. K., 284
Orford, J., 469
Orgass, B., 293
Orom, H., 201
Ortony, A., 16
Osborn, C., 203
Ouellette, J. A., 471
Owen, A. M., 73
Owens, E. B., 333, 334, 341
Ozer, E. M., 195

P

Pagani, L., 361
Pagano, R., 477
Pagnoni, G., 234
Pak, H. J., 190, 225
Palfai, T. P., 344, 467, 471
Pandya, D. N., 66, 67
Panksepp, J., 287, 359
Pantelis, C., 75
Paradise, A. W., 386
Paradiso, S., 234
Parasuraman, R., 294
Pardo, P. J., 295
Parekh, P. I., 246

Park, C. L., 472
Park, D. C., 214
Parker, A. M., 435
Parker, E. S., 467, 476
Parker, L. E., 412
Parkinson, B., 40, 41, 42, 47, 49, 53, 54
Parritz, R. H., 330
Parrott, D. J., 457, 474
Parrott, W. G., 22, 42, 240
Parsons, T., 538
Paruchuri, S., 176
Passingham, R. E., 236, 237
Passler, M. A., 315
Pastorelli, C., 190, 192
Paternoster, R., 543
Patrick, C. J., 437, 438, 477
Patterson, C. J., 115, 122, 349
Patterson, C. M., 261, 422, 423, 430, 431, 436
Patterson, G. R., 541
Patti, E. T., 131
Paulus, M. P., 69
Paus, T., 68, 69, 237
Pavese, A., 293
Payton, D. W., 25
Peake, P. K., 108, 114, 115, 191, 192, 262, 364, 265, 341
Peasley, C., 202
Pedlow, R., 361
Peirce, R., 416
Pelham, B. W., 396
Pellegrini, D. S., 301
Pennebaker, J. W., 46, 373
Pennington, B. F., 302, 315, 344, 346
Pennington, G. L., 174
Perkins, H. W., 468
Perlick, D., 456
Pernanen, K., 437, 476
Perrett, D. I., 235, 289
Perri, M. G., 131
Perrott, M. A., 450, 453, 457, 477
Person, D., 202
Perusse, D., 346
Pervin, L. A., 14, 188
Pessoa, L., 245, 424
Petersen, S. E., 69
Peterson, B. S., 236
Peterson, C., 520
Peterson, J. B., 479
Peterson, K., 71
Peterson, R. A., 417
Petit, L., 69
Petrides, M., 70, 237
Petruzzello, S. J., 48
Petry, N. M., 108
Pettit, G. S., 342, 346, 347, 361

Petty, R. E., 50
Pezzuti, L., 192
Pfaff, D. M., 283
Pham, L. B., 225
Phelps, E. A., 234, 236
Phillips, C. M., 45
Phillips, D. A., 276, 344
Phillips, K. A., 518
Phillips, L. H., 85
Phillips, M., 375, 467
Phillips, M. L., 236
Phillips, R. G., 428
Piasecki, T. M., 449
Pickering, A. D., 261
Picton, T. W., 62
Pidada, S., 275
Pien, D. L., 263
Pierce, C. S., 307
Pierce, E. W., 341
Pierce, G. R., 192
Pierce, K., 295
Pihl, R. O., 417, 476, 479, 480
Pillon, B., 64
Pinderhughes, E. E., 275, 350
Pinker, S., 309
Piotrowski, N. A., 191
Piper, M. E., 449
Piquero, A. R., 542
Piron, F., 513
Pittman, N. L., 28
Pittman, T. S., 28
Pliszka, S. R., 361
Polakowski, M., 548
Polan, H. J., 329
Polivy, J., 403, 452, 493, 495, 497, 499, 500, 501, 503, 504
Pollock, V. E., 474
Pomerantz, E. M., 26, 27
Poncet, M., 66
Ponesse, J. S., 263
Pope, H. J., Jr., 517
Pösl, I., 223
Posner, M. I., 68, 69, 70, 116, 232, 236, 245, 259, 260, 261, 262, 263, 264, 283, 284, 285, 286, 287, 288, 289, 290, 291, 292, 293, 294, 295, 335, 345, 360, 362, 363, 364, 422
Post, R. M., 246
Postle, B. R., 65
Potts, M. K., 301, 315
Poulos, C. X., 460, 474
Power, T. G., 275
Powers, R. B., 304
Powers, W. T., 14, 16, 84
Pozo, C., 118
Prentice-Dunn, S., 31

Presson, C. C., 138
Prevor, M. V., 346
Pribram, K. H., 14
Price, D. D., 287
Price, J. L., 235, 237
Priester, J. R., 183
Prigogene, I., 32
Prior, M., 269, 272, 316, 361
Prizmic, Z., 50, 52, 54, 55
Prochaska, J. O., 131, 132, 134
Pryor, J., 157
Puca, R. M., 221, 222, 224
Pulkkinen, L., 54, 268
Purcell, R., 75
Puri, R., 514
Purvis, K. L., 301
Putnam, K. M., 231, 287
Putnam, S. P., 273

Q

Quadland, M. C., 526
Quamma, J. P., 276
Quanty, M. B., 45
Quay, H. C., 315
Quigley, B. M., 474, 480
Quinn, E. P., 450
Quinn, J. M., 132
Quinsey, V. L., 387

R

Raab, G., 519
Rachlin, H., 108
Rafnsson, F. D., 467
Ragland, D. R., 468
Raichle, M. E., 69, 72, 237, 284, 285
Raine, A., 361, 362
Rainville, P., 287
Rajkowski, J., 427
Rakowski, W., 131
Ramachandran, V. S., 64
Ramsay, D. S., 28
Ramsey, S. E., 470
Randall, C., 415, 418
Randall, P. K., 472
Rappley, M. D., 302
Rapus, T., 344
Raskin, R., 384
Rather, B. C., 470
Ratliff, K., 416
Raver, C. C., 265, 268, 344, 345, 346
Rawsthorne, L., 198
Raymond, P., 157
Raz, A., 290

Raz, N., 248
Read, D., 108
Read, J. P., 471
Read, S. J., 14, 30, 32, 101, 158
Reason, J. T., 63
Rebello-Britto, P., 341
Redfern, B. B., 65
Reed, G. M., 51
Reed, M., 263
Reed, M. A., 116, 121, 261, 361, 362, 364
Reed, M. B., 26, 27
Reeder, G. D., 401
Rees, G., 439
Reilly, N., 40, 42, 49, 52, 480
Reiman, E. M., 235, 236, 237, 295
Reinsch, S., 106
Reis-Bergan, M., 471
Reisch, L. A., 519
Reiser, M., 41, 116, 121, 260, 275, 365
Reiss, A. L., 69
Reisz, L., 500
Remington, R. E., 141
Reno, R. R., 131
Rensink, R. A., 284
Repertinger, S., 517
Resnick, H. S., 473
Reuter-Lorenz, P. A., 248
Reynolds, C., 361
Reynolds, C. A., 248
Reynolds, S., 40
Reznick, J. S., 314, 361
Reznik, I., 157
Rhodewalt, F., 101, 384, 395
Richards, J. M., 53, 117, 155, 232
Richeson, J. A., 402, 405
Richman, J. A., 468
Richmond, B. J., 70
Richter, L., 93
Rickards, S., 529, 530
Rickman, R. L., 533
Ridderinkhof, K. R., 291
Ridge, B., 342
Ridley, Mark, 311
Ridley, Matt, 310, 312
Riese, M. L., 264
Ringholz, G. M., 66
Rippere, V., 42
Rison, R. A., 428
Risser, A. H., 304
Rist, F., 292
Rivkin, I. D., 225, 347
Robbins, T. W., 237
Roberts, A. C., 237
Roberts, L. J., 474
Roberts, M. A., 301

Roberts, R. D., 54
Roberts, R. J., 71, 344
Robertson, D. H., 512
Robertson, J., 527
Robins, C., 202
Robins, R. W., 385, 387
Robinson, J., 345
Robinson, T. E., 454
Rodier, P. M., 295
Rodin, G. C., 144
Rodin, J., 106, 498
Rodriguez, M. L., 104, 108, 110, 114, 116, 119, 265, 269, 303, 327, 342, 344, 348, 364, 467, 503
Roehrich, L., 471
Roese, N. J., 174
Rogers, R. D., 68
Rogers, R. W., 31, 131, 132
Roghfleisch, J., 479
Rohner, R., 530
Rolls, E. T., 67, 234, 235, 236, 242, 427
Roman, R. J., 171
Rompa, D., 531
Roney, C., 172
Ronis, D. L., 130
Rook, D. W., 513, 514, 515, 516
Roozendaal, B., 427
Rosay, A. B., 542
Rose-Krasnor, L., 333
Rosenberg, E. L., 457, 458
Rosenberg, M., 382, 386
Rosenblatt, M., 454
Rosenhan, D. L., 51
Rosenthal, T. L., 141
Rosovsky, H., 473
Rospenda, K. M., 468
Ross, L. T., 47, 161, 475
Ross, M., 399
Rosseaux, M., 308
Roth, D. A., 493
Roth, Z., 467
Rothbart, M. K., 68, 69, 116, 259, 260, 261, 262, 263, 264, 265, 266, 267, 270, 283, 285, 288, 289, 290, 291, 325, 326, 335, 342, 345, 350, 357, 358, 359, 360, 361, 362, 363, 364, 365, 366, 422
Rothman, A. J., 130, 131, 132, 133, 134, 137, 139, 142
Rousseaux, M., 73
Rowe, A. C., 153
Rozin, R., 374
Rubin, K. H., 324, 333, 342, 349
Rubonis, A., 417

Ruderman, A. J., 190, 499
Rueda, M. R., 289, 291, 296, 362, 364
Ruff, C., 69
Ruff, H. A., 263, 285, 326
Rumbaugh, D. M., 296
Rumelhart, D. E., 101
Rusbult, C. E., 118, 533
Rushworth, M. F., 237
Russell, M., 415, 416, 470, 472
Rusting, C. L., 48, 54, 412
Ryan, R. M., 33, 143, 144, 151, 198, 378
Ryding, E., 304, 314
Rypma, B., 248

S

Saarni, C., 247
Sadava, S. W., 468
Saks, A. M., 191
Salovey, P., 48, 51, 54, 131, 132, 133, 136, 140, 154, 178
Saltzman, H., 261
Saltzman, J. L., 381
Samaras, M. R., 304, 314
Sampson, R., 538, 540, 543
Samuels, R., 374
Sanderson, C. A., 190, 201
Sandler, I. N., 260, 261, 269
Sandman, P. M., 141
Sandy, J. M., 472
Sanitioso, R., 171
Sannibale, C., 418
Sanson, A., 361
Sarason, B. R., 192
Sarason, I. G., 192
Sarter, M., 427
Saunders, B. E., 473
Sayette, M. A., 448, 450, 451, 452, 453, 454, 455, 456, 457, 458, 459, 460, 467, 477, 479
Scabini, D., 73
Schaal, B., 159, 160, 216
Schachar, R. J., 263
Schachter, S., 456, 498
Schaefer, S., 41
Schafer, J., 473
Schafer, L. C., 141
Schaffer, H. R., 361
Scheier, L. M., 471
Scheier, M. F., 2, 13, 14, 15, 16, 17, 21, 22, 23, 28, 29, 30, 31, 32, 52, 84, 100, 133, 164, 196, 211, 373, 376, 426, 435, 502
Scher, S. J., 199

Scherer, K. R., 230, 231, 234, 235
Scheres, A., 316
Scherhorn, G., 519, 520
Schildbach, S., 530
Schilling, E. M., 270
Schippers, G. M., 467
Schlosser, S. S., 517, 519, 520, 530
Schmager, C., 530
Schmalt, H. D., 221
Schmeichel, B. J., 2, 4, 91, 92, 94, 394, 401, 458, 515, 516
Schmidt, N. B., 468
Schmitt, W. A., 429, 431, 436
Schmitz, S., 345
Schneider, D. J., 72, 90, 117
Schneider, W., 85
Schnetter, K., 190, 225
Schnur, E., 342, 348
Schoenbach, C., 382
Schoenbaum, G., 235
Scholl, B. J., 425
Schon, F., 64
Schonberg, M. A., 272, 332
Schooler, C., 382
Schooler, J. W., 153
Schore, A. N., 329
Schorr, A., 230
Schreck, C. J., 548
Schreindorfer, L. S., 382
Schröger, E., 73
Schultz, D., 341
Schulz, R., 29, 533
Schulze, D., 471
Schwartz, G. E., 237
Schwartz, M. F., 64, 65
Schwartz, S. S., 343
Schwarz, N., 22, 23, 133, 199, 200, 214
Schwarzer, R., 132, 141, 195
Schweizer, T. A., 476
Scott, J., 435
Scott, K. D., 473, 474
Scott, W. D., 199, 200
Sealy, J. R., 529
Searle, J. R., 189
Sears, P. S., 199
Secco, W. P., 533
Sedikides, C., 201, 399, 401
Seeley, E. A., 393
Segarra, P., 436
Seidner, M. L., 106
Seligman, M. E. P., 41, 49, 106
Semcesen, T. K., 345
Semrud-Clikeman, M., 296
Sena, D., 429
Sene'cal, C., 198

Serdaru, M., 64
Sergeant, J. A., 262, 270, 316, 470
Servan-Schreiber, D., 427
Sethi, A., 116, 265, 273, 274, 327, 348, 364
Seto, M., 387
Shack, J. R., 246
Shackelford, T. K., 309
Shadel, W. G., 201
Shah, J. Y., 19, 101, 157, 158, 159, 160, 163, 172, 173, 174, 176, 183, 196, 197, 198
Shah, P., 154
Shallice, T., 24, 63, 64, 65, 69, 70, 72, 73, 85, 93, 422
Shapiro, I. J., 513
Shapiro, J. R., 343
Sharkansky, E. J., 470, 471
Sharp, M. J., 472
Shastri, L., 31
Shaw, D. S., 272, 332, 333, 334, 335, 341, 347
Shaw, J. M., 141
Shea, C. A., 141
Sheeran, P., 132, 214, 215, 219
Sheldon, K. M., 197, 198
Shelton, C. M., 50
Shelton, N. J., 402, 405
Shepard, S. A., 263, 267, 268, 270, 365
Sheppard, D. M., 75
Sher, K. J., 415, 435, 469, 470, 476
Sherer, M., 196
Sherman, D. A., 171
Sherman, S. J., 138
Sherwood, N. E., 139
Shiaw, W. T., 51
Shidara, M., 70
Shiffman, S., 139, 141, 449, 450, 451, 452, 454, 455, 456, 458
Shiffrin, R. M., 85, 159, 165
Shimamura, A. P., 72, 304
Shin, L. M., 235
Shinar, O., 472
Shinsako, S. A., 468
Shisler, R. J., 71
Shoda, Y., 14, 100, 101, 102, 104, 108, 110, 114, 115, 116, 119, 191, 262, 265, 269, 271, 303, 327, 341, 348, 364, 503
Shonkoff, J. P., 276, 344
Shrooder, K., 195
Shulman, G. L., 69, 71, 73, 284, 286

Sicoly, F., 399
Siegel, R. A., 431
Siegel, S., 460
Siegel, S. J., 415
Sigelman, J. D., 21
Siladi, M., 201
Silva, P. A., 268, 341, 361
Silver, R., 497
Silverman, I. W., 273
Silverstein, B., 456
Simmel, C., 302
Simmons, R. G., 51
Simon, H. A., 23, 24, 25, 28, 202, 290, 296
Simons, D. J., 425
Simons-Morton, B., 470
Simpson, J. A., 533
Simpson, J. R., Jr., 237
Simpson, T., 472
Sinclair, L., 383
Singer, J. A., 48
Singer, S. I., 539
Singleton, E. G., 467
Sirigu, A., 304
Sirota, L., 347
Sivers, H., 357
Sjöberg, L., 474
Sjoeholm, B. A., 469
Skilling, T. A., 478
Skinner, B. F., 106, 156, 303
Skinner, E. A., 190
Skinner, J. B., 470
Skutle, A., 470
Sloan, L., 475
Slochower, J. A., 504
Sloman, S. A., 31
Smart, L., 384
Smelser, N. J., 376
Smith, A. M., 69
Smith, C., 326
Smith, C. A., 234
Smith, C. L., 261, 272, 333
Smith, D. W., 477
Smith, E. E., 154, 232, 235
Smith, E. R., 31, 159, 160
Smith, G. T., 470, 471
Smith, J. A., 471
Smith, J. M., 517
Smith, M., 324
Smith, R., 100
Smith, R. E., 195
Smith, R. S., 96
Smith, Y. S., 301
Snel, J., 469
Snider, N. A., 269
Snidman, N., 361
Snyder, A. Z., 237
Snyder, C. R., 50
Sobell, M. B., 474

Sohlberg, M. M., 293, 296
Sommer, K. L., 401
Sommer, T., 290
Sorrow, D. L., 384
Sousa, L., 413
Southwick, L., 477
Spector, I. P., 531
Speltz, M. L., 334
Spence, S. A., 65, 75
Spencer, J. A., 499
Spencer, K., 471
Spencer, S. J., 155, 161
Spiegel, S., 180, 181, 184
Spielberger, C. D., 436
Spinhoven, P., 53
Spinner, H., 64
Spinnler, H., 64
Spinrad, T. L., 261
Spratke, K. L., 467
Spreen, O., 304
Sprengelmeyer, R., 234
Spritz, B. L., 273
Squire, L. R., 304
Sroufe, A. L., 325, 327, 328, 331
Srull, T. K., 153
Stack, D. M., 314
Stacy, A. W., 470, 471
Staiger, P. K., 467
Staines, W. R., 232
Stajkovic, A. D., 192
Stankov, L., 54
Stanley, S. A., 304
Stattin, H., 545, 547
Staub, E., 105
Staudinger, U. M., 193
Steele, C. M., 31, 437, 451, 453, 477, 478, 504
Steele, D. J., 133
Stein, J. A., 140, 542
Stein, K. D., 471
Steinberg, L., 531
Steketee, G., 529
Steller, B., 212, 221
Stenger, V. A., 65, 69, 287
Stengers, I., 32
Stern, H., 512, 513
Sternberg, C., 230
Stevens, A. A., 54
Stevens, M. J., 48
Stevenson, J., 316
Stevenson, J. F., 471
Stewart, B. L., 199, 203
Stewart, S. H., 417, 471, 472
Stice, E., 271
Stifter, C. A., 24, 273, 324, 325, 327, 330
Still, G. F., 302, 315
Stillwell, A. M., 394
Stock, J., 197

Stokes, T. F., 301
Stone, A. A., 51, 139, 457
Stone, V. E., 67
Stone-Elander, S., 71, 237
Stoner, S. A., 475
Stoolmiller, M., 467
Stouthamer-Loeber, M., 266, 270
Strack, F., 133, 157, 184
Strahan, E. J., 161
Strakowski, S. M., 517
Strange, B. A., 246
Strathman, A., 470
Strausser, K. S., 380
Strecher, V. J., 131
Strelau, J., 358, 359
Stritzke, W. G. K., 437, 438
Stroop, J. R., 426, 427, 432
Strubbe, J. H., 427
Stuart, R. B., 503
Sturm, W., 293, 296
Stuss, D. T., 62, 64, 65, 67, 70, 72, 75, 302, 304, 308, 313
Styles, E. A., 85
Suh, M. E., 248
Sullivan, M. W., 28
Suls, J., 16, 47, 139
Sumner, M., 219
Sunderland, T., 294
Sutherland, E. H., 538
Sutton, S. K., 246
Sutton, S. R., 134
Suwazono, S., 235
Swanson, H. L., 247
Swanson, J. M., 283, 293, 294, 295, 357
Swearingen, L., 334, 341
Swendsen, J. D., 416, 468
Swets, J. A., 177
Swick, D., 232, 287
Szpiler, J. A., 106
Szumowski, E. K., 341

T

Tambor, E., 374, 376, 381
Tamminga, C. A., 70
Tamres, L. K., 41, 46
Tanner, W. P., Jr., 177
Tannock, R., 263, 301
Tarbox, A. R., 470
Target, M., 283, 285
Tate, S. R., 470
Taylor, C., 292, 344, 362, 543
Taylor, C. B., 192
Taylor, E., 346
Taylor, J. R., 459
Taylor, S. E., 51, 106, 117, 136, 221, 222, 223, 225, 383, 387

Taylor, S. F., 236, 237
Taylor, S. P., 437, 474, 476, 478
Taylor, T. H., 476
Teasdale, J. D., 235
Teicher, M., 529
Tein, J., 260
Tellegen, A., 19, 20, 435
Tennen, H., 46, 117, 471
Terdal, S., 374
Tesser, A., 22, 26, 27, 101, 165
Testa, A., 101, 114
Testa, M., 475, 478
Teti, L. O., 261
Thaler, R., 179
Thayer, J. F., 422
Thayer, R. E., 41, 42, 48, 53, 54, 55
Thomas, A., 359
Thomas, K. M., 247, 292
Thomason, M., 75
Thompson, E. P., 171
Thompson, J., 296
Thompson, R. A., 40, 324, 325, 327
Thompson, S. C., 106
Thorndike, E. L., 296
Thornquist, M. H., 430
Tice, D. M., 2, 31, 49, 85, 88, 89, 91, 95, 142, 152, 217, 373, 382, 394, 403, 447, 448, 466, 501, 504, 511, 512, 515, 518
Tiffany, S. T., 448, 449, 452, 453, 454, 456, 457, 460, 467
Tillema, J., 199
Timmer, S., 416
Titchener, E. B., 284
Tittle, C. R., 542
Tjebkes, T. L., 264, 265, 345
Tobin, R. M., 101
Toby, J., 539
Tolman, E. C., 152
Tomarken, A. J., 499
Tomich, P., 335
Toni, I., 236
Tooby, J., 309, 310, 373, 374
Torgesen, J. K., 302
Torp, N., 265, 344
Torrubia, R., 436
Totterdell, P., 40, 42, 53, 54, 55
Tournier, P., 510
Tracy, J. I., 476
Tracy, P. E., 539
Tranel, D., 67, 74, 234, 287
Travis, T., 459
Trebilcock, M., 314
Tremblay, R. E., 346, 361
Trick, L. M., 290
Trilling, L., 122

Trimpop, R. M., 474
Troiden, R. R., 526
Tronick, E. Z., 345
Trope, Y., 26, 27, 31, 108, 109, 177
Trötschel, R., 85, 156, 218, 219
Troutman, B. R., 192
Trower, P., 377
Trull, T. J., 435
Trzebinski, J., 158
Tucker, D. M., 290
Tucker, K. L., 47, 413
Tuer, M., 468
Tuholski, S. W., 71
Tulving, E., 313
Turchi, J., 427
Turcotte, N., 471
Turk, D. J., 75
Turken, A. U., 287
Turner, S., 542
Tversky, A., 513
Twenge, J. M., 91, 403, 515
Twisk, J. W. R., 469
Twomey, H., 203
Tyssen, R., 472

U

Uggen, C., 537
Ullman, S. E., 475
Ungerleider, L. G., 69, 245, 424
Urbszat, D., 499
Urrows, S., 117
Ursprung, A., 417
Usher, M., 427

V

Vaccaro, D., 467
Vagg, P. R., 436
Vaglum, P., 472
Vaidya, C. J., 75
Vaidya, J., 19
Vaillant, G. E., 51
Vakili, S., 474
Vallacher, R. R., 16, 26, 30, 31, 32, 101
Vancouver, J. B., 14
Vandegeest, K. A., 285, 365
van der Molen, M. W., 291
Van der Staak, C. P. F., 467
Van Hoesen, G. W., 66
Van Horn, J. D., 72
Van Landuyt, L. M., 48
Vanman, E. J., 32
Van Mechelen, I., 101
Van Treuren, R. R., 476, 478

van Veen, V., 292, 293
Vasconcellos, J., 376
Vasey, M. W., 270, 362
Vaughn, B. E., 343
Vaughn, L. J., 433
Vaux, A., 383
Vega, W. A., 382
Velez-Blasini, C. J., 469
Velicer, W. F., 132
Venables, P. H., 361, 362
Ventner, J. C., 285
Veroff, J., 416
Vik, P. W., 470
Vitale, J. E., 429
Vitaro, F., 361
Vogel, R., 202
Vogel-Sprott, M., 470, 476, 478, 479, 480
Vogt, B. A., 69
Vohs, K. D., 2, 6, 7, 15, 31, 44, 48, 91, 92, 94, 95, 142, 143, 373, 387, 393, 394, 399, 400, 401, 403, 405, 452, 458, 468, 504, 509, 512, 515, 516, 518
Volkow, N. D., 67, 459
von Hippel, W., 202
Von Restorff, H., 73
Vondra, J. I., 333, 334, 341
Vorst, H., 531
Voss, W. D., 431
Vowell, P. R., 547
Vygotsky, L. S., 307

W

Wade, D., 67, 235
Wagner, E. H., 144
Wakefield, J. C., 309
Wall, A. M., 469, 471
Wall, S., 328
Wallace, H. M., 89
Wallace, J. F., 429, 434, 435
Wallis, J. D., 237
Walsch, K. W., 64
Wan, C. K., 533
Wang, Y., 275
Ward, A., 413, 504
Ward, D. A., 474
Ware, J., 202
Warheit, G. J., 382
Warren, L., 474
Wasel, W., 159
Washburn, D. A., 296
Waters, A. J., 454, 458
Waters, E., 328, 331
Watson, D., 19, 20, 359, 413, 435

Watt, J. D., 531
Watts, W., 66
Webb, T. L., 215, 219
Webster, D. M., 93
Wechsler, H., 466, 468, 475
Wegener, D. T., 50
Wegner, D. M., 16, 33, 72, 85, 90, 117, 155, 159, 373, 533
Weimer, B., 335
Weinberg, M. K., 345
Weinberg, P., 513, 515
Weingardt, K. R., 470
Weinstein, N. D., 131, 132, 134, 139, 140, 141, 142
Weiss, E. L., 529
Weiss, F., 457
Weitlauf, J., 195, 196
Welch, M. C., 285
Weller, A., 347
Wells, S., 466, 473
Wells-Parker, E., 467
Welsh, M. C., 302, 315, 342
Welte, J. W., 474
Wentzel, M., 267
Wertz, J. M., 450, 453, 454, 456, 457, 467, 477
West, P., 466, 473
West, R. L., 192, 194
West, S. G., 131, 260, 269
Westdorp, A., 69, 234
Westerberg, H., 296
Whalen, P. J., 234, 427
Wheatman, S., 386
Wheeler, L., 47
Wheeler, M. A., 313
Whitaker, D., 386
White, C. D., 69
White, D., 198
White, G. L., 383
White, H. R., 473
White, J., 203
White, J. L., 266, 270
White, K., 203, 348
White, L. C., 530
White, T. L., 20, 21, 90, 117
Whitfield, S. L., 357
Wicklund, R. A., 217, 519
Widaman, K., 347
Widiger, T. A., 435
Wiederman, M. W., 531, 532, 533

Wiener, N., 14
Wiers, R. W., 470
Wikler, A., 449
Wilde, G. J. S., 474
Willett, R. P., 512
Williams, B. R., 263
Williams, G. C., 144, 311, 312, 313
Williams, J. M. G., 435, 454
Williams, L. L., 362
Williams, L. M., 529
Williams, M., 362
Williams, M. T., 467
Williams, S., 51
Williams, S. L., 192
Williamson, S., 431
Willis, S. L., 193
Willmes, K., 293
Wills, T. A., 16, 271, 467, 472
Wilsnack, R., 415
Wilsnack, S., 415
Wilson, B., 70
Wilson, B. J., 346
Wilson, E. O., 307
Wilson, G. T., 449, 460, 477, 479
Wilson, P. H., 141
Wilson, P., 314
Wilson, R. S., 264
Wilson, T. D., 90, 457
Wincze, J. P., 531
Windle, M., 271, 417, 470
Wingood, G. M., 534
Winquist, J., 528
Winsler, A., 301, 315
Winslow, E. B., 333
Winston, J. S., 246
Wise, S. P., 314
Wolfe, C. T., 155
Wolfer, J. A., 117
Wolff, C., 73
Wolfgang, M., 539
Wood, J. V., 16, 106, 459
Wood, M., 415
Wood, M. D., 471
Wood, P. K., 415, 469
Wood, R., 192, 198
Wood, W., 130, 132, 138
Woodward, C. K., 131
Woodward, T., 69
Woody, E. Z., 499
Wortman, C. B., 28, 29

Wright, J., 114, 119
Wright, P. M., 195
Wright, R., 303
Wrosch, C., 29
Wu, Y., 294
Wulfert, E., 108, 467, 533
Wyatt, R. J., 476
Wyer, R. S., Jr., 153
Wyland, C. L., 69, 72

Y

Yaeger, A. M., 472
Yates, J. F., 130
Ye, R. M., 259, 350, 360
Yen, Y., 101
Yeomans, F., 530
Yniguez, R. M., 469
Youn, S., 513
Young, R. D., 476, 477
Youngstrom, E. A., 341
Yum, K. S., 478

Z

Zacks, R. T., 85
Zahn-Waxler, C., 345, 414
Zajac, D. M., 197
Zakocs, R. C., 466
Zald, D. H., 235, 237, 242
Zambon, A., 466
Zanakos, S., 155
Zanarini, M. C., 530
Zanna, M. P., 161, 451, 477, 478
Zawacki, T., 475
Zayas, V., 101
Zeichner, A., 474, 476
Zeigarnik, B., 179
Zeiss, A. R., 107, 113
Zelazo, P. D., 344, 345, 479
Zelazo, P. R., 314
Zentall, S. S., 301
Zhao, Z., 234
Zhou, Q., 275
Ziaie, H., 264, 325
Zimmerman, R. S., 382
Zinser, M. C., 457, 458
Zuckerman, M., 359, 430
Zuroff, D. C., 41
Zywiak, W. H., 467

Subject Index

Absent-minded lapses, 449
Absorption, 520
Abstinence, 454
Acceptance, 378
Accommodation, 398
Acquiescence, 455, 515
Activity substitution, 179
Addiction, 447
Affect, 13, 40, 449, 456, 477
    and action 18
Affect regulation, 415
Affect specificity, 56
Aggression, 333, 366, 437, 473
Alcohol, 94, 415, 437, 466, 501, 549
    abuse and dependence, 417
    motives, 472
    myopia, 477, 504
    social drinkers, 416
    use disorder, 415
Alien hand syndrome, 64
Altering, 286
Altruism, 50, 310
Amygdalae, 234, 427
Anterior cingulate cortex, 68, 116, 236
Antisocial personality disorder (APD), 387, 429
Anxiety, 411, 434, 519
    disorder, 418
Appraisal efficacy, 176
Appraisal processes, 189, 458
Arousal, 287, 501, 517
Attachment, 539

Attachment styles, 327, 401
Attention, 71, 153, 245, 284, 342, 422–423, 437, 454, 476
    allocation, 425
    disorders, 293
    shifting, 263
    supervisory system, 63
Attentional capacity, 432
Attentional control, 114, 270, 283
Attention-deficit/hyperactivity disorder (ADHD), 295, 301, 315
Attitudes, 450
Autism, 295
Automaticity, 106, 115, 151, 160, 212
    in smoking, 452
Autonomy, 273, 331

B

Bargaining strategies, 514
Behavior change, 130
    methodological considerations, 139
Behavior initiation, 130
Behavior maintenance, 130
    phases of, 134
    table of, 135
Behavior regulation, 155
Behavioral approach, 359
Behavioral inhibition, 359

Behavioral loops, 17
Beliefs, 539
Belongingness, 374
Biased inferences, 222
Binge eating, 503
Borderline personality disorder (BPD), 294, 530
Bulimia nervosa, 500

C

Catharsis, 44
Cerebral novelty network, 73
Childhood, 359
Childhood abuse, 529
Childrearing model, 541
Choice, 74
Closed-mindedness, 222
Coalition formation, 310
Coasting, 22
Cognition, 476
Cognitive conflict, 288
    control, 342
    narrowing, 519
    reappraisal, 46, 117
    restructuring, 503
    tuning, 221
Cognitive-affective processing system, 99, 102
    diagram of, 103, 120
Commitment, 539
Comparator, 15
Competence, 268
Compliance 265

Compulsive buying, 516, 519
Compulsive sexuality, 526
Conditioning models, 460
Condom use, 142, 533
Confidence, 30
Conflict, 30
Conformity, 161, 403
Conscience, 266, 289
Contention scheduling system, 63
Control, 105, 413
Cool systems, 108
Cooling strategies, 117
Coping, 47
    emotion-focused, 47
    problem-focused, 47
    resources, 458
    responses, 454
    skills, 454
    strategies, 512
    styles, 472
Counterfactual thinking, 174
Crime, 537
    and age, 544
    in childhood, 544
Criminology, 537
Cues, dominant and nondominant, 422, 438
Cultural deviance, 538
Culture, 349
Cybernetic theory, 2

D

Decision making, 74, 90, 133
Delay of gratification, 99, 107, 265, 342, 502
    diagnosticity of, 108
    distraction strategies, 112, 117
Delay tactics, 514
Delinquency, 270
Depression, 134, 366, 411, 519
Desire, 504
Deviance, 548
Dieting, 94, 403, 494
Discounting principle, 176
Discriminative facility, 114
Disinhibition, 478, 499
Distraction, 44, 216
Dominant response set, 423
Dorsolateral prefrontal cortex, 65

Drugs
    cravings, 467
    environmental factors, 468
    treatment, 460
    use, 454
Dynamic systems, 30–32
Dysexecutive syndrome, 70
Dysregulation, 434

E

Eating, 48, 492
    disorders, 434
    social influences on, 496
Effortful attention, 342
Effortful control, 99, 259, 362
    development of, 262
    individual differences in, 99
Ego depletion, 95, 155, 219, 516
Emotion, 40, 375, 431
Emotion regulation, 40, 116, 154, 230, 259, 287, 518
    definition of, 324
    development of, 325
    efficacy in, 54
    in adulthood, 247
    in childhood, 247
    individual differences in, 53, 246
    models of, 52
    neuroscience of, 229
    physical and mental health, 41
    strategies, 42, 231, 324
    styles of, 55
Emotion suppression, 45, 117
Emotional expressivity, 51, 264
Emotional responding, 246
Emotions, 25, 230
    positive, 245
Empathy, 267, 289
Error detection, 290
Error signal, 15
Evolutionary theories, 301, 309, 377
Executive control function, 70, 286
Executive function, 302, 479
    model of, 306
Exercise, 48
Exit, 398
Expectancies, 173, 469
Extended-now state, 94
Extraversion, 358, 435

F

Facial expressivity, 457
False hope syndrome, 452
Fasting, 495
Fear, 361
Feedback control, 16
Feedback loops, 14–17
Feeling tones, 40
Flexibility, 218
Flexible attention deployment, 114
Food, capacity for, 500
Free will, 75
Frontal lobes, 63
    and crime, 63
Functional magnetic resonance imaging (fMRI), 237

G

Gains, 513
Gambling, 431
Gender, 345, 411
Genetic inheritance, 294, 364, 414
Goals, 14, 25, 111, 152
    activation, 157-161
    approach and avoidance, 197
    attainment, 28, 162
    conflict, 163
    contagion, 157
    dimensions, 197
    implementation, 212
    inhibition, 163
    looms larger effect, 179
    priorities, 25
    pursuit, 178, 215
    setting, 192
    shielding theory, 163
    strength and disruption, 162
    types, 213
Gratitude, 50
Group membership, 402

H

Habits, 138
Hippocampus, 428
Home, 346
Homunculus, 101
Hope, 136
Hot and cold processing, 108, 455

Humor, 51
Hunger, 493
Hypomania, 27

I

Iconic representations, 113
Ideation, hot and cool, 119
If–then plans, 212
Imagery, 113
Imitation, 310
Implementation intentions, 115, 160, 213
  strength of, 215
Impulse buying, 512
Impulse control, 230, 400, 532
Impulsivity, 31, 261
Inertia, 453
Infancy, 343, 359, 493
Informal social control theory, 538
Information processing, 32, 423, 436
Inhibition, 71, 302
  conflict, 477
Input function, 15
Interpersonal behavior, 373, 392
Involvement, 539
Isolation, 49

J

Judgmental processes, 171–181

K

Knowledge, 189

L

Lateral prefrontal cortex, 235
Laughter, 51
Losses, 513
Loyalty, 398

M

Macroenvironment, 349
Magical thinking, 520
Mania, 27

Martial conflict, 418
Mealtimes, 494
Medial prefrontal cortex, 237
Mental illness, 294, 309
Metacognition, 302
Microenvironment, 346
Minimal and maximal goals, 178
Mismatch negativity (MMN), 73
Misregulation, 447, 517
Mixed anxiety–depression syndrome, 413
Mixed-race interactions, 402
Moderation mediation model, 471
Monitoring, 164, 374, 451
Mood, 40, 164, 199, 448, 514
  disorders, 418
Moral judgments, 182
Morality, 266
Motivated cognition, 171
Motivation, 104, 155, 173, 198, 224, 308, 457, 498
  chronic, 159
  internal and external, 143
  success and failure, 180

N

Narcissism, 384
Neglect, 398
Neighborhoods, 349
Neuroticism, 359, 435
Norms, 515
Novelty, 72

O

Object substitution, 179
Obsessive–compulsive disorder (OCD), 70, 527
Opportunistic shifting, 27
Oppositional defiant disorder (ODD), 333
Optimism, 136, 223
Orbitofrontal cortex, 235, 236
Orbitofrontal syndrome, 67
Orienting, 286
Ostracism, 402
Ought self, 176, 435
Outcome expectancies, 133
Output function, 15

P

Palatability, 500
Parental influence, 546
Passivity, 431
Peers, 348
Perception, 155
Person specificity, 56
Personality, 188, 358
Phenylketonuria, 346
Planning, 211, 224, 498
  changing, 179
Power, 157
Prefrontal cortex, 232, 427
Prejudice, 216
Preloading, 499
Preschool, 343
Priming, 153, 161, 398
Priority adjustment, 28
Priority management, 24
Probability estimates, 176
Promotion-prevention-pride, 172
  strategies, 171, 396
Prosocial behavior, 267
Proximity, 513
  physical, 514
  temporal, 514
Psychoanalytic framework, 285
Psychopathy, 429
Purchasing behavior, 509

R

Reactive systems, 261
Reactivity, 357
Reappraisal, 229, 246
Rebound effects, 218
Reference values, 15
Regulatory fit, 181
Regulatory focus, 173, 396
Rejection, 374, 401–403
  sensitivity, 118, 383
Relational value, 374
Relaxation, 48
Reprioritization, 25
Resistance, 395
Response bias, 177
Response inhibition, 303
Response modulation hypothesis, 422
Rewards, 111
Risk-taking, 474, 548
Rumination, 44, 411

S

Satiety, 493
Satisficing, 23
Savoring, 457
Schizophrenia, 295
Seizing and freezing, 93
Self, 377
  definition of, 86
Self-awareness, 480, 518
Self-control, 144
  definition of, 86, 303
  purpose of, 303
  theory, 540
Self-disclosure, 401
Self-discrepancy theory, 435
Self-efficacy, 28, 89, 105, 132,
  140, 188, 200–202, 454,
  467
  and age, 194
Self-esteem, 26, 155, 373, 376,
  517
  illusions in, 387
  private, 379
  trait, 381
Self-evaluations, 165
Self-gifting, 509
Self-knowledge, 200
Self-organization, 31–32
Self-play, 308
Self-presentation, 394
Self-regulation, 13
  anterior cingulate cortex,
  69
  as a schema, 87
  as a skill, 88
  automaticity in, 85, 152
  cognitive neuroscience of, 62
  definition of, 2, 86
  development of, 104, 340
  executive functioning, 85
  failures in, 426, 447, 497
  impact of environment on,
  340
  individual differences, 115,
  340
  limited resource model, 27,
  84, 394

passivity, 89
practice, 159
processes of, 100
strength, 84, 142, 452,
  504
Self-reward, 47
Self-schemas, 201
Self-serving bias, 398
Sexual addiction, 526
  behavior, 475, 525
  harassment, 433
  self-control, 530
Shyness, 365
Situational norms, 160
Skill learning, 32
Smoking, 447
  cravings, 450
  quitting, 451
  relapse, 449
  withdrawal, 452
Snowballing, 517
Social behavior, 175
Social bonding theory, 538
Social comparison, 46
Social control theory, 538
Social disorganization theory,
  538
Social functioning, 260
Social inference, 396
Social learning theories, 538
Social norms, 161, 496
Social orientation, 393
Socialization, 272
Socializing, 49
Social-loafing, 217
Societal influence, 546
Sociometer, 373
Somatic markers, 122
Speed–accuracy tradeoffs,
  178
Standards, 199, 378, 449
Stereotypes, 216, 404
Stimulus control, 106
Stopping, 303
Strain theories, 538
Stress, 110, 504
Striatum, 234
Subjective well-being, 41

Sunk costs effect, 179
Supervisory attentional system
  (SAS), 63

T

Temperament, 260, 289, 345,
  357, 363, 414
Temporal, discounting, 108, 305
  perception, 458
Test-operate-test-exit (TOTE)
  system, 84, 164
Theory of mind, 290
Think-aloud assessments, 202
Thought suppression, 72
Time, experience of, 94
Toddlerhood, 343
Transcendence, 118, 451, 519

U

Underregulation, 447
Utilization behavior, 64

V

Value transfer, 181
Venting, 44
Ventromedial prefrontal cortex,
  66
Visuospatial sketchpad, 307
Voice, 398
Von Restorff effect, 73

W

Warning system, 374
Weight control, 448, 493
What-the-hell effect, 498
Willpower, 84, 99, 106, 514
Withdrawal, 49
Working memory, 71, 154,
  285, 307
Workplace problems, 468